PLAYING THE MA… BUSINESS—BUT *S*… DOESN'T HAVE TO BE!

Whether you stop by the corner deli or shop at a 24-hour megasupermarket, whether you handpick your vegetables at the greengrocer or log on for on-line shopping, you can take the uncertainty out of choosing the best buys available with *THE FOOD SHOPPING COUNTER.* In this all-new revised edition of *The Supermarket Nutrition Counter,* bestselling authors Annette B. Natow and Jo-Ann Heslin provide more than 20,000 entries in more than 350 food categories, making this essential guide to smart food shopping more comprehensive than ever before. Also included are food storage tips, shopping strategies for navigating the typical supermarket, the top three reasons why a consumer selects a food, how men and women differ when shopping the aisles, and other information to help you get more for your money every time you shop.

Books by Annette B. Natow and Jo-Ann Heslin

The Antioxidant Vitamin Counter
The Calorie Counter
The Cholesterol Counter (Fifth Edition)
The Diabetes Carbohydrate and Calorie Counter
Eating Out Food Counter
The Fat Attack Plan
The Fat Counter (Fourth Edition)
The Food Shopping Counter
Megadoses
No-Nonsense Nutrition for Kids
The Pocket Encyclopedia of Nutrition
The Pocket Fat Counter (Second Edition)
The Pocket Protein Counter
The Pregnancy Nutrition Counter
The Protein Counter
The Sodium Counter
The Supermarket Nutrition Counter (Second Edition)

Published by POCKET BOOKS

THE FOOD SHOPPING COUNTER

ANNETTE B. NATOW, Ph.D., R.D.
and JO-ANN HESLIN, M.A., R.D.

POCKET BOOKS
New York London Toronto Sydney Tokyo Singapore

Originally published in 1995 by Pocket Books as *The Supermarket Counter.*

POCKET BOOKS, a division of Simon & Schuster Inc.
1230 Avenue of the Americas, New York, NY 10020

ISBN: 0-671-00452-2

First Pocket Books printing of this revised edition January 1999

10 9 8 7 6 5 4

POCKET and colophon are registered trademarks of Simon & Schuster Inc.

Cover photo by Beery Photography / Stock Food

Printed in the U.S.A.

To our families who support us through every project: Harry, Allen, Irene, Sarah, Meryl, Laura, Marty, George, Emily, Steven, Joe, Kristen, and Karen.

ACKNOWLEDGMENTS

Without the tireless cooperation of Steven Natow, M.D., and Stephen Llano, *The Food Shopping Counter* would never have been completed. Our thanks to the National Live Stock and Meat Board and the Food Marketing Institute for providing research material and resources. Special thanks to our agent, Nancy Trichter; our editor, Jane Cavolina; and her assistant, Brett Freese.

We are all inclined to think the foods which we like are good for us, and appearance and flavor attract or repel very quickly; but as far as real nourishment goes, these things are second hand and the [shopper] must be able to discriminate between real nutritive value and other factors, in order to spend . . . money to the best advantage.

Mary Swartz Rose, Ph.D.
Feeding the Family
The Macmillan Company, 1919

SOURCES OF DATA

Values in this counter have been obtained from the Composition of Foods, United States Department of Agriculture, Agricultural Handbooks: No. 8-1, Dairy and Egg Products; No. 8-2, Spices and Herbs; No. 8-3, Baby Foods; No. 8-4, Fats and Oils; No. 8-5, Poultry Products; No. 8-6, Soups, Sauces and Gravies; No. 8-7, Sausages and Luncheon Meats; No. 8-8, Breakfast Cereals; No. 8-9, Fruit and Fruit Juices; No. 8-10, Pork Products; No. 8-11, Vegetables and Vegetable Products; No. 8-12, Nut and Seed Products; No. 8-13, Beef Products; No. 8-14, Beverages; No. 8-15, Finfish and Shellfish Products; No. 8-16, Legumes and Legume Products; No. 8-17, Lamb, Veal and Game Products; No. 8-18, Baked Products; No. 8-19, Snacks and Sweets; No. 8-20, Cereal Grains and Pasta; No. 8-21, Fast Foods; Supplements 1989, 1990, 1991, 1992.

"Nutritive Value of Foods." United States Department of Agriculture. Home and Garden Bulletin No. 72.

J. Davies and J. Dickerson. *Nutrient Content of Food Portions.* Cambridge, UK: Royal Society of Chemistry, 1991.

G. A. Leveille, M. E. Zabik, K. J. Morgan. *Nutrients in Foods.* Cambridge, MA: Nutrition Guild, 1983.

A. Moller, E. Saxholt, B. E. Mikkelsen. *Food Composition Tables: Amino Acids, Carbohydrates and Fatty Acids in Danish Foods,* 1991.

Souci, Fachmann, and Kraut. *Food Composition and Nutrition Tables.* Stuttgart: Wissenschaftliche Verlagsgesellschaft MbH, 1989.

Information from food labels, manufacturers, and processors. The values are based on research conducted through the first half of 1998. Manufacturers' ingredients are subject to change and may vary in different regions, so current values may differ from those listed in this book.

INTRODUCTION

It's hard to believe, but the average supermarket carries 30,000 separate items and more than half of these are foods. No wonder grocery shopping takes so long. And when you try to compare the nutrients in different products to ensure the healthiest menu, it takes even longer. Recent surveys show that over 90% of Americans are concerned about the nutritional value in the foods they eat. Fat is the greatest concern, followed by salt, cholesterol, and sugar. You want to make good choices but you may not have enough time to compare the labels of five or more pasta sauces, rice mixes, or frozen dinners. That's where *The Food Shopping Counter* lends a hand. Now you have a chance to compare these products before you get near the food store.

The Food Shopping Counter will show you how to navigate the food market to find the best choices in each section as you push your cart up and down the aisles. You'll also learn how to interpret the nutrition facts on labels, use cents-off coupons, make use of storage tips to preserve the nutrients in the foods you buy, and stock your kitchen so you will always have a quick something to eat.

Fast fact

A total of 2,076 new lowfat and reduced fat products were introduced in 1996, more than twice the number in 1993. In fact, reduced fat items made up almost 16% of all food

products introduced in 1996. It is projected that by 2001, sales of reduced fat foods will total nearly $32 billion.

Fast fact

In the United States there are 127,000 grocery stores with over $425 billion in sales.

TRAVELING THROUGH THE FOOD MARKET

The first step to efficient, healthy shopping is getting to know the layout of the food market where you shop. Grocery stores tend to have similar layouts, and there are a few tricks to getting the most out of your shopping time. Wheel your cart around the outside aisles first. You'll pass the fresh dairy products, fruits, vegetables, breads, and meat, fish, and poultry. These foods are the ones that are emphasized in the Food Guide Pyramid (see page xxix). Fill your basket with these.

Navigating the Food Market Aisles

Food markets are set up to encourage shoppers to buy more. For instance, milk, which is usually bought on every shopping trip, is placed in the rear of the store to encourage spontaneous shopping on the way to the dairy case. Marketers know we expect to find sale items at the end of the aisle. Placing not-on-sale items here or at the checkout counter results in increased sales. Salad dressings placed near the lettuce in the produce section are more likely to be bought than others shelved separately, as are items placed at eye level on store shelves. Studies show that placing a product at eye level can increase sales by

50%. Being aware of these practices can start you on the road to savvy shopping.

Fast fact

A food market shopping cart travels 30,000 miles in its lifetime and on an average shopping trip carries 20 items, with an average cost of $19.20.

Fast fact

According to a Food Marketing Institute survey, taste, convenience, and nutrition are the basic selling points for new food products. Over 90% were variations on existing products, such as new flavors. Fewer than 10% were truly new items. The failure rate among new products runs between 80 and 94%.

TRENDS: What's New in Food Shopping

- Large food markets now offer shoppers many amenities, including fitness centers, cooking schools, and services such as driver's license renewals and baby-sitting.
- Sales of organic foods have increased, totaling $872 million in 1996.
- The vegetarian market is booming, with sales close to $300 million. Vegetarians are getting younger and now include about 15% of college students.
- More specialty foods are available by mail order, and all kinds of nonperishable foods are available via the Internet.

Food Shopping on the Internet

If you'd rather not wait in line at a food store, why not try online shopping instead? NetGrocer (www.netgrocer.com) allows consumers to shop for food by computer. Just point and click your mouse through a menu of nonperishable grocery items and they'll be delivered by FedEx within two to four business days. There is a shipping charge, but items cost less than at food stores. This can be a wonderful time-saver. Experts believe that in less than ten years, 15% of groceries will be sold through the Internet.

Shopping Strategies

Shop with a list whenever you can. Surveys show that 55% of shoppers make a list before going grocery shopping. They tend to buy twice as many items as are on their list, but the list reminds them of needed items and helps to direct purchases.

Larger sizes are usually, but not always, a better value. A half gallon of milk costs less than two one-quart containers, but it's a bargain only if you'll use it up before it spoils.

Prices on store brands may be as much as 50% less than the least expensive brand-name competitor. Check this out by comparing the unit cost (price per ounce or per pound) of the store brand to that of your favorite brand. Also check out the quality of store brands. You may find them improved over the last time you used them.

Watch out for sale items, especially in the case of produce. You may not be able to use them before they spoil. Sale items with freshness dates may be near the end of their shelf life.

Get familiar with the layout of the store you shop in most often. Grocery shoppers spend an average of $1.33 for every minute they remain in the store. Up to a point, the more time you spend looking for an item, the more money you spend.

It pays to stoop down to lower shelves when grocery shopping. The high-profit items are at eye level; you'll find the lower markup products down below.

Cents-off coupons can save you money if they don't encourage you to buy items you wouldn't ordinarily use. Manufacturers offer cents-off coupons to promote their products. If you use them when the food market doubles the coupons' value or when an item is on sale, you can save even more. You will be seeing more and more point of purchase coupons. Look for them in shelf dispensers or at the checkout counter. Preferred-customer cards, available from some supermarket chains, offer additional savings.

Remember that you pay for convenience. Unsliced Italian bread costs less than bread that is sliced and has a garlic flavored spread. You may be willing to pay for preparation time saved, or you may prefer to slice and flavor the bread yourself and save money.

Convenience foods like canned vegetables, frozen juice concentrates, and packaged mixes for muffins and cakes can be real time-savers. They also make it unnecessary to keep supplies of ingredients that you rarely use.

Fast fact

The greatest number of coupons distributed are for cereals and other breakfast foods. Grocery shoppers saved $4.2 billion in 1994 by redeeming coupons. Even though only a small percentage of coupons are redeemed, a recent study showed that merely seeing a coupon in a newspaper insert can boost sales. Cents-off coupons you get as inserts in newspapers have a redemption rate of 2 to 3%. The coupons you get from shelf dispensers have redemption rates of up to 17%. In 1997, almost 25% of consumers used cou-

pons nearly every time they shopped. In 1988 the number was 40%.

Fast fact

Food stores are moving from the business of selling ingredients to selling meals. Sales of lunch and dinner meal items are growing. In 1997 about 22% of all take-out food was bought at food markets, up from 12% in 1996.

Fast fact

More than a quarter of all food produced in the United States is wasted, according to a Department of Agriculture study. In 1995 about 96 billion pounds of food (22%) were lost at the retail, consumer, and food service levels. This did not include pre-harvest, on-the-farm, or farm-to-retail and wholesale losses.

Sex in the Food Market

While male shoppers in food markets are still in the minority, their numbers are increasing. *Progressive Grocer* magazine reported that 19% of the men surveyed said they were the primary grocery shopper, compared with 14% in 1988. Other studies report that as many as a third of the weekend shoppers are men.

Men and women tend to buy different items. Men—especially younger ones—buy beer, cupcakes, ice cream, and hot dogs. Women buy more cottage cheese, yogurt, and salad dressing. Single males and men who head families grocery shop more times a week than women. They also tend to shop at the last minute and when they are hungry, so they are more susceptible to impulse buying. And men are less likely to use cents-off coupons.

FOOD LABELING

In May 1994 the current food labeling law took effect, but Americans have always been label conscious. According to a survey done by the Calorie Control Council, 62% of adults said they always try to check nutrition labels of foods to determine the fat content. Almost as many check for calorie content. In 1996 Trends: Consumer Attitudes and the Supermarket, a survey conducted by the Food Marketing Institute, half of all food market shoppers said they always read the nutrition label when they buy a food for the first time. About 90% of shoppers found the information on the nutrition labels useful.

A "Nutrition Facts" label is found on almost all packaged foods (see page xx). These labels are designed to show how a food fits into the daily diet. They also make it easier to compare one food with another. The number of calories in a serving

Food Label at a Glance

Serving sizes are now more consistent across product lines, are stated in both household and metric measures, and reflect the amounts people actually eat.

New title signals that the label contains the newly required information.

Calories from fat are now shown on the label to help consumers meet dietary guidelines that recommend people get no more than 30 percent of the calories in their overall diet from fat.

% Daily Value shows how a food fits into the overall daily diet.

The **list of nutrients** covers those most important to the health of today's consumers, most of whom need to worry about getting <u>too much</u> of certain nutrients (fat, for example), rather than too few vitamins or minerals, as in the past.

Nutrition Facts

Serving Size 1 cup (228g)
Servings Per Container 2

Amount Per Serving

Calories 260 Calories from Fat 120

	% Daily Value*
Total Fat 13g	**20%**
Saturated Fat 5g	**25%**
Cholesterol 30mg	**10%**
Sodium 660mg	**28%**
Total Carbohydrate 31g	**10%**
Dietary Fiber 0g	**0%**
Sugars 5g	
Protein 5g	

Vitamin A 4% • Vitamin C 2%
Calcium 15% • Iron 4%

* Percent Daily Values are based on a 2,000 calorie diet. Your daily values may be higher or lower depending on your calorie needs:

	Calories:	2,000	2,500
Total Fat	Less than	65g	80g
Sat Fat	Less than	20g	25g
Cholesterol	Less than	300mg	300mg
Sodium	Less than	2,400mg	2,400mg
Total Carbohydrate		300g	375g
Dietary Fiber		25g	30g

Calories per gram:
Fat 9 • Carbohydrate 4 • Protein 4

Daily Values are also something new. Some are maximums, as with fat (65 grams <u>or less</u>); others are minimums, as with carbohydrate (300 grams <u>or more</u>). The daily values for a 2,000- and 2,500-calorie diet must be listed on the label of larger packages.

The label of larger packages may now tell the number of calories per gram of fat, carbohydrate, and protein.

This label is only a sample. Exact specifications are in the final rules.
Source: Food and Drug Administration, 1994

(serving size closely reflects the amounts people actually eat) and the calories from fat are given in numbers. Total fat, cholesterol, sodium, total carbohydrate, and dietary fiber are given both as numbers and as percentages of Daily Value (DV).

Daily Values are the label reference numbers. These numbers are set by the government and are based on current nutrition recommendations. The percent daily values are based on a 2,000 calorie diet; values can also be given for an optional 2,500 calorie diet. While these calorie levels cover the average intake of most people, they do not cover everybody. The nutrients listed on the label are the ones that are important for good health; too much of some and too little of others may lead to increased risk for certain diseases. It really isn't necessary to worry about nutrition values for each food you eat or even each meal you eat. What you should aim for most of the time is those foods that give you more carbohydrate, vitamins, and minerals and less sodium, fat, saturated fat, and cholesterol.

The Daily Values for total fat, saturated fat, cholesterol, and sodium set upper limits on the amount to eat each day to stay healthy. Other DVs help you identify the best levels to aim for each day. This applies to total carbohydrate, fiber, vitamins, and minerals.

Loopholes in the Labels

Although the labels can help guide consumers in making better food choices, they are not perfect. Many issues were involved in formulating labels that accurately represent the nutritional value of different foods, but even with the concerted effort of experts, there remain some gray areas:

1. Two percent milk may no longer be called "lowfat." The approved term now is "reduced fat." A glass of 2% milk contains up to 5 grams of fat, which is more than the Food

and Drug Administration's definition of "lowfat"—3 grams of fat in a serving.

2. Trans fatty acids are formed when liquid oils are hardened (hydrogenated) to form solid shortenings. These trans fatty acids are found in margarine, chips, crackers, cookies, and other processed foods. Trans fats are included in the "total fat" category on nutrition labels. Under the labeling law, the manufacturer must list the amount of total fat, saturated fat, and cholesterol in a food, but not the amount of trans fat. Recent research suggests that trans fat could be responsible for 30,000 deaths from heart disease each year in the United States because it raises blood cholesterol the same way saturated fats do. Some experts, however, believe that more studies are needed to clarify the dangers of trans fatty acids.
3. Fruits and vegetables and fresh meats and poultry are not required to have individual nutrition labels. However, the meat industry is participating in a voluntary program in which food markets will display posters showing nutrition information on the most popular cuts. In 1996 some 78% of raw fruits and vegetables were labeled, as was 74% of raw fish.
4. Rules about the use of the word "healthy" on food labels went into effect in 1996. To be labeled "healthy," foods will have to contain low levels of fat and saturated fat, limited amounts of sodium and cholesterol, and at least some amount of a beneficial nutrient, like vitamin C.
5. Businesses that produce 600,000 or fewer units of food a year are exempt from nutrition labeling rules. These are generally local businesses like a cider mill or small regional bakery. That number will drop to 100,000 units in a few years.
6. Foods in small packages, like Lifesavers and snack-size candies, don't need nutrition labels but must list a tele-

phone number or address where consumers can get the required information. Also exempt are food products like coffee, tea, some spices, and flavorings that contain no significant amounts of any nutrient. Take-out foods and ready-to-eat foods prepared on site at a deli or bakery also do not need labeling.

What the Label Claims Really Mean

The FDA required labels mean you'll no longer have to guess what it means when you see a nutrition claim like "low sodium" or "fat free" on a package. These claims can be made only when the food meets strict government definitions.

LABEL LANGUAGE

Label Claim	Definition*
Calorie Free	Less than 5 calories
Low Calorie	40 calories or less
Light or Lite	50% or less fat content than previous standard for the product; fat content must be reduced by 50% or more
Light in Sodium	50% less sodium than previous standard for the product
Less Sodium or Reduced in Sodium	25% less sodium than previous standard for the product
Fat Free	Less than ½ gram fat
Low Fat	3 grams or less fat
Reduced Fat	25% less fat than previous standard for the product
Cholesterol Free	Less than 2 milligrams cholesterol and 2 grams or less saturated fat
Low Cholesterol	20 milligrams or less cholesterol and 2 grams or less saturated fat
Sodium Free and Salt Free	Less than 5 milligrams sodium
Very Low Sodium	35 milligrams or less sodium
Low Sodium	140 milligrams or less sodium

Label Claim	Definition*
High Fiber	5 grams or more fiber
Excellent or High source of a nutrient	Must supply at least 20% of the Daily Value of the nutrient
Good source of a nutrient	Must supply between 10 and 19% of the Daily Value of the nutrient
Lean meat, poultry, seafood, packaged meals	Less than 10 grams fat, 4 grams saturated fat, 95 milligrams cholesterol
Extra lean meat, poultry, seafood, packaged meals	Less than 5 grams fat, 2 grams saturated fat, 95 milligrams cholesterol

*Per Reference Amount (standard serving size). Some claims have higher nutrient levels for main dish products and meal products such as frozen entrées and dinners.

The Food and Drug Administration has proposed a new policy for food labels on foods that require refrigeration.

Group A foods, which are actually hazardous if not kept cold, will carry this label:

IMPORTANT: Must be refrigerated to maintain safety.

Group B foods, which are shelf stable until opened, will carry this label:

IMPORTANT:
Must be refrigerated after opening to maintain safety.

Group C foods are not hazardous if unrefrigerated after opening, but they may deteriorate in quality. Manufacturers may decide whether or not to label these products.

Health Claims

In the past you may have seen health claims on labels suggesting that a product could help prevent a specific disease. Today health claims on food labels are regulated. A food must meet certain nutrient levels to make a health claim. At this time, only the following health claims are allowed, and they may be made only when research supports a link between the nutrient and the disease.

HEALTH CLAIMS ALLOWED ON LABELS

Calcium and osteoporosis (adult bone loss)
Sodium and high blood pressure (hypertension)
Dietary fat and cancer
Dietary saturated fat and cholesterol and risk of coronary heart disease
Fruits and vegetables and cancer
Fiber-containing grain products, fruits, and vegetables and cancer
Fruits, vegetables, and grain products that contain fiber and risk of coronary heart disease
Adequate folate and reduced risk of having a child with a brain or spinal cord birth defect

A label may not make a health claim for a specific nutrient in a food if the food also contains other nutrients that would lessen the health benefits. So that while a container of fat free milk can make a health claim for its calcium content, a container of whole milk cannot, because even though it contains calcium, it also has a lot of fat, which increases the risk for other diseases. Foods that have more than 13 grams of fat, 4 grams of saturated fat, 60 milligrams of cholesterol, or 480 milligrams of sodium per serving and have a nutrient claim for a different nutrient must carry the following statement: "See [appropriate panel] for information about [nutrient requiring disclosure] and other nutrients." Because of the complex rules governing these health claims, experts believe they will not be widely used.

Summing Up: While the new food labels may not be perfect, they are beneficial. Many foods will now be required to display them, and serving sizes are now standardized to make comparisons easier. Rather than trying to interpret every fact, concentrate on what is important. The values for carbohydrate, fiber, vitamins A and C, calcium, and iron should be high, while the values for total fat, saturated fat, cholesterol, and sodium should be low.

Fast fact

The American Dietetic Association's National Center for Nutrition and Dietetics has a consumer hotline for food labeling information and materials. Call 1-800-366-1655.

FOOD MARKET SECTIONS

The Bread Box

Experts urge us to eat whole grains. They have all the vitamins, minerals, and fiber originally found in grain. Many of these important nutrients are lost when the grains are refined. Some nutrients—vitamins B_1 (thiamin), B_2 (riboflavin), niacin, folic acid, and the mineral iron—are added to refined grains, which are then called "enriched." Refined, enriched wheat is the kind usually used to make white bread.

You can't always tell by the color whether or not bread is made with whole grains. Some wheat breads look toasty brown, but the color is not from whole wheat flour. Caramel (browned sugar), molasses, or raisin juice can add rich brown color. The ingredient list on the label will tell you which grains are in the bread. The one listed first is the major grain in the bread, cereal, or cracker.

Bread labeled "100% whole wheat" contains only whole wheat flour. But even a bread that is not 100% whole wheat can be nutritious. Wheat germ, cracked wheat, oatmeal, sprouted wheat, bran breads, and enriched breads are also good sources of nutrients. You may enjoy the flavor of pumpernickel and rye breads, which are mixtures of white flour and smaller amounts of whole grains.

What Kinds of Bread Do We Use?

A recent study shows that half of U.S. households use white bread. This is down from three-fourths just ten years ago. Americans have expanded their taste in bread:

49.2% use white bread
43.8% use whole wheat
16.4% use 100% whole grain
16.4% use French or Italian
12.2% use low calorie or light
11.9% use rye or pumpernickel
10.6% use raisin
10.5% use sourdough
9.3% use fiber or high fiber
8.7% use oat or oat bran

Tortillas are becoming part of the mainstream American diet; sales totaled $2.87 billion in 1996. This is more than the total sales of all other ethnic and specialty breads combined, including bagels, croissants, muffins, and pita. About 60% of tortillas are eaten by non-Latinos. Tortillas are the fastest growing segment of the U.S. baking industry.

Cereals

Cereals can be hot—cooked in a pan or in the microwave—or cold and ready to eat. They are rich in nutrients, fill you up, and are usually low in fat too. If your favorite has a lot of added sugar (you can tell when you see sugar listed as one of the first ingredients), mix it with a cereal that contains less sugar, or use it as a snack instead of cookies.

Note: Some cereals that contain fruit or fruit juice and have more than 4 grams (1 teaspoon) of sugar in a serving may still be good choices. They may look like they're high in sugar, but the sugar in the dried fruit or juice is included on the label, with the added sugar.

Crackers

The cracker shelf is one of the largest and most varied in the supermarket. For a healthy snack, try some of the new reduced fat and fat free varieties, like cracked pepper, which are flavorful without fat. Rice cakes (the chocolate ones are great), bagel chips, breadsticks, saltines, and soda crackers are usually good lowfat choices, but don't forget old-fashioned graham crackers for a sweet treat.

Other Grains

Many delicious grains are now available. Besides regular enriched white rice, you'll find long grain, short grain, wild rice (not really rice at all), barley, buckwheat (kasha), bulgur, cracked wheat, millet, cornmeal, and quinoa, to name some of the more common grains available. Package labels give cooking directions.

Summing Up: The Food Guide Pyramid, the USDA guide for choosing a good diet (see page xxix), recommends eating six to eleven servings from the Bread and Cereal Group each day. In 1996 only 12% of Americans ate the recommended six servings. The average intake of grains is three to four servings a day; only

FOOD GUIDE PYRAMID

A Guide to Daily Food Choices

The Pyramid is an outline of what to eat each day. It's not a rigid prescription, but a general guide that lets you choose a healthful diet that's right for you. The Pyramid calls for eating a variety of foods to get the nutrients you need and at the same time the right amount of calories to maintain a healthy weight.

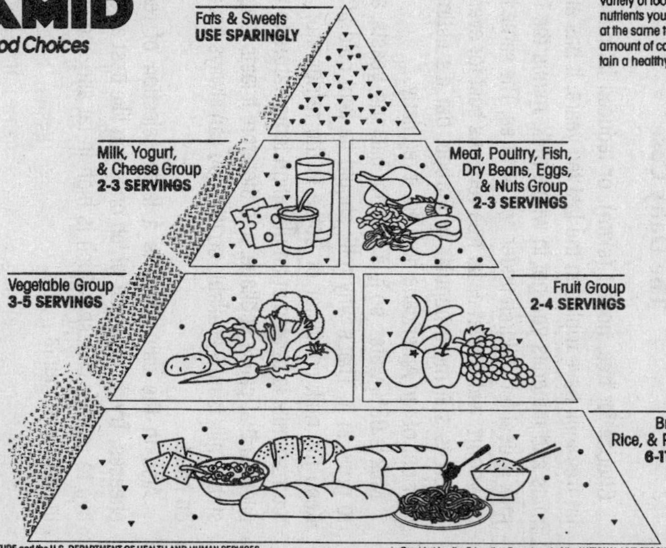

The Food Guide Pyramid emphasizes foods from the five food groups shown in the three lower sections of the Pyramid.

Each of these food groups provides some, but not all, of the nutrients you need. Foods in one group can't replace those in another. No one food group is more important than another—for good health, you need them all.

Source: U.S. DEPARTMENT OF AGRICULTURE and the U.S. DEPARTMENT OF HEALTH AND HUMAN SERVICES.

Provided by: the Education Department of the NATIONAL LIVE STOCK AND MEAT BOARD.

5% eat the minimum six grain servings. A serving is 1 slice of bread, 4 crackers, 1 ounce of ready-to-eat cereal, or ½ cup of hot cereal, pasta, rice, bulgur, or other grains.

The Dairy Case

Choose fat free, nonfat (skim), or reduced fat milk. Sales of fat free milk have tripled in the last ten years. It has all the vitamins and minerals you get in whole milk, minus the fat. Whole milk is best for children under two or three. The same holds true for yogurt, with lowfat or fat free versions best for everyday use. Yogurt is still more popular in Europe, but it's estimated that four out of ten Americans now eat it regularly.

Milk is 93% water, so it is easy for bacteria, yeasts, and molds to grow in it. That's why milk should be kept cold at all times. Keep the milk container or bottle in the refrigerator. Ultrapasteurized milk is treated at an ultrahigh temperature to kill off the bacteria that cause spoilage, and therefore it lasts longer. Shelf-stable milk is now available so that you can always have a supply on hand.

Also in the dairy case is a large selection of reduced fat cheeses. Try them to see which ones you like best as an alternative to regular cheese, which is high in fat and should be used in smaller amounts.

Summing Up: The Food Guide Pyramid recommends two to three servings from the Milk, Yogurt & Cheese Group. Teens, young adults, and women who are pregnant or breast-feeding need three servings. The average American has only one serving a day. A serving is 1 cup of milk, buttermilk, or yogurt; 1½ cups reduced fat ice cream; 1½ ounces hard cheese; or 2 ounces processed cheese. It takes 2 cups of cottage cheese to equal the calcium in 1 cup of milk, so it's not an equal milk replacement.

Pick Up Some Culture

Bacterial cultures cause milk to ferment and make yogurt yogurt. Research suggests that yogurt containing live bacteria has health benefits. These bacteria seem to boost the immune system and help to prevent colon cancer. Yogurt has also been shown to help prevent diarrhea and canker sores. The types with active cultures are a good source of calcium and are well tolerated by some people who cannot handle lactose, the sugar in milk. Some yogurt makers pasteurize yogurt after the bacteria is added, killing the cultures and eliminating the live bacteria. If you want live cultures, look for a label that states "active yogurt cultures," "live yogurt cultures," or "cultured after pasteurization."

Fruits and Vegetables

Even though fresh fruits and vegetables account for only about 10% of grocery sales, surveys show that customers often decide where to shop based on the quality of the produce section. Twenty years ago food markets stocked 30 to 40 produce items; now there are 350 to 400 items. Fruits and vegetables are no longer seasonal. Now you can buy almost any kind year-round. At any one time your food market may stock apples from New Zealand, grapes from Chile, melons from Israel, and mangoes from Peru.

But remember, buying fruits and vegetables in season means lower prices and better quality. Medium-size fruits are a better buy than larger fruits, and you pay a premium price for jumbo because they are scarce.

Prepared produce—like cut-up melons, washed salad ingredients, and celery and carrot sticks—costs much more. A pound of whole carrots may cost as little as 35 cents. The price of carrot sticks climbs to almost $2.00 a pound, but the time saved may be worth the cost.

Note: The Nutrition Facts Panel on dried fruit may lead you to believe that prunes, for example, contain a lot of added sugar. In fact, there is no added sugar. The 11 grams of sugar (almost 3 teaspoons) in 6 prunes is all natural sugar. The nutrition label does not distinguish between added sugar and natural sugar. Read the ingredient listing to see if there is any sugar added. When no sugar is listed, all the sugar is natural to the food.

Fruit and vegetable juices are good sources of vitamins and minerals, but they do not contain all the fiber in the original fruit. They are available as frozen concentrates, ready to use from the dairy case, and in shelf-stable containers (box drinks). Don't confuse pure juice with juice drinks. They are not the same. Pure juice is 100% fruit juice, while juice drinks can contain as little as 10 to 30% real juice. In addition, these drinks contain water and added sugar.

The federal labeling law requires that the percentage of actual fruit juice or vegetable juice in a drink, punch, ade, or cocktail be shown on the label. You will find it on the side nutrition panel of juice packages. Because it is not on the front and it may be in small print, you may have to look carefully to find it, but don't let that stop you. Higher percentages of fruit and vegetable juices mean a healthier beverage that is richer in vitamins and minerals and has less water and usually fewer sweeteners. Many juice drinks cost the same as or even more than pure (100%) juice even though sugar and water cost less.

Note: Some 100% juice drinks contain a large percentage of apple or grape juice in addition to more exotic juices like guava or papaya that lend their names to the beverage.

Fast fact

Kids' favorite fruits and vegetables, in order of popularity, are bananas, apples, grapes, oranges, plums, carrots, lettuce, tomatoes, and broccoli.

Summing Up: The Food Guide Pyramid recommends five or more servings of fruit and vegetables a day. Some surveys suggest that many Americans do not eat even one. Only 25% of Americans eat the recommended five or more servings a day, and even this may be an overestimate. The United Fresh Fruit and Vegetable Association found that people frequently overestimate the amount eaten by 33%. Men eat fewer fruits and vegetables than women. It is much easier to meet this guideline if you stock up on ready-to-use fruits and vegetables when you shop.

A serving of fruit is ½ grapefruit; 1 medium apple, banana, or orange; 1 peach or pear; 2 plums; 12 cherries; 2 raw figs; ½ cup cooked or canned fruit; ½ cup berries, pineapple, or melon chunks; ¼ cup dried fruit; or ¾ cup fruit juice.

A serving of vegetables is 1 small potato, ½ cup cooked vegetables, 1 small ear of corn, 1 cup raw leafy vegetables, or ¾ cup vegetable juice.

Does Sex Really Matter?

You may have heard that some eggplants are female and others male. The sex is determined by the shape of the scarlike depression on the blossom end of the vegetable, opposite the stem end. If the scar is round, the eggplant is male; if it's elongated, the eggplant is female. Don't bother examining your eggplant, because experts say that sex has no effect on the quality of the vegetable.

Variety in the Salad Bowl

Food markets now stock a variety of salad greens. Washed greens are available in bags and in salad bars, and heads of lettuce are sold in the produce department. Iceberg lettuce has always been popular because of its crispness, but if you want greener, leafier, or tastier choices that are more nutrient rich, try arugula, Belgian endive, butterhead, radicchio, romaine, chicory, escarole, spinach, or watercress.

Arugula: slender green leaves with a peppery flavor; younger, smaller leaves are milder.

Belgian endive: not really a green, since bullet-shaped heads are yellow; crisp, mildly sharp, and flavorful.

Butterhead: includes Boston and Bibb; soft, buttery texture with a mild, sweet flavor.

Radicchio: colorful red leaves that look like little red cabbages; not as crisp as endive, which it stars with in tricolored salads.

Chicory: also called curly endive, its thin, curly leaves are fairly bitter; can be used raw or cooked.

Escarole: leaves are wider and flatter than chicory; slightly bitter, but the inner leaves tend to be milder; popular in soups; can be used raw.

Romaine: very nutritious green often used in Caesar salads.

Watercress: small, dark green leaves with a sharp, peppery flavor; used in salads and sandwiches, and as a garnish.

Meat Case (and Beans Too)

The meat group in the Food Guide Pyramid includes meat, poultry, fish, dry beans, eggs, and nuts. Protein is found in all the foods in this group, as are iron and other minerals and vitamins. Animal protein foods also supply vitamin B_{12}, while beans are a good source of fiber.

Four ounces of lean, boneless meat, fish, or poultry will give three ounces cooked, about the size of a deck of cards. That's plenty, even though it's less than you usually get in a restaurant.

Chickens Up

Americans almost doubled their annual intake of chicken between 1975 and 1992. We eat about 48 pounds of chicken a year. It is estimated that this will increase to 94 pounds by the year 2005.

In 1994, according to the Department of Agriculture, Americans ate, per person:

63.7 pounds of beef
49.5 pounds of pork
48.2 pounds of chicken
14.9 pounds of fish and shellfish
14.3 pounds of turkey
0.9 pounds of lamb
0.8 pounds of veal

Poultry is often thought of as low in fat, but some types, like goose, are high in fat and should be eaten only occasionally. While chicken is low in fat, the skin is loaded with it. Research shows that cooking chicken with the skin on keeps the meat moist without adding fat, but always remove the skin before you eat the chicken.

Choosing Lower Fat Protein Foods

High fat option	Low fat option
Porterhouse steak	Flank steak
Rib roast	Eye round
Regular hamburger	Ground meat, 10% or less fat
Spareribs	Center-cut pork loin
Frozen breaded fish	Frozen plain fish
Sardines packed in oil	Sardines in mustard sauce
Tuna packed in oil	Tuna packed in water
Refried beans	Plain beans with salsa
Bluefish, mackerel	Scrod, halibut, tuna
Fried chicken	Baked chicken

Note: You can find reduced fat bologna, salami, hot dogs, and bacon, but the original varieties are high in fat and salt. Both types, regular and reduced fat, usually contain nitrites that combine with substances found naturally in some foods and in the stomach to form carcinogens (cancer-causing substances) called nitrosamines. Use these kinds of processed meats only once in a while. Nuts and seeds, other members of the meat group, are good sources of protein but they are high in fat. Eat small amounts of these.

Summing Up: The Food Guide Pyramid recommends two to three servings from the Meat, Poultry, Fish, Dry Beans, Eggs & Nuts Group. The average American eats more than two servings a day from the meat group. A serving is equal to 3 ounces of cooked lean meat, fish, or poultry. One-half cup cooked beans or lentils, 2 ounces tofu, 2 tablespoons peanut butter, ⅓ cup nuts, or 1 egg can fill in for 1 ounce of meat.

Fast fact

A survey conducted by Kraft Foods found that 37% of men were unwilling to give up red meat, and 42% of women felt the same way about sweets.

Fast fact

The average American ate 14.9 pounds of seafood in 1994. Tuna remained the favorite. The other top nine in order of consumption were shrimp, Alaska pollack (surimi), salmon, cod, catfish, clams, flatfish, crabs, and scallops.

Why Not Try Tofu?

Ounce for ounce, tofu has just as much protein as meat, and it's cholesterol free and very low in saturated fat. Because tofu is made from soybeans, it has the same cholesterol lowering and cancer preventing properties of soy that scientists are beginning to learn about.

Tofu can be found in most supermarkets and greengrocers. It is versatile, picking up the flavors of foods it's cooked with. Soft tofu—called silken on the package—can be mashed and used as a substitute for cottage cheese, or it can be blended until creamy in a food processor or blender and then substituted for sour cream or mayonnaise in dips. Firm tofu can be sliced and marinated in soy sauce, garlic, sesame oil, and ginger (try 2 tablespoons of reduced salt soy sauce, 1 teaspoon of sesame oil, 1 minced garlic clove, and a sprinkle of ginger) and then stir-fried or—even tastier—broiled for a flavorful meat substitute.

Note: Packaged tofu is usually pasteurized and will be labeled as such. Tofu sold in blocks from water-filled basins usually isn't; eating it may put you at risk of *E. coli* food poisoning.

Snacks

Many snacks fall into the Fats & Sweets Group, which includes oils. This group makes up the tip, the smallest part of the Food Guide Pyramid. Instead of a recommended number of servings, the advice given is to use these foods sparingly. Most of us enjoy high sugar, high fat snacks like soda, chips, cookies, cake, ice cream, and candy. Considered fun foods, they are often used as a treat or reward, as a cure for boredom, or as a quick way to satisfy hunger. Americans are such eager snackers that over three hundred new snack items are introduced every year!

Eating these foods is not the issue; the amount you eat is. Have a snack-size candy bar, not a regular size. Try an ice cream bar or a small cup instead of a soup bowl full of ice cream. Reach for an individual bag of chips rather than the giant economy size. Eat a cupcake instead of a large slice of cake.

Chips and pretzels are popular snack foods. In 1994, Americans ate, on average, 22 pounds of salty snacks like potato chips, popcorn, pretzels, and tortilla chips. Pretzels usually are lower in fat than regular chips and are also available lightly salted or unsalted, but Americans prefer chips, eating three times as many potato chips and twice as many tortilla chips as pretzels.

Choose cookies that snap instead of bend or fruit bars for lowfat choices; buy air-popped corn or pretzels rather than chips. Lower fat and no fat versions of your favorite chips are becoming available, so look for them.

Americans love candy. We each eat an average of 24 pounds a year! Try some licorice, jelly beans, candy corn, or marshmallows. These are all sweet lowfat treats. Hard candies and lollipops provide long-lasting, lowfat, sweet snacking.

Ice cream should be a "sometimes" food. While it does contain some calcium, it also has lots of fat, saturated fat, and cholesterol. Look for lower fat or fat free varieties. Or look for lower fat frozen desserts like sorbet, ices, or frozen yogurt.

Pastries such as pies, Danish pastries, croissants, and doughnuts can be very high in fat. They're all "once in a while" snacks. Even muffins, often thought of as a healthy substitute for pastries, can be high in fat. Look for muffins that are labeled lowfat, or have a bagel with jelly instead.

Americans drink a lot of soda—nearly 9 ounces of carbonated soft drinks a day. One ounce of soda contains about 1 teaspoon of sugar, so the usual 12-ounce can contains 12 teaspoons.

Colas, the most popular soda, and some fruit-flavored sodas often contain caffeine too. Instead of soda, try plain sparkling water (mixed half and half with fruit juice), mineral water, or iced tea for a change.

Deep Freeze

Frozen fruits and vegetables are a quick and convenient way to add vitamins and minerals to meals. Most of the time, stay away from those that are sauced, buttered, or sugared. You can add your own flavorings and toppings, as little or as much as you like, suiting your taste and saving money at the same time. Frozen potatoes are popular, but label reading is important, because many are high in fat and should be reserved for occasional use.

Instead of complete dinners, use frozen entrées—pasta dishes, pizza, tacos, chicken, fish, pancakes, or waffles—convenience foods you can use as the base for a quick meal. Simply add a salad or fresh fruit, some bread, and a beverage.

SO THAT THERE'S ALWAYS SOMETHING TO EAT

Sometimes you just may be too tired to eat out or even order in. Even though there are no leftovers from yesterday, you can easily put together a quick, satisfying meal when you keep your refrigerator and cabinets stocked with foods we used to call staples.

Use the following list for a start, adding your own special favorites. You'll never have to complain again about there being nothing to eat.

Freezer

Bread: sliced loaf, tortillas, pita

Made in minutes: bagel pizza, salad pita, grilled cheese

Vegetables: green peas, mixed vegetables, corn
  Made in minutes: peas and pasta
Fruit: strawberries, raspberries
  Made in minutes: fruit cup, topping for angel food cake
Frozen juice and juice drinks
Frozen lowfat or fat free yogurt
Meat and poultry: hamburger or turkey patties, chicken pieces, boneless chicken breast
  Made in minutes: creamed chicken (use canned cream soup)

Refrigerator

Cheese: your favorite hard cheese, grated cheese
Eggs
Butter or other spread
Vegetables: onions, carrots

Cupboard

Canned tomatoes: crushed, stewed, sauce
Pasta, rice
Canned beans: chickpeas, black beans, blackeye peas, baked beans
Oil: olive oil and another vegetable oil, like corn or canola
Vinegar: try flavored*
Ketchup
Soy sauce
Salsa*
Anchovy or sun-dried tomato paste*
Bread crumbs
Dried fruit: raisins, prunes, apricots
Nuts: walnuts or your favorites

---

*A small amount of these will add a punch of flavor.

Milk: shelf-stable or evaporated
Dried mushrooms*
Spices: cinnamon, ginger, oregano, paprika, curry powder, dried garlic, seasoned pepper
Bouillon cubes or powder
Canned soup: chicken broth, cream soup*
Cereal: Oatmeal and ready-to-eat
Jam or jelly
Sugar
Popcorn, unpopped
Tea
Coffee

Fast fact

A Whirlpool Corporation survey found that 80% of the respondents had milk in their refrigerators, 37% had eggs, 36% had juice and soda, 26% had butter, and 11% had cheese.

Fast fact

For a healthful meal, fill three-quarters of your plate with vegetables, beans, lentils, bread, pasta, rice, grains, and fruits, and fill the other quarter with lean meat, fish, poultry, or a protein alternative like nuts, eggs, or tofu.

Fast fact

Forget the myth that dishes prepared with mayonnaise are more likely to spoil in the heat. These foods are actually safer because of the high acid level of mayonnaise.

HANDLING FOOD SAFELY

To keep food at its best in flavor and nutrition and to avoid food poisoning, you must handle and store it carefully. When you're loading your cart in the supermarket, it's a good idea to pick up cold and frozen foods last. Cold foods should feel cold, and frozen foods should be solid. Pack them together in one double bag so they have less chance to thaw out on the way home. And go home quickly. Canned foods should be free of dents, rust, cracks, and bulges, which can indicate food spoilage. Look for the use-by date on packaged foods, and don't buy any that you can't use by the time listed.

Be sure that your refrigerator and freezer are kept cold enough. Refrigerators should be at 40°F, as cold as possible without freezing milk or vegetables. The freezer should be at 0°F, keeping the contents frozen hard. Unpack and refrigerate or freeze your food as soon as you get home. If you can't use meat, poultry, or fish within two days, freeze it.

There is a time limit for storage of all foods. Even canned foods that look as if they will last forever are best when used within one year. Rotate canned and frozen foods so that the older ones are used up first. You may have noticed that more packaged foods now show a date on their label. Sometimes only a date appears, as on milk and juice containers; other times the statement "Best when purchased by (date)" or "Sell by (date)" is on condiments, salad dressings, and baked goods. "Use by" is on box drinks, jellies and cereals. Some products have expiration dates that indicate the end of their shelf life. Fewer than 5% of shoppers pay attention to these dates. Depending on the product, there is a reasonable time to use it after the sell date before it gets stale or spoils. Of course, the way the food has been handled before it is sold in the store will affect the length of time it remains usable. It's always best to buy food in a store that has a rapid turnover of products.

A good food rule is, "When in doubt, throw it out." When you see mold on soft cheese, sour cream, yogurt, bread, cake, or cooked beans, toss them. Small moldy spots can be cut away from hard cheese or firm fruits and vegetables. Cut at least one inch around and below the spot of mold. Store the food in a clean container and use it as soon as you can. You can also scoop out tiny spots of mold from jellies. Be careful to scoop out a larger amount around the mold. *Pure* maple syrup that has become moldy can simply be boiled and used.

The high temperatures of cooking will kill most of the bacteria that cause food-borne illness. While steaks can be served very pink in the center (medium rare), all poultry and ground meat should be thoroughly cooked. *Ground meat must be cooked until it is gray, not pink, in the middle, particularly if children, elderly persons, or people with compromised immune systems will be eating the meat.* Several deaths of children have been reported recently due to eating undercooked ground meat from cattle carrying a deadly strain of *E. coli* bacteria. Thorough cooking of the ground meat will kill the bacteria.

Once cooked, keep the food hot (above 140°F) until it is served. Put cooked meat and poultry on a clean platter, not the raw meat platter. Don't keep cooked foods at room temperature for longer than two hours. Don't allow leftovers to cool on the kitchen counter before refrigerating. Thaw perishable foods in the refrigerator or microwave, not at room temperature.

Do not eat raw seafood unless it is prepared by a trained sushi chef. Fish and shellfish need special handling, as they deteriorate quickly. Fresh fish should be frozen immediately if it will not be used in a day or two. During some times of the year, eating oysters may pose a problem for people with suppressed immune systems. Viruses that can cause fever, nausea, and occasionally death may be found even in oysters that have been steamed for thirty minutes. These viruses will not harm most healthy adults.

Always wash fruit before eating it, even when you will peel it. Use clean running water and no soap. Soap can leave a residue.

Here's how you can keep your kitchen sponge or dishcloth free of harmful bacteria: simply rinse it, wring it out, put it in the microwave, and zap it at full power for thirty seconds. This will make it virtually sterile.

If you have specific questions about safe food handling, you can call these numbers:

- USDA's Meat and Poultry Hotline: 1-800-535-4555 (10:00 A.M. to 4:00 P.M. Eastern Standard Time, weekdays)
- Centers for Disease Control and Prevention, Food-borne Illness Line: 1-404-332-4597 (twenty-four-hour recorded information)
- Your local health department
  Extension home economists or department of public health (listed in phone book)

Fast fact

Hot (spicy) seafood cocktail sauce was found to disinfect the raw oysters on which it was served. Horseradish and lemon juice also killed off some bacteria but were not as effective as Tabasco and other hot sauces.

SAFE TIME LIMITS FOR REFRIGERATOR OR FREEZER STORAGE

Food	Cabinet	Refrigerator	Freezer
Berries		1–2 days	
Brownie and cake mixes	9 months		
Canned foods	12 months		
Chicken, fresh		1–2 days	9 months

(continued)

Food	Cabinet	Refrigerator	Freezer
Dried peas and beans	12 months		
Egg substitutes, opened		3 days	Do not freeze
Eggs		3 weeks	Do not freeze
Fish (cod, sole)		1–2 days	6 months
Fish (salmon)		1–2 days	2–3 months
Flour	6–8 months		
Frozen dinners			3–4 months
Ground meat		1–2 days	3–4 months
Half & half		10 days	
Ham slices		3–4 days	1–2 months
Herbs, dried	6 months		
Hot dogs, luncheon meat, unopened		1 week	1–2 months
Jellies			
Unopened	12 months		
Opened		3 months	
Mayonnaise			
Unopened	2–3 months		
Opened		2 months	
Meat leftovers		3–4 days	
Milk		5 days	
Pasta	2 years		
Popcorn kernels	2 years		
Potatoes	2–3 months		
Rice, white	2 years		
Salad dressing			
Unopened	10–12 months		
Opened		3 months	
Salad oil, opened	1–3 months		

Food	Cabinet	Refrigerator	Freezer
Sauce and gravy mix	6–12 months		
Shrimp			
Fresh		1 day	
Frozen			12 months
Soups and stews		3–4 days	2–3 months
Spices and herbs (basil, cinnamon, thyme, chili powder, parsley flakes, paprika, etc.)	1 year		
Steaks, chops		3–5 days	6–9 months
Sugar			
White	2 years		
Brown	4 months		
Syrup	12 months		
Tea bags	18 months		

Food Poisoning

Every year more than 7 million Americans suffer from food poisoning. Symptoms include nausea, vomiting, diarrhea, fever, and cramps. These symptoms can begin anywhere from thirty minutes to as long as two weeks after the food was eaten, but most times they occur within four to forty-eight hours. Sometimes symptoms are very severe. If the person is elderly, very young, pregnant, or already ill, call a doctor or go to an emergency room right away.

Most cases of food-related illness can be prevented by safe food handling. The Partnership for Food Safety Education, a coalition of industry, government, and consumer groups, has initiated a nationwide food safety campaign known as *Fight* BAC!

You'll be seeing *Fight* BAC! information displayed in many places.

Safe Handling Instructions for Fresh Meat and Poultry

The Department of Agriculture requires fresh meat and poultry to be labeled with safe-handling instructions. The safe-handling instruction label was developed to help consumers prevent food-borne illness at home. It covers four safety guidelines: safety, cross-contamination, cooking, and handling leftovers.

USING YOUR FOOD SHOPPING COUNTER

Shoppers average just over two trips a week to the food market. It doesn't matter whether you shop at Safeway, Kroger, A&P, Publix, Associated, Winn-Dixie, Wild Oats, Grand Union, or Bal-

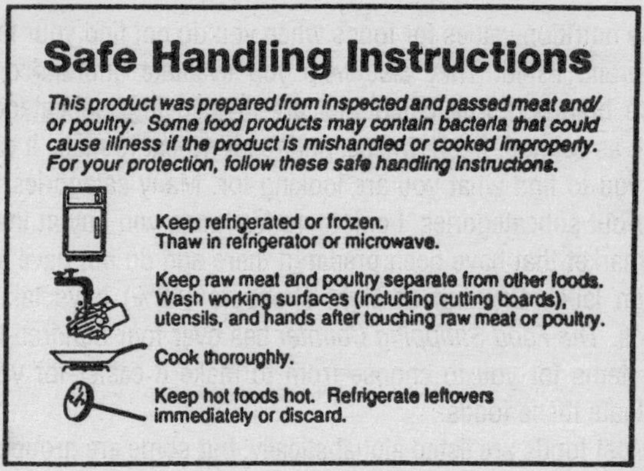

Safe Handling Instructions

This product was prepared from inspected and passed meat and/ or poultry. Some food products may contain bacteria that could cause illness if the product is mishandled or cooked improperly. For your protection, follow these safe handling instructions.

Keep refrigerated or frozen.
Thaw in refrigerator or microwave.

Keep raw meat and poultry separate from other foods.
Wash working surfaces (including cutting boards), utensils, and hands after touching raw meat or poultry.

Cook thoroughly.

Keep hot foods hot. Refrigerate leftovers immediately or discard.

ducci's in New York, this book lists the calories, fat, cholesterol, sodium, and fiber of most of the 20,000 foods you'll find there. For the first time, information about these nutrient values is at your fingertips. Now you will find it easy to follow a healthy diet. Before *The Food Shopping Counter,* it was impossible to compare so many foods at one time. For example, when you want to select bread, look up the bread category on page 53. You will find over 430 different breads listed, so you can see which one is the best source of carbohydrate and fiber.

The Food Shopping Counter lists the calories, fat, carbohydrate, sodium, and fiber values. These are key nutrients for good health. Fat and sodium should be limited, while carbohydrate and fiber should be increased. The food labeling act established guidelines for nutrient intake. It recommends that a diet of 2,000 calories a day include at least 300 grams of carbohydrate and 25 grams of dietary fiber and less than 65 grams of total fat and 2,400 milligrams of sodium.

In *The Food Shopping Counter* foods are listed alphabetically. For each group, you will find nonbranded (generic) foods listed first in alphabetical order, followed by an alphabetical listing of brand-name food. The nonbranded listings will help you determine nutrition values for foods when you do not find your favorite brand listed. They also help you evaluate unbranded and store brands. Large categories are divided into subcategories such as canned, fresh, frozen, and ready-to-eat to make it easier for you to find what you are looking for. Many categories have take-out subcategories. Look there for foods you buy at the supermarket that have been prepared there and do not have a nutrition label. One out of eight shoppers (12%) buys take-out foods. *The Food Shopping Counter* has over four hundred take-out items for you to choose from to make it easier for you to evaluate these foods.

Most foods are listed alphabetically, but some are grouped by category. For example, pasta dinners, like spaghetti and meat balls, lasagna, and manicotti, are all found under the category "Pasta Dishes." Other group categories include the following:

Fast fact

Although Sara Lee is a real person, as were the late Orville Redenbacher and Duncan Hines, there is no Betty Crocker, Mrs. Paul, or Chef Boyardee.

DEFINITIONS

as prep (as prepared): refers to food that has been prepared according to package directions

home recipe: describes homemade dishes; those included can be used as a guide to the nutrient values of similar products you may prepare or take-out food you buy ready-to-eat

lean and fat: describes meat with some fat on its edges that is not cut away before cooking or poultry prepared with skin and fat as purchased

lean only: lean portion, trimmed of all visible fat

shelf stable: refers to prepared products found on the supermarket shelf that are ready to be heated or eaten and do not require refrigeration

take-out: describes prepared dishes that you purchase ready-to-eat; those included serve as a guide to the nutrient and calorie values of similar products you may purchase

(tr) trace: value used when a food contains less than one calorie, less than one gram (g) of fat, carbohydrate or fiber, or less than one milligram (mg) of sodium

ABBREVIATIONS

avg	=	average
diam	=	diameter
fl	=	fluid
frzn	=	frozen
g	=	gram
in	=	inch
lb	=	pound
<	=	less than
lg	=	large
med	=	medium
mg	=	milligram
oz	=	ounce
pkg	=	package
prep	=	prepared
pt	=	pint
qt	=	quart
reg	=	regular
sec	=	second
serv	=	serving
sm	=	small
sq	=	square
tbsp	=	tablespoon
tr	=	trace
tsp	=	teaspoon
w/	=	with
w/o	=	without

EQUIVALENT MEASURES

1 tablespoon	=	3 teaspoons
4 tablespoons	=	¼ cup
8 tablespoons	=	½ cup
12 tablespoons	=	¾ cup
16 tablespoons	=	1 cup
1,000 milligrams	=	1 gram
28 grams	=	1 ounce

Liquid Measures

2 tablespoons	=	1 ounce
¼ cup	=	2 ounces
½ cup	=	4 ounces
¾ cup	=	6 ounces
1 cup	=	8 ounces
2 cups	=	1 pint
4 cups	=	1 quart

Dry Measures

4 ounces	=	¼ pound
8 ounces	=	½ pound
12 ounces	=	¾ pound
16 ounces	=	1 pound

NOTES

Discrepancies in figures are due to rounding, product reformulation, and reevaluation. Labeling law allows rounding of values. Because most of the data are analysis data, obtained directly from manufacturers, not from labels, in some cases our values may not be exactly the same as label information because they have not been rounded.

All total fat, carbohydrate (CARB.) and fiber* (FIB.) values are given in grams (g).

All sodium (SOD.) values are given in milligrams (mg).

A dash (—) indicates data not available.

*All fiber values are dietary fiber. Except for sweets, foods that are high in carbohydrate (pasta, bread, cereals, fruit, and vegetables) also provide dietary fiber. Animal products—eggs, milk, cheese, meat, fish, poultry—are not sources of fiber. The fiber values indicated for these foods come from added ingredients.

THE FOOD SHOPPING COUNTER

FOOD	PORTION	CAL.	FAT	SOD.	CARB.	FIB.
ABALONE						
fresh fried	3 oz	161	6	502	9	—
raw	3 oz	89	1	255	5	—
ACEROLA						
fresh	1	2	tr	0	tr	—
ACEROLA JUICE						
juice	1 cup	51	1	7	12	—
ADZUKI BEANS						
CANNED						
sweetened	1 cup	702	tr	646	163	—
Eden						
Organic	½ cup (4.1 oz)	100	0	10	18	5
DRIED						
cooked	1 cup	294	tr	18	57	—
READY-TO-EAT						
yokan sliced	3¼ in slices	112	tr	36	26	—
AKEE						
fresh	3½ oz	223	20	—	5	—
ALE						
(*see* BEER AND ALE, *and* MALT)						
ALFALFA						
sprouts	1 tbsp	1	tr	0	tr	—
sprouts	1 cup	40	tr	2	1	—
ALLIGATOR						
tail cooked	3½ oz	143	3	—	1	—
ALLSPICE						
ground	1 tsp	5	tr	1	1	—
ALMONDS						
almond butter honey & cinnamon	1 tbsp	96	8	2	4	—
almond butter w/ salt	1 tbsp	101	9	75	3	—
almond butter w/o salt	1 tbsp	101	10	2	3	—
almond meal	1 oz	116	5	2	8	—
almond paste	1 oz	127	8	3	12	—
dried blanched	1 oz	166	15	3	5	—
dried unblanched	1 oz	167	15	3	6	—
dry roasted unblanched	1 oz	167	15	3	7	—
dry roasted unblanched salted	1 oz	167	15	260	7	—

FOOD	PORTION	CAL.	FAT	SOD.	CARB.	FIB.
oil roasted blanched	1 oz	174	16	3	5	3
oil roasted blanched salted	1 oz	174	16	3	5	—
oil roasted unblanched	1 oz	176	16	3	5	—
toasted unblanched	1 oz	167	14	3	7	3
Beer Nuts						
Almonds	1 pkg (1 oz)	180	14	51	7	—
Dole						
Blanched Slivered	1 oz	170	14	4	5	—
Blanched Whole	1 oz	170	14	4	5	—
Chopped Natural	1 oz	170	14	4	5	—
Sliced Natural	1 oz	170	14	4	5	—
Whole Natural	1 oz	170	14	4	5	—
Erewhon						
Almond Butter	1 tbsp (16 g)	90	8	18	2	—
Hain						
Almond Butter Natural Raw	2 tbsp	190	18	120	3	—
Almond Butter Toasted	2 tbsp	220	19	210	3	—
Lance						
Smoked	1 pkg (0.7 oz)	120	11	130	3	—
Nutella						
Spread	1 tbsp (0.5 oz)	85	5	5	9	—
Planters						
Almonds	1 oz	170	15	0	5	3
Gold Measure Slivered	1 pkg (2 oz)	340	31	0	11	4
Honey Roasted	1 oz	160	14	190	7	2

AMARANTH

(*see also* CEREAL, COOKIES)

FOOD	PORTION	CAL.	FAT	SOD.	CARB.	FIB.
cooked	½ cup	59	tr	14	3	—
uncooked	½ cup	366	6	21	65	—
Arrowhead						
Seeds	¼ cup (1.6 oz)	170	2	0	29	3
Health Valley						
Amaranth Cereal With Bananas	½ cup (1 oz)	110	2	5	20	4
Amaranth Crunch With Raisins	¼ cup (1 oz)	110	3	10	20	3
Amaranth Flakes 100% Organic	½ cup (1 oz)	90	tr	5	21	3
Fast Menu Amaranth With Garden Vegetables	7½ oz	140	3	140	16	8

ANASAZI BEANS

FOOD	PORTION	CAL.	FAT	SOD.	CARB.	FIB.
Arrowhead						
Dried	¼ cup (1.5 oz)	150	1	0	27	9

FOOD	PORTION	CAL.	FAT	SOD.	CARB.	FIB.
Bean Cuisine						
Dried	½ cup	115	1	5	—	5
ANCHOVY						
CANNED						
in oil	5	42	2	734	0	—
in oil	1 can (1.6 oz)	95	4	1651	0	—
FRESH						
fillets	3 (0.4 oz)	21	1	—	tr	—
raw	3 oz	62	4	88	0	—
ANGLERFISH						
raw	3½ oz	72	1	109	0	—
ANISE						
seed	1 tsp	7	tr	tr	1	—
ANTELOPE						
roasted	3 oz	127	2	46	0	—
APPLE						
CANNED						
sliced sweetened	1 cup	136	1	7	34	—
Luck's						
Fried Apples	8 oz	190	0	—	—	—
White House						
Escalloped Apples	4 oz	120	0	10	28	1
Sliced	4 oz	55	0	10	15	1
Spiced Apple Rings	1 ring	25	0	0	6	tr
DRIED						
cooked w/ sugar	½ cup	116	tr	27	29	—
cooked w/o sugar	½ cup	172	tr	26	20	—
rings	10	155	tr	56	42	—
Del Monte						
Sliced	⅓ cup (1.4 oz)	80	0	310	23	5
Mariani						
Apples	¼ cup	150	0	—	—	—
Sonoma						
Pieces	10-12 pieces (1.4 oz)	110	0	0	29	4
FRESH						
apple	1	81	tr	1	21	3
w/o skin sliced	1 cup	62	tr	0	16	2
w/o skin sliced & cooked	1 cup	91	tr	1	23	—
w/o skin sliced & microwaved	1 cup	96	tr	1	25	—

FOOD	PORTION	CAL.	FAT	SOD.	CARB.	FIB.
Dole						
Apple	1	80	1	0	18	5
Tastee						
Candy Apple	1 (3 oz)	160	5	20	26	4
Caramel Apple	1 (3 oz)	160	5	20	26	4
FROZEN						
sliced w/o sugar	½ cup	41	tr	3	11	—
Mrs. Paul's						
Apple Fritters	2	270	9	500	35	—
Stouffer's						
Escalloped	1 cup (6 oz)	180	3	70	37	3
APPLE JUICE						
frzn as prep	1 cup	111	tr	17	28	—
frzn not prep	6 oz	349	1	54	87	—
juice	1 cup	116	tr	7	29	tr
After The Fall						
Organic	1 bottle (10 oz)	110	0	25	28	—
Vermont Apple	1 bottle (8 oz)	90	0	20	22	—
Vermont Apple	1 bottle (10 oz)	110	0	24	27	—
Vermont Harvest Moon Sparkling Apple Cider	8 fl oz	110	0	5	27	—
Apple & Eve						
Cider	6 fl oz	80	0	0	16	—
Juice	6 fl oz	80	0	0	16	—
Nothin' But Juice	6 fl oz	78	0	0	18	—
Bruce						
Lite	½ cup	88	0	25	20	—
Everfresh						
Apple Juice	1 can (8 oz)	110	0	10	29	0
Hi-C						
Jammin' Apple	8 fl oz	130	0	30	31	—
Hood						
Select Cider	1 cup (8 oz)	120	0	2	30	—
Juice Works						
Juice	6 oz	100	0	—	—	—
Minute Maid						
Box	8.45 fl oz	120	0	30	29	—
Juices To Go	1 can (11.5 fl oz)	160	0	40	40	—
Juices To Go	1 bottle (10 fl oz)	140	0	35	35	—
Juices To Go	1 bottle (16 fl oz)	110	0	30	28	—
Naturals	8 fl oz	110	0	30	28	—
Mott's						
From Concentrate as prep	8 fl oz	120	0	20	29	0

FOOD	PORTION	CAL.	FAT	SOD.	CARB.	FIB.
Mott's (CONT.)						
Fruit Basket Cocktail as prep	8 fl oz	120	0	5	29	0
Natural	8 fl oz	120	0	20	29	0
Ocean Spray						
Juice	8 fl oz	110	0	35	28	0
Odwalla						
Live Apple	8 fl oz	140	0	25	34	0
Red Cheek						
From Concentrate	8 fl oz	120	0	20	29	0
Natural	8 fl oz	120	0	20	29	0
S&W						
100% Unsweetened	6 oz	85	0	5	20	—
Seneca						
Clarified frzn, as prep	8 fl oz	120	0	24	30	0
Granny Smith frzn as prep	8 fl oz	120	0	24	30	0
Natural frzn as prep	8 fl oz	120	0	24	30	0
Sippin' Pak						
100% Pure	8.45 fl oz	110	0	25	28	—
Sipps						
Juice	8.45 oz	130	0	—	—	—
Snapple						
Apple Crisp	10 fl oz	140	0	30	36	—
Tree Of Life						
East Coast Apple	8 fl oz	120	0	25	30	—
Tree Top						
Cider	6 oz	90	0	10	22	—
Cider frzn as prep	6 oz	90	0	10	22	—
Frzn, as prep	6 oz	90	0	10	22	—
Juice	6 oz	90	0	10	22	—
Sparkling Juice	6 oz	90	0	—	22	—
Unfiltered	6 oz	90	0	10	22	—
Unfiltered frzn as prep	6 oz	90	0	10	22	—
w/ Vitamin C	6 oz	90	0	10	22	—
Tropicana						
Season's Best	1 container (6 fl oz)	80	0	5	21	—
Season's Best	1 container (8 fl oz)	110	0	10	28	—
Season's Best	1 container (10 fl oz)	140	0	15	35	—
Season's Best	8 fl oz	110	0	10	28	—
Season's Best	1 bottle (10 fl oz)	140	0	15	35	—
Season's Best	1 bottle (7 fl oz)	100	0	10	24	—
Season's Best	1 can (11.5 fl oz)	160	0	25	40	—

FOOD	PORTION	CAL.	FAT	SOD.	CARB.	FIB.
Veryfine						
100%	8 oz	107	0	<10	27	—
White House						
Juice	6 oz	90	0	0	22	0
APPLESAUCE						
sweetened	½ cup	97	tr	4	25	2
unsweetened	½ cup	53	tr	2	14	2
Eden						
Applesauce	½ cup (4.3 oz)	50	0	15	15	2
Mott's						
Chunky	5 oz	110	0	0	26	2
Cinnamon	5 oz	120	0	0	29	1
Fruit Snacks Apple Spice	4 oz	70	0	0	18	1
Fruit Snacks Cinnamon	4 oz	90	0	0	23	1
Fruit Snacks Strawberry	4 oz	80	0	5	19	1
Fruit Snacks Sweetened	4 oz	90	0	0	22	1
Sweetened	5 oz	110	0	0	28	1
S&W						
Diet	½ cup	55	0	10	14	—
Gravenstein Sweetened	½ cup	90	0	10	24	—
Gravenstein Unsweetened	½ cup	55	0	5	14	—
Sweetened	½ cup	55	0	10	14	—
Unsweetened	½ cup	25	2	5	2	—
Seneca						
Cinnamon	½ cup	100	0	0	24	3
Golden Delicious	½ cup	100	0	0	24	3
McIntosh	½ cup	100	0	0	24	3
Natural	½ cup	60	0	0	15	3
Regular	½ cup	100	0	0	24	3
Tree Of Life						
Applesauce	½ cup (4.3 oz)	50	0	15	15	2
Tree Top						
Cinnamon	½ cup	80	0	0	21	—
Natural	½ cup	60	0	0	15	—
Original	½ cup	80	0	0	21	—
White House						
Chunky	4 oz	80	0	5	22	1
Cinnamon	4 oz	100	0	5	25	1
Natural Packed w/ Apple Juice	4 oz	60	0	5	14	1
Regular	4 oz	80	0	5	22	1
Unsweetened	4 oz	50	0	0	12	2

FOOD	PORTION	CAL.	FAT	SOD.	CARB.	FIB.
APRICOT JUICE						
nectar	1 cup	141	tr	9	36	2
Del Monte						
Nectar	8 fl oz	140	0	15	35	1
Kern's						
Nectar	6 fl oz	110	0	0	27	—
Libby						
Nectar	1 can (11.5 fl oz)	220	0	10	52	—
S&W						
Nectar	6 oz	35	0	20	12	—
APRICOTS						
CANNED						
halves heavy syrup pack w/ skin	1 cup (9.1 oz)	214	tr	10	55	—
halves water pack w/ skin	1 cup (8.5 oz)	65	tr	7	16	—
halves water pack w/o skin	1 cup (8 oz)	51	tr	25	12	—
heavy syrup w/ skin	3 halves	70	tr	3	18	—
juice pack w/ skin	3 halves	40	tr	3	10	—
light syrup w/ skin	3 halves	54	tr	3	14	—
puree from heavy syrup pack w/ skin	¾ cup (9.1 oz)	214	tr	10	55	—
puree from light pack w/ skin	¾ cup (8.9 oz)	160	tr	10	42	—
puree from water pack w/ skin	¾ cup (8.5 oz)	65	tr	7	16	—
puree juice pack w/ skin	1 cup (8.7 oz)	119	tr	9	31	—
water pack w/ skin	3 halves	22	tr	2	5	—
water pack w/o skin	4 halves	20	tr	10	5	—
Del Monte						
Halves Unpeeled In Heavy Syrup	½ cup (4.5 oz)	100	0	10	26	1
Halves Unpeeled Lite	½ cup (4.3 oz)	60	0	10	16	1
Libby						
Halves Unpeeled Lite	½ cup (4.4 oz)	60	0	10	13	1
S&W						
Halves Diet	½ cup	35	0	5	9	—
Halves Unpeeled In Heavy Syrup	½ cup	110	0	15	28	—
Halves Unsweetened	½ cup	35	0	5	9	—
Whole Peeled Diet	½ cup	28	0	5	7	—
Whole Peeled In Heavy Syrup	½ cup	100	0	15	26	—
DRIED						
halves	10	83	tr	3	22	3

FOOD	PORTION	CAL.	FAT	SOD.	CARB.	FIB.
halves cooked w/o sugar	½ cup	106	tr	4	27	—
Del Monte						
Sun Dried	⅓ cup (1.4 oz)	80	0	5	25	6
Mariani						
Apricots	¼ cup	140	0	—	—	—
Sonoma						
Dried	10 pieces (1.4 oz)	120	0	0	31	1
FRESH						
apricots	3	51	tr	1	12	—
FROZEN						
sweetened	½ cup	119	tr	5	30	—
ARROWHEAD						
fresh boiled	1 med (⅓ oz)	9	tr	2	2	—
ARROWROOT						
flour	1 cup	457	tr	2	113	4
ARTICHOKE						
CANNED						
Progresso						
Hearts	2 pieces (2.9 oz)	35	0	240	6	1
Hearts Marinated	⅓ cup (3 oz)	160	14	290	6	1
S&W						
Hearts Marinated	½ cup	225	26	15	6	—
FRESH						
boiled	1 med (4 oz)	60	tr	114	13	—
hearts cooked	½ cup	42	tr	80	9	—
Dole						
Large Whole	1	23	tr	65	5	3
FROZEN						
cooked	1 pkg (9 oz)	108	1	127	22	—
Birds Eye						
Hearts Deluxe	½ cup	30	0	40	7	3
ARUGULA						
raw	½ cup	2	tr	3	tr	—
ASIAN FOOD						
(*see also* DINNER, EGG ROLLS, PASTA, SUSHI)						
CANNED						
chow mein chicken	1 cup	95	tr	725	18	—
La Choy						
Bi-Pack Beef Pepper	¾ cup	80	2	950	10	2
Bi-Pack Chow Mein Chicken	¾ cup	80	3	970	8	1

FOOD	PORTION	CAL.	FAT	SOD.	CARB.	FIB.
La Choy (CONT.)						
Bi-Pack Chow Mein Pork	¾ cup	80	4	950	7	2
Bi-Pack Chow Mein Shrimp	¾ cup	70	1	860	6	1
Bi-Pack Sweet & Sour Chicken	¾ cup	120	2	440	18	2
Bi-Pack Teriyaki Chicken	¾ cup	85	2	850	8	1
Dinner Chow Mein Chicken	¾ pkg	300	17	1800	29	2
Entree Beef Pepper Oriental	¾ cup	100	4	1340	12	2
Entree Chow Mein Beef	¾ cup	40	2	960	5	2
Entree Chow Mein Chicken	¾ cup	70	4	850	2	4
Entree Chow Mein Meatless	¾ cup	25	tr	860	5	2
Entree Chow Mein Shrimp	¾ cup	35	1	940	4	2
Entree Sweet & Sour Chicken	¾ cup	240	2	1420	47	1
Entree Sweet & Sour Pork	¾ cup	250	4	1540	48	1
FRESH						
wonton wrappers	1	23	tr	46	5	—
Azumaya						
Won Ton Wraps	1 (8 g)	23	tr	50	5	—
FROZEN						
Banquet						
Chow Mein Chicken	1 pkg (9 oz)	400	7	850	28	3
Birds Eye						
Easy Recipe Chicken Teriyaki not prep	½ pkg	160	4	600	28	4
Easy Recipe Oriental Beef not prep	½ pkg	100	7	620	11	8
Internationals Chinese Stir Fry not prep	3.3 oz	35	0	125	6	2
Japanese Stir Fry International not prep	3.3 oz	30	0	310	5	2
Chun King						
Beef Pepper Steak	1 pkg (13 oz)	300	4	1670	50	5
Chow Mein Chicken	1 pkg (13 oz)	370	14	2010	45	4
Imperial Chicken	1 pkg (13 oz)	460	10	1670	59	5
Sweet & Sour Pork	1 pkg (13 oz)	450	6	1180	66	4
Walnut Chicken	1 pkg (13 oz)	460	19	1820	56	5

FOOD	PORTION	CAL.	FAT	SOD.	CARB.	FIB.
Lean Cuisine						
Chicken Chow Mein With Rice	1 pkg (9 oz)	220	5	560	33	3
Chicken Oriental w/ Vegetables & Vermicelli	1 pkg (9 oz)	250	6	530	30	4
Oriental Style Dumplings	1 pkg (9 oz)	300	6	520	51	2
Teriyaki Stir Fry	1 pkg (10 oz)	290	4	590	48	4
Luigino's						
Chicken & Almonds With Rice	1 pkg (8 oz)	250	8	770	33	3
Chop Suey Pork With Rice	1 pkg (8.5 oz)	210	4	980	34	2
Lo Mein Chicken	1 pkg (8 oz)	320	5	950	35	3
Lo Mein Shrimp	1 pkg (8 oz)	190	3	980	31	4
Oriental Beef & Peppers With Rice	1 pkg (8 oz)	230	5	820	38	2
Pasta Favorites						
Chicken Lo Mein	1 pkg (10.5 oz)	270	6	1060	43	5
Rice Gourmet						
Chicken Teriyaki Rice Bowl	1 bowl (10.9 oz)	430	6	1210	77	1
Stouffer's						
Chicken Chow Mein w/ Rice	1 pkg (10.6 oz)	260	5	1090	40	3
Tyson						
Stir Fry Kit With Yoshida Oriental Sauce	10.6 oz	330	10	1740	37	—
Sweet & Sour Kit With Sweet & Sour Sauce	14.85 oz	440	9	1300	71	—
Weight Watchers						
Smart Ones Chicken Chow Mein	1 pkg (9 oz)	200	2	570	34	3
Smart Ones Hunan Style Rice & Vegetables	1 pkg (10.34 oz)	250	7	630	39	8
Smart Ones King Pao Noodles & Vegetables	1 pkg (10 oz)	260	10	690	35	5
Smart Ones Spicy Szechuan Style Vegetables & Chicken	1 pkg (9 oz)	220	2	730	39	3
MIX						
Kikkoman						
Chow Mein Seasoning	1⅛ oz pkg	98	tr	—	—	—
Teriyaki Baste & Glaze	1 tbsp	24	tr	310	5	—

FOOD	PORTION	CAL.	FAT	SOD.	CARB.	FIB.
La Choy						
Dinner Classics Egg Foo Young	2 patties + 3 oz sauce	170	7	1390	20	1
Dinner Classics Pepper Steak	¾ cup	180	9	760	9	1
Dinner Classics Sweet & Sour	¾ cup	310	6	860	30	tr
TAKE-OUT						
cha siu bao steamed buns w/ chicken filling	1 (2.3 oz)	160	3	300	26	tr
chicken teriyaki	¾ cup	399	27	2190	7	—
chicken teriyaki w/ rice	1 serv (11 oz)	430	6	1210	77	1
chop suey w/ beef & pork	1 cup	300	17	1053	13	—
chop suey w/ pork	1 cup	375	29	1378	29	2
chow mein chicken	1 cup	255	10	718	10	—
chow mein pork	1 cup	425	24	1673	21	3
chow mein shrimp	1 cup	221	10	1658	21	3
chow mein vegetable	1 serv (8 oz)	90	3	1010	15	4
fried rice	6.6 oz	249	6	—	48	2
fried rice w/ egg	6.7 oz	395	20	—	49	2
spring roll deep fried	3.5 oz	202	9	—	24	—
sweet & sour pork	1 serv (8 oz)	250	8	1500	37	2
szechuan chicken w/ lo mein	1 cup (5.3 oz)	190	1	560	35	0
wonton fried	½ cup (1 oz)	111	8	147	8	1
wonton soup	1 cup	205	3	322	26	1

ASPARAGUS

FOOD	PORTION	CAL.	FAT	SOD.	CARB.	FIB.
CANNED						
spears	½ cup	24	1	—	3	—
Del Monte						
Salad Tips Tender Green	½ cup (4.4 oz)	20	0	420	3	1
Spears Cut Tender Green	½ cup (4.4 oz)	20	0	420	3	1
Spears Extra Long Tender Green	½ cup (4.4 oz)	20	0	420	3	1
Spears Tender Green	½ cup (4.4 oz)	20	0	420	3	1
Tips Tender Green	½ cup (4.4 oz)	20	0	420	3	1
Owatonna						
Spears Cut	½ cup	20	0	—	—	—
S&W						
Points Water Pack	½ cup	17	0	10	3	—
Spears Colossal Fancy	½ cup	20	0	320	4	—
Spears Fancy	½ cup	18	0	320	3	—
Seneca						
Asparagus	½ cup	20	0	264	3	2

FOOD	PORTION	CAL.	FAT	SOD.	CARB.	FIB.
FRESH						
cooked	½ cup	22	tr	10	4	—
cooked	4 spears	14	tr	7	3	—
raw	½ cup	16	tr	2	3	—
raw	4 spears	14	tr	1	3	—
Dole						
Spears	5	18	0	0	2	2
FROZEN						
cooked	4 spears	17	tr	2	3	—
cooked	1 pkg (10 oz)	82	1	12	14	—
Big Valley						
Spears	5-6 (3 oz)	20	0	0	3	1
Birds Eye						
Cut	½ cup	23	0	5	4	—
Spears	½ cup	25	0	0	4	—
Green Giant						
Harvest Fresh Cuts	½ cup	25	0	60	4	2
ATEMOYA						
fresh	½ cup	94	1	2	24	—
AVOCADO						
FRESH						
avocado	1	324	31	21	15	—
mashed	1 cup	370	35	24	17	—

BABY FOOD

Nutritional guidelines for infants are different from those recommended for older children and adults. Check with a pediatrician for advice on feeding children under the age of 2.

FOOD	PORTION	CAL.	FAT	SOD.	CARB.	FIB.
BAKED SELECTIONS						
Gerber						
Chunky Animal Cookies	2 (0.5 oz)	60	2	—	10	—
Chunky Biter Biscuits	1 (0.4 oz)	50	1	—	9	—
Chunky Zwieback Toast	2 (0.5 oz)	70	2	—	10	—
Graduates Animal Crackers Cinnamon	2 (0.2 oz)	30	1	—	5	—
Graduates Arrowroot Cookies	2 (0.4 oz)	50	2	—	8	—
Graduates Pretzels	2 (0.4 oz)	45	0	—	10	—
CEREAL						
Beech-Nut						
Stage 1 Barley	½ oz	60	0	10	12	1
Stage 1 Oatmeal	½ oz	60	2	15	11	1
Stage 1 Oatmeal & Apples	1 jar (4 oz)	70	0	0	16	1

FOOD	PORTION	CAL.	FAT	SOD.	CARB.	FIB.
Beech-Nut (CONT.)						
Stage 1 Rice	½ oz	60	0	0	13	0
Stage 2 Mixed	½ oz	50	1	10	12	tr
Stage 2 Mixed & Apples	1 jar (4 oz)	70	0	0	16	1
Stage 2 Oatmeal & Chiquita Bananas	½ oz	60	1	0	12	1
Stage 2 Rice & Apples	1 jar (4 oz)	70	0	0	16	1
Stage 2 Rice & Chiquita Bananas	½ oz	60	0	0	13	0
Stage 2 Rice & Golden Delicious Apples	½ oz	60	0	0	14	0
Earth's Best						
Brown Rice	5 tbsp (0.5 oz)	60	0	0	12	—
Mixed Grain	5 tbsp (0.5 oz)	60	0	0	11	—
Peach Oatmeal Banana	1 jar (4.5 fl oz)	60	0	10	12	—
Prunes & Oatmeal	1 jar (4.5 fl oz)	100	0	20	24	—
Gerber						
1st Foods Barley	4 tbsp (0.5 oz)	60	1	—	11	—
1st Foods Oatmeal	4 tbsp (0.5 oz)	50	1	—	9	—
1st Foods Rice	4 tbsp (0.5 oz)	60	1	—	11	—
2nd Foods High Protein	4 tbsp (0.5 oz)	50	1	—	6	—
2nd Foods Mixed	4 tbsp (0.5 oz)	60	1	—	11	—
2nd Foods Mixed With Applesauce & Bananas	1 jar (4 oz)	90	1	—	20	—
2nd Foods Mixed With Banana	4 tbsp (0.5 oz)	60	1	—	11	—
2nd Foods Oatmeal With Applesauce & Bananas	1 jar (4 oz)	90	1	—	20	—
2nd Foods Oatmeal With Bananas	4 tbsp (0.5 oz)	60	1	—	10	—
2nd Foods Rice With Applesauce & Bananas	1 jar (4 oz)	90	0	—	21	—
2nd Foods Rice With Bananas	4 tbsp (0.5 oz)	60	1	—	11	—
3rd Foods Mixed With Applesauce & Bananas	1 jar (6 oz)	140	1	—	31	—
3rd Foods Oatmeal With Applesauce & Bananas	1 jar (6 oz)	140	1	—	28	—
3rd Foods Rice With Mixed Fruit	1 jar (6 oz)	130	0	—	31	—

FOOD	PORTION	CAL.	FAT	SOD.	CARB.	FIB.
Gerber (CONT.)						
Tropical Foods Corn Cereal	4 tbsp (0.5 oz)	60	1	—	12	—
Tropical Foods Rice With Mango	4 tbsp (0.5 oz)	50	0	—	12	—
Health Valley						
Brown Rice 100% Organic	1 tbsp (0.5 oz)	60	1	5	10	1
Sprouted Baby Cereal 100% Organic	1 tbsp (0.5 oz)	60	1	5	10	—
DESSERT						
Beech-Nut						
Stage 2 Apple & Strawberry Dessert	1 jar (4 oz)	100	0	0	23	1
Stage 2 Apple Peach & Strawberry Dessert	1 jar (4 oz)	100	0	0	22	1
Stage 2 Apple Yogurt Dessert	1 jar (4 oz)	100	1	25	22	0
Stage 2 Banana Pineapple Dessert	1 jar (4 oz)	100	0	15	23	0
Stage 2 Banana Pudding (Spanish Label)	1 jar (4 oz)	110	0	0	26	0
Stage 2 Banana Yogurt Dessert	1 jar (4 oz)	120	2	25	24	0
Stage 2 Cottage Cheese With Pears Dessert	1 jar (4 oz)	120	1	15	24	1
Stage 2 Dutch Apple Dessert	1 jar (4 oz)	100	0	10	22	0
Stage 2 Flan De Banana	1 jar (4 oz)	110	0	0	26	0
Stage 2 Flan De Vanilla	1 jar (4 oz)	120	3	60	23	0
Stage 2 Fruit Dessert	1 jar (4 oz)	80	0	0	19	1
Stage 2 Frutas Islenas Dessert	1 jar (4 oz)	100	0	10	23	0
Stage 2 Guava Tropical Fruit Dessert	1 jar (4 oz)	90	0	10	22	2
Stage 2 Mango Tropical Fruit Dessert	1 jar (4 oz)	110	0	10	26	1
Stage 2 Mixed Fruit Yogurt Dessert	1 jar (4 oz)	100	0	15	21	1
Stage 2 Papaya Tropical Fruit Dessert	1 jar (4 oz)	100	0	10	22	0
Stage 2 Vanilla Custard Pudding	1 jar (4 oz)	120	3	60	23	0
Stage 3 Cottage Cheese With Pears	1 jar (6 oz)	180	2	20	37	1

FOOD	PORTION	CAL.	FAT	SOD.	CARB.	FIB.
Beech-Nut (CONT.)						
Stage 3 Fruit Dessert	1 jar (6 oz)	120	0	0	28	2
Stage 3 Mixed Fruit Yogurt Dessert	1 jar (6 oz)	170	0	30	39	1
Stage 3 Vanilla Custard Pudding	1 jar (6 oz)	190	6	85	32	0
Gerber						
2nd Foods Banana Apple Dessert	1 jar (4 oz)	80	0	—	19	—
2nd Foods Banana Yogurt Dessert	1 jar (4 oz)	90	0	—	21	—
2nd Foods Cherry Vanilla Pudding	1 jar (4 oz)	80	0	—	19	—
2nd Foods Dutch Apple	1 jar (4 oz)	100	2	—	20	—
2nd Foods Fruit Dessert	1 jar (4 oz)	100	0	—	23	—
2nd Foods Hawaiian Delight	1 jar (4 oz)	90	0	—	22	—
2nd Foods Mixed Fruit Yogurt Dessert	1 jar (4 oz)	90	0	—	21	—
2nd Foods Peach Cobbler	1 jar (4 oz)	90	0	—	21	—
2nd Foods Peach Yogurt Dessert	1 jar (4 oz)	90	0	—	21	—
2nd Foods Vanilla Custard Pudding	1 jar (4 oz)	100	1	—	21	—
3rd Foods Dutch Apple	1 jar (6 oz)	130	2	—	29	—
3rd Foods Fruit Dessert	1 jar (6 oz)	120	0	—	30	—
3rd Foods Hawaiian Delight	1 jar (6 oz)	150	0	—	35	—
3rd Foods Peach Cobbler	1 jar (6 oz)	130	0	—	31	—
3rd Foods Vanilla Custard Pudding	1 jar (6 oz)	150	2	—	31	—
Tropical Foods Banana Vanilla Dessert	1 jar (4 oz)	100	1	—	21	—
Tropical Foods Guava With Tapioca	1 jar (4 oz)	80	0	—	21	—
Tropical Foods Mango Banana Passion Fruit	1 jar (4 oz)	80	0	—	20	—
Tropical Foods Mango With Tapicoa	1 jar (4 oz)	80	0	—	21	—
Tropical Foods Papaya Pineapple Dessert	1 jar (4 oz)	90	0	—	22	—
Tropical Foods Papaya With Tapioca	1 jar (4 oz)	70	0	—	17	—

FOOD	PORTION	CAL.	FAT	SOD.	CARB.	FIB.
Gerber (CONT.)						
Tropical Foods Peaches Mango	1 jar (4 oz)	80	0	—	19	—
Tropical Foods Pineapple Banana Dessert	1 jar (4 oz)	90	0	—	22	—
Tropical Foods Tropical Fruits Medley	1 jar (4 oz)	70	0	—	18	—
DINNER						
Beech-Nut						
Stage 2 Beef & Egg Noodle	1 jar (4 oz)	100	6	50	8	2
Stage 2 Beef Supreme	1 jar (4 oz)	130	9	45	8	1
Stage 2 Chicken & Rice	1 jar (4 oz)	80	3	70	9	1
Stage 2 Chicken Noodle	1 jar (4 oz)	70	4	45	7	2
Stage 2 Chicken Soup	1 jar (4 oz)	90	4	50	8	1
Stage 2 Turkey Supreme	1 jar (4 oz)	90	4	45	9	1
Stage 2 Vegetable Beef	1 jar (4 oz)	80	4	45	8	1
Stage 2 Vegetable Chicken	1 jar (4 oz)	80	4	40	8	1
Stage 2 Vegetable Ham	1 jar (4 oz)	80	3	30	9	1
Stage 2 Vegetable Lamb	1 jar (4 oz)	80	3	55	9	1
Stage 2 Vegetable Turkey Rice	1 jar (4 oz)	70	3	50	8	1
Stage 3 Beef & Egg Noodle	1 jar (6 oz)	130	6	50	13	2
Stage 3 Chicken Noodle	1 jar (6 oz)	110	4	55	14	1
Stage 3 Macaroni & Beef	1 jar (6 oz)	130	6	60	14	2
Stage 3 Spaghetti & Beef	1 jar (6 oz)	130	6	70	16	1
Stage 3 Turkey Rice	1 jar (6 oz)	100	3	60	13	2
Stage 3 Vegetable Beef	1 jar (6 oz)	130	6	60	14	2
Stage 3 Vegetable Chicken	1 jar (6 oz)	110	4	55	14	1
Table Time Chicken & Stars	1 bowl (6 oz)	150	6	170	17	1
Table Time Macaroni & Cheese	1 bowl (6 oz)	200	12	320	21	0
Table Time Seashells In Tomato Sauce	1 bowl (6 oz)	150	4	170	25	1
Table Time Spaghetti Rings In Meat Sauce	1 bowl (6 oz)	160	6	180	20	0
Table Time Turkey Stew With Rice	1 bowl (6 oz)	150	4	200	14	1
Table Time Vegetable Stew With Beef	1 bowl (6 oz)	110	3	170	16	1

FOOD	PORTION	CAL.	FAT	SOD.	CARB.	FIB.
Earth's Best						
Corn Rice & Cheese Dinner	1 jar (4.5 fl oz)	120	5	45	13	—
Macaroni & Cheese	1 jar (4.5 oz)	100	4	10	12	—
Pasta Dinner	1 jar (4.5 fl oz)	90	3	20	13	—
Potato & Green Bean Dinner	1 jar (4.5 fl oz)	100	3	25	13	—
Rice & Lentil Dinner	1 jar (4.5 fl oz)	80	2	25	13	—
Summer Vegetable Dinner	1 jar (4.5 oz)	90	3	15	12	—
Gerber						
2nd Foods Apples & Chicken	1 jar (4 oz)	70	2	—	12	—
2nd Foods Apples & Ham	1 jar (4 oz)	70	1	—	14	—
2nd Foods Apples & Turkey	1 jar (4 oz)	80	2	—	13	—
2nd Foods Beef Egg Noodle	1 jar (4 oz)	80	3	—	10	—
2nd Foods Broccoli & Chicken	1 jar (4 oz)	50	2	—	4	—
2nd Foods Carrots & Beef	1 jar (4 oz)	70	3	—	7	—
2nd Foods Chicken Noodle	1 jar (4 oz)	70	2	—	11	—
2nd Foods Green Beans & Turkey	1 jar (4 oz)	70	2	—	9	—
2nd Foods Macaroni Cheese	1 jar (4 oz)	80	3	—	10	—
2nd Foods Macaroni Tomato Beef	1 jar (4 oz)	70	2	—	11	—
2nd Foods Turkey Rice	1 jar (4 oz)	70	3	—	9	—
2nd Foods Vegetable Bacon	1 jar (4 oz)	90	5	—	10	—
2nd Foods Vegetable Beef	1 jar (4 oz)	70	3	—	10	—
2nd Foods Vegetable Chicken	1 jar (4 oz)	70	2	—	11	—
2nd Foods Vegetable Ham	1 jar (4 oz)	70	3	—	10	—
2nd Foods Vegetable Turkey	1 jar (4 oz)	60	2	—	9	—
3rd Foods Beef Egg Noodle	1 jar (6 oz)	110	4	—	15	—

FOOD	PORTION	CAL.	FAT	SOD.	CARB.	FIB.
Gerber (CONT.)						
3rd Foods Chicken Noodle	1 jar (6 oz)	100	3	—	15	—
3rd Foods Macaroni Tomato Beef	1 jar (6 oz)	110	2	—	19	—
3rd Foods Spaghetti Tomato Sauce Beef	1 jar (6 oz)	120	3	—	19	—
3rd Foods Turkey Rice	1 jar (6 oz)	100	3	—	14	—
3rd Foods Vegetable Bacon	1 jar (6 oz)	130	6	—	17	—
3rd Foods Vegetable Beef	1 jar (6 oz)	120	4	—	16	—
3rd Foods Vegetable Chicken	1 jar (6 oz)	100	3	—	15	—
3rd Foods Vegetable Ham	1 jar (6 oz)	110	4	—	16	—
3rd Foods Vegetable Turkey	1 jar (6 oz)	100	3	—	15	—
Chunky Homestyle Noodles & Beef	1 jar (6 oz)	150	6	—	18	—
Chunky Macaroni Alphabets With Beef & Sauce	1 jar (6.3 oz)	140	4	—	20	—
Chunky Noodles & Chicken With Carrots & Peas	1 jar (6 oz)	110	3	—	16	—
Chunky Rice With Beef & Tomato Sauce	1 jar (6.3 oz)	140	4	—	21	—
Chunky Saucy Rice With Chicken	1 jar (6 oz)	120	3	—	19	—
Chunky Spaghetti Tomato Sauce Beef	1 jar (6.3 oz)	150	4	—	22	—
Chunky Vegetables & Beef	1 jar (6.3 oz)	130	5	—	16	—
Chunky Vegetables & Chicken	1 jar (6.3 oz)	140	5	—	17	—
Chunky Vegetables & Ham	1 jar (6.3 oz)	130	5	—	16	—
Chunky Vegetables & Turkey	1 jar (6.3 oz)	110	3	—	15	—
Graduates Chicken Stew With Noodles	1 bowl (6 oz)	120	4	—	15	—
Graduates Macaroni And Beef in Sauce	1 bowl (6 oz)	150	4	—	20	—

FOOD	PORTION	CAL.	FAT	SOD.	CARB.	FIB.
Gerber (CONT.)						
Graduates Spaghetti With Mini Meatballs & Sauce	1 bowl (6 oz)	160	5	—	21	—
Graduates Tomato Sauce With Beef Ravioli	1 bowl (6 oz)	170	4	—	28	—
Graduates Tomato Sauce With Cheese Ravioli	1 bowl (6 oz)	170	4	—	28	—
Graduates Turkey Stew With Rice	1 bowl (6 oz)	100	2	—	13	—
Graduates Vegetable Stew With Beef	1 bowl (6 oz)	130	3	—	15	—
Tropical Foods Beans & Rice	1 jar (4 oz)	60	2	—	9	—
Tropical Foods Chicken & Rice	1 jar (4 oz)	60	2	—	8	—
FRUIT						
Beech-Nut						
Stage 1 Applesauce Golden Delicious	1 jar (4 oz)	70	0	0	15	1
Stage 1 Applesauce Golden Delicious	1 jar (2.5 oz)	50	0	0	12	1
Stage 1 Bananas Chiquita	1 jar (4 oz)	110	0	0	24	1
Stage 1 Bananas Chiquita	1 jar (2.5 oz)	70	0	0	16	1
Stage 1 Chiquita Bananas With Pears & Apples	1 jar (4 oz)	90	0	0	21	1
Stage 1 Peaches Yellow Cling	1 jar (4 oz)	70	0	0	14	3
Stage 1 Peaches Yellow Cling	1 jar (2.5 oz)	45	0	0	11	2
Stage 1 Pears Bartlett	1 jar (2.5 oz)	50	0	0	12	2
Stage 1 Pears Bartlett	1 jar (4 oz)	70	0	0	18	3
Stage 2 Apples & Apricots	1 jar (4 oz)	70	0	0	17	1
Stage 2 Apples & Bananas	1 jar (4 oz)	60	0	0	14	1
Stage 2 Apples & Blueberries	1 jar (4 oz)	70	0	0	17	1
Stage 2 Apples & Cherries	1 jar (4 oz)	80	0	0	18	1
Stage 2 Apples Pears & Bananas	1 jar (4 oz)	90	0	0	20	1

FOOD	PORTION	CAL.	FAT	SOD.	CARB.	FIB.
Beech-Nut (CONT.)						
Stage 2 Apricots With Pears & Apples	1 jar (4 oz)	90	0	0	20	2
Stage 2 Bartlett Pears & Pineapple	1 jar (4 oz)	70	0	0	17	3
Stage 2 Peaches & Bananas	1 jar (4 oz)	70	0	0	15	3
Stage 2 Plums With Apples & Rice	1 jar (4 oz)	90	0	10	18	1
Stage 2 Prunes With Pears	1 jar (4 oz)	110	0	10	24	3
Stage 3 Apples & Bananas	1 jar (6 oz)	90	0	0	21	1
Stage 3 Apples & Cherries	1 jar (6 oz)	110	0	0	26	1
Stage 3 Applesauce	1 jar (6 oz)	100	0	0	23	2
Stage 3 Apricots With Pears & Apples	1 jar (6 oz)	130	0	0	32	—
Stage 3 Bananas Chiquita	1 jar (6 oz)	160	0	0	33	3
Stage 3 Peaches	1 jar (6 oz)	100	0	0	21	4
Stage 3 Pears Bartlett	1 jar (6 oz)	110	0	0	27	5
Earth's Best						
Apples	1 jar (4.5 oz)	70	0	10	17	—
Apples & Apricots	1 jar (4.5 fl oz)	70	0	5	17	—
Apples & Blueberries	1 jar (4.5 fl oz)	70	0	10	17	—
Apples & Plums	1 jar (4.5 fl oz)	70	0	10	17	—
Bananas	1 jar (4.5 oz)	90	0	0	20	—
Pear	1 jar (4.5 fl oz)	60	0	10	14	—
Plums Bananas & Rice	1 jar (4.5 fl oz)	90	1	10	19	—
Gerber						
1st Foods Applesauce	1 jar (2.5 oz)	25	0	—	9	—
1st Foods Bananas	1 jar (2.5 oz)	70	0	—	17	—
1st Foods Peaches	1 jar (2.5 oz)	30	0	—	7	—
1st Foods Pears	1 jar (2.5 oz)	40	0	—	10	—
1st Foods Prunes	1 jar (2.5 oz)	70	0	—	17	—
2nd Foods Apple Blueberry	1 jar (4 oz)	50	0	—	13	—
2nd Foods Applesauce	1 jar (4 oz)	60	0	—	14	—
2nd Foods Applesauce Apricot	1 jar (4 oz)	60	0	—	14	—
2nd Foods Apricots With Tapioca	1 jar (4 oz)	80	0	—	19	—
2nd Foods Banana With Pineapple & Tapioca	1 jar (4 oz)	60	0	—	14	—

FOOD	PORTION	CAL.	FAT	SOD.	CARB.	FIB.
Gerber (CONT.)						
2nd Foods Banana With Tapioca	1 jar (4 oz)	90	0	—	21	—
2nd Foods Peaches	1 jar (4 oz)	70	0	—	17	—
2nd Foods Pear Pineapple	1 jar (4 oz)	60	0	—	15	—
2nd Foods Pears	1 jar (4 oz)	60	0	—	15	—
2nd Foods Plums With Tapioca	1 jar (4 oz)	80	0	—	20	—
2nd Foods Prunes With Tapioca	1 jar (4 oz)	90	0	—	21	—
JUICE						
Beech-Nut						
Stage 1 Apple	4 fl oz	60	0	10	15	0
Stage 1 Pear	4 fl oz	60	0	0	15	0
Stage 1 White Grape	4 fl oz	100	0	10	23	0
Stage 2 Apple Banana	4 fl oz	70	0	0	16	0
Stage 2 Apple Cherry	4 fl oz	70	0	10	17	0
Stage 2 Apple Cranberry	4 fl oz	60	0	10	15	0
Stage 2 Apple Grape	4 fl oz	70	0	15	18	0
Stage 2 Juice Plus Grape	4 fl oz	100	0	10	23	0
Stage 2 Mango Nectar (Spanish Label)	4 fl oz	80	0	0	18	0
Stage 2 Mixed Fruit	4 fl oz	70	0	10	15	0
Stage 2 Papaya Nectar (Spanish Label)	4 fl oz	80	0	10	20	0
Stage 2 Tropical Blend	4 fl oz	90	0	5	15	0
Stage 2 Tropical Blend Nectar (Spanish Label)	4 fl oz	90	0	5	19	0
Stage 3 Orange	4 fl oz	60	0	0	15	0
Earth's Best						
Apple	1 bottle (4.2 fl oz)	60	0	20	14	—
Apple Banana	1 bottle (4.2 fl oz)	60	0	20	14	—
Apple Grape	1 bottle (4.2 fl oz)	60	0	15	14	—
Apples & Bananas	1 jar (4.5 fl oz)	80	0	20	18	—
Pear	1 bottle (4.2 fl oz)	60	0	0	15	—
Gerber						
1st Foods Apple	4 fl oz	60	0	—	14	—
1st Foods Pear	4 fl oz	60	0	—	14	—
1st Foods Red Grape	4 fl oz	80	0	—	20	—
1st Foods White Grape	4 fl oz	80	0	—	19	—
2nd Foods Apple Banana	4 fl oz	60	0	—	15	—
2nd Foods Apple Cherry	4 fl oz	60	0	—	14	—

FOOD	PORTION	CAL.	FAT	SOD.	CARB.	FIB.
Gerber (CONT.)						
2nd Foods Apple Grape	4 fl oz	60	0	—	15	—
2nd Foods Apple Peach	4 fl oz	60	0	—	14	—
2nd Foods Apple Plum	4 fl oz	60	0	—	15	—
2nd Foods Apple Prune	4 fl oz	60	0	—	16	—
2nd Foods Apple With Yogurt	4 fl oz	100	2	—	18	—
2nd Foods Banana With Yogurt	4 fl oz	110	2	—	21	—
2nd Foods Mixed Fruit	4 fl oz	60	0	—	14	—
2nd Foods Mixed Fruit with Yogurt	4 fl oz	100	2	—	18	—
2nd Foods Orange	4 fl oz	60	0	—	13	—
2nd Foods Pear Peach With Yogurt	4 fl oz	90	1	—	18	—
3rd Foods Apple Carrot	4 fl oz	50	0	—	12	—
3rd Foods Apple Sweet Potato	4 fl oz	60	0	—	14	—
3rd Foods Orange Carrot	4 fl oz	50	0	—	12	—
3rd Foods Pineapple Carrot	4 fl oz	60	0	—	13	—
Graduates Apple	4 fl oz	80	0	—	21	—
Graduates Apple Banana	4 fl oz	90	0	—	23	—
Graduates Apple Cherry	4 fl oz	80	0	—	21	—
Graduates Apple Grape	4 fl oz	90	0	—	22	—
Tropical Foods Guava With Mixed Fruit	4 fl oz	70	0	—	18	—
Tropical Foods Mango With Mixed Fruit	4 fl oz	70	0	—	18	—
Tropical Foods Papaya With Mixed Fruit	4 fl oz	70	0	—	18	—
MEAT						
Beech-Nut						
Stage 1 Beef & Broth	1 jar (2.5 oz)	90	6	40	0	0
Stage 1 Chicken & Broth	1 jar (2.5 oz)	70	3	55	0	0
Stage 1 Lamb & Broth	1 jar (2.5 oz)	60	3	50	0	0
Stage 1 Turkey & Broth	1 jar (2.5 oz)	90	6	40	0	0
Stage 1 Veal & Broth	1 jar (2.5 oz)	60	2	50	0	0
Gerber						
2nd Foods Beef	1 jar (2.5 oz)	80	4	—	0	—
2nd Foods Chicken	1 jar (2.5 oz)	90	6	—	0	—
2nd Foods Egg Yolks	1 jar (2.5 oz)	130	11	—	1	—
2nd Foods Ham	1 jar (2.5 oz)	90	6	—	0	—
2nd Foods Lamb	1 jar (2.5 oz)	80	4	—	0	—

FOOD	PORTION	CAL.	FAT	SOD.	CARB.	FIB.
Gerber (CONT.)						
2nd Foods Turkey	1 jar (2.5 oz)	80	5	—	0	—
2nd Foods Veal	1 jar (2.5 oz)	70	4	—	0	—
3rd Foods Beef	1 jar (2.5 oz)	80	4	—	0	—
3rd Foods Chicken	1 jar (2.5 oz)	90	6	—	0	—
3rd Foods Ham	1 jar (2.5 oz)	90	6	—	0	—
3rd Foods Turkey	1 jar (2.5 oz)	90	5	—	0	—
3rd Foods Veal	1 jar (2.5 oz)	80	4	—	0	—
Graduates Chicken Sticks	1 jar (2.5 oz)	110	7	—	2	—
Graduates Meat Sticks	1 jar (2.5 oz)	110	7	—	2	—
Graduates Turkey Sticks	1 jar (2.5 oz)	120	8	—	2	—
VEGETABLE						
Beech-Nut						
Stage 1 Butternut Squash	1 jar (2.5 oz)	30	0	10	7	2
Stage 1 Butternut Squash	1 jar (4 oz)	50	0	10	11	3
Stage 1 Carrots Sweet Tender	1 jar (4 oz)	50	0	100	10	4
Stage 1 Carrots Tender Sweet	1 jar (2.5 oz)	30	0	80	7	2
Stage 1 Green Beans (Spanish Label)	1 jar (2.5 oz)	20	0	0	4	2
Stage 1 Green Beans Tender Young	1 jar (4 oz)	35	0	0	6	3
Stage 1 Peas Tender Sweet	1 jar (4 oz)	60	0	0	11	5
Stage 1 Peas Tender Sweet	1 jar (2.5 oz)	40	0	0	7	3
Stage 1 Sweet Potatoes Tender Golden	1 jar (4 oz)	80	0	10	17	0
Stage 1 Sweet Potatoes Tender Golden	1 jar (2.5 oz)	50	0	10	10	0
Stage 2 Carrots & Peas	1 jar (4 oz)	50	0	25	10	3
Stage 2 Creamed Corn	1 jar (4 oz)	90	0	20	18	2
Stage 2 Garden Vegetables	1 jar (4 oz)	50	0	10	9	3
Stage 2 Mixed Vegetables	1 jar (4 oz)	45	0	10	9	3
Stage 3 Carrots	1 jar (6 oz)	70	0	240	15	5
Stage 3 Green Beans	1 jar (6 oz)	50	0	0	10	4
Stage 3 Sweet Potatoes	1 jar (6 oz)	110	0	15	25	1
Earth's Best						
Carrots	1 jar (4.5 fl oz)	40	0	70	8	—

FOOD	PORTION	CAL.	FAT	SOD.	CARB.	FIB.
Earth's Best (CONT.)						
Carrots & Parsnips	1 jar (4.5 fl oz)	60	0	30	14	—
Corn & Butternut Squash	1 jar (4.5 fl oz)	90	2	0	15	—
Garden Vegetables	1 jar (4.5 fl oz)	70	0	15	15	—
Green Beans & Rice	1 jar (4.5 fl oz)	40	1	15	6	—
Peas & Brown Rice	1 jar (4.5 fl oz)	80	0	10	16	—
Spinach & Potatoes	1 jar (4.5 fl oz)	60	2	25	8	—
Sweet Potatoes	1 jar (4.5 fl oz)	60	1	15	12	—
Winter Squash	1 jar (4.5 fl oz)	50	0	10	12	—
Gerber						
1st Foods Carrots	1 jar (2.5 oz)	25	0	—	5	—
1st Foods Green Beans	1 jar (2.5 oz)	25	0	—	5	—
1st Foods Peas	1 jar (2.5 oz)	30	0	—	6	—
1st Foods Squash	1 jar (2.5 oz)	25	0	—	5	—
1st Foods Sweet Potatoes	1 jar (2.5 oz)	45	0	—	10	—
2nd Foods Beets	1 jar (4 oz)	45	0	—	10	—
2nd Foods Carrots	1 jar (4 oz)	30	0	—	7	—
2nd Foods Creamed Corn	1 jar (4 oz)	80	1	—	15	—
2nd Foods Creamed Spinach	1 jar (4 oz)	50	1	—	8	—
2nd Foods Garden Vegetables	1 jar (4 oz)	45	1	—	7	—
2nd Foods Green Beans	1 jar (4 oz)	35	0	—	7	—
2nd Foods Mixed Vegetables	1 jar (4 oz)	50	1	—	9	—
2nd Foods Peas	1 jar (4 oz)	60	1	—	9	—
2nd Foods Squash	1 jar (4 oz)	35	0	—	8	—
2nd Foods Sweet Potatoes	1 jar (4 oz)	70	0	—	16	—
3rd Foods Broccoli Carrots Cheese	1 jar (6 oz)	80	2	—	12	—
3rd Foods Carrots	1 jar (6 oz)	50	0	—	11	—
3rd Foods Creamed Green Beans	1 jar (6 oz)	80	1	—	16	—
3rd Foods Mixed Vegetables	1 jar (6 oz)	70	0	—	15	—
3rd Foods Peas	1 jar (6 oz)	80	1	—	14	—
3rd Foods Squash	1 jar (6 oz)	60	1	—	12	—
3rd Foods Sweet Potatoes	1 jar (6 oz)	100	0	—	24	—
Graduates Carrots	1 jar (4.5 oz)	30	0	—	6	—

FOOD	PORTION	CAL.	FAT	SOD.	CARB.	FIB.
Gerber (CONT.)						
Graduates Green Beans	1 jar (4.5 oz)	30	0	—	6	—
Graduates Peas	1 jar (4.5 oz)	60	0	—	11	—
Graduates Potatoes	1 jar (4.5 oz)	50	0	—	11	—
BACON						
(*see also* BACON SUBSTITUTES)						
breakfast strips cooked	3 strips (34 g)	156	12	—	—	—
breakfast strips beef cooked	3 strips (34 g)	153	12	766	tr	—
cooked	3 strips	109	9	303	tr	—
gammon lean & fat grilled	4.2 oz	274	15	—	0	0
grilled	2 slices (1.7 oz)	86	4	719	1	—
Armour						
Lower Salt cooked	1 strip	38	3	—	—	—
Star cooked	1 strip	38	3	185	—	—
Black Label						
Center Cut cooked	3 slices (0.5 oz)	70	6	240	0	0
Cooked	2 slices (0.5 oz)	80	7	330	0	0
Low Salt cooked	2 slices (0.5 oz)	80	7	210	0	0
Hillshire						
Bacon	1 slice	120	12	150	tr	—
Hormel						
Bacon Bits	1 tsp (7 g)	30	2	250	0	0
Bacon Pieces	1 tsp (7 g)	25	2	170	0	0
Microwave cooked	2 slices (0.5 oz)	70	5	230	0	0
Jones						
Sliced	1 slice	130	13	150	tr	—
Nathan's						
Beef cooked	3 slices	100	7	310	tr	—
Old Smokehouse						
Cooked	2 slices (0.5 oz)	80	7	280	0	0
Oscar Mayer						
Bacon Bits	1 tbsp (7 g)	25	2	220	0	0
Center Cut cooked	3 slices (0.5 oz)	70	6	320	tr	0
Cooked	2 slices (0.4 oz)	60	5	290	0	0
Lower Sodium cooked	2 slices (0.5 oz)	60	5	180	0	0
Thick Cut cooked	1 slice (0.4 oz)	50	4	250	0	0
Range Brand						
Cooked	2 slices (0.7 oz)	100	9	460	0	0
Red Label						
Cooked	2 slices (0.5 oz)	80	7	330	0	0
Shannon						
Irish	1 oz	70	5	—	0	—

FOOD	PORTION	CAL.	FAT	SOD.	CARB.	FIB.
BACON SUBSTITUTES						
bacon substitute	1 strip	25	2	117	1	—
Bac-Os						
Pieces	1½ tbsp	30	1	130	2	0
Harvest Direct						
Bacon Bits	3.5 oz	320	15	2000	24	17
Lightlife						
Fakin' Bacon	3 strips (2 oz)	79	3	233	6	—
Louis Rich						
Turkey Bacon	1 slice (0.5 oz)	30	3	190	0	0
McCormick						
Bac'n Pieces	2 tsp	20	tr	140	1	—
Morningstar Farms						
Breakfast Strips	3 (25 g)	80	6	350	4	—
Mr. Turkey						
Slice	1	25	2	170	0	—
Worthington						
Stripples	4 strips (33 g)	120	9	460	6	—
BAGEL						
FRESH						
cinnamon raisin	1 (3½ in)	194	1	229	39	—
cinnamon raisin toasted	1 (3½ in)	194	1	229	39	—
egg	1 (3½ in)	197	2	359	38	—
egg toasted	1 (3½ in)	197	2	358	38	—
oat bran	1 (3½ in)	181	1	360	38	—
oat bran toasted	1 (3½ in)	181	1	360	38	—
onion	1 (3½ in)	195	1	379	38	2
plain	1 (3½ in)	195	1	379	38	2
plain toasted	1 (3½ in)	195	1	379	38	2
poppy seed	1 (3½ in)	195	1	379	38	2
Alvarado St. Bakery						
Sprouted Wheat	1 (3.3 oz)	260	1	400	54	2
Sprouted Wheat Cinnamon/Raisin	1 (3.3 oz)	280	1	270	59	3
Sprouted Wheat Onion/ Poppyseed	1 (3.3 oz)	320	2	410	66	2
Sprouted Wheat Sesame	1 (3.3 oz)	320	4	410	64	2
FROZEN						
Great Starts						
Ham & Cheese On A Bagel	3 oz	240	8	600	28	—
Lender's						
Cinnamon'N Raisin	1 (2.5 oz)	200	1	310	40	1

FOOD	PORTION	CAL.	FAT	SOD.	CARB.	FIB.
Lender's (CONT.)						
Egg	1 (2 oz)	150	1	360	29	—
Onion	1 (2 oz)	160	1	290	31	1
Plain	1 (2 oz)	150	1	320	30	—
Sara Lee						
Cinnamon & Raisin	1 (3 oz)	240	2	280	48	—
Cinnamon Raisin	1 (2.5 oz)	200	2	230	39	—
Egg	1 (2.5 oz)	200	2	360	38	—
Egg	1 (3 oz)	250	2	450	48	—
Oat Bran	1 (2.5 oz)	180	1	360	38	—
Oat Bran	1 (3 oz)	220	1	450	47	—
Onion	1 (3 oz)	230	1	560	45	—
Onion	1 (2.5 oz)	190	1	450	37	—
Plain	1 (3 oz)	230	1	580	46	—
Plain	1 (2.5 oz)	190	1	460	38	—
Poppy Seed	1 (3 oz)	230	1	560	46	—
Poppy Seed	1 (2.5 oz)	190	1	450	37	—
Sesame Seed	1 (3 oz)	240	2	550	46	—
Sesame Seed	1 (2.5 oz)	190	1	440	37	—
Tree Of Life						
Onion	1 (3 oz)	210	0	115	44	0
Plain	1 (3 oz)	210	0	115	44	0
Poppy	1 (3 oz)	210	0	115	44	0
Raisin	1 (3 oz)	210	0	115	45	tr
Sesame	1 (3 oz)	210	0	115	44	0
BAKING POWDER						
baking powder	1 tsp	2	0	488	1	—
low sodium	1 tsp	5	0	4	2	—
Calumet						
Baking Powder	¼ tsp (1 g)	0	0	100	0	0
Clabber Girl						
Baking Powder	1 tsp	0	0	435	1	—
Davis						
Baking Powder	1 tsp	6	0	450	2	—
Watkins						
Baking Powder	¼ tsp (1 g)	0	0	150	0	0
BAKING SODA						
baking soda	1 tsp	0	0	1259	0	—
Arm & Hammer						
Baking Soda	1 tsp	0	0	1368	0	—
BALSAM PEAR						
leafy tips cooked	½ cup	10	tr	4	2	—

FOOD	PORTION	CAL.	FAT	SOD.	CARB.	FIB.
leafy tips raw	½ cup	7	tr	3	1	—
pods cooked	½ cup	12	tr	4	3	—
BAMBOO SHOOTS						
CANNED						
sliced	1 cup	25	1	9	4	—
Empress						
Sliced	2 oz	14	0	10	3	—
Ka-Me						
Sliced	½ cup (4.5 oz)	15	0	10	3	1
La Choy						
Sliced	¼ cup	6	tr	2	1	tr
FRESH						
cooked	½ cup	15	tr	5	2	—
raw	½ cup	21	tr	3	1	—
BANANA						
banana chips	1 oz	147	10	2	17	2
DRIED						
powder	1 tbsp	21	tr	0	5	—
Rainforest Farms						
Slices	5 slices (1.3 oz)	60	0	10	12	—
FRESH						
banana	1	105	tr	1	27	2
mashed	1 cup	207	1	2	53	4
Chiquita						
Fresh	1 (3½ oz)	110	0	—	—	—
Dole						
Banana	1	120	1	0	28	3
BANANA JUICE						
Libby						
Nectar	1 can (11.5 fl oz)	190	0	35	47	—
BARBECUE SAUCE						
(*see also* SAUCE)						
barbecue	1 cup	188	5	2038	32	—
Bull's Eye						
Original	2 tbsp	50	0	—	—	—
Hain						
Honey	1 tbsp	14	1	120	1	—
Healthy Choice						
Hickory	2 tbsp (1.1 oz)	26	0	229	6	tr
Hot & Spicy	2 tbsp (1.1 oz)	25	0	229	6	tr
Original	2 tbsp (1.1 oz)	25	0	229	6	tr

FOOD	PORTION	CAL.	FAT	SOD.	CARB.	FIB.
Heinz						
Select	1 oz	40	0	275	9	—
Select Hickory	1 oz	35	0	260	8	—
Thick & Rich Cajun Style	1 oz	35	0	360	8	—
Thick & Rich Chunky	1 oz	30	0	380	6	—
Thick & Rich Hawaiian Style	1 oz	40	0	210	10	—
Thick & Rich Hickory Smoke	1 oz	35	0	380	8	—
Thick & Rich Mesquite Smoke	1 oz	30	0	380	7	—
Thick & Rich Mushroom	1 oz	30	0	460	6	—
Thick & Rich Old Fashioned	1 oz	35	0	350	8	—
Thick & Rich Onion	1 oz	30	0	420	7	—
Thick & Rich Original	1 oz	35	0	390	8	—
Thick & Rich Texas Hot	1 oz	30	0	390	7	—
House Of Tsang						
Hong Kong	1 tbsp (0.6 oz)	10	0	150	2	0
Hunt's						
Barbeque	¼ cup (2.2 oz)	57	tr	887	14	1
Bold Hickory	2 tbsp (1.2 oz)	47	tr	283	11	1
Bold Original	2 tbsp (1.2 oz)	46	tr	315	11	1
Hickory	2 tbsp (1.2 oz)	38	tr	410	9	1
Hickory & Brown Sugar	2 tbsp (1.3 oz)	75	tr	382	18	1
Honey Hickory	2 tbsp (1.2 oz)	38	tr	410	9	1
Honey Mustard	2 tbsp (1.2 oz)	48	tr	450	12	1
Hot & Spicy	2 tbsp (1.2 oz)	48	tr	450	12	1
Light	2 tbsp (1.2 oz)	23	tr	169	6	1
Mesquite Barbecue	2 tbsp (1.2 oz)	40	tr	361	9	1
Mild	2 tbsp (1.2 oz)	41	tr	381	10	1
Mild Dijon	2 tbsp (1.2 oz)	39	tr	400	9	tr
Original	2 tbsp (1.2 oz)	39	tr	399	9	1
Teriyaki	2 tbsp (1.2 oz)	46	tr	351	11	1
Kraft						
Char-Grill	2 tbsp (1.3 oz)	60	0	460	13	0
Extra Rich Original	2 tbsp (1.2 oz)	50	0	440	12	0
Hickory Smoke	2 tbsp (1.2 oz)	40	0	420	9	0
Hickory Smoke Onion Bits	2 tbsp (1.2 oz)	45	0	360	11	0
Honey	2 tbsp (1.3 oz)	50	0	360	13	0
Honey Hickory	2 tbsp (1.3 oz)	60	0	370	14	0
Honey Mustard	2 tbsp (1.3 oz)	60	0	300	13	0
Hot	2 tbsp (1.2 oz)	40	0	520	9	0

FOOD	PORTION	CAL.	FAT	SOD.	CARB.	FIB.
Kraft (CONT.)						
Hot Hickory Smoke	2 tbsp (1.2 oz)	40	0	380	9	0
Kansas City Style	2 tbsp (1.2 oz)	50	0	310	11	0
Mesquite Smoke	2 tbsp (1.2 oz)	40	0	420	9	0
Molasses	2 tbsp (1.3 oz)	70	0	390	16	0
Onion Bits	2 tbsp (1.2 oz)	45	0	360	11	0
Original	2 tbsp (1.2 oz)	40	0	420	9	0
Roasted Garlic	2 tbsp (1.2 oz)	50	0	360	12	0
Spicy Honey	2 tbsp (1.3 oz)	60	0	360	14	0
Teriyaki	2 tbsp (1.3 oz)	60	1	440	12	0
Thick 'N Spicy Brown Sugar	2 tbsp (1.2 oz)	60	0	350	15	0
Thick 'N Spicy Hickory Bacon	2 tbsp (1.2 oz)	60	1	570	13	0
Thick 'N Spicy Hickory Smoke	2 tbsp (1.2 oz)	50	0	450	12	0
Thick 'N Spicy Honey	2 tbsp (1.3 oz)	60	0	360	13	0
Thick 'N Spicy Honey Mustard	2 tbsp (1.3 oz)	60	0	310	14	0
Thick'N Spicy Hickory Smoke	2 tbsp (1.2 oz)	50	0	440	12	0
Thick'N Spicy Honey	2 tbsp (1.2 oz)	60	0	350	13	0
Thick'N Spicy Kansas City Style	2 tbsp (1.3 oz)	60	0	310	14	0
Thick'N Spicy Mesquite Smoke	2 tbsp (1.2 oz)	50	0	440	12	0
Thick'N Spicy Original	2 tbsp (1.2 oz)	50	0	440	12	0
Lawry's						
Dijon Honey	¼ cup	203	1	1768	27	tr
Maull's						
Beer Non-Alcholic	3.5 oz	128	2	—	—	—
Regular	3.5 oz	123	2	—	—	—
Smoky	3.5 oz	124	tr	—	—	—
Sweet-N-Mild	3.5 oz	167	2	—	—	—
Sweet-N-Smoky	3.5 oz	160	tr	—	—	—
With Onion Bits	3.5 oz	126	2	—	—	—
Red Wing						
"K" Sauce	2 tbsp (1.2 oz)	45	0	410	9	0
Watkins						
Bold	2 tsp (0.4 oz)	25	0	290	5	0
Honey	2 tsp (0.4 oz)	25	0	290	6	0
Mesquite	2 tsp (0.4 oz)	25	0	300	5	0
Original	2 tsp (0.4 oz)	25	0	300	5	0
Smokehouse	2 tsp (0.4 oz)	25	0	300	5	0

FOOD	PORTION	CAL.	FAT	SOD.	CARB.	FIB.
BARLEY						
pearled cooked	½ cup	97	tr	2	30	—
pearled uncooked	½ cup	352	1	9	78	16
Arrowhead						
Barley	¼ cup (1.7 oz)	170	1	0	37	6
Hulless	¼ cup (1.6 oz)	140	1	0	35	6
Quaker						
Medium Pearled	¼ cup	172	1	0	36	5
Quick Pearled	¼ cup	172	1	0	36	5
Scotch						
Medium Pearled	¼ cup	172	1	0	36	5
Quick Pearled	¼ cup	172	1	0	36	5
BASIL						
fresh chopped	2 tbsp	1	tr	0	tr	—
ground	1 tsp	4	tr	tr	1	—
leaves fresh	5	1	tr	0	tr	—
Watkins						
Liquid Spice	1 tbsp (0.5 oz)	120	14	0	0	0
BASS						
freshwater raw	3 oz	97	3	59	0	—
sea cooked	3 oz	105	2	74	0	—
sea raw	3 oz	82	2	58	0	—
striped baked	3 oz	105	3	75	0	—
BAY LEAF						
crumbled	1 tsp	2	tr	tr	tr	—
Watkins						
Bay Leaves	¼ tsp (0.5 g)	0	0	0	0	0
BEAN SPROUTS						
(*see also individual bean names*)						
La Choy						
Bean Sprouts	⅔ cup	8	tr	20	1	tr
BEANS						
(*see also individual names*)						
CANNED						
baked beans plain	½ cup	118	1	504	26	10
baked beans vegetarian	½ cup	118	1	504	26	10
baked beans w/ beef	½ cup	161	5	632	22	—
baked beans w/ franks	½ cup	182	8	551	20	9
baked beans w/ pork	½ cup	133	2	522	25	7
baked beans w/ pork & sweet sauce	½ cup	140	2	423	26	7

FOOD	PORTION	CAL.	FAT	SOD.	CARB.	FIB.
baked beans w/ pork & tomato sauce	½ cup	123	1	554	24	7
refried beans	½ cup	134	1	534	23	—
Allen						
Baked	½ cup (4.5 oz)	150	1	350	29	8
B&M						
99% Fat Free Baked Beans	½ cup (4.6 oz)	160	1	220	31	7
Baked With Honey	½ cup (4.7 oz)	170	2	450	30	8
Barbeque Baked Beans	½ cup (4.7 oz)	170	2	360	32	6
Brick Oven Baked	½ cup (4.6 oz)	180	2	390	32	7
Extra Hearty Baked	½ cup (4.6 oz)	190	2	450	36	8
Brick Oven						
Baked Beans	½ cup	160	2	560	28	—
Brown Beauty						
Mexican Beans With Jalapeno	½ cup (4.5 oz)	120	1	370	21	7
Bush's						
Baked	½ cup (4.6 oz)	150	1	550	29	7
Baked With Onions	½ cup (4.6 oz)	150	2	500	26	6
Homestyle Baked	½ cup (4.6 oz)	160	2	480	28	8
Vegetarian	½ cup (4.6 oz)	140	1	550	24	6
Campbell						
Barbecue Beans	½ can (7⅞ oz)	210	4	900	43	—
Home Style Beans	½ can (8 oz)	220	4	820	48	—
Hot Chili Beans	½ can (7¾ oz)	180	4	870	38	—
Old Fashioned Beans In Molasses & Brown Sugar Sauce	½ can (8 oz)	230	3	730	49	—
Pork & Beans In Tomato Sauce	½ can (8 oz)	200	3	770	43	—
Vegetarian	½ can (7¾ oz)	170	1	780	40	—
Casa Fiesta						
Refried	3.5 oz	110	2	299	17	—
Chi-Chi's						
Ranchero Beans	½ cup (4.3 oz)	100	1	540	18	1
Refried	½ cup (4.2 oz)	130	6	570	16	4
Crest Top						
Pork And Beans	½ cup (4.5 oz)	130	1	330	21	6
Friend's						
Maple Baked	8 oz	240	2	890	52	11
Original Baked	½ cup (4.6 oz)	170	1	390	32	7
Gebhardt						
Chili	4 oz	115	1	580	21	5

FOOD	PORTION	CAL.	FAT	SOD.	CARB.	FIB.
Gebhardt (CONT.)						
Refried	4 oz	100	2	490	20	7
Refried Jalapeno	4 oz	115	2	270	19	7
Green Giant						
Pork And Beans In Tomato Sauce	½ cup	90	1	420	21	6
Three Bean Salad	½ cup	70	tr	470	18	3
Hanover						
Four Bean Salad	½ cup	80	0	—	—	—
Health Valley						
Boston Baked	7½ oz	190	tr	300	41	5
Boston Baked No Salt Added	7.5 oz	190	tr	20	41	5
Fast Menu Honey Baked Organic Beans With Tofu Weiner	7½ oz	150	4	140	15	16
Vegetarian With Miso	7½ oz	180	1	60	38	5
Heartland						
Iron Kettle Baked	½ cup (4.6 oz)	150	1	400	29	5
Hormel						
Beans & Wieners	1 can (7.5 oz)	290	13	1270	32	6
Hunt's						
Big John's Beans & Fixin's	½ cup (4.7 oz)	127	4	590	23	6
Pork & Beans	½ cup (4.5 oz)	130	1	516	28	4
Kid's Kitchen						
Beans & Weiners	1 cup (7.5 oz)	310	13	760	37	8
Little Pancho						
Refried & Green Chili	½ cup	80	0	330	15	—
Luck's						
Cut Green & Shelled Beans Seasoned w/ Pork	7.25 oz	200	6	—	—	—
Mixed Beans Seasoned w/ Pork	7.25 oz	200	5	—	—	—
McIlhenny						
Spicy	1 oz	7	tr	19	1	1
Old El Paso						
Mexe-Beans	½ cup (4.6 oz)	110	1	630	19	7
Refried	½ cup (4.2 oz)	110	2	500	17	5
Refried Fat Free	½ cup (4.4 oz)	110	0	480	20	6
Refried Spicy	½ cup (4.3 oz)	140	3	560	22	6
Refried Vegetarian	½ cup (4.1 oz)	100	1	490	16	6
Refried With Cheese	½ cup (4.2 oz)	130	4	500	18	6

FOOD	PORTION	CAL.	FAT	SOD.	CARB.	FIB.
Old El Paso (CONT.)						
Refried With Green Chilies	½ cup (4.3 oz)	110	1	720	19	6
Refried With Sausage	½ cup (4.1 oz)	200	13	360	14	8
Rosarita						
Refried	4 oz	100	2	480	18	6
Refried Spicy	4 oz	100	2	500	19	6
Refried Vegetarian	4 oz	100	2	480	18	6
Refried With Bacon	4 oz	110	2	560	20	6
Refried With Green Chilies	4 oz	90	2	460	18	6
Refried With Nacho Cheese	4 oz	110	2	490	20	6
Refried With Onions	4 oz	110	2	490	21	6
S&W						
Barbecue Beans Texas Style	½ cup	135	1	550	24	—
Maple Sugar Beans	½ cup	150	1	586	28	—
Mixed Bean Salad Marinated	½ cup	90	1	730	17	—
Pork 'N Beans	½ cup	130	2	135	22	—
Smokey Ranch	½ cup	130	2	569	20	—
Taco Bell						
Home Originals Fat Free Refried Beans	½ cup (4.6 oz)	110	0	460	21	6
Home Originals Fat Free Refried Beans w/ Mild Chilies	½ cup (4.5 oz)	110	0	480	20	5
Home Originals Refried Beans	½ cup (4.7 oz)	140	3	530	23	7
Trappey						
Mexi-Beans With Jalapeno	½ cup (4.5 oz)	130	2	460	22	8
Pork And Beans	½ cup (4.5 oz)	110	1	710	21	7
Pork And Beans With Jalapeno	½ cup (4.5 oz)	130	2	610	24	6
Van Camp's						
Baked Beans Fat Free	½ cup (4.6 oz)	130	0	430	28	5
Baked Beans Premium	½ cup (4.6 oz)	140	1	520	29	5
Beanee Weenee	1 cup (9 oz)	320	14	1240	35	8
Beanee Weenee Baked Flavor	1 cup (9 oz)	410	14	1210	58	10
Beanee Weenee Barbeque	1 cup (9 oz)	340	14	1150	43	8

FOOD	PORTION	CAL.	FAT	SOD.	CARB.	FIB.
Van Camp's (CONT.)						
Brown Sugar Beans	½ cup (4.6 oz)	170	3	410	31	6
Mexican Style Chili Beans	½ cup (4.6 oz)	110	2	430	21	8
Pork And Beans	½ cup (4.6 oz)	110	2	490	24	6
Vegetarian In Tomato Sauce	½ cup (4.6 oz)	110	1	400	23	5
Wagon Master						
Pork And Beans	½ cup (4.5 oz)	110	1	710	21	7
FROZEN						
Hanover						
Romano Bean Medley	½ cup	25	0	—	—	—
MIX						
Bean Cuisine						
Florentine Beans With Bow Ties	½ cup	199	7	450	27	—
Pasta & Beans Country French With Gemelli	½ cup	214	8	369	27	—
TAKE-OUT						
baked beans	½ cup	190	6	532	27	—
barbecue beans	3.5 oz	120	tr	460	26	—
four bean salad	3.5 oz	100	tr	280	20	—
refried beans	½ cup	43	2	104	5	—
three bean salad	¾ cup	230	11	500	31	1

BEAR

simmered	3 oz	220	11	—	0	—

BEAVER

roasted	3 oz	140	6	50	0	—
simmered	3 oz	141	5	39	0	—

BEECHNUTS

dried	1 oz	164	14	—	10	—

BEEF

(*see also* BEEF DISHES, VEAL)

(FAST FACT: In 1996, the per capita consumption of beef was 64 pounds.)

CANNED						
corned beef	3 oz	85	5	—	0	—
corned beef	1 oz	71	4	—	—	—
Armour						
Chopped Beef	2 oz	170	15	810	2	—
Corned Beef	2 oz	120	7	490	1	—
Potted Meat	¼ cup (2.2 oz)	90	6	600	0	—

FOOD	PORTION	CAL.	FAT	SOD.	CARB.	FIB.
Armour (CONT.)						
Potted Meat	1 can (3 oz)	120	8	820	0	—
Tripe	3 oz	90	2	100	0	—
Hormel						
Corned Beef	2 oz	120	7	490	0	0
Potted Meat	4 tbsp (2 oz)	60	7	580	1	0
Treet						
50% Less Fat	2 oz	120	8	750	4	—
Beef	2 oz	150	12	770	4	—
Underwood						
Roast Beef	2.08 oz	140	11	360	tr	—
Roast Beef Mesquite Smoked	2.08 oz	126	11	300	tr	—
Roast Beef Light	2.08 oz	90	6	210	2	—
DRIED						
Hormel						
Pillow Pack	10 slices (1 oz)	45	1	810	1	0
Sliced	10 slices (1 oz)	50	2	1240	1	0
FRESH						
bottom round lean & fat trim 0 in Choice roasted	3 oz	172	8	56	0	—
bottom round lean & fat trim 0 in Select braised	3 oz	171	6	43	0	—
bottom round lean & fat trim 0 in Select roasted	3 oz	150	24	56	0	—
bottom round lean & fat trim 0 in braised	3 oz	193	26	43	0	—
bottom round lean & fat trim ¼ in Choice braised	3 oz	241	15	42	0	—
bottom round lean & fat trim ¼ in Choice roasted	3 oz	221	14	53	0	—
bottom round lean & fat trim ¼ in Select braised	3 oz	220	13	42	0	—
bottom round lean & fat trim ¼ in Select roasted	3 oz	199	11	54	0	—
brisket flat half lean & fat trim 0 in braised	3 oz	183	8	53	0	—
brisket flat half lean & fat trim ¼ in braised	3 oz	309	24	48	0	—
brisket point half lean & fat trim 0 in braised	3 oz	304	24	57	0	—
brisket point half lean & fat trim ¼ in braised	3 oz	343	29	55	0	—
brisket whole lean & fat trim 0 in braised	3 oz	247	17	55	0	—

FOOD	PORTION	CAL.	FAT	SOD.	CARB.	FIB.
brisket whole lean & fat trim ¼ in braised	3 oz	327	27	52	0	—
chuck arm pot roast lean & fat trim 0 in braised	3 oz	238	14	53	0	—
chuck arm pot roast lean & fat trim ¼ in braised	3 oz	282	20	51	0	—
chuck blade roast lean & fat trim 0 in braised	3 oz	284	21	56	0	—
chuck blade roast lean & fat trim ¼ in braised	3 oz	293	22	55	0	—
corned beef brisket cooked	3 oz	213	16	964	tr	—
eye of round lean & fat trim 0 in Choice roasted	3 oz	153	5	53	0	—
eye of round lean & fat trim 0 in Select roasted	3 oz	137	4	53	0	—
eye of round lean & fat trim ¼ in Choice roasted	3 oz	205	12	50	0	—
eye of round lean & fat trime ¼ in Select roasted	3 oz	184	10	51	0	—
flank lean & fat trim 0 in braised	3 oz	224	14	60	0	—
flank lean & fat trim 0 in broiled	3 oz	192	11	69	0	—
ground extra lean broiled medium	3 oz	217	14	59	0	—
ground extra lean broiled well done	3 oz	225	14	70	0	—
ground extra lean fried medium	3 oz	216	14	59	0	—
ground extra lean fried well done	3 oz	224	14	69	0	—
ground extra lean raw	4 oz	265	19	75	0	—
ground lean broiled medium	3 oz	231	16	65	0	—
ground lean broiled well done	3 oz	238	15	76	0	—
ground regular broiled medium	3 oz	246	18	70	0	—
ground regular broiled well done	3 oz	248	17	79	0	—
ground low-fat w/ carrageenan raw	4 oz	160	7	70	tr	—

FOOD	PORTION	CAL.	FAT	SOD.	CARB.	FIB.
porterhouse steak lean & fat trim ¼ in Choice broiled	3 oz	260	19	52	0	—
porterhouse steak lean only trim ¼ in Prime broiled	3 oz	185	9	56	0	—
rib eye small end lean & fat trim 0 in Choice broiled	3 oz	261	19	54	0	—
rib large end lean & fat trim 0 in roasted	3 oz	300	24	55	0	—
rib large end lean & fat trim ¼ in broiled	3 oz	295	24	54	0	—
rib large end lean & fat trim ¼ in roasted	3 oz	310	25	54	0	—
rib small end lean & fat trim 0 in broiled	3 oz	252	18	54	0	—
rib small end lean & fat trim ¼ in broiled	3 oz	285	22	53	0	—
rib small end lean & fat trim ¼ in roasted	3 oz	295	24	53	0	—
rib whole lean & fat trim ¼ in Choice broiled	3 oz	306	25	53	0	—
rib whole lean & fat trim ¼ in Choice roasted	3 oz	320	27	53	0	—
rib whole lean & fat trim ¼ in Prime roasted	3 oz	348	30	54	0	—
rib whole lean & fat trim ¼ in Select broiled	3 oz	274	21	54	0	—
rib whole lean & fat trim ¼ in Select roasted	3 oz	286	23	54	0	—
shank crosscut lean & fat trim ¼ in Choice simmered	3 oz	224	12	52	0	—
short loin top loin lean & fat trim 0 in Choice broiled	3 oz	193	10	57	0	—
short loin top loin lean & fat trim 0 in Choice broiled	1 steak (5.4 oz)	353	19	104	0	—
short loin top loin lean & fat trim 0 in Select broiled	1 steak (5.4 oz)	309	14	104	0	—
short loin top loin lean & fat trim ¼ in Choice braised	3 oz	253	18	54	0	—

FOOD	PORTION	CAL.	FAT	SOD.	CARB.	FIB.
short loin top loin lean & fat trim ¼ in Choice broiled	1 steak (6.3 oz)	536	38	114	0	—
short loin top loin lean & fat trim ¼ in Prime broiled	1 steak (6.3 oz)	582	43	114	0	—
short loin top loin lean & fat trim ¼ in Select broiled	1 steak (6.3 oz)	473	31	114	0	—
short loin top loin lean only trim 0 in Choice broiled	1 steak (5.2 oz)	311	14	101	0	—
short loin top loin lean only trim ¼ in Choice broiled	1 steak (5.2 oz)	314	15	100	0	—
shortribs lean & fat Choice braised	3 oz	400	36	43	0	—
t-bone steak lean & fat trim ¼ in Choice broiled	3 oz	253	18	52	0	—
t-bone steak lean only trim ¼ in Choice broiled	3 oz	182	9	56	0	—
tenderloin lean & fat trim 0 in Select broiled	3 oz	194	11	52	0	—
tenderloin lean & fat trim ¼ in Choice broiled	3 oz	259	19	50	0	—
tenderloin lean & fat trim ¼ in Choice roasted	3 oz	288	22	55	0	—
tenderloin lean & fat trim ¼ in Choice broiled	3 oz	208	12	52	0	—
tenderloin lean & fat trim ¼ in Prime broiled	3 oz	270	20	50	0	—
tenderloin lean & fat trim ¼ in Select roasted	3 oz	275	21	48	0	—
tenderloin lean only trim 0 in Select broiled	3 oz	170	7	54	0	—
tenderloin lean only trim ¼ in Choice broiled	3 oz	188	10	54	0	—
tenderloin lean only trim ¼ in Select broiled	3 oz	169	7	54	0	—
tip round lean & fat trim 0 in Choice roasted	3 oz	170	8	54	0	—
tip round lean & fat trim 0 in Select roasted	3 oz	158	6	55	0	—
tip round lean & fat trim ¼ in Choice roasted	3 oz	210	13	53	0	—
tip round lean & fat trim ¼ in Prime roasted	3 oz	233	15	53	0	—

FOOD	PORTION	CAL.	FAT	SOD.	CARB.	FIB.
tip round lean & fat trim ¼ in Select roasted	3 oz	191	10	53	0	—
top round lean & fat trim 0 in Choice braised	3 oz	184	6	38	0	—
top round lean & fat trim 0 in Select braised	3 oz	170	5	38	0	—
top round lean & fat trim ¼ in Choice braised	3 oz	221	11	38	0	—
top round lean & fat trim ¼ in Choice broiled	3 oz	190	9	51	0	—
top round lean & fat trim ¼ in Choice fried	3 oz	235	13	58	0	—
top round lean & fat trim ¼ in Prime broiled	3 oz	195	9	51	0	—
top round lean & fat trim ¼ in Select braised	3 oz	175	7	51	0	—
top round lean & fat trim ¼ in Select braised	3 oz	199	8	38	0	—
top sirloin lean & fat trim 0 in Choice broiled	3 oz	194	10	55	0	—
top sirloin lean & fat trim 0 in Select broiled	3 oz	166	6	55	0	—
top sirloin lean & fat trim ¼ in Choice broiled	3 oz	228	14	53	0	—
top sirloin lean & fat trim ¼ in Choice fried	3 oz	277	19	59	0	—
top sirloin lean & fat trim ¼ in Select broiled	3 oz	208	12	54	0	—
tripe raw	4 oz	111	4	52	0	—
Dakota Lean						
Chuck Roast raw	3 oz	80	2	—	1	—
Eye Round raw	3 oz	80	2	—	0	—
Flank Steak raw	3 oz	80	1	—	1	—
Ground raw	3 oz	88	2	—	0	—
Outside Round raw	3 oz	80	1	—	0	—
Ribeye raw	3 oz	90	2	—	1	—
Sirloin Tip raw	3 oz	90	3	—	1	—
Strip Loin raw	3 oz	90	2	—	1	—
Tenderloin raw	3 oz	70	1	—	1	—
Top Round raw	3 oz	80	1	—	1	—
Double J						
Filet	3.5 oz	130	4	54	—	—
NY Strip	3.5 oz	133	4	57	—	—
Rib Eye	3.5 oz	134	5	55	—	—

FOOD	PORTION	CAL.	FAT	SOD.	CARB.	FIB.
Double J (CONT.)						
Top Butt	3.5 oz	136	5	55	—	—
Healthy Choice						
Ground Extra Lean	4 oz	130	4	230	2	0
Laura's Lean						
Eye Of Round	4 oz	150	5	85	0	—
Flank Steak	4 oz	160	7	75	0	—
Ground	4 oz	180	10	75	0	—
Ground Round	4 oz	160	7	75	0	—
Ribeye Steak	4 oz	150	5	60	0	—
Sirloin Tip Round	4 oz	140	5	65	0	—
Sirloin Top Butt	4 oz	140	5	90	0	—
Strip Steak	4 oz	150	5	85	0	—
Tenderloins	4 oz	150	6	75	0	—
Top Round	4 oz	140	4	80	0	—
Maverick Ranch						
Ground Round Extra Lean	4 oz	130	4	65	0	—
FROZEN						
patties broiled medium	3 oz	240	17	66	0	—
READY-TO-EAT						
Healthy Choice						
Deli-Thin Roast Beef	6 slices (2 oz)	60	2	520	1	0
Fresh-Trak Roast Beef	1 slice (1 oz)	30	1	260	0	0
Jordan's						
Healthy Trim 97% Fat Free Roast Beef Medium	1 slice (1 oz)	30	1	130	0	0
Healthy Trim 97% Fat Free Roast Beef Rare	1 slice (1 oz)	30	1	130	0	0
Oscar Mayer						
Deli-Thin Roast Beef	4 slices (1.8 oz)	60	2	530	1	0
Weight Watchers						
Deli Thin Oven Roasted Cured	5 slices (⅓ oz)	10	tr	85	tr	—
TAKE-OUT						
roast beef medium	2 oz	70	2	210	0	—
roast beef rare	2 oz	70	2	210	0	—

BEEF DISHES

FOOD	PORTION	CAL.	FAT	SOD.	CARB.	FIB.
CANNED						
corned beef hash	3 oz	155	10	—	9	—
Armour						
Corned Beef Hash	1 cup (8.3 oz)	440	30	840	23	—

FOOD	PORTION	CAL.	FAT	SOD.	CARB.	FIB.
Armour (CONT.)						
Roast Beef Hash	1 cup (8.4 oz)	400	25	1460	23	—
Roast Beef In Gravy	½ cup (4.6 oz)	150	4	640	3	—
Stew	1 cup (8.6 oz)	220	12	1250	21	—
Dinty Moore						
Meatball Stew	1 cup (8.4 oz)	250	15	1120	17	2
Stew	1 cup (8.2 oz)	230	14	950	16	2
Hormel						
Beef Goulash	1 can (7.5 oz)	230	11	1040	19	3
Corned Beef Hash	1 cup (8.3 oz)	390	24	930	22	2
Roast Beef Hash	1 cup (8.3 oz)	390	24	790	22	2
Roast Beef With Gravy	2 oz	60	2	280	1	0
Mary Kitchen						
Corned Beef Hash	1 can (7.5 oz)	350	22	850	19	2
Roast Beef Hash	1 can (7.5 oz)	348	21	707	21	2
Wolf Brand						
Beef Stew	1 cup	179	8	1043	18	—
FROZEN						
Chefwich						
Beef w/ Barbecue Sauce	1	340	10	—	—	—
Hot Pocket						
Stuffed Sandwich Barbecue	1 (4.5 oz)	340	12	850	45	1
Stuffed Sandwich Beef & Cheddar	1 (4.5 oz)	360	18	830	36	tr
Stuffed Sandwich Beef Fajita	1 (4.5 oz)	360	17	780	39	5
Lean Pockets						
Stuffed Sandwich Beef & Broccoli	1 (4.5 oz)	250	7	710	37	7
Luigino's						
Creamed Sauce Shaved Cured Beef With Croutons	1 pkg (8 oz)	360	20	810	29	3
Egg Noodles Rich Gravy Swedish Meatballs	1 cup (7.5 oz)	280	12	690	30	3
Egg Noodles Rich Gravy Swedish Meatballs	1 pkg (9 oz)	340	15	820	36	3
Ovenstuffs						
Beef/Cheddar Deli Melt	1 (4.75 oz)	390	22	820	28	—
Tyson						
Microwave BBQ Sandwich	1 sandwich	200	3	600	29	—
MIX						
Casbah						
Gyro as prep	1 patty (2 oz)	145	5	456	12	tr

FOOD	PORTION	CAL.	FAT	SOD.	CARB.	FIB.
Hamburger Helper						
BBQ Beef as prep	1 cup	320	10	760	37	1
Beef Pasta as prep	1 cup	270	10	910	26	tr
Beef Romanoff as prep	1 cup	280	10	920	27	0
Beef Stew as prep	1 cup	250	10	750	26	2
Beef Taco as prep	1 cup	310	11	930	31	1
Beef Teriyaki as prep	1 cup	290	10	990	34	2
Cheddar 'n Bacon as prep	1 cup	350	16	890	28	tr
Cheddar Melt as prep	1 cup	310	12	900	31	tr
Cheddar Spirals Reduced Sodium as prep	1 cup	320	14	650	27	1
Cheeseburger Macaroni as prep	1 cup	360	16	1000	31	tr
Cheesy Italian as prep	1 cup	330	14	920	29	tr
Cheesy Shells as prep	1 cup	340	14	850	30	tr
Chili Macaroni as prep	1 cup	290	10	870	30	tr
Fettuccine Alfredo as prep	1 cup	310	13	850	26	1
Four Cheese Lasagne as prep	1 cup	330	14	860	31	0
Italian Herb Reduced Sodium as prep	1 cup	270	10	650	29	2
Italian Rigatoni as prep	1 cup	280	10	870	29	1
Lasagne as prep	1 cup	280	10	990	30	0
Meat Loaf as prep	1/6 loaf	270	14	580	11	0
Mushroom & Wild Rice as prep	1 cup	310	12	880	30	2
Nacho Cheese as prep	1 cup	320	13	930	30	tr
Pizza Pasta as prep	1 cup	290	10	760	31	0
Pizzabake as prep	1/6 pie	270	10	720	28	tr
Potatoes Au Gratin as prep	1 cup	290	14	820	24	2
Potatoes Stroganoff as prep	1 cup	270	12	870	25	2
Ravioli as prep	1 cup	280	10	840	30	1
Rice Oriental as prep	1 cup	310	10	1050	35	0
Salisbury as prep	1 cup	270	10	790	26	tr
Southwestern Beef Reduced Sodium as prep	1 cup	300	10	650	32	2
Spaghetti as prep	1 cup	300	11	940	29	tr
Stroganoff as prep	1 cup	320	13	830	30	0

FOOD	PORTION	CAL.	FAT	SOD.	CARB.	FIB.
Hamburger Helper (CONT.)						
Swedish Meatballs as prep	1 cup	300	14	780	24	tr
Three Cheeses as prep	1 cup	340	15	830	32	tr
Zesty Italian as prep	1 cup	320	11	890	34	tr
Zesty Mexican as prep	1 cup	300	11	730	32	1
SHELF-STABLE						
Dinty Moore						
Microwave Cup Corned Beef Hash	1 cup (7.5 oz)	350	22	850	19	1
Microwave Cup Hearty Burger Stew	1 cup (7.5 oz)	240	13	930	19	3
Microwave Cup Stew	1 cup (7.5 oz)	190	10	900	15	2
Lunch Bucket						
Beef Stew	1 pkg (7.5 oz)	180	11	870	13	—
Micro Cup Meals						
Beef Stew	1 cup (7.5 oz)	180	9	880	15	2
TAKE-OUT						
bubble & squeak	5 oz	186	13	—	16	3
cornish pasty	1 (8 oz)	847	52	—	79	3
irish stew	1 cup (7 oz)	280	16	—	10	—
kebab indian	1 (5.4 oz)	553	40	—	2	—
kheena	6.7 oz	781	71	—	1	tr
koftas	5	280	22	—	3	tr
roast beef sandwich plain	1	346	14	792	33	—
roast beef sandwich w/ cheese	1	402	18	1634	27	—
roast beef submarine sandwich w/ tomato lettuce & mayonnaise	1	411	13	845	44	—
samosa	2 (4 oz)	652	62	—	20	2
shepherd's pie	6 oz	196	10	—	15	1
steak & kidney pie w/ top crust	1 slice (5 oz)	400	26	—	23	1
steak sandwich w/ tomato lettuce salt & mayonnaise	1	459	14	798	52	—
stew	6 oz	208	13	—	6	1
stew w/ vegetables	1 cup	220	11	292	15	—
stroganoff	¾ cup	260	19	503	43	—
swiss steak	4.6 oz	214	9	139	10	2
toad in the hole	1 (4.7 oz)	383	29	—	23	1

BEEFALO

FOOD	PORTION	CAL.	FAT	SOD.	CARB.	FIB.
roasted	3 oz	160	5	70	0	—

FOOD	PORTION	CAL.	FAT	SOD.	CARB.	FIB.
BEER AND ALE						
alcohol free beer	7 fl oz	50	tr	3	11	—
ale brown	10 oz	77	0	—	8	0
ale pale	10 oz	88	0	—	12	0
beer light	12 oz can	100	0	10	5	—
beer regular	12 oz can	146	0	19	13	—
lager	10 oz	80	0	—	4	0
pilsener lager beer	7 fl oz	85	tr	4	13	—
stout	10 oz	102	0	—	6	0
Amstel						
Light	12 oz	95	0	—	—	—
Anheuser Busch						
Natural Light	12 oz	110	0	—	—	—
Bud						
Light	12 oz	108	0	—	—	—
Coors						
Beer	12 oz	132	0	10	30	—
Extra Gold	12 oz	147	0	10	32	—
Light	12 oz	101	0	10	13	—
Guinness						
Kaliber nonalcoholic	12 oz	43	0	—	—	—
Hamm's						
Beer	12 oz	137	0	—	12	—
Nonalcoholic	12 oz	55	0	—	12	—
Killian's						
Beer	12 oz	212	0	10	29	—
Kingsbury						
Nonalcoholic	12 fl oz	60	0	—	—	—
Michelob						
Light	12 oz	134	0	—	—	—
Miller						
Lite	12 oz	96	0	—	—	—
Molson						
Light	12 oz	109	0	—	—	—
Old Milwaukee						
Beer	12 oz	145	0	25	13	—
Light	12 oz	122	0	18	9	—
Olympia						
Beer	12 oz	143	0	—	12	—
Pabst						
Beer	12 oz	143	0	—	12	—
Nonalcoholic	12 oz	55	0	—	12	—
Piels						
Light	12 oz	136	0	—	—	—

FOOD	PORTION	CAL.	FAT	SOD.	CARB.	FIB.
Schaefer						
Beer	12 oz	138	0	23	13	—
Light	12 oz	111	0	16	8	—
Schlitz						
Beer	12 oz	145	0	23	13	—
Light	12 oz	99	0	9	3	—
Schmidts						
Light	12 oz	96	0	—	—	—
Signature						
Beer	12 oz	150	0	21	13	—
Spirit						
Nonalcoholic	12 oz	80	0	—	16	—
Stroh						
Beer	12 oz	142	0	23	13	—
Light	12 oz	115	0	11	7	—
Winterfest						
Beer	12 oz	167	0	11	38	—

BEET JUICE

FOOD	PORTION	CAL.	FAT	SOD.	CARB.	FIB.
juice	3½ oz	36	0	200	8	—

BEETS

FOOD	PORTION	CAL.	FAT	SOD.	CARB.	FIB.
CANNED						
harvard	½ cup	89	tr	199	22	—
pickled	½ cup	75	tr	301	19	—
sliced	½ cup	27	tr	—	6	—
Del Monte						
Pickled Crinkle Style Sliced	½ cup (4.5 oz)	80	0	380	19	2
Sliced	½ cup (4.3 oz)	35	0	290	8	2
Whole	½ cup (4.3 oz)	35	0	290	8	2
Whole Tiny	½ cup (4.3 oz)	35	0	290	8	2
S&W						
Diced Tender	½ cup	40	0	270	9	—
Julienne French Style	½ cup	40	0	270	9	—
Pickled Whole Extra Small	½ cup	70	0	215	16	—
Pickled w/ Red Wine Vinegar Sliced	½ cup	70	0	215	16	—
Sliced Small Premium	½ cup	40	0	270	9	—
Sliced Water Pack	½ cup	35	0	40	9	—
Whole Small	½ cup	40	0	270	9	—
Seneca						
Cut	½ cup	35	0	264	9	2
Diced	½ cup	35	0	264	9	2

FOOD	PORTION	CAL.	FAT	SOD.	CARB.	FIB.
Seneca (CONT.)						
Harvard	½ cup	90	0	144	21	1
Pickled	2 tbsp	20	0	48	6	0
Pickled With Onions	2 tbsp	20	0	48	6	0
Sliced	½ cup	35	0	264	9	2
Whole	½ cup	35	0	264	9	2
FRESH						
greens cooked	½ cup	20	tr	173	4	—
greens raw	½ cup	4	tr	38	1	—
greens raw chopped	½ cup	4	tr	38	1	—
raw sliced	½ cup (2.4 oz)	29	tr	53	7	—
sliced cooked	½ cup (3 oz)	38	tr	65	9	—
whole cooked	2 (3.5 oz)	44	tr	77	10	—
whole raw	2 (5.7 oz)	70	tr	126	16	—

BEVERAGES

(*see* BEER AND ALE, CHAMPAGNE, COFFEE, DRINK MIXERS, FRUIT DRINKS, ICED TEA, LIQUOR/LIQUEUR, MALT, MILKSHAKE, MINERAL/BOTTLED WATER, SODA, SPORTS DRINKS, TEA/HERBAL TEA, WINE, WINE COOLER)

BISCUIT

FOOD	PORTION	CAL.	FAT	SOD.	CARB.	FIB.
FROZEN						
Great Starts						
Egg Canadian Bacon & Cheese	5.2 oz	420	22	1845	37	—
Sausage	4.7 oz	410	22	1180	36	—
Jimmy Dean						
Chicken Twin	2 (3.2 oz)	280	13	870	32	2
Sausage Twin	2 (3.4 oz)	330	21	900	25	2
Steak Twin	2 (3.2 oz)	270	13	660	26	2
Rudy's Farm						
Ham Twin	2 (3 oz)	160	3	790	23	1
Sausage & Cheese Twin	2 (3 oz)	290	18	570	22	1
Sausage Twin	2 (2.7 oz)	296	18	580	22	1
HOME RECIPE						
buttermilk	1 (2 oz)	212	10	348	27	—
oatcakes	2 (4 oz)	115	5	—	16	1
plain	1 (2 oz)	212	10	348	27	—
MIX						
buttermilk	1 (2 oz)	191	7	544	28	1
plain	1 (2 oz)	191	7	544	28	1
Arrowhead						
Biscuit Mix	¼ cup (1.2 oz)	120	1	200	23	3
Bisquick						
Mix	½ cup (2 oz)	240	8	700	37	—

FOOD	PORTION	CAL.	FAT	SOD.	CARB.	FIB.
Bisquick (CONT.)						
Reduced Fat	½ cup (2 oz)	210	4	660	39	—
Health Valley						
Buttermilk Biscuit Mix not prep	1 oz	100	1	170	20	3
Jiffy						
As prep	1	150	7	384	30	2
Biscuit	¼ cup (1.1 oz)	130	5	320	22	1
Buttermilk as prep	1	170	4	380	29	tr
READY-TO-EAT						
Arnold						
Old Fashioned	1	60	3	100	8	—
REFRIGERATED						
buttermilk	1 (1 oz)	98	4	341	14	—
plain	1 (1 oz)	98	4	341	14	tr
1869 Brand						
Baking Powder	1	100	5	310	12	—
Butter Tastin'	1	100	5	300	12	—
Buttermilk	1	100	5	310	12	—
Ballard						
Ovenready	1	50	1	180	10	—
Ovenready Buttermilk	1	50	1	180	10	—
Big Country						
Southern Style	1	100	4	320	14	—
Hungry Jack						
Butter Tastin' Flaky	1	90	4	280	11	—
Buttermilk Flaky	1	90	4	300	12	—
Buttermilk Fluffy	1	90	4	280	12	—
Extra Rich Buttermilk	1	50	1	180	9	—
Flaky	1	80	4	300	12	—
Honey Tastin' Flaky	1	90	4	290	13	—
Pillsbury						
Big Country Butter Tastin'	1	100	4	320	14	—
Big Country Buttermilk	1	100	4	320	14	—
Butter	1	50	1	180	10	—
Buttermilk	1	50	1	180	10	—
Country	1	50	1	180	10	—
Deluxe Heat N' Eat Buttermilk	2	170	5	530	27	—
Good'N Buttery Fluffy	1	90	5	270	11	—
Hearty Grains Multi-Grain	1	80	2	230	15	—
Hearty Grains Oatmeal Raisin	1	90	2	210	16	—

FOOD	PORTION	CAL.	FAT	SOD.	CARB.	FIB.
Pillsbury (CONT.)						
Heat N' Eat Big Premium	2	280	15	610	32	—
Tender Layer Buttermilk	1	50	1	170	9	—
Roman Meal						
Biscuit	2 (2.4 oz)	180	4	456	34	1
Honey Nut Oat Bran	1 (1.5 oz)	131	5	278	21	1
TAKE-OUT						
buttermilk	1	127	6	368	17	—
plain	1 (35 g)	276	34	584	13	—
w/ egg	1	315	20	655	24	—
w/ egg & bacon	1	457	31	999	29	—
w/ egg & sausage	1	582	39	1142	41	—
w/ egg & steak	1	474	28	888	37	—
w/ egg cheese & bacon	1	477	31	1261	33	—
w/ ham	1	387	18	1433	44	—
w/ sausage	1	485	32	1071	40	—
w/ steak	1	456	26	795	44	—
BISON						
roasted	3 oz	122	2	48	0	—
BLACK BEANS						
CANNED						
Allen						
Seasoned	½ cup (4.5 oz)	120	2	410	20	7
Eden						
Organic	½ cup (4.3 oz)	100	0	15	17	6
Health Valley						
Fast Menu Organic Black Beans With Tofu Weiners	7½ oz	150	1	170	20	15
Fast Menu Western Black Beans With Garden Vegetable	7½ oz	160	5	250	14	14
Old El Paso						
Black Beans	½ cup (4.6 oz)	100	1	400	17	7
Refried	½ cup (4.2 oz)	120	2	340	18	6
Progresso						
Black Beans	½ cup (4.6 oz)	100	1	400	17	7
Trappey						
Seasoned	½ cup (4.5 oz)	120	2	410	20	7
DRIED						
cooked	1 cup	227	1	1	41	—
MIX						
Bean Cuisine						
Black Turtle	½ cup	115	1	5	—	5

FOOD	PORTION	CAL.	FAT	SOD.	CARB.	FIB.
Bean Cuisine (CONT.)						
Pasta & Beans Black Beans With Fusilli	½ cup	174	4	453	27	—
Mahatma						
Black Beans & Rice	1 cup	200	2	850	39	6
BLACKBERRIES						
CANNED						
in heavy syrup	½ cup	118	tr	3	30	—
Allen-Wolco						
Blackberries	½ cup (5.3 oz)	60	1	20	13	9
FRESH						
blackberries	½ cup	37	tr	0	9	3
FROZEN						
unsweetened	1 cup	97	1	2	24	—
Big Valley						
Blackberries	⅔ cup (4.9 oz)	70	0	0	15	4
BLACKBERRY JUICE						
Kool-Aid						
Scary Blackberry Ghoul-Aid Drink as prep w/ sugar	1 serv (8 oz)	100	0	0	25	0
BLACKEYE PEAS						
CANNED						
w/pork	½ cup	199	4	840	40	—
Allen						
Blackeye Peas	½ cup (4.5 oz)	110	1	340	18	4
Fresh Shell	½ cup (4.4 oz)	120	1	350	21	6
With Bacon	½ cup (4.5 oz)	105	2	390	20	5
With Snaps	½ cup (4.4 oz)	120	1	420	20	5
Dorman						
Fresh Shell	½ cup (4.4 oz)	120	1	350	21	6
East Texas Fair						
Blackeye Peas	½ cup (4.5 oz)	110	1	340	18	4
Fresh Shell	½ cup (4.4 oz)	120	1	350	21	6
With Snaps	½ cup (4.4 oz)	120	1	420	20	5
Homefolks						
Fresh Shell	½ cup (4.4 oz)	120	1	350	21	6
With Jalapeno	½ cup (4.4 oz)	120	1	580	20	5
With Snaps	½ cup (4.4 oz)	120	1	420	20	5
Luck's						
Seasoned w/ Pork	7.25 oz	200	6	—	—	—
Sunshine						
With Bacon	½ cup (4.5 oz)	105	2	390	20	5

FOOD	PORTION	CAL.	FAT	SOD.	CARB.	FIB.
Trappey						
With Bacon	½ cup (4.5 oz)	120	2	350	19	5
With Bacon & Jalapeno	½ cup (4.4 oz)	110	2	470	19	5
DRIED						
cooked	1 cup	198	1	6	36	16
FROZEN						
Fresh Like	3.5 oz	138	1	6	24	1
BLINTZE						
Empire						
Apple	2 (4.4 oz)	220	6	260	36	5
Blueberry	2 (4.4 oz)	190	4	260	36	2
Cheese	2 (4.4 oz)	200	6	310	29	3
Cherry	2 (4.4 oz)	200	4	280	38	3
Potato	2 (4.4 oz)	190	6	530	32	3
Golden						
Apple Raisin	1 (2.25 oz)	80	2	145	16	—
Blueberry	1 (2.25 oz)	90	1	150	18	—
Cheese	1 (2.25 oz)	80	2	135	13	—
Cherry	1 (2.25 oz)	95	1	145	18	—
Potato	1 (2.25 oz)	90	4	170	15	—
TAKE-OUT						
cheese	2	186	6	268	18	tr
BLUEBERRIES						
CANNED						
in heavy syrup	1 cup	225	1	9	56	—
S&W						
In Heavy Syrup	½ cup	111	0	—	30	—
DRIED						
Sonoma						
Dried	¼ cup (1.3 oz)	140	0	0	33	5
FRESH						
blueberries	1 cup	82	1	9	20	—
FROZEN						
unsweetened	1 cup	78	1	1	19	—
Big Valley						
Blueberries	¾ cup (4.9 oz)	70	0	0	12	4
BLUEBERRY JUICE						
After The Fall						
Maine Coast	1 cup (8 oz)	90	0	20	25	0
BLUEFIN						
fillet baked	4.1 oz	186	6	90	0	—

FOOD	PORTION	CAL.	FAT	SOD.	CARB.	FIB.
BLUEFISH						
fresh baked	3 oz	135	5	65	0	—
BOAR						
wild roasted	3 oz	136	4	—	0	—
BOK CHOY						
Dole						
Shredded	½ cup	5	tr	23	1	—
BONIATO						
fresh	½ cup	90	tr	7	20	—
BORAGE						
fresh chopped cooked	3½ oz	25	1	88	4	—
raw chopped	½ cup	9	tr	35	1	—
BOYSENBERRIES						
in heavy syrup	1 cup	226	tr	9	57	—
unsweetened frzn	1 cup	66	tr	2	16	—
BOYSENBERRY JUICE						
Smucker's						
Juice	8 oz	120	0	10	30	—
Juice Sparkler	10 oz	130	tr	5	31	—
BRAINS						
beef pan-fried	3 oz	167	13	134	0	—
beef simmered	3 oz	136	11	102	0	—
lamb braised	3 oz	124	9	114	0	—
lamb fried	3 oz	232	19	133	0	—
pork braised	3 oz	117	8	77	0	—
veal braised	3 oz	115	8	133	0	—
veal fried	3 oz	181	14	150	0	—
Armour						
Pork Brains In Milk Gravy	⅔ cup (5.5 oz)	150	5	550	10	—
BRAN						
corn	⅓ cup	56	tr	2	21	21
oat cooked	½ cup	44	tr	1	13	—
oat dry	½ cup	116	3	1	31	7
rice dry	⅓ cup	88	6	1	14	6
wheat dry	½ cup	65	1	1	19	13
Arrowhead						
Oat Bran	⅓ cup (1.4 oz)	150	3	0	23	7
Wheat Bran	¼ cup (0,6 oz)	30	1	0	7	6

FOOD	PORTION	CAL.	FAT	SOD.	CARB.	FIB.
Good Shepherd						
Wheat Bran	1 oz	80	1	5	18	3
H-O						
Super Bran	⅓ cup	110	2	0	18	3
Health Valley						
Fast Menu Oat Bran Pilaf With Garden Vegetables	7½ oz	210	7	330	30	15
Hodgson Mill						
Oat	¼ cup (1.3 oz)	120	3	3	23	6
Wheat	¼ cup (0.5 oz)	30	1	0	10	7
Kretschmer						
Toasted Wheat Bran	⅓ cup	57	2	2	15	3
Mother's						
Oat Bran	½ cup	150	3	0	24	6
Quaker						
Oat Bran	½ cup	150	3	0	24	6
Unprocessed	2 tbsp	8	tr	0	4	3
Roman Meal						
Oat	1 oz	94	3	3	13	5
Stone-Buhr						
Oat	⅓ cup (1 oz)	90	2	0	20	4

BRAZIL NUTS

dried unblanched	1 oz	186	19	0	4	—

BREAD

(*see also* BAGEL, BISCUIT, BREADSTICK, CROISSANT, ENGLISH MUFFIN, MUFFIN, ROLL, SCONE)

CANNED						
boston brown	1 slice (1.6 oz)	88	1	284	20	2
B&M						
Brown Bread	½ in slice (2 oz)	130	1	390	29	2
Brown Bread Raisins	½ in slice (2 oz)	130	1	360	29	2
S&W						
Brown Bread New England Recipe	2 slices	76	0	172	17	—
FROZEN						
Kineret						
Challah	⅛ loaf (2 oz)	150	4	220	25	1
HOME RECIPE						
banana	1 slice (2 oz)	195	6	181	33	—
cornbread as prep w/ 2% milk	1 piece (2.3 oz)	173	5	428	28	—
cornbread as prep w/ whole milk	1 piece (2.3 oz)	176	5	428	28	—

FOOD	PORTION	CAL.	FAT	SOD.	CARB.	FIB.
datenut	½ in slice	92	3	63	15	—
irish soda bread	1 slice (2 oz)	174	3	239	34	—
pita whole wheat	1-6 in	247	1	—	—	—
pumpkin	1 slice (1 oz)	94	4	89	15	—
white as prep w/ nonfat dry milk	1 slice	78	1	95	15	—
white as prep w/ 2% milk	1 slice	81	2	104	14	—
white as prep w/ whole milk	1 slice	82	2	104	14	—
whole wheat	1 slice	79	2	98	15	—
MIX						
cornbread	1 piece (2 oz)	189	6	467	29	1
Aunt Jemima						
Corn Bread Easy Mix	⅓ cup (1.3 oz)	150	4	450	26	1
Ballard						
Corn Bread	⅛ bread	140	3	570	25	—
Dromedary						
Corn Bread	1 piece (2 in x 2 in)	130	3	480	20	—
Natural Ovens						
Cracked Wheat	2 slices (2.4 oz)	140	1	140	38	4
English Muffin Bread	2 slices (2.4 oz)	140	1	140	35	2
Executive Fitness Sunny Millet	2 slices (2.6 oz)	160	2	70	37	4
Garden Bread	1 oz	50	1	100	14	1
Glorious Cinnamon & Raisin Fat Free	2 slices (2.1 oz)	110	1	140	30	3
Honey 'N Flax	2 slices (2.5 oz)	140	1	140	30	4
Hunger Filler Bread	2 slices (2.1 oz)	110	2	140	28	5
Light Wheat	2 slices (2.2 oz)	84	1	140	30	5
Nutty Natural Wheat Bread	2 slices (2.5 oz)	140	2	140	32	6
Seven Grain Herb	2 slices (2.5 oz)	140	1	140	30	4
Soft Hearth Whole Wheat	2 slices (2 oz)	100	2	140	30	4
Soft Sandwich Very Low Fat	2 slices (2.3 oz)	110	1	140	26	2
Stay Slim	2 slices (2 oz)	100	2	140	20	4
Zia Foods						
Cornbread Blue Cornmeal	1 piece (1.2 oz)	110	6	—	—	—
READY-TO-EAT						
cracked wheat	1 slice	65	1	135	12	1
egg	1 slice (1.4 oz)	115	2	197	19	—
french	1 slice (1 oz)	78	1	172	15	1

FOOD	PORTION	CAL.	FAT	SOD.	CARB.	FIB.
french	1 loaf (1 lb)	1270	18	2633	230	—
gluten	1 slice	47	tr	104	8	—
italian	1 loaf (1 lb)	1255	4	2656	256	—
italian	1 slice (1 oz)	81	1	175	15	1
navajo fry	1 (5 in diam)	296	9	625	48	—
navajo fry	1 (10.5 in diam)	527	15	1112	85	—
oat bran	1 slice	71	1	122	12	1
oat bran reduced calorie	1 slice	46	1	81	10	—
oatmeal	1 slice	73	1	162	13	1
oatmeal reduced calorie	1 slice	48	1	89	10	—
pita	1 reg (2 oz)	165	1	322	33	1
pita	1 sm (1 oz)	78	tr	152	16	1
pita whole wheat	1 sm (1 oz)	76	1	151	16	2
pita whole wheat	1 reg (2 oz)	170	2	340	35	5
protein	1 slice	47	tr	104	8	—
pumpernickel	1 slice	80	1	215	15	2
raisin	1 slice	71	1	101	14	—
rice bran	1 slice	66	1	119	12	—
rye	1 slice	83	1	211	16	2
rye reduced calorie	1 slice	47	1	93	9	—
seven grain	1 slice	65	1	127	12	2
sourdough	1 slice (1 oz)	78	1	172	15	1
vienna	1 slice (1 oz)	78	1	172	15	1
wheat reduced calorie	1 slice	46	1	117	10	3
wheat berry	1 slice	65	1	132	12	1
wheat bran	1 slice	89	1	175	17	3
wheat germ	1 slice	74	1	157	14	—
white	1 slice	67	1	135	12	1
white reduced calorie	1 slice	48	1	104	10	2
white toasted	1 slice	67	1	136	13	—
white cubed	1 cup	80	1	154	15	—
whole wheat	1 slice	70	1	149	13	2
Alvarado St. Bakery						
Barley	1 slice (1.2 oz)	70	1	140	15	2
California Style	1 slice (1.2 oz)	60	1	150	10	2
French	1 slice (1.2 oz)	80	1	125	15	2
Multi-Grain	1 slice (1.2 oz)	60	1	160	11	2
Multi-Grain No-Salt	1 slice (1.2 oz)	60	1	0	11	2
Oat Berry	1 slice (1.2 oz)	70	1	150	13	2
Raisin	1 slice (1.1 oz)	80	1	105	15	2
Rye Seed	1 slice (1.2 oz)	60	1	150	11	2
Sourdough	1 slice (1.2 oz)	80	1	125	15	2
Wheat	1 slice (1.3 oz)	90	1	170	18	3

FOOD	PORTION	CAL.	FAT	SOD.	CARB.	FIB.
America's Own						
Wheat Cottage	1 slice	70	1	—	—	—
White Cottage	1 slice	70	1	—	—	—
Arnold						
12 Grain Natural	1 slice (0.8 oz)	60	0	100	10	1
Augusto Pan De Aqua	1 oz	80	1	150	14	1
Bran'nola Country Oat	1 slice (1.3 oz)	90	3	130	16	3
Bran'nola Dark Wheat	1 slice (1.3 oz)	90	3	150	15	3
Bran'nola Hearty Wheat	1 slice (1.3 oz)	100	3	160	15	3
Bran'nola Nutty Grains	1 slice (1.3 oz)	90	2	120	14	3
Bran'nola Original	1 slice (1.3 oz)	90	2	150	16	3
Cinnamon Chip	1 slice	80	2	90	13	tr
Cinnamon Raisin	1 slice (0.9 oz)	70	1	85	13	1
Country Bran Bakery Light	1 slice (0.8 oz)	40	tr	80	7	3
Cranberry	1 slice (0.9 oz)	70	1	80	14	1
French Twin Loaves Francisco	2 slices (2 oz)	150	2	280	27	—
French Stick Francisco	1 slice (1 oz)	70	2	110	12	—
French Stick Savoni	1 oz	80	tr	—	15	1
Italian Bakery Light	1 slice (0.7 oz)	40	tr	90	7	2
Italian Francisco	1 slice (1 oz)	70	1	110	12	—
Italian Stick Francisco	1 oz	90	1	110	17	—
Oatmeal Bakery	1 slice	60	1	95	12	2
Oatmeal Bakery Light	1 slice	40	tr	100	8	2
Oatmeal Raisin	1 slice (0.9 oz)	60	tr	90	12	2
Pita Wheat	½ pocket (1 oz)	71	0	—	16	—
Pita White	½ pocket (0.5 oz)	71	0	—	16	—
Pumpernickel	l slice (1.1 oz)	70	1	200	15	1
Rye Bakery Soft Light	1 slice (1.1 oz)	40	tr	90	7	2
Rye Bakery Soft Seeded	1 slice (1.1 oz)	70	1	170	14	1
Rye Bakery Soft Unseeded	1 slice (1.1 oz)	70	1	170	14	1
Rye Dill	1 slice (1.1 oz)	60	1	140	10	1
Rye Real Jewish Dijon	1 slice	70	tr	210	15	1
Rye Real Jewish Melba Thin	1 slice (0.7 oz)	40	tr	95	9	1
Rye Real Jewish Unseeded	1 slice	80	tr	180	16	1
Rye Real Jewish With Caraway	1 slice	70	tr	150	13	1
Rye Real Jewish Without Seeds	1 slice (1.1 oz)	70	tr	150	15	1
Sourdough Francisco	1 slice	90	1	250	19	1

FOOD	PORTION	CAL.	FAT	SOD.	CARB.	FIB.
Arnold (CONT.)						
Wheat Brick Oven	1 slice (0.8 oz)	60	2	100	9	2
Wheat Golden Light	1 slice (0.8 oz)	40	tr	90	7	2
Wheat Natural	1 slice (1.3 oz)	80	1	180	15	2
Wheat Berry Honey	1 slice (1.1 oz)	80	2	140	13	2
White Brick Oven	1 slice (0.8 oz)	60	1	130	11	1
White Country	1 slice (1.3 oz)	100	2	200	18	1
White Extra Fiber Brick Oven	1 slice (0.9 oz)	50	tr	90	10	2
White Light Brick Oven	1 slice (0.8 oz)	40	tr	95	10	2
White Premium Light	1 slice	40	tr	90	7	2
White Thin Sliced Brick Oven	1 slice	40	tr	75	7	tr
Whole Wheat 100% Light Brick Oven	1 slice (0.8 oz)	40	tr	85	6	3
Whole Wheat 100% Stoneground	1 slice (0.8 oz)	50	1	100	8	2
August Bros.						
Pumpernickel	1 slice	80	1	210	14	1
Rye Onion	1 slice	80	1	210	14	1
Rye Thin Unseeded	1 slice	40	—	110	8	1
Rye With Seeds	1 slice (1 lb loaf)	80	1	210	14	1
Rye Without Seeds	1 slice	80	1	210	14	1
Rye N' Pump	1 slice	90	1	220	18	1
Beefsteak						
Pumpernickel	1 slice (1 oz)	70	1	180	13	1
Rye Hearty	1 slice (1 oz)	70	1	170	13	1
Rye Light	2 slices (1.6 oz)	70	1	250	17	5
Rye Mild	2 slices (1.4 oz)	90	1	240	18	2
Rye Soft	1 slice (1 oz)	70	1	180	13	1
Wheat Hearty	1 slice (1 oz)	70	1	160	13	1
Wheat Soft	1 slice (1 oz)	70	1	150	13	tr
White Robust	1 slice (1 oz)	70	1	140	13	tr
Bread Du Jour						
Austrian Wheat	3 in slice (1 oz)	130	2	280	26	2
French	3 in slice (1 oz)	130	1	300	26	1
Brownberry						
Bran'nola Country Oat	1 slice	90	2	166	18	3
Bran'nola Hearty Wheat	1 slice	88	2	197	17	3
Bran'nola Nutty Grains	1 slice	85	2	144	17	3
Bran'nola Original	1 slice	85	1	137	18	3
Health Nut	1 slice	71	3	158	12	3
Oatmeal Natural	1 slice	63	1	144	13	1
Oatmeal Soft	1 slice	48	1	82	10	2

FOOD	PORTION	CAL.	FAT	SOD.	CARB.	FIB.
Brownberry (CONT.)						
Raisin Bran	1 slice	61	1	108	12	2
Raisin Cinnamon	1 slice	66	1	107	12	1
Raisin Walnut	1 slice	68	3	96	11	2
Wheat Apple Honey	1 slice	69	2	148	11	2
Wheat Soft	1 slice	74	2	127	12	1
Cedar's						
Mountain Bread Six Grain	1 piece (2.4 oz)	200	4	380	35	4
Damascus Bakeries						
Mountain Shepard Lahvash	⅓ loaf (2 oz)	135	0	90	28	2
Dicarlo's						
Foccaccia	⅛ bread (2 oz)	130	2	260	25	1
French Parisian	2 slices (1 oz)	70	1	150	14	tr
Freihofer's						
Country Potato	1 slice (1.3 oz)	100	1	200	19	1
Country White	1 slice (1.3 oz)	100	1	220	19	tr
Wheat	1½ slices	70	1	—	—	—
Wheat Light	1 slice (1.6 oz)	80	0	180	17	4
White Light	2 slices (1.6 oz)	80	1	210	18	4
Whole Wheat 100%	1 slice (1.3 oz)	90	2	160	16	2
Home Pride						
Hearty Buttermilk & Biscuit White	1 slice (1.3 oz)	100	2	280	18	tr
Hearty Deli Rye	1 slice (2 oz)	140	2	350	26	3
Hearty Golden Honey Wheat	1 slice (1.3 oz)	90	2	210	18	2
Hearty Honey Oats & Cracked Wheat	1 slice (1.4 oz)	100	2	210	19	2
Hearty Seven Grain Multi Grain	1 slice (1.3 oz)	100	2	200	17	2
Honey Wheat	1 slice (1 oz)	70	1	150	13	1
Seven Grain	1 slice (0.9 oz)	60	1	130	12	1
Wheat	1 slice (0.9 oz)	70	1	140	13	1
Wheat Light	3 slices (2.1 oz)	110	2	300	25	6
White	1 slice (0.9 oz)	70	1	160	13	0
White Grain	1 slice (1 oz)	60	1	140	13	2
White Light	3 slices (0.9 oz)	110	2	320	25	6
Whole Wheat Hearty 100% Stoneground	1 slice (1.4 oz)	90	2	250	18	3
Malsovit						
Bread	1 slice	66	1	146	12	4
Raisin	1 slice	77	1	146	12	3

FOOD	PORTION	CAL.	FAT	SOD.	CARB.	FIB.
Matthew's						
9 Grain & Nut	1 slice	80	3	100	9	2
Cinnamon	1 slice	70	1	100	13	2
Golden	1 slice	70	1	125	14	1
Oat Bran	1 slice	65	0	110	12	2
Pita Whole Wheat	1	210	2	390	45	7
Sodium Free	1 slice	70	2	<5	12	2
Whole Wheat	1 slice	70	1	130	12	2
Mediterranean Magic						
Focaccia	⅕ loaf (1.8 oz)	140	2	550	27	tr
Monks' Bread						
Hi-Fibre	1 slice	50	1	110	13	—
Raisin	1 slice	70	2	85	10	—
Sunflower & Bran	1 slice	70	1	80	12	2
White	1 slice	60	1	95	10	—
Whole Wheat 100% Stoneground	1 slice	70	1	110	13	—
Parisian						
French Stick Extra Sour	2 oz	150	1	311	27	—
French Stick Sweet	2 oz	154	2	331	27	—
Pepperidge Farm						
7 Grain Hearty Slice	2 slices	180	2	340	36	2
Cinnamon	1 slice	90	3	110	15	2
Cracked Wheat	1 slice	70	1	140	13	1
Crunchy Oat 1½ lb Loaf	2 slices	190	4	290	34	3
Date Walnut	1 slice	90	3	110	14	2
French Fully Baked	2 oz	150	2	320	28	1
French Twin	1 oz	80	1	160	15	0
Honey Bran	1 slice	90	1	160	18	1
Italian Brown & Serve	1 oz	80	1	150	14	0
Italian Sliced	1 slice	70	1	125	12	—
Oatmeal	1 slice	70	1	160	12	1
Oatmeal 1½ lb Loaf	1 slice	90	1	200	17	1
Oatmeal Light	1 slice	45	0	95	9	1
Oatmeal Very Thin Sliced	1 slice	40	1	80	8	—
Pumpernickel Family	1 slice	80	1	230	15	2
Pumpernickel Party	4 slices	60	1	160	12	1
Raisin With Cinnamon	1 slice	90	2	100	16	1
Rye Dijon	1 slice	50	1	180	9	1
Rye Dijon Thick Sliced	1 slice	70	1	260	15	2
Rye Family	1 slice (32 g)	80	1	220	16	2
Rye Party	4 slices	60	1	250	12	1
Rye Seedless Family	1 slice	80	1	210	16	2
Rye Soft	1 slice	70	1	120	12	—

FOOD	PORTION	CAL.	FAT	SOD.	CARB.	FIB.
Pepperidge Farm (CONT.)						
Sesame Wheat	2 slices	190	3	340	36	3
Sprouted Wheat	1 slice	70	2	100	11	2
Vienna Light	1 slice	45	0	100	10	1
Vienna Thick Sliced	1 slice	70	1	125	13	0
Wheat 1½ lb Loaf	1 slice	90	2	190	18	2
Wheat Family	1 slice	70	1	130	13	2
Wheat Light	1 slice	45	0	90	9	1
Wheat Very Thin Sliced	1 slice	35	0	75	7	0
White Country	2 slices	190	2	340	38	2
White Large Family Thin Slice	1 slice	70	1	150	13	0
White Sandwich	2 slices	130	2	260	24	0
White Thin Slice	1 slice	80	2	130	14	0
White Toasting	1 slice	90	1	200	17	1
White Very Thin Sliced	1 slice	40	0	80	8	0
Whole Wheat Thin Slice	1 slice	60	1	110	12	2
Roman Meal						
Brown & Serve Mini Loaf	½ loaf (2 oz)	136	2	275	24	1
Cracked Wheat	1 slice (1.4 oz)	92	2	129	15	2
Hearty Wheat Light	1 slice (0.8 oz)	42	tr	102	7	2
Honey Nut Oat Bran	1 slice (1 oz)	72	2	129	11	1
Honey Oat Bran	1 slice (1 oz)	70	1	132	12	1
Oat	1 slice (1 oz)	69	1	100	12	1
Oat Bran	1 slice (1 oz)	68	1	136	12	1
Oat Bran Light	1 slice (0.8 oz)	42	tr	100	7	2
Round Top	1 slice (1 oz)	67	1	142	12	1
Sandwich	1 slice (0.8 oz)	55	1	115	10	1
Seven Grain	1 slice (1 oz)	67	1	142	12	1
Seven Grain Light	1 slice (0.8 oz)	42	1	101	7	3
Sourdough Light	1 slice (0.8 oz)	41	tr	115	7	3
Sourdough Whole Grain Light	1 slice (0.8 oz)	40	tr	104	7	3
Sun Grain	1 slice (1 oz)	70	2	135	11	1
Twelve Grain	1 slice (1 oz)	70	2	140	11	1
Twelve Grain Light	1 slice (0.8 oz)	42	tr	104	7	3
Wheat Light	1 slice (0.8 oz)	41	tr	102	7	3
Wheatberry Honey	1 slice (1 oz)	67	1	139	12	1
Wheatberry Light	1 slice (0.8 oz)	42	tr	102	7	2
White Light	1 slice (0.8 oz)	41	tr	105	7	3
Whole Grain 100%	1 slice (1.4 oz)	91	1	198	16	2
Whole Grain Sourdough	1 slice (1 oz)	66	1	141	12	1
Whole Wheat 100%	1 slice (1 oz)	64	1	141	11	2
Whole Wheat 100% Light	1 slice (0.8 oz)	42	tr	102	7	2

FOOD	PORTION	CAL.	FAT	SOD.	CARB.	FIB.
Sahara						
Pita Oat Bran	½ pocket (1 oz)	66	tr	163	14	2
Pita White	½ pocket	78	1	147	16	—
Stroehmann						
White Whole Special Recipe	1 slice	70	1	160	13	—
White Whole Special Recipe Kids	1 slice	60	tr	150	12	—
Sunmaid						
Raisin	1 slice	70	tr	85	13	1
Tree Of Life						
100% Spelt	1 slice (1.8 oz)	130	3	290	22	3
Millet	1 slice (1.8 oz)	130	2	240	25	2
Rye Sour Dough	1 slice (1.8 oz)	110	0	30	24	5
Sprouted Seven Grain	1 slice (1.8 oz)	110	2	140	20	2
Wonder						
Calcium Enriched	1 slice (1 oz)	70	1	150	12	tr
Cinnamon Raisin	1 slice (1 oz)	70	1	100	14	tr
Cracked Wheat	1 slice (1 oz)	70	1	150	14	1
French	1 slice (1 oz)	80	2	160	15	tr
French Light	2 slices (1.6 oz)	80	1	210	18	5
Granola	1 slice (1.5 oz)	100	2	210	19	2
Honey Bran Light	2 slices (1.6 oz)	80	1	190	18	6
Italian	1 slice (1.1 oz)	80	1	190	15	tr
Italian Family	1 slice (1 oz)	70	1	170	13	tr
Italian Light	2 slices (1.6 oz)	80	1	230	18	5
Kid	1 slice (0.9 oz)	70	1	150	13	tr
Light Calcium Enriched	2 slices (1.6 oz)	80	1	240	18	5
Nine Grain Light	2 slices (1.6 oz)	80	1	230	18	6
Oatmeal Light	2 slices (1.6 oz)	90	0	230	19	4
Rye	1 slice (1 oz)	70	1	170	13	1
Rye Light	2 slices (1.6 oz)	70	1	220	17	5
Sourdough	1 slice (1.2 oz)	90	2	180	17	tr
Sourdough Light	2 slices (1.6 oz)	80	1	250	18	5
Texas Toast	1 slice (1.4 oz)	100	1	220	19	1
Vienna	1 slice (1 oz)	70	1	170	13	tr
Wheat Calcium Light	2 slices (1.6 oz)	80	1	240	18	6
Wheat Family	1 slice (0.9 oz)	70	1	150	13	tr
Wheat Golden Country Style	2 slices (1.4 oz)	100	2	220	19	1
Wheat Light	2 slices (1.6 oz)	80	1	230	18	6
White	1 slice (0.9 oz)	70	1	150	13	tr
White Calcium	2 slices (1.6 oz)	100	1	240	20	1
White Calcium Light	2 slices (1.6 oz)	80	1	260	18	5

FOOD	PORTION	CAL.	FAT	SOD.	CARB.	FIB.
Wonder (CONT.)						
White Light	2 slices (1.6 oz)	80	1	230	18	5
White With Buttermilk	1 slice (1 oz)	80	1	180	14	tr
Whole Wheat 100%	1 slice (1 oz)	70	1	180	12	2
Whole Wheat 100% Soft	2 slices (1.6 oz)	110	2	240	21	1
Whole Wheat 100% Stoneground	1 slice (1.2 oz)	80	2	190	14	2
ZA						
Pit-Za Hearty Multi-Grain	1/9 bread (2 oz)	130	2	210	25	2
Pit-Za Salt-Free Garlic Whole Wheat	1/9 bread (2 oz)	150	1	10	28	3
REFRIGERATED						
Pillsbury						
Crusty French Loaf	1 in slice	60	tr	120	11	—
Hearty Grains Country Oatmeal Twists	1	80	2	120	15	—
Hearty Grains Cracked Wheat Twists	1	80	2	120	14	—
Pipin'Hot Wheat Loaf	1 in slice	70	2	170	12	—
Pipin'Hot White Loaf	1 in slice	70	2	170	12	—
Roman Meal						
Loaf	1 slice (1 oz)	85	3	199	13	1
Stefano's						
Stuffed Bread Broccoli & Cheese	1/2 bread (6 oz)	450	17	830	54	7
TAKE-OUT						
chapatis as prep w/ fat	1 bread (1.6 oz)	95	2	180	18	3
chapatis as prep w/o fat	1 (2½ oz)	141	1	—	31	5
cornbread	2 in x 2 in (1.4 oz)	107	2	276	18	—
cornstick	1 (1.3 oz)	101	4	195	13	tr
focaccia onion	1 piece (4.6 oz)	282	10	536	43	2
focaccia rosemary	1 piece (3.5 oz)	251	7	535	40	2
focaccia tomato olive	1 piece (4.7 oz)	270	8	683	42	2
garlic bread	2 slices (2 oz)	190	8	290	27	1
naan	1 bread (3.5 oz)	286	9	546	43	2
papadums fried	2 (1.5 oz)	81	4	—	9	2
paratha	1 bread (2.1 oz)	201	10	268	23	2

BREAD COATING

FOOD	PORTION	CAL.	FAT	SOD.	CARB.	FIB.
Don's Chuck Wagon						
All Purpose Mix	1/4 cup (1 oz)	100	0	580	20	1
Fish & Chips Mix	1/4 cup (1 oz)	100	0	740	21	1
Fish Mix	1/4 cup (1 oz)	95	0	940	21	1
Frying Mix Chicken	1/4 cup (1 oz)	95	0	850	21	1

FOOD	PORTION	CAL.	FAT	SOD.	CARB.	FIB.
Don's Chuck Wagon (CONT.)						
Frying Mix Seafood Seasoned	¼ cup (1 oz)	95	1	990	21	1
Mushroom Mix	¼ cup (1 oz)	95	0	990	21	1
Onion Ring Mix	¼ cup (1 oz)	100	0	690	21	1
Golden Dipt						
Breading Frying Mix	1 oz	90	0	630	20	—
Chicken Frying Mix	1 oz	90	0	1430	20	—
Onion Ring Mix	1 oz	100	0	570	22	—
Ka-Me						
Tempura Batter Mix	1 oz	100	0	5	22	0
Little Crow						
Fryin' Magic	0.5 oz	43	tr	542	8	—
Mrs. Dash						
Crispy Coating	2 tbsp (0.6 oz)	65	1	3	10	—
Oven Fry						
Extra Crispy For Chicken	⅛ pkg (0.5 oz)	60	1	420	10	0
Extra Crispy For Pork	⅛ pkg (0.5 oz)	60	2	340	11	0
Shake 'N Bake						
Buffalo Wings	1/10 pkg (0.4 oz)	40	1	300	8	0
Classic Italian Chicken or Pork	⅛ pkg (0.4 oz)	40	1	270	7	0
Country Mild Recipe	⅛ pkg (0.3 oz)	35	2	240	5	0
Glazes Barbecue Chicken Or Pork	⅛ pkg (0.4 oz)	45	1	410	9	0
Glazes Honey Mustard Chicken Or Pork	⅛ pkg (0.4 oz)	45	1	300	9	0
Glazes Tangy Honey Chicken Or Pork	⅛ pkg (0.4 oz)	45	1	300	9	0
Home Style Flour Recipe For Chicken	⅛ pkg (0.4 oz)	40	1	470	7	0
Hot & Spicy Chicken Or Pork	⅛ pkg (0.4 oz)	40	1	170	7	0
Original For Chicken	⅛ pkg (0.4 oz)	40	1	220	7	0
Original For Fish	¼ pkg (0.7 oz)	80	2	350	14	tr
Original For Pork	⅛ pkg (0.4 oz)	45	1	230	8	0
BREAD MACHINE MIX						
Dromedary						
Country White	½ in slice (2 oz)	140	1	230	28	1
Italian Herb	½ in slice (1.8 oz)	140	3	250	25	1
Stoneground Wheat	½ in slice (1.8 oz)	140	2	200	26	2
Pillsbury						
Cracked Wheat	1/12 pkg (1.3 oz)	130	2	260	25	2

FOOD	PORTION	CAL.	FAT	SOD.	CARB.	FIB.
Sassafras						
Apricot Oatmeal	1 slice (1.4 oz)	140	1	190	29	2
Wanda's						
Dried Tomato Cheddar	¼ cup mix per serv (1.2 oz)	140	0	230	22	3
European White	¼ cup mix per serv (1.2 oz)	130	0	115	26	1
Oatmeal	¼ cup mix per serv (1.2 oz)	120	0	350	24	1
Oatmeal Cinnamon	¼ cup mix per serv (1.2 oz)	120	0	280	19	1
Old World Rye	¼ cup mix per serv (1.9 oz)	90	0	300	27	3
Onion	¼ cup mix per serv (1.2 oz)	120	0	270	25	1
Orange Cinnamon	¼ cup mix per serv (1.3 oz)	130	0	90	28	1
Oregano Garlic	¼ cup mix per serv (1.2 oz)	130	1	270	25	2
Rosemary Basil	¼ cup mix per serv (1.2 oz)	130	0	250	26	1
Rye	¼ cup mix per serv (1.2 oz)	120	0	270	25	1
Rye Caraway	¼ cup mix per serv (1.2 oz)	120	0	270	25	1
Sourdough	¼ cup mix per serv (1.2 oz)	120	0	160	25	1
Sunflower Sesame Poppyseed	¼ cup mix per serv (1.2 oz)	120	0	310	25	2
Ten Grain	¼ cup mix per serv (1.4 oz)	140	0	160	27	3
Wheat	¼ cup mix per serv (1.2 oz)	130	0	270	26	2
White	¼ cup mix per serv (1.2 oz)	130	0	250	26	1
Whole Wheat	¼ cup mix per serv (1.3 oz)	130	0	330	26	4
BREADCRUMBS						
dry	1 cup	426	6	930	78	5
dry seasoned	1 cup (4 oz)	441	3	3180	85	5
fresh	⅔ cup	76	1	153	14	1
4C						
Salt Free	1 tbsp (0.5 oz)	50	1	0	10	—

FOOD	PORTION	CAL.	FAT	SOD.	CARB.	FIB.
4C (CONT.)						
Seasoned	1 tbsp (.5 oz)	50	1	270	10	—
Toasted	1 tbsp (0.5 oz)	50	1	110	10	—
Toasted Salt Free	1 tbsp (0.5 oz)	50	1	0	10	—
Arnold						
Italian	½ oz	50	tr	200	8	tr
Plain	½ oz	50	tr	80	8	tr
Contadina						
Plain	⅓ cup	100	2	700	19	1
Devonsheer						
Italian Style	1 oz	104	1	408	20	1
Plain	1 oz	108	1	272	21	1
Friday's						
Seasoned	1 oz	56	tr	—	—	—
Jaclyn's						
Organic Whole Wheat Italian Style	½ oz	28	1	5	13	—
Organic Whole Wheat Plain	½ oz	28	1	5	13	—
Progresso						
Italian Style	¼ cup (1 oz)	110	2	430	20	1
Lemon Herb	¼ cup (0.9 oz)	100	1	480	20	2
Plain	¼ cup (1 oz)	100	2	210	19	1
Tomato Basil	¼ cup (1.1 oz)	120	2	750	22	2

BREADFRUIT

breadfruit	3.5 oz	109	tr	—	—	—
fresh	¼ small	99	tr	2	26	—
seeds cooked	1 oz	48	1	—	9	—
seeds raw	1 oz	54	2	—	8	—
seeds roasted	1 oz	59	tr	—	11	—

BREADNUTTREE SEEDS

dried	1 oz	104	tr	—	23	—

BREADSTICKS

onion poppyseed home recipe	1	64	1	69	11	—
plain	1	41	1	66	7	—
plain	1 sm	25	1	66	4	—
Angonoa						
Cheese	5 (1 oz)	120	3	270	20	1
Cheese Mini	16 (1 oz)	120	3	120	20	1
Garlic	6 (1 oz)	120	2	390	21	1
Italian Style Plain	5 (1 oz)	120	3	280	20	1

FOOD	PORTION	CAL.	FAT	SOD.	CARB.	FIB.
Angonoa (CONT.)						
Low Sodium With Sesame Seed	6 (1 oz)	130	4	65	19	2
Onion	6 (1 oz)	120	2	200	21	2
Pizza Mini	26 (1 oz)	120	2	180	21	1
Sesame Mini	16 (1 oz)	130	4	220	19	2
Sesame Royale	6 (1 oz)	130	4	210	18	2
Whole Wheat Mini	14 (1 oz)	130	4	220	19	3
Bread Du Jour						
Italian	1 (1.9 oz)	130	2	280	25	1
Sourdough	1 (1.9 oz)	130	1	280	25	1
J.J. Cassone						
Garlic	1 (1.6 oz)	150	3	—	26	2
Keebler						
Garlic	2	30	tr	20	6	—
Onion	2	30	tr	25	6	—
Plain	2	30	tr	30	6	—
Sesame	2	30	1	30	5	—
Lance						
Cheese	2	20	0	40	4	—
Garlic	2	30	0	40	5	—
Plain	2	30	0	50	5	—
Sesame	2	30	0	50	4	—
Pillsbury						
Soft Bread Sticks	1	100	2	230	17	—
Roman Meal						
Brown & Serve Soft	1 (2.7 oz)	181	3	275	32	3
Refrigerated	1 (1.4 oz)	117	4	274	18	1
Stella D'Oro						
Deli Garlic Fat Free	5	60	0	120	12	—
Deli Original Fat Free	5	60	0	130	12	—
Garlic	1	35	1	55	6	—
Grissini Garlic Fat Free	3	60	0	120	12	—
Grissini Original Fat Free	3	60	0	130	12	—
Onion	1	40	1	38	6	—
Regular	1	40	1	40	7	—
Regular Sodium Free	2	80	2	0	14	—
Sesame Low Fat	2	70	1	90	14	—
Sesame Sodium Free	1	50	3	0	7	—
Traditional Garlic Fat Free	2	70	0	150	15	—
Traditional Original Fat Free	2	70	0	150	15	—

FOOD	PORTION	CAL.	FAT	SOD.	CARB.	FIB.
Stella D'Oro (CONT.)						
Wheat	1	40	1	20	6	—

BREAKFAST BAR

(*see also* BREAKFAST DRINKS, NUTRITIONAL SUPPLEMENTS)

FOOD	PORTION	CAL.	FAT	SOD.	CARB.	FIB.
Carnation						
Chewy Chocolate Chip	1 (1.26 oz)	150	6	80	22	tr
Chewy Peanut Butter Chocolate Chip	1 (1.26 oz)	140	5	90	21	tr
Glenny's						
Sunrise Bee Pollen	1 (1.5 oz)	190	8	—	22	—
Sunrise Ginseng	1 (1.5 oz)	160	7	—	24	—
Sunrise Spirulina	1 (1.5 oz)	140	5	—	21	—
Nutri-Grain						
Apple Cinnamon	1 (1.3 oz)	140	3	60	27	1
Blueberry	1 (1.3 oz)	140	3	60	27	1
Peach	1 (1.3 oz)	140	3	60	27	1
Raspberry	1 (1.3 oz)	140	3	60	27	1
Strawberry	1 (1.3 oz)	140	3	60	27	1

BREAKFAST DRINKS

(*see also* BREAKFAST BAR, NUTRITIONAL SUPPLEMENTS)

FOOD	PORTION	CAL.	FAT	SOD.	CARB.	FIB.
orange drink powder	3 rounded tsp	93	0	4	24	—
orange drink powder as prep w/water	6 oz	86	0	9	22	—
Carnation						
Instant Breakfast Cafe Mocha	1 pkg	130	1	100	28	1
Instant Breakfast Cafe Mocha	1 pkg + skim milk (9 fl oz)	220	1	216	39	1
Instant Breakfast Cafe Mocha	1 can (10 fl oz)	220	3	210	35	0
Instant Breakfast Classic Chocolate Malt	1 pkg + skim milk (9 fl oz)	220	1	240	39	1
Instant Breakfast Classic Chocolate Malt	1 pkg	130	2	130	26	1
Instant Breakfast Creamy Milk Chocolate	1 pkg + skim milk (9 fl oz)	220	1	240	39	1
Instant Breakfast Creamy Milk Chocolate	1 pkg	130	1	100	28	1

FOOD	PORTION	CAL.	FAT	SOD.	CARB.	FIB.
Carnation (CONT.)						
Instant Breakfast Creamy Milk Chocolate	8 fl oz	220	3	220	36	1
Instant Breakfast Creamy Milk Chocolate	1 can (10 fl oz)	220	3	230	37	1
Instant Breakfast French Vanilla	1 pkg + skim milk	220	1	240	39	0
Instant Breakfast French Vanilla	1 pkg	130	0	110	27	0
Instant Breakfast No Sugar Added Classic Chocolate	1 pkg + skim milk (9 fl oz)	160	2	240	24	1
Instant Breakfast No Sugar Added Classic Chocolate	1 pkg	70	2	120	11	1
Instant Breakfast No Sugar Added Creamy Milk Chocolate	1 pkg + skim milk (9 fl oz)	160	1	216	24	1
Instant Breakfast No Sugar Added Creamy Milk Chocolate	1 pkg	70	1	90	12	1
Instant Breakfast No Sugar Added French Vanilla	1 pkg	70	0	90	12	0
Instant Breakfast No Sugar Added French Vanilla	1 pkg + skim milk (9 fl oz)	150	1	216	24	0
Instant Breakfast No Sugar Added Strawberry Creme	1 pkg	70	0	90	12	0
Instant Breakfast No Sugar Added Strawberry Creme	1 pkg + skim milk (9 fl oz)	150	1	216	24	0
Instant Breakfast Strawberry Creme	1 pkg + skim milk	220	1	288	39	0
Instant Breakfast Strawberry Creme	1 pkg	130	0	160	28	0
Pillsbury						
Instant Breakfast Chocolate Malt as prep w/ milk	1 serv	290	9	310	38	—
Instant Breakfast Chocolate as prep w/ milk	1 serv	290	9	310	38	—

FOOD	PORTION	CAL.	FAT	SOD.	CARB.	FIB.
Pillsbury (CONT.)						
Instant Breakfast Strawberry as prep w/ milk	1 serv	290	9	300	39	—
Instant Breakfast Vanilla as prep w/ whole milk	1 serv	300	9	330	41	—
BROAD BEANS						
canned	1 cup	183	1	1161	32	—
dried cooked	1 cup	186	1	8	33	—
fresh cooked	3½ oz	56	tr	41	10	—
BROCCOFLOWER						
fresh raw	½ cup (1.8 oz)	16	tr	12	3	—
Dole						
Fresh	⅕ head	35	0	30	7	—
BROCCOLI						
FRESH						
chopped cooked	½ cup	22	tr	20	4	2
raw chopped	½ cup	12	tr	12	2	1
Dole						
Spear	1 med	40	1	75	4	5
FROZEN						
chopped cooked	½ cup	25	tr	22	5	—
spears cooked	10 oz pkg	69	tr	60	13	4
spears cooked	½ cup	25	tr	22	5	3
Big Valley						
Chopped	¾ cup (3 oz)	25	0	20	4	2
Cuts	¾ cup (3 oz)	25	0	20	4	2
Birds Eye						
Baby Spears Deluxe	⅔ cup	30	0	15	5	3
Chopped	¾ cup (3 oz)	25	0	20	4	2
Farm Fresh Spears	¾ cup	30	0	25	7	2
Florets Deluxe	½ cup	25	0	20	5	3
Polybag Cuts	½ cup	25	0	25	4	3
Polybag Deluxe Florets	⅔ cup	25	0	15	4	3
Spears	⅔ cup	25	0	20	5	3
With Cheese Sauce	½ pkg	110	5	520	9	1
Fresh Like						
Spear	3.5 oz	26	tr	32	5	1
Green Giant						
Cut	½ cup	16	0	95	3	2
Cuts	½ cup	12	0	15	3	2
Harvest Fresh Spears	½ cup	20	0	115	4	2
In Butter Sauce	½ cup	40	2	350	6	—

FOOD	PORTION	CAL.	FAT	SOD.	CARB.	FIB.
Green Giant (CONT.)						
In Cheese Sauce	½ cup	60	2	530	9	2
Mini Spears Select	4-5 spears	18	0	25	5	3
One Serve Cuts In Butter Sauce	1 pkg	45	2	10	7	3
Valley Combinations Broccoli Fanfare	½ cup	80	2	340	14	—
Hanover						
Cut	½ cup	25	0	—	—	—
Florets	½ cup	30	0	—	—	—
Pepperidge Farm						
Broccoli With Cheese In Pastry	1	230	16	380	18	—
Stouffer's						
Au Gratin	1 serv (4 oz)	100	4	450	10	2
Tree Of Life						
Broccoli	1 cup (3.1 oz)	25	0	20	4	2

BROWNIE

FOOD	PORTION	CAL.	FAT	SOD.	CARB.	FIB.
FROZEN						
Pepperidge Farm						
Monterey Hot Fudge Chocolate Chunk Brownie	1	480	26	200	56	—
Newport Hot Fudge Brownie	1	400	20	160	50	—
Weight Watchers						
Brownie A La Mode	1 (3.14 oz)	190	4	170	34	2
Double Fudge Brownie Parfait	1 (5.3 oz)	190	3	170	39	2
HOME RECIPE						
plain	1 (0.8 oz)	112	7	82	12	1
w/nuts	1 (0.8 oz)	95	6	51	11	—
MIX						
plain	1 (1.2 oz)	139	7	83	20	1
plain low calorie	1 (0.8 oz)	84	2	21	16	1
Betty Crocker						
Brownie With Hot Fudge MicroRave Single	1	350	12	260	55	—
Frosted MicroRave	1	180	7	120	21	—
Fudge Family Size	1	150	5	100	22	—
Fudge Light	1	100	1	90	21	—
Fudge MicroRave	1	150	6	110	22	—
Fudge Regular Size	1	150	6	105	23	—

FOOD	PORTION	CAL.	FAT	SOD.	CARB.	FIB.
Betty Crocker (CONT.)						
Supreme Caramel	1	120	4	115	21	—
Supreme Frosted	1	160	6	120	26	—
Supreme German Chocolate	1	160	7	110	24	—
Supreme Original	1	140	6	80	21	—
Supreme Party	1	160	6	110	26	—
Supreme Walnut	1	140	7	80	18	—
Walnut MicroRave	1	160	7	95	21	—
Estee						
Lite	2	100	4	0	23	1
Jiffy						
Fudge as prep	1	160	4	150	28	tr
Pillsbury						
Deluxe Family-Size Fudge Brownie	2 in sq	150	7	95	20	—
Deluxe Fudge Brownie	2 in sq	150	6	100	21	—
Deluxe Fudge Brownie With Walnuts	2 in sq	150	8	90	19	—
Fudge Microwave	1	190	9	105	25	—
The Ultimate Carmel Fudge Chunk Brownie	2 in sq	170	7	105	25	—
The Ultimate Chunky Triple Fudge Brownie	2 in sq	170	7	105	25	—
The Ultimate Double Fudge Brownie	2 in sq	160	6	105	24	—
The Ultimate Rockey Road Fudge Brownie	2 in sq	170	8	95	24	—
READY-TO-EAT						
plain	1 sm (1 oz)	115	5	88	18	1
plain	1 lg (2 oz)	227	9	175	36	1
w/ nuts	1 (1 oz)	100	4	59	16	—
w/o nuts	1 (2 oz)	243	10	153	39	—
Frito Lay						
Fudge Nut	3 oz	360	14	225	56	—
Greenfield						
Brownie HomeStyle	1 (1.4 oz)	120	0	65	29	1
Hostess						
Brownie Bites	5 (2 oz)	260	14	125	32	2
Brownie Bites Walnut	5 (2 oz)	270	15	140	31	2
Lance						
Brownie	1 pkg (78 g)	320	12	210	52	—
Little Debbie						
Fudge	1 pkg (2.1 oz)	270	13	170	39	1

FOOD	PORTION	CAL.	FAT	SOD.	CARB.	FIB.
Little Debbie (CONT.)						
Fudge	1 pkg (2.5 oz)	310	15	190	44	1
Fudge	1 pkg (2.9 oz)	360	17	230	52	1
Fudge	1 pkg (3.6 oz)	450	21	280	65	2
Pepperidge Farm						
Charlotte Fudgey Brownie	1	220	11	105	28	2
Tahoe Milk Chocolate Pecan	1	210	10	100	30	1
Westport Fudgey Brownies w/ Walnuts	1	220	11	105	28	2
Sweet Rewards						
Double Fudge	1 (1.1 oz)	110	0	100	25	tr
Fat Free Brownie	1 bar (1 oz)	90	0	90	21	<1
Tastykake						
Brownie	1 (85 g)	340	14	220	53	5

BRUSSELS SPROUTS

FOOD	PORTION	CAL.	FAT	SOD.	CARB.	FIB.
FRESH						
cooked	½ cup	30	tr	17	7	3
cooked	1 sprout	8	tr	4	2	—
raw	1 sprout	8	tr	5	2	1
raw	½ cup	19	tr	11	4	—
Dole						
Sprouts	½ cup	19	tr	11	4	2
FROZEN						
cooked	½ cup	33	tr	18	6	—
Big Valley						
Whole	5-8 pieces (3 oz)	35	0	9	6	1
Birds Eye						
Brussels Sprouts	½ cup	35	0	15	7	3
Fresh Like						
Sprouts	3.5 oz	37	tr	21	7	1
Green Giant						
In Butter Sauce	½ cup	40	1	280	8	—
Sprouts	½ cup	25	0	10	6	2
Hanover						
Brussels Sprouts	½ cup	40	0	—	—	—

BUCKWHEAT

FOOD	PORTION	CAL.	FAT	SOD.	CARB.	FIB.
flour whole groat	1 cup	402	4	—	85	—
groats roasted cooked	½ cup	91	tr	4	20	—
groats roasted uncooked	½ cup	283	2	9	61	—
Wolff's						
Brown Groats Roasted	1 cup (8 oz)	900	4	—	188	—

FOOD	PORTION	CAL.	FAT	SOD.	CARB.	FIB.
Wolff's (CONT.)						
Flour	1 cup (8 oz)	860	5	—	170	—
Kasha Coarse cooked	¼ cup (1.6 oz)	170	2	10	35	2
Kasha Fine cooked	¼ cup (1.6 oz)	170	2	10	35	2
Kasha Medium cooked	¼ cup (1.6 oz)	170	2	10	35	2
Kasha Whole cooked	¼ cup (1.6 oz)	170	2	10	35	2
White Grits	1 cup (8 oz)	840	3	—	173	—
BUFFALO						
water buffalo roasted	3 oz	111	2	48	0	—
BULGUR						
cooked	½ cup	76	tr	5	17	—
uncooked	½ cup	239	tr	12	53	—
Casbah						
Pilaf Mix as prep	1 cup	200	1	450	42	4
Salad Mix as prep	⅔ cup	90	tr	350	20	1
Good Shepherd						
Bulgur	¼ cup (43 g)	150	1	0	33	1
Hodgson Mill						
Bulgur	¼ cup (1.4 oz)	120	1	0	24	1
BURBOT (FISH)						
fresh baked	3 oz	98	1	106	0	—
BURDOCK ROOT						
cooked	1 cup	110	tr	5	26	—
raw	1 cup	85	tr	6	20	—
BUTTER						
(*see also* BUTTER BLENDS, BUTTER SUBSTITUTES, MARGARINE)						
clarified butter	3½ oz	876	99	—	0	—
stick	1 pat (5 g)	36	4	41	tr	—
stick	1 stick (4 oz)	813	92	937	tr	—
whipped	1 pat (4 g)	27	3	31	tr	—
whipped	4 oz	542	61	625	tr	—
Cabot						
Stick	1 tsp	35	4	41	0	—
Unsalted Stick	1 tsp	35	4	0	0	—
Crystal						
Salted Stick	1 tbsp (0.5 oz)	102	11	89	tr	0
Unsalted Stick	1 tbsp (0.5 oz)	102	11	1	tr	0
Hotel Bar						
Stick	1 tsp	35	4	35	0	—
Keller's						
Stick	1 tsp	35	4	35	0	—

FOOD	PORTION	CAL.	FAT	SOD.	CARB.	FIB.
Land O'Lakes						
Light Stick	1 tbsp	50	6	70	0	—
Light Unsalted Stick	1 tbsp	50	6	5	0	—
Stick	1 tbsp (0.5 oz)	100	11	85	0	—
Unsalted Stick	1 tbsp (0.5 oz)	100	11	0	0	—
Unsalted Tub	1 tbsp	60	7	0	0	—
Whipped	1 tbsp (0.3 oz)	70	7	55	0	—
BUTTER BEANS						
CANNED						
Allen						
Baby	½ cup (4.5 oz)	120	1	460	22	6
Large	½ cup (4.5 oz)	120	1	290	20	7
Hanover						
Butter Beans	½ cup	80	0	—	—	—
In Sauce	½ cup	100	0	—	—	—
Luck's						
Speckled Seasoned w/ Pork	7.5 oz	230	8	—	—	—
S&W						
Tender Cooked	½ cup	100	0	440	19	—
Sunshine						
Butter Beans	½ cup (4.5 oz)	120	1	370	23	8
Trappey						
Baby White With Bacon	½ cup (4.5 oz)	130	2	350	21	6
Large White With Bacon	½ cup (4.5 oz)	110	1	300	21	6
Van Camp's						
Butter Beans	½ cup	110	1	430	22	7
BUTTER BLENDS						
(*see also* BUTTER, BUTTER SUBSTITUTES, MARGARINE)						
stick	1 stick	811	91	1013	1	—
Blue Bonnet						
Better Blend Stick	1 tbsp	90	11	95	0	—
Better Blend Tub	1 tbsp	90	11	95	0	—
Better Blend Unsalted Stick	1 tbsp	90	11	0	0	—
Country Morning						
Blend Light Stick	1 tbsp (0.5 oz)	50	6	110	0	—
Blend Light Tub	1 tbsp (0.5 oz)	50	6	90	0	—
Blend Stick	1 tbsp	100	11	90	0	—
Blend Tub	1 tbsp	100	11	80	0	—
Blend Unsalted Stick	1 tbsp	100	11	0	0	—
Downey's						
Cinnamon Honey-Butter Tub	1 tbsp	52	1	5	—	—

FOOD	PORTION	CAL.	FAT	SOD.	CARB.	FIB.
Downey's (CONT.)						
Original Honey-Butter Tub	1 tbsp	52	1	5	—	—
Le Slim Cow						
Tub	1 tbsp	40	4	15	—	—
Touch Of Butter						
Tub	1 tbsp (0.5 oz)	60	7	110	0	0
BUTTER SUBSTITUTES						
(*see also* BUTTER BLENDS, MARGARINE)						
Brummel & Brown						
Spread Made With Yogurt	1 tbsp (0.5 oz)	50	5	95	0	—
Butter Buds						
Mix	1 tsp (2 g)	5	0	75	2	—
Sprinkles	1 tsp (2 g)	5	0	120	2	—
Molly McButter						
Cheese	1 tsp	5	0	125	1	—
Light Sodium	1 tsp	5	0	90	1	—
Natural Butter	1 tsp	5	0	180	1	—
Roasted Garlic	1 tsp	5	0	125	1	—
Mrs. Bateman's						
Butterlike Baking Butter	1 tbsp (0.5 oz)	36	1	20	8	0
Butterlike Saute Butter	1 tbsp (0.5 oz)	40	2	60	8	0
Watkins						
Butter Sprinkles	1 tsp (2 g)	5	0	170	1	0
Imitation Butter Flavored Mist	1 tbsp (0.5 oz)	120	14	0	0	0
BUTTERBUR						
canned fuki chopped	1 cup	3	tr	5	tr	—
fresh fuki raw	1 cup	13	tr	7	3	—
BUTTERFISH						
baked	3 oz	159	9	97	0	—
fillet baked	1 oz	47	3	29	0	—
BUTTERNUTS						
dried	1 oz	174	16	0	3	—
BUTTERSCOTCH						
(*see also* CANDY)						
Nestle						
Morsels Butterscotch	1 tbsp	80	4	15	10	—
CABBAGE						
(*see also* COLESLAW)						
FRESH						
chinese pak-choi raw shredded	½ cup	5	tr	23	1	—

FOOD	PORTION	CAL.	FAT	SOD.	CARB.	FIB.
chinese pak-choi shredded cooked	½ cup	10	tr	29	2	—
chinese pe-tsai raw shredded	1 cup	12	tr	7	2	—
chinese pe-tsai shredded cooked	1 cup	16	tr	11	3	—
danish raw	1 head (2 lbs)	228	2	164	49	18
danish raw shredded	½ cup (1.2 oz)	9	tr	6	2	tr
danish shredded cooked	½ cup (2.6 oz)	17	tr	6	3	1
green raw	1 head (2 lbs)	228	2	164	49	18
green raw shredded	½ cup (1.2 oz)	9	tr	6	2	tr
green shredded cooked	½ cup (2.6 oz)	17	tr	6	3	1
red raw shredded	½ cup	10	tr	4	2	1
red shredded cooked	½ cup	16	tr	6	3	—
savoy raw shredded	½ cup	10	tr	10	2	—
savoy shredded cooked	½ cup	18	tr	17	4	—
Dole						
Cabbage	1/12 med head	18	0	30	3	2
Napa shredded	½ cup	6	tr	3	1	tr
Fresh Express						
Cole Slaw	1½ cups (3 oz)	25	0	25	6	2
HOME RECIPE						
coleslaw w/ dressing	¾ cup	147	11	267	13	—
TAKE-OUT						
stuffed cabbage	1 (6 oz)	373	22	1007	18	—
sweet & sour red cabbage	4 oz	61	3	—	8	3
vinegar & oil coleslaw	3.5 oz	150	9	480	16	—

CAKE

(*see also* BROWNIE, CAKE MIX, COOKIE, DANISH PASTRY, DOUGHNUT, PIE) (FAST FACT: Toaster pastries are the fastest-growing breakfast food. Consumption has tripled since they were introduced in 1964.)

FOOD	PORTION	CAL.	FAT	SOD.	CARB.	FIB.
angelfood	1 cake (11.9 oz)	876	3	2548	197	5
angelfood home recipe	1/12 cake (1.9 oz)	142	tr	96	32	1
apple crisp home recipe	1 recipe 6 serv (29.6 oz)	1377	31	1537	273	—
bakewell tart	1 slice (3 oz)	410	27	—	39	2
battenburg cake	1 slice (2 oz)	204	10	—	28	1
boston cream pie frzn	1/6 cake (3.2 oz)	232	8	132	40	1
carrot w/ cream cheese icing home recipe	1 cake 10 in diam	6175	328	4470	775	—
cheesecake	1 cake 9 in diam	3350	213	2464	317	—

FOOD	PORTION	CAL.	FAT	SOD.	CARB.	FIB.
cheesecake	1/6 cake (2.8 oz)	256	18	165	20	2
cheesecake home recipe	1/12 cake (4.5 oz)	456	9	362	32	—
cherry fudge w/ chocolate frosting	1/8 cake (2.5 oz)	187	9	160	27	—
chocolate cupcake creme filled w/ frosting home recipe	1 (1.8 oz)	188	7	213	30	—
chocolate w/o frosting home recipe	1/12 cake (3.3 oz)	340	14	299	51	—
chocolate w/o frosting home recipe	2 layers (39.9 oz)	4067	172	3581	608	—
coffeecake creme-filled chocolate frosting home recipe	1/6 cake (3.2 oz)	298	10	290	49	2
coffeecake crumb topped cinnamon home recipe	1/12 cake (2.1 oz)	240	12	233	30	2
coffeecake fruit	1/8 cake (1.8 oz)	156	5	192	26	—
cream puff shell home recipe	1 (2.3 oz)	239	17	368	15	—
crumpets toasted	2 (4 oz)	119	1	—	26	2
devil's food cupcake w/ chocolate frosting	1	120	4	92	20	—
devil's food w/ creme filling	1 (1 oz)	105	4	105	17	—
eccles cake	1 slice (2 oz)	285	16	—	36	1
eclair	1 (1.4 oz)	149	10	—	15	tr
eclair home recipe	1 (3 oz)	262	16	337	24	—
fruitcake	1 piece (1.5 oz)	139	4	116	27	—
fruitcake dark home recipe	1 cake 7½ in x 2¼ in	5185	228	2123	738	—
madeira cake	1 slice (1 oz)	98	4	—	15	1
pound	1 cake 8½ x 3½ x 3 in	1935	94	1857	257	—
pound	1/10 cake (1 oz)	117	6	119	15	—
pound fat free	1 cake (12 oz)	961	4	1158	208	—
pound cake home recipe	1 loaf 8½ in x 3½ in	1935	94	1645	265	—
sheet cake w/ white frosting home recipe	1 cake 9 in sq	4020	129	2488	694	—
sheet cake w/o frosting home recipe	1 cake 9 in sq	2830	108	2331	434	—
sheet cake w/o frosting home recipe	1/9 cake	315	12	258	48	—
shortcake home recipe	1 (2.3 oz)	225	9	329	32	—
sour cream pound	1/10 cake (1 oz)	117	5	120	16	tr
sponge	1/12 cake (1.3 oz)	110	1	93	23	—

FOOD	PORTION	CAL.	FAT	SOD.	CARB.	FIB.
sponge home recipe	1/12 cake (2.2 oz)	140	2	107	27	—
sponge w/ creme filling	1 (1.5 oz)	155	5	155	27	—
tiramisu	1 cake (4.4 lbs)	5732	421	1107	439	3
toaster pastry apple	1 (1¾ oz)	204	5	218	37	—
toaster pastry blueberry	1 (1¾ oz)	204	5	218	37	—
toaster pastry brown sugar cinnamon	1 (1¾ oz)	206	7	212	34	—
toaster pastry cherry	1 (1¾ oz)	204	5	218	37	—
toaster pastry strawberry	1 (1¾ oz)	204	5	218	37	—
treacle tart	1 slice (2.5 oz)	258	10	—	42	1
vanilla slice	1 slice (2½ oz)	248	13	—	30	1
white w/ coconut frosting home recipe	1/12 cake (3.9 oz)	399	12	318	71	—
white w/o frosting home recipe	1/12 cake (2.6 oz)	264	9	242	42	—
white w/ white frosting	1/16 cake	260	9	176	42	—
white w/ white frosting	1 cake 9 in diam	4170	148	2827	670	—
yellow w/ chocolate frosting	1/8 cake (2.2 oz)	242	11	216	36	1
yellow w/ chocolate frosting	1 cake 9 diam	3895	175	3080	620	—
yellow w/o frosting home recipe	1/12 cake (2.4 oz)	245	10	233	36	—
yellow w/o frosting home recipe	2 layers (28.7 oz)	2947	119	2803	433	—
Baby Watson						
Cheesecake	1 slice (3.8 oz)	390	30	330	23	2
Cheesecake Light	1/16 cake (3.9 oz)	280	16	270	24	3
Baker Maid						
Creole Royal Pineapple Apricot	3 slices (5 oz)	270	3	230	61	4
Creole Royal Pineapple Apricot	1 slice (1.7 oz)	90	1	75	20	1
Carousel						
New York Cheese Cake	1 cake (3 oz)	250	19	180	16	1
Drake's						
Coffee Cake	1 (1.1 oz)	140	6	90	18	—
Coffee Cake Chocolate Crumb	1 (2.5 oz)	245	9	206	38	—
Coffee Cake Cinnamon Crumb	1/12 cake (1.3 oz)	150	6	110	22	—
Coffee Cake Small	1 (2 oz)	220	9	160	33	—
Devil Dog	1 (1.5 oz)	160	6	135	24	—
Funny Bones	1 (1.25 oz)	150	8	110	18	—

FOOD	PORTION	CAL.	FAT	SOD.	CARB.	FIB.
Drake's (CONT.)						
Light & Fruity Apple	1 (1.2 oz)	90	1	110	20	—
Light & Fruity Blueberry	1 (1.2 oz)	90	1	95	20	—
Light & Fruity Cinnamon Raisin	1 (1.2 oz)	90	1	105	19	—
Mini Coffee Cakes	4 (1.83 oz)	220	9	140	33	1
Pound Cake	1	110	5	70	16	—
Ring Ding	1 (1.5 oz)	180	10	115	23	—
Ring Ding Mint	1 (1.5 oz)	190	11	115	22	—
Sunny Doodle	1 (1 oz)	100	3	100	16	—
Yankee Doodle	1 (1 oz)	100	4	110	16	—
Yodel's	1 (1 oz)	150	9	65	16	—
Dutch Mill						
Dessert Shells Chocolate Covered	1 (0.5 oz)	80	5	—	8	0
Entenmann's						
Apple Puffs	1 (3 oz)	280	13	320	39	—
Apple Strudel Old Fashioned	1 serv (1.5 oz)	120	5	110	17	—
Cheese Topped Buns	1 (2.3 oz)	240	12	240	29	—
Cinnamon Buns	1 (2.1 oz)	230	10	200	31	—
Cinnamon Filbert Ring	1 serv (1.5 oz)	190	12	160	19	—
Coffee Cake Cheese	1 serv (1.6 oz)	150	7	140	20	—
Coffee Cake Cheese Filled Crumb	1 serv (1.4 oz)	130	6	140	18	—
Coffee Cake Crumb	1 serv (1.3 oz)	160	7	160	21	—
Danish Ring	1 serv (1.5 oz)	180	10	160	18	—
Danish Ring Pecan	1 serv (1.5 oz)	190	12	130	19	—
Danish Ring Walnut	1 serv (1.5 oz)	190	12	130	19	—
Danish Twist Lemon	1 serv (1.2 oz)	140	7	140	17	—
Danish Twist Raspberry	1 serv (1.2 oz)	140	7	120	18	—
Devil's Food Cake Fudge Iced	1 serv (1.2 oz)	130	5	120	19	—
French Crumb Cake All Butter	1 serv (1.6 oz)	180	8	220	26	—
Louisiana Crunch Cake	1 serv (1.7 oz)	180	8	180	27	—
Pound Loaf All Butter	1 serv (1 oz)	110	5	150	15	—
Pound Loaf Sour Cream	1 serv (1 oz)	120	7	90	14	—
Thick Fudge Golden Cake	1 serv (1.2 oz)	130	6	120	20	—
Freihofer's						
Angel Food	⅕ cake (2 oz)	150	0	410	35	0
Cinnamon Swirl Buns	1 (2.8 oz)	290	9	250	47	1
Coffee Cake Cinnamon Pecan	⅛ cake (2 oz)	220	9	160	33	1

FOOD	PORTION	CAL.	FAT	SOD.	CARB.	FIB.
Freihofer's (CONT.)						
Crumb	1/8 cake (2 oz)	240	11	260	33	1
Homestyle Golden Loaf	1/8 cake (1.8 oz)	200	9	190	28	0
Pound	1/5 cake (2.8 oz)	330	17	330	41	0
Greenfield						
Blondie Apple Spice	1 (1.4 oz)	120	0	65	28	0
Blondie Chocolate Chip	1 (1.4 oz)	120	0	65	29	0
Hostess						
Angel Food Ring	1/6 cake (1.6 oz)	150	3	220	29	0
Apple Twist	1 (2.5 oz)	220	4	270	42	tr
Baseball Yellow Cakes	1 (1.6 oz)	160	3	160	32	0
Choco Licious	1 (1.5 oz)	170	6	190	28	1
Choco-Diles	1 (1.8 oz)	210	10	160	31	1
Cinnaminis Original	5 (2.4 oz)	300	17	230	37	2
Cinnamon Roll	1 (2.3 oz)	220	6	260	39	1
Crumb Cake	1 (1.9 oz)	210	8	135	33	1
Cup Cakes Chocolate	1 (1.6 oz)	170	5	160	28	tr
Cup Cakes Chocolate Light	1 (1.4 oz)	120	2	170	26	tr
Cup Cakes Orange	1 (1.5 oz)	160	5	160	28	0
Dessert Cups	1 (1 oz)	90	2	170	18	0
Ding Dongs	1 (1.3 oz)	160	9	110	21	tr
Fruit Cake Holiday	1/6 cake (5.3 oz)	490	14	410	93	3
Fruit Loaf	1 (3.8 oz)	350	10	290	67	2
Ho Ho's	1 (1 oz)	130	6	75	17	tr
Holiday Cakes	1 (1.6 oz)	160	3	160	32	0
Honey Bun Glazed	1 (2.7 oz)	320	19	90	35	2
Honey Bun Iced	1 (3.4 oz)	390	20	220	49	2
Hopper Cakes	1 (1.6 oz)	160	3	160	32	0
Lights Low Fat Cinnamon Crumb Cake	1 (1 oz)	90	1	100	19	0
Lil Angels	1 (1 oz)	90	2	130	17	0
Pecan Spinners	1 (1 oz)	110	5	65	15	tr
Pound Cake	1/5 cake (3.2 oz)	350	16	360	48	1
Sno Balls	1 (1.6 oz)	160	5	180	29	1
Suzy Q's	1 (2 oz)	220	9	270	35	2
Suzy Q's Banana	1 (2 oz)	220	10	280	32	tr
Swirls Caramel Pecan	1 (2 oz)	140	15	55	25	1
Tiger Tails	1 (1.5 oz)	160	6	150	26	tr
Twinkies	1 (1.4 oz)	140	4	180	25	0
Twinkies Banana	2 (2.7 oz)	300	13	370	42	tr
Twinkies Devil Food	2 (2.7 oz)	300	12	360	47	2
Twinkies Lights	1 (1.4 oz)	120	2	200	24	0

FOOD	PORTION	CAL.	FAT	SOD.	CARB.	FIB.
Hostess (CONT.)						
Twinkies Strawberry Fruit 'n Creme	1 (1.6 oz)	150	3	200	30	tr
Jell-O						
Cheesecake Snack Original	1 (3.3 oz)	160	6	130	23	0
Cheesecake Snack Strawberry	1 (3.3 oz)	150	5	125	26	0
Kellogg's						
Pop-Tarts Apple Cinnamon	1 (1.8 oz)	210	5	170	38	1
Pop-Tarts Blueberry	1 (1.8 oz)	210	7	210	36	1
Pop-Tarts Brown Sugar Cinnamon	1 (1.8 oz)	220	9	210	32	1
Pop-Tarts Cherry	1 (1.8 oz)	200	5	220	37	1
Pop-Tarts Chocolate Graham	1 (1.8 oz)	210	6	220	36	1
Pop-Tarts Frosted Blueberry	1 (1.8 oz)	200	5	210	37	1
Pop-Tarts Frosted Brown Sugar Cinnamon	1 (1.8 oz)	210	7	180	34	1
Pop-Tarts Frosted Cherry	1 (1.8 oz)	200	5	220	37	1
Pop-Tarts Frosted Chocolate Vanilla Creme	1 (1.8 oz)	200	5	230	37	1
Pop-Tarts Frosted Chocolate Fudge	1 (1.8 oz)	200	5	220	37	1
Pop-Tarts Frosted Grape	1 (1.8 oz)	200	5	200	38	1
Pop-Tarts Frosted Raspberry	1 (1.8 oz)	210	6	210	37	1
Pop-Tarts Frosted S'mores	1 (1.8 oz)	200	5	200	37	1
Pop-Tarts Frosted Strawberry	1 (1.8 oz)	200	5	170	38	1
Pop-Tarts Strawberry	1 (1.8 oz)	200	5	180	37	1
Pop-Tarts Minis Frosted Chocolate	1 pkg (1.5 oz)	170	4	200	30	1
Pop-Tarts Minis Frosted Grape	1 pkg (1.5 oz)	170	4	180	32	0
Pop-Tarts Minis Frosted Strawberry	1 pkg (1.5 oz)	170	4	180	32	0
Rice Krispies Treats	1 (0.8 oz)	90	2	75	18	0
Lance						
Apple Oatmeal	1 pkg (51 g)	200	9	210	35	—

FOOD	PORTION	CAL.	FAT	SOD.	CARB.	FIB.
Lance (CONT.)						
Dunking Sticks	1 (39 g)	190	10	130	22	—
Fig Cake	1 pkg (60 g)	210	3	90	43	—
Honey Buns	1 (85 g)	330	14	210	48	—
Oatmeal Cake	1 (57 g)	240	11	250	35	—
Pecan Twirls	1 pkg (57 g)	220	8	190	34	—
Raisin Cake	1 (57 g)	230	10	200	35	—
Little Debbie						
Apple Delights	1 pkg (1.2 oz)	140	5	115	24	1
Apple-Roos	1 pkg (1.5 oz)	150	3	80	32	1
Banana Nut Muffin Loaves	1 pkg (1.9 oz)	210	9	210	30	1
Banana Twins	1 pkg (2.2 oz)	250	10	180	40	0
Be My Valentine	1 pkg (2.2 oz)	280	14	150	39	1
Cherry Cordials	1 pkg (1.3 oz)	160	8	100	23	1
Choc-o-Jel	1 pkg (1.2 oz)	150	7	95	21	1
Choco-Cakes	1 pkg (2.1 oz)	250	13	170	35	1
Choco-Cakes	1 pkg (2.2 oz)	240	12	180	35	1
Chocolate	1 pkg (3 oz)	360	17	220	52	1
Chocolate Chip	1 pkg (2.4 oz)	290	15	190	42	1
Chocolate Twins	1 pkg (2.4 oz)	240	9	280	42	1
Christmas Tree Cakes	1 pkg (1.5 oz)	190	9	90	27	0
Coconut	1 pkg (2.1 oz)	270	13	180	38	1
Coconut	1 pkg (2.4 oz)	300	14	200	42	0
Coconut Rounds	1 pkg (1.2 oz)	140	7	85	22	1
Coffee Cake Apple	1 pkg (1.9 oz)	220	7	190	36	1
Coffee Cake Apple Streusel	1 pkg (2 oz)	220	7	200	37	1
Devil Cremes	1 pkg (1.6 oz)	190	8	160	28	0
Devil Cremes	1 pkg (3.2 oz)	380	17	310	57	1
Devil Squares	1 pkg (2.2 oz)	260	13	180	39	1
Easter Basket Cakes	1 pkg (2.5 oz)	310	15	180	44	1
Fancy Cakes	1 pkg (2.4 oz)	300	15	160	42	0
Fudge Crispy	1 pkg (1.1 oz)	170	10	50	20	1
Fudge Round	1 pkg (2.5 oz)	290	12	170	49	2
Fudge Round	1 pkg (3 oz)	350	14	210	59	2
Fudge Rounds	1 pkg (1.2 oz)	140	5	80	23	1
Golden Cremes	1 pkg (1.5 oz)	170	7	180	25	0
Golden Cremes	1 pkg (3 oz)	330	15	350	50	0
Holiday Cake Chocolate	1 pkg (2.4 oz)	290	14	180	43	1
Holiday Cake Vanilla	1 pkg (2.5 oz)	310	15	180	44	1
Honey Bun	1 pkg (3 oz)	380	23	190	39	4
Honey Bun	1 pkg (4 oz)	510	31	250	53	5
Jelly Rolls	1 pkg (2.1 oz)	230	7	160	41	0

FOOD	PORTION	CAL.	FAT	SOD.	CARB.	FIB.
Little Debbie (CONT.)						
Lemon Stix	1 pkg (1.5 oz)	210	10	45	30	1
Marshmallow Supremes	1 pkg (1.1 oz)	130	5	70	22	1
Mint Sprints	1 pkg (1.5 oz)	230	13	70	28	1
Nutty Bar	1 pkg (2 oz)	290	17	115	34	1
Pecan Twins	1 pkg (2 oz)	220	9	200	32	1
Pumpkin Delights	1 pkg (1.1 oz)	130	5	115	21	1
Smiley Faces Cherry	1 pkg (1.2 oz)	140	5	115	23	1
Smiley Faces Pumpkin	1 pkg (1 oz)	130	5	215	20	1
Snack Cake Chocolate	1 pkg (2.5 oz)	300	15	180	43	1
Snack Cake Vanilla	1 pkg (2.6 oz)	320	16	180	45	1
Spice	1 pkg (2.5 oz)	300	15	230	43	1
Star Crunch	1 pkg (1.1 oz)	140	6	85	21	1
Star Crunch	1 pkg (2.6 oz)	330	14	240	51	1
Swiss Rolls	1 pkg (2.1 oz)	250	12	160	38	1
Swiss Rolls	1 pkg (3.2 oz)	380	18	250	57	1
Swiss Rolls	1 pkg (2.7 oz)	320	15	210	47	1
Teddy Berries	1 pkg (1.2 oz)	130	4	105	23	1
Vanilla	1 pkg (3 oz)	370	18	210	53	0
Vanilla Cremes	1 pkg (1.4 oz)	170	7	125	25	0
Zebra Cakes	1 pkg (2.6 oz)	150	16	180	45	1
Nabisco						
Frosted Strawberry	1 (1.7 oz)	190	5	190	35	1
Pepperidge Farm						
Amhurst Apple Crumb Coffee Cake	1	220	11	150	30	—
Apple 'N Spice Bake Dessert Lights	1 piece (4¼ oz)	170	2	105	37	—
Apple Turnover	1	300	17	210	34	—
Berkshire Apple Crisp	1	250	8	130	43	1
Blueberry Turnovers	1	310	19	230	32	—
Boston Cream Supreme	1 piece (2⅞ oz)	290	14	190	39	—
Butter Pound	1 slice (1 oz)	130	7	150	16	—
Carrot Classic	1 cake	260	16	280	32	—
Carrot w/ Cream Cheese Icing	1 slice (1½ oz)	150	9	160	19	—
Charleston Peach Melba Shortcake	1	220	5	170	41	—
Cherries Supreme Dessert Lights	1 piece (3¼ oz)	170	11	35	38	—
Cherry Turnover	1	310	19	280	32	—
Chocolate Supreme	1 piece (2⅞ oz)	300	16	140	37	—
Chocolate Fudge Large Layer	1 slice (1⅝ oz)	180	10	140	23	—

FOOD	PORTION	CAL.	FAT	SOD.	CARB.	FIB.
Pepperidge Farm (CONT.)						
Chocolate Fudge Strip Large Layer	1 piece (1⅝ oz)	170	9	140	20	—
Chocolate Mousse Cake Dessert Lights	1 piece (2½ oz)	190	9	260	25	—
Cholesterol Free Pound	1 slice (1 oz)	110	6	85	13	—
Coconut Classic	1 cake	230	11	160	31	—
Coconut Large Layer	1 slice (1⅝ oz)	180	8	120	24	—
Devil's Food Large Layer	1 slice (1⅝ oz)	180	9	135	24	—
Double Chocolate Classic	1 cake	250	13	180	31	—
Fruit Squares Apple	1	220	12	170	27	—
Fruit Squares Cherry	1	230	12	180	28	—
Fudge Golden Classic	1 cake	260	14	160	34	—
German Chocolate Classic	1 cake	250	13	230	29	—
German Chocolate Large Layer	1 slice (1⅝ oz)	180	10	170	22	—
Golden Large Layer	1 slice (1⅝ oz)	180	9	110	24	—
Lemon Cake Supreme Dessert Lights	1 piece (2¾ oz)	170	5	100	26	—
Lemon Coconut Classic Cake	3 oz	280	13	—	—	—
Lemon Coconut Supreme	1 piece (3 oz)	280	13	220	38	—
Lemon Cream Supreme	1 piece (1⅝ oz)	170	9	120	21	—
Manhattan Strawberry Cheesecake	1	300	9	250	49	—
Peach Melba Supreme	1 (3⅛ oz)	270	7	135	50	—
Peach Parfait Dessert Lights	1 piece (4¼ oz)	150	5	70	24	—
Peach Turnover	1	310	18	260	34	—
Pineapple Cream Supreme	1 piece (2 oz)	190	7	130	28	—
Raspberry Turnovers	1	310	17	260	36	—
Raspberry Vanilla Swirl Dessert Lights	1 piece (3¼ oz)	160	5	140	25	—
Strawberry Shortcake Dessert Lights	1 piece (3 oz)	170	5	50	30	
Strawberry Cream Supreme	1 piece (2 oz)	190	7	120	30	
Strawberry Strip Large Layer	1 piece (1½ oz)	160	8	120	21	
Toaster Tart Apple Cinnamon	1	170	7	120	25	-

FOOD	PORTION	CAL.	FAT	SOD.	CARB.	FIB.
Pepperidge Farm (CONT.)						
Toaster Tart Cheese	1	190	10	180	22	—
Toaster Tart Strawberry	1	190	7	120	28	—
Vanilla Fudge Swirl Classic	1 cake	250	11	160	33	—
Vanilla Large Layer	1 slice (1⅝ oz)	190	8	120	25	—
Perugina						
Pannettone Au Beurre	⅙ cake (2.9 oz)	310	12	140	47	2
Pet-Ritz						
Cobbler Apple	⅙ cake (4.33 oz)	290	9	—	50	—
Cobbler Blackberry	⅙ cake (4.33 oz)	250	10	—	39	—
Cobbler Blueberry	⅙ cake (4.33 oz)	270	12	—	50	—
Cobbler Cherry	⅙ cake (4.33 oz)	280	10	—	46	—
Cobbler Peach	⅙ cake (4.33 oz)	260	10	—	46	—
Cobbler Strawberry	⅙ cake (4.33 oz)	290	9	—	50	—
Pillsbury						
Apple Turnovers	1	170	8	330	23	—
Cherry Turnovers	1	170	8	320	23	—
Coffee Cake Cinnamon Swirl	⅛ of cake	180	9	170	22	—
Coffee Cake Pecan Streusel	⅛ of cake	180	9	170	21	—
Pastry Pockets	1	240	13	520	25	—
Sara Lee						
All Butter Pound Snack Cake	1	200	11	190	23	—
Apple Crisp Light	1 (3 oz)	150	2	130	31	—
Banana Single Layer Iced	1 slice (1.7 oz)	170	6	160	28	—
Black Forest Light	1 (3.6 oz)	170	5	85	34	—
Black Forest Two Layer	1 slice (2.5 oz)	190	8	100	28	—
Carrot Light	1 (2.5 oz)	170	4	75	30	—
Carrot Single Layer Iced	1 slice (2.4 oz)	250	13	240	30	—
Cheesecake Original Strawberry	1 slice (3.2 oz)	222	8	171	34	—
Cheesecake Original Cherry	1 slice (3.2 oz)	243	8	184	35	—
Cheesecake Original Plain	1 slice (2.8 oz)	230	11	153	27	—
Chocolate Free & Light	1 slice (1.7 oz)	110	0	140	26	—
Chocolate Fudge Snack Cake	1	190	10	125	24	—
Classic Snack Cheesecake	1	200	14	150	16	—

FOOD	PORTION	CAL.	FAT	SOD.	CARB.	FIB.
Sara Lee (CONT.)						
Coffee Cake All Butter Streusel	1 slice (1.4 oz)	160	7	160	20	—
Coffee Cake All Butter Cheese	1 slice (2 oz)	210	11	220	25	—
Coffee Cake All Butter Pecan	1 slice (1.4 oz)	160	8	180	19	—
Coffee Cake Cheese Reduced Fat	⅙ cake (2 oz)	180	6	230	28	0
Coffee Cake Raspberry	⅙ cake (1.9 oz)	200	8	220	27	tr
Deluxe Carrot Snack Cake	1	180	7	200	26	—
Double Chocolate Light	1 (2.5 oz)	150	5	85	23	—
Double Chocolate Three Layer	1 slice (2.2 oz)	220	11	130	26	—
French Cheese	1 slice (2.9 oz)	250	16	120	23	—
Lemon Cream Light	1 (3.2 oz)	180	6	60	29	—
Pound Free & Light	1 slice (1 oz)	70	0	105	17	—
Pound All Butter Family Size	1 slice (1 oz)	130	7	85	14	—
Pound All Butter Original	1 slice (1 oz)	130	7	85	14	—
Pound Cake Reduced Fat	1 slice (1 oz)	100	4	125	15	0
Snack Coffee Cake Apple Cinnamon	1	290	13	270	40	—
Snack Coffee Cake Butter Streusel	1	230	12	270	27	—
Snack Coffee Cake Pecan	1	280	16	270	30	—
Strawberry French Cheesecake Light	1 (3.5 oz)	150	2	65	29	—
Strawberry Shortcake Two Layer	1 slice (2.5 oz)	190	8	90	26	—
Strawberry Yogurt Dessert Free & Light	1 slice (2.2 oz)	120	1	90	26	—
Sinbad						
Baklava	1 piece (2 oz)	337	20	153	44	2
Tastykake						
Butter Cream Cream Filled Cupcake	1 (32 g)	120	4	120	20	1
Chocolate Cream Filled Cupcake	1 (34 g)	130	5	130	21	1
Chocolate Cupcake	1 (30 g)	100	3	120	19	1
Creamies Banana Treat	1	138	3	—	—	—
Creamies Chocolate	1	174	7	—	—	—

FOOD	PORTION	CAL.	FAT	SOD.	CARB.	FIB.
Tastykake (CONT.)						
Creamies Vanilla	1	182	8	—	—	—
Honeybun Glazed	1 pkg (92 g)	360	20	220	42	4
Honeybun Iced	1 pkg (92 g)	350	15	250	50	1
Junior Chocolate	1 pkg (94 g)	340	12	220	57	4
Junior Coconut	1 pkg (94 g)	300	6	300	60	3
Junior Lemon	1 pkg (94 g)	310	7	330	75	1
Junior Orange	1 pkg (94 g)	340	9	240	61	1
Kandy Kake Chocolate	1 (19 g)	80	3	35	13	1
Kandy Kake Coconut	1 (19 g)	80	4	40	11	1
Kandy Kake Peanut Butter	1 (19 g)	90	4	40	11	1
Koffee Kake Cream Filled	1 (29 g)	110	4	80	18	0
Koffee Kake Junior	1 pkg (71 g)	260	8	210	44	1
Kreme Kup	1 (25 g)	90	3	115	15	1
Krimpet Butterscotch	1 (28 g)	100	1	85	19	0
Krimpet Jelly	1 (28 g)	90	1	80	19	1
Krimpet Strawberry	1 (28 g)	100	2	85	20	0
Pastry Pocket Apple	1 (85 g)	320	18	220	38	—
Pastry Pocket Cheese	1 (85 g)	330	19	230	38	1
Pastry Pocket Cherry	1 (85 g)	330	17	230	41	1
Pecan Twirls	1 (28 g)	110	1	75	17	—
Royale Chocolate Cupcake	1 (46 g)	170	7	130	28	2
Tasty Too Chocolate Cream Filled Cupcake	1 (32 g)	100	1	115	21	1
Tasty Too Vanilla Cream Filled Cupcake	1 (32 g)	100	1	120	21	1
Tasty Twists	1 (4 g)	18	1	—	3	—
Thomas'						
Date Nut Loaf	1 oz	90	2	170	18	1
Toast-R-Cakes						
Blueberry	1	110	3	158	18	—
Bran	1	103	3	163	18	—
Corn	1	120	4	142	19	—
Toastettes						
Frosted Blueberry	1 (1.7 oz)	190	5	190	45	1
Frosted Brown Sugar Cinnamon	1 (1.7 oz)	190	5	180	35	1
Frosted Cherry	1 (1.7 oz)	190	5	190	35	1
Frosted Fudge	1 (1.7 oz)	190	5	280	34	3
Strawberry	1 (1.7 oz)	190	5	200	35	1
Weight Watchers						
Chocolate Raspberry Royale	1 (3.5 oz)	190	3	190	39	2

FOOD	PORTION	CAL.	FAT	SOD.	CARB.	FIB.
Weight Watchers (CONT.)						
Chocolate Chip Cookie Dough Sundae	1 (2.64 oz)	180	4	115	33	2
Chocolate Eclair	1 (2.1 oz)	150	5	160	25	2
Coffee Cake Apple Cinnamon Danish	1 piece (1.9 oz)	160	3	170	30	1
Coffee Cake Cheese Danish	1 piece (1.9 oz)	160	3	200	29	1
Coffee Cake Cinnamon Streusel	1 (2.25 oz)	190	2	190	35	2
Coffee Cake Raspberry Danish	1 piece (1.9 oz)	160	3	170	30	1
Double Fudge	1 piece (2.75 oz)	190	5	200	36	2
French Style Cheesecake	1 piece (3.9 oz)	180	5	230	28	2
New York Style Cheesecake	1 piece (2.5 oz)	150	5	140	21	0
Strawberry Parfait Royale	1 (5.24 oz)	180	2	100	35	0
Triple Chocolate Eclair	1 (2.14 oz)	160	5	190	25	1
Well-Bred Loaf						
Banana Bread	1 slice (3.5 oz)	330	11	380	52	tr
Banana Nut	1 slice (4.3 oz)	440	19	350	59	2
Blueberry	1 slice (4.3 oz)	440	16	330	69	1
Carrot	1 slice (4.3 oz)	480	24	125	64	2
Carrot Traditional	1 slice (4.3 oz)	440	16	280	71	2
Chocolate Chip	1 slice (4.3 oz)	490	19	320	74	2
Cinnamon Walnut	1 slice (4.3 oz)	480	18	340	72	1
Coconut Rum	1 slice (4.3 oz)	490	23	330	64	tr
Cranberry	1 slice (4.3 oz)	460	15	320	77	1
Marble	1 slice (4.3 oz)	530	18	390	83	1
Pound All Butter	1 slice (4.3 oz)	470	17	360	73	tr
Pound Mandarin Orange	1 slice (4 oz)	460	18	310	68	tr
Raisin	1 slice (4.3 oz)	460	15	310	76	2
TAKE-OUT						
angelfood	1/12 cake (1 oz)	73	tr	212	16	1
apple crisp	½ cup (5 oz)	230	5	257	46	—
baklava	1 oz	126	9	78	10	1
boston cream pie	1/6 cake (3.3 oz)	293	12	309	43	1
carrot w/ cream cheese icing	1/12 cake (3.9 oz)	484	29	273	52	—
cheesecake w/ cherry topping	1/12 cake (5 oz)	359	23	254	33	—
chocolate w/ chocolate frosting	1/8 cake (2.2 oz)	235	11	213	35	2

FOOD	PORTION	CAL.	FAT	SOD.	CARB.	FIB.
coffeecake cheese	1/6 cake (2.7 oz)	258	12	257	38	1
coffeecake crumb topped cheese	1/6 cake (2.7 oz)	258	12	257	38	1
coffeecake crumb topped cinnamon	1/9 cake (2.2 oz)	263	15	221	29	2
cream puff w/ custard filling	1 (4.6 oz)	336	20	444	30	—
eclair w/ chocolate icing & custard filling	1	205	10	—	—	—
fruitcake	1/36 cake (2.9 oz)	302	10	121	54	3
gingerbread	1/9 cake (2.6 oz)	264	12	242	36	2
panettone dal forno	1/9 cake (1.9 oz)	212	8	120	31	0
pineapple upside down	1/9 cake (4 oz)	367	14	367	58	—
pound fat free	1 oz	80	tr	96	17	—
pound cake	1 slice (1 oz)	120	5	96	15	—
sheet cake w/ white frosting	1/9 cake	445	14	275	77	—
strudel apple	1 piece (2½ oz)	195	8	191	29	2
tiramisu	1 piece (5.1 oz)	409	30	79	31	tr
trifle w/ cream	6 oz	291	16	—	34	1
yellow w/ vanilla frosting	1/8 cake (2.2 oz)	239	9	220	38	—
CAKE ICING						
chocolate as prep w/ butter	1 box (13.7 oz)	1908	65	754	357	—
chocolate as prep w/ butter	1/12 box (1.5 oz)	161	6	63	30	—
chocolate as prep w/ butter home recipe	1 recipe (21.1 oz)	2409	69	1144	467	—
chocolate as prep w/ butter home recipe	1/12 recipe (1.8 oz)	200	6	95	39	—
chocolate as prep w/ margarine	1 box (13.7 oz)	1909	65	819	357	—
chocolate as prep w/ margarine	1/12 box (1.5 oz)	161	6	69	30	—
chocolate as prep w/ margarine home recipe	1 recipe (21.1 oz)	2411	69	1235	468	—
chocolate as prep w/ margarine home recipe	1/12 recipe (1.8 oz)	200	6	103	39	—
chocolate ready-to-use	1/12 pkg (1.3 oz)	151	7	70	24	—
chocolate ready-to-use	1 pkg (16 oz)	1834	81	845	292	—
coconut ready-to-use	1/12 pkg (1.3 oz)	157	9	74	20	—
coconut ready-to-use	1 pkg (16 oz)	1903	111	899	244	—
cream cheese ready-to-use	1/12 pkg (1.3 oz)	157	7	90	25	—

FOOD	PORTION	CAL.	FAT	SOD.	CARB.	FIB.
cream cheese ready-to-use	1 pkg (16 oz)	1906	80	1094	308	—
glaze home recipe	1/12 recipe (1 oz)	97	2	25	20	—
glaze home recipe	1 recipe (11.5 oz)	1173	26	307	240	—
seven minute home recipe	1/12 recipe (1.1 oz)	102	0	55	26	—
seven minute home recipe	1 recipe (13.6 oz)	1231	0	859	312	—
sour cream ready-to-use	1/12 pkg (1.3 oz)	157	7	78	26	—
sour cream ready-to-use	1 pkg (16 oz)	1904	80	943	312	—
vanilla as prep w/ butter	1/12 pkg (1.5 oz)	182	7	90	30	—
vanilla as prep w/ butter	1 pkg (14.5 oz)	2188	86	1082	366	—
vanilla as prep w/ butter home recipe	1 recipe (20.1 oz)	1972	24	366	448	—
vanilla as prep w/ butter home recipe	1/12 recipe (1.7 oz)	165	2	31	38	—
vanilla as prep w/ margarine	1/12 pkg (1.5 oz)	182	7	96	30	—
vanilla as prep w/ margarine	1 pkg (14.5 oz)	2190	86	1149	366	—
vanilla as prep w/ margarine home recipe	1 recipe (20.1 oz)	2326	62	1175	454	—
vanilla as prep w/ margarine home recipe	1/12 recipe (1.7 oz)	195	5	98	38	—
vanilla ready-to-use	1 pkg (16 oz)	1936	78	418	321	—
vanilla ready-to-use	1/12 pkg (1.3 oz)	159	6	34	26	—
white as prep w/ water	1 pkg (11.1 oz)	770	0	490	197	—
white as prep w/ water	1/12 pkg (0.9 oz)	64	0	40	16	—
Betty Crocker						
Butter Pecan Ready-to-Spread	1/12 tub	170	7	50	26	—
Cherry Ready-to-Spread	1/12 tub	160	6	50	27	—
Chocolate Ready-to-Spread	1/12 tub	160	7	60	24	—
Chocolate Chip Ready-to-Spread	1/12 tub	170	7	30	27	—
Chocolate Fudge as prep	1/12 mix	180	6	70	30	—
Chocolate Light Ready-to-Spread	1/12 tub	130	2	60	28	—
Chocolate With Candy Coated Chocolate Chips Ready-to-Spread	1/12 tub	160	7	60	24	—
Chocolate With Dinosaurs Ready-to-Spread	1/12 tub	160	7	60	24	—

FOOD	PORTION	CAL.	FAT	SOD.	CARB.	FIB.
Betty Crocker (CONT.)						
Chocolate With Turbo Racers Ready-to-Spread	1/12 tub	160	7	60	24	—
Coconut Pecan Ready-to-Spread	1/12 tub	160	9	80	20	—
Coconut Pecan as prep	1/12 mix	180	8	50	19	—
Cream Cheese Ready-to-Spread	1/12 tub	170	7	70	26	—
Creamy Milk Chocolate as prep	1/12 mix	170	5	40	29	—
Creamy Vanilla as prep	1/12 mix	170	5	50	32	—
Dark Dutch Fudge Ready-to-Spread	1/12 tub	160	7	70	22	—
Lemon Ready-to-Spread	1/12 tub	170	6	70	28	—
Milk Chocolate Light Ready-to-Spread	1/12 tub	140	2	50	29	—
Milk Chocolate Ready-to-Spread	1/12 tub	160	6	55	25	—
Rainbow Chip Ready-to-Spread	1/12 tub	170	7	30	27	—
Sour Cream Chocolate Ready-to-Spread	1/12 tub	160	7	100	23	—
Sour Cream White Ready-to-Spread	1/12 tub	160	6	50	27	—
Vanilla Ready-to-Spread	1/12 tub	160	6	30	27	—
Vanilla Light Ready-to-Spread	1/12 tub	140	2	30	30	—
Vanilla With Teddy Bears Ready-to-Spread	1/12 tub	160	6	25	27	—
White Fluffy as prep	1/12 mix	70	0	40	16	—
Duncan Hines						
Chocolate Creamy Homestyle	1 oz	130	5	95	20	2
Milk Chocolate Creamy Homestyle	1 oz	130	5	95	20	1
Vanilla Creamy Homestyle	1 oz	140	5	60	22	1
Estee						
Lite Frosting as prep	3 tbsp (0.7 oz)	100	3	0	20	0
Jiffy						
Fudge	1/4 cup (1.2 oz)	150	4	150	28	tr
White	1/4 cup (1.2 oz)	150	5	150	27	0

FOOD	PORTION	CAL.	FAT	SOD.	CARB.	FIB.
Pillsbury						
Cake & Cookie Decorator Chocolate	1 tbsp	60	2	0	11	—
Cake & Cookie Decorator all colors except chocolate	1 tbsp	70	2	0	12	—
Chocolate Fudge	for 1/8 cake	110	5	65	17	—
Coconut Almond Frosting Mix	for 1/12 cake	160	10	85	16	—
Coconut Pecan Frosting Mix	for 1/12 cake	150	7	105	20	—
Fluffy White Frosting Mix	for 1/12 cake	60	0	65	15	—
Frost It Hot Chocolate	for 1/8 cake	50	0	50	12	—
Frost It Hot Fluffy White	for 1/8 cake	50	0	50	12	—
Frosting Supreme Caramel Pecan	for 1/12 cake	160	8	70	21	—
Frosting Supreme Chocolate Chip	for 1/12 cake	150	5	70	27	—
Frosting Supreme Chocolate Fudge	for 1/12 cake	150	6	80	24	—
Frosting Supreme Chocolate Mint	for 1/12 cake	150	7	80	24	—
Frosting Supreme Coconut Almond	for 1/12 cake	150	9	60	17	—
Frosting Supreme Coconut Pecan	for 1/12 cake	160	10	60	17	—
Frosting Supreme Cream Cheese	for 1/12 cake	160	6	115	26	—
Frosting Supreme Double Dutch	for 1/12 cake	140	6	45	22	—
Frosting Supreme Lemon	for 1/12 cake	160	6	80	26	—
Frosting Supreme Milk Chocolate	for 1/12 cake	150	6	60	23	—
Frosting Supreme Mocha	for 1/12 cake	150	6	60	24	—
Frosting Supreme Sour Cream Vanilla	for 1/12 cake	160	6	80	27	—
Frosting Supreme Strawberry	for 1/12 cake	160	6	75	26	—
Frosting Supreme Vanilla	for 1/12 cake	160	6	75	26	—
Funfetti Chocolate Fudge	1/12 can	140	6	80	22	—
Funfetti Vanilla Pink	1/12 can	150	6	70	24	—

FOOD	PORTION	CAL.	FAT	SOD.	CARB.	FIB.
Pillsbury (CONT.)						
Funfetti Vanilla White	1/12 can	150	6	70	24	—
Vanilla	for 1/8 cake	120	5	60	19	—
CAKE MIX						
(*see also* CAKE)						
angelfood	10 in cake (20.9 oz)	1535	2	3036	350	9
angelfood	1/12 cake (1.8 oz)	129	tr	255	29	1
carrot w/o frosting	1/12 cake (2.5 oz)	239	11	249	33	—
carrot w/o frosting	2 layers (29.6 oz)	2886	133	3001	395	—
cheesecake no-bake	1/8 cake (3.5 oz)	271	13	377	35	2
chocolate pudding type w/o frosting	2 layers (32.4 oz)	3234	172	4815	409	—
chocolate pudding type w/o frosting	1/12 cake (2.7 oz)	270	14	402	34	—
chocolate w/o frosting	2 layers (26.8 oz)	2393	92	4464	384	—
chocolate w/o frosting	1/12 cake (2.3 oz)	198	8	370	32	—
chocolate w/o frosting low sodium	1/10 cake (1.3 oz)	116	3	130	23	—
coffeecake crumb topped cinnamon	1/8 cake (2 oz)	178	5	236	30	2
devil's food w/o frosting	1/12 cake (2.3 oz)	198	8	370	32	—
devil's food w/ chocolate frosting	1 cake 9 in diam	3755	136	2900	645	—
devil's food w/ chocolate frosting	1/16 cake	235	8	181	40	—
fudge w/o frosting	1/12 cake (2.3 oz)	198	8	370	32	—
german chocolate pudding type w/ coconut nut frosting	1/12 cake (3.9 oz)	404	21	369	55	—
gingerbread	1 cake 8 in sq	1575	39	1733	291	—
gingerbread	1/9 cake (2.4 oz)	207	7	307	34	2
lemon w/o frosting no sugar low sodium	1/10 cake (1.3 oz)	118	3	83	23	—
marble pudding type w/o frosting	2 layers (30.6 oz)	3021	148	2884	412	—
marble pudding type w/o frosting	1/12 cake (2.6 oz)	253	12	242	35	—
white pudding type w/o frosting	1/12 cake (2.4 oz)	244	10	305	36	—
white pudding type w/o frosting	2 layers (29 oz)	2915	123	3654	427	—
white w/o frosting	1/12 cake (2.2 oz)	190	5	301	34	—
white w/o frosting	2 layer cake (26 oz)	2265	57	3593	410	—

FOOD	PORTION	CAL.	FAT	SOD.	CARB.	FIB.
white w/o frosting no sugar low sodium	1/10 cake (1.3 oz)	118	3	83	23	—
yellow pudding-type w/o frosting	2 layers (31 oz)	3084	139	3800	421	—
yellow pudding-type w/o frosting	1/12 cake (2.6 oz)	257	12	317	35	—
yellow w/ chocolate frosting	1/16 cake	235	8	157	40	—
yellow w/o frosting	2 layers (26.5 oz)	2415	71	3580	411	—
yellow w/o frosting	1/12 cake (2.2 oz)	202	6	299	34	—
yellow w/ chocolate frosting	1 cake 9 in diam	3895	175	3080	620	—
Aunt Jemima						
Coffee Cake Easy Mix	1/3 cup (1.4 oz)	170	5	240	30	1
Betty Crocker						
Angel Food Confetti	1/12 cake	150	0	300	34	—
Angel Food Traditional	1/12 cake	130	0	170	30	—
Angel Food White	1/12 cake	150	0	300	34	—
Angel Food Lemon Custard	1/12 cake	150	0	300	34	—
Apple Streusel MicroRave	1/6 cake	240	11	190	33	—
Apple Streusel MicroRave No Cholesterol Recipe	1/6 cake	210	8	200	33	—
Butter Chocolate	1/12 cake	280	14	400	35	—
Butter Pecan No Cholesterol Recipe	1/12 cake	220	7	320	35	—
Butter Pecan SuperMoist	1/12 cake	250	11	320	35	—
Butter Yellow	1/12 cake	260	11	340	37	—
Carrot	1/12 cake	250	10	300	36	—
Carrot No Cholesterol Recipe	1/12 cake	210	6	300	36	—
Cherry Chip	1/12 cake	190	3	270	37	—
Chocolate Chocolate Chip	1/12 cake	260	12	400	34	—
Chocolate Pudding Classic Dessert	1/6 cake	230	5	250	44	—
Chocolate Chip	1/12 cake	290	15	300	35	—
Chocolate Chip No Cholesterol Recipe	1/12 cake	220	8	300	35	—
Chocolate Fudge	1/12 cake	260	12	450	35	—
Cinnamon Pecan Streusel Microwave	1/6 cake	280	12	220	40	—

FOOD	PORTION	CAL.	FAT	SOD.	CARB.	FIB.
Betty Crocker (CONT.)						
Cinnamon Pecan Streusel Microwave No Cholesterol	1/6 cake	230	7	220	40	—
Devil's Food	1/12 cake	260	12	430	35	—
Devil's Food Chocolate Frosting MicroRave	1/6 cake	310	17	250	37	—
Devil's Food No Cholesterol Recipe	1/12 cake	220	7	430	35	—
Devils Food SuperMoist Light	1/12 cake	200	4	340	36	—
Devils Food SuperMoist Light No Cholesterol Recipe	1/12 cake	180	3	370	36	—
Devils Food With Chocolate Frosting MicroRave Single	1	440	18	480	64	—
German Chocolate	1/12 cake	260	12	420	35	—
German Chocolate Chocolate Frosting MicroRave	1/6 cake	320	18	250	37	—
German Chocolate No Cholesterol Recipe	1/12 cake	220	8	420	35	—
Gingerbread Classic Dessert	1/9 cake	22	7	330	35	—
Gingerbread Classic Dessert No Cholesterol Recipe	1/9 cake	210	6	330	35	—
Golden Pound Classic Dessert	1/12 cake	200	9	170	28	—
Golden Vanilla	1/12 cake	280	14	270	36	—
Golden Vanilla No Cholesterol Recipe	1/12 cake	220	7	270	36	—
Golden Vanilla Rainbow Chip Frosting MicroRave	1/6 cake	320	18	230	40	—
Lemon	1/12 cake	260	11	280	37	—
Lemon Chiffon Classic Dessert	1/12 cake	200	5	200	36	—
Lemon No Cholesterol Recipe	1/12 cake	220	7	280	37	—
Lemon Pudding Classic Dessert	1/6 cake	230	5	270	45	—
Marble	1/12 cake	260	11	290	36	—

FOOD	PORTION	CAL.	FAT	SOD.	CARB.	FIB.
Betty Crocker (CONT.)						
Marble No Cholesterol Recipe	1/12 cake	220	7	290	36	—
Milk Chocolate	1/12 cake	260	12	340	34	—
Milk Chocolate No Cholesterol Recipe	1/12 cake	210	7	340	34	—
Pineapple Upsidedown Classic Dessert	1/9 cake	250	10	210	39	—
Rainbow Chip	1/12 cake	250	11	320	35	—
Sour Cream Chocolate	1/12 cake	260	12	430	35	—
Sour Cream Chocolate No Cholesterol Recipe	1/12 cake	220	8	430	35	—
Sour Cream White	1/12 cake	180	3	290	36	—
Spice	1/12 cake	260	11	320	36	—
Spice No Cholesterol Recipe	1/12 cake	220	7	320	36	—
White	1/12 cake	240	9	270	36	—
White No Cholesterol Recipe	1/12 cake	220	7	270	36	—
White SuperMoist Light	1/12 cake	180	3	330	37	—
Yellow	1/12 cake	260	11	300	36	—
Yellow Chocolate Frosting MicroRave	1/6 cake	300	17	220	36	—
Yellow No Cholesterol Recipe	1/12 cake	220	7	300	36	—
Yellow SuperMoist Light	1/12 cake	200	4	310	37	—
Yellow SuperMoist Light No Cholesterol Recipe	1/12 cake	190	3	330	37	—
Yellow With Chocolate Frosting MicroRave Single	1	440	19	500	64	—
Bisquick						
Mix	1/2 cup (2 oz)	240	8	700	37	—
Reduced Fat	1/2 cup (2 oz)	210	4	660	39	—
Dromedary						
Carrot	1/12 cake	232	15	292	23	—
Cobbler Apple Crumb	1/8 cake	237	6	490	41	—
Cobbler Cherry Crumb	1/8 cake	231	6	160	42	—
Date Nut	1/12 cake	183	8	248	26	—
Date Nut Roll	1/2 in slice	80	2	160	13	—
Gingerbread	1 piece (2 in x 2 in)	100	2	190	19	—
Pound	1/2 in slice	150	6	160	21	—
Duncan Hines						
Angel Food	1/12 pkg (1.3 oz)	140	0	115	30	1

FOOD	PORTION	CAL.	FAT	SOD.	CARB.	FIB.
Duncan Hines (CONT.)						
Cupcake Yellow With Chocolate Frosting	1	180	0	140	29	—
Devil's Food Moist Deluxe	1/12 cake (1.5 oz)	290	15	390	34	1
French Vanilla Moist Deluxe	1/12 cake (1.5 oz)	250	11	270	36	0
Fudge Marble Moist Deluxe	1/12 cake (1.5 oz)	250	11	270	36	0
Lemon Supreme Moist Deluxe	1/12 cake (1.5 oz)	250	11	270	36	0
Yellow Moist Deluxe	1/12 cake (1.5 oz)	250	11	270	36	—
Estee						
Lite White as prep	1/5 cake (1.7 oz)	200	4	170	38	tr
Lite Chocolate	1/5 cake (1.7 oz)	190	4	264	36	1
Lite Pound as prep	1/5 cake (1.7 oz)	200	4	170	38	tr
Hain						
Whole Wheat Baking Mix	1½ oz	150	1	680	30	5
Jell-O						
No Bake Cherry Cheesecake as prep	1/8 cake (4.8 oz)	340	12	400	52	tr
No Bake Double Layer Chocolate as prep	1/8 cake (4.4 oz)	260	12	410	34	1
No Bake Double Layer Cookies And Creme as prep	1/8 cake (4.5 oz)	390	19	480	51	1
No Bake Double Layer Lemon as prep	1/8 cake (4.4 oz)	260	12	370	36	tr
No Bake Homestyle Cheesecake as prep	1/6 cake (4.6 oz)	360	15	550	50	tr
No Bake Peanut Butter Cup as prep	1/8 cake (3.8 oz)	380	23	380	41	1
No Bake Reduced Fat Strawberry Swirl Cheesecake as prep	1/8 cake (4 oz)	250	6	430	44	0
No Bake Strawberry Cheesecake as prep	1/8 cake (4.8 oz)	340	12	400	52	tr
Real Cheesecake as prep	1/8 cake (4.6 oz)	360	16	510	47	1
Jiffy						
Devil's Food as prep	1/5 cake	220	6	528	40	1
Golden Yellow as prep	1/5 cake	220	5	340	41	1
White as prep	1/5 cake	210	5	320	41	tr
Pillsbury						
Apple Cinnamon Coffee Cake	1/8 cake	240	7	150	40	—

FOOD	PORTION	CAL.	FAT	SOD.	CARB.	FIB.
Pillsbury (CONT.)						
Banana Quick Bread	1/12 loaf	170	6	200	27	—
Blueberry Nut Quick Bread	1/12 loaf	150	4	150	26	—
Butter Recipe	1/12 cake	260	12	370	34	—
Cherry Nut Quick Bread	1/12 loaf	180	5	150	29	—
Chocolate Chip	1/12 cake	270	14	290	33	—
Chocolate Microwave	1/8 cake	210	12	260	23	—
Chocolate With Chocolate Frosting	1/8 cake	300	17	310	35	—
Chocolate With Vanilla Frosting	1/8 cake	300	17	300	36	—
Cranberry Quick Bread	1/12 loaf	160	4	200	30	—
Date Quick Bread	1/12 loaf	160	2	150	32	—
Devil's Food	1/12 cake	270	14	370	32	—
Double Chocolate Supreme Microwave	1/8 cake	330	19	340	39	—
Double Lemon Supreme Microwave	1/8 cake	300	15	210	40	—
Fudge Marble	1/12 cake	270	12	300	36	—
German Chocolate	1/12 cake	250	11	—	—	—
Gingerbread	3 in sq	190	4	310	36	—
Lemon	1/12 cake	250	11	290	34	—
Lemon Microwave	1/8 cake	220	13	180	23	—
Lemon With Lemon Frosting	1/8 cake	300	17	220	37	—
Nut Quick Bread	1/12 loaf	170	6	190	28	—
Strawberry	1/12 cake	260	11	300	37	—
Streusel Swirl Cinnamon	1/16 cake	260	11	200	38	—
Streusel Swirl Cinnamon Microwave	1/8 cake	240	11	180	33	—
Streusel Swirl Lemon	1/16 cake	270	11	340	39	—
Tunnel of Fudge Bundt	1/16 cake	270	12	—	—	—
Tunnel of Fudge Bundt Microwave	1/8 cake	290	17	320	36	—
White	1/12 cake	240	10	290	35	—
Yellow	1/12 cake	260	12	300	36	—
Yellow Microwave	1/8 cake	220	13	170	23	—
Yellow With Chocolate Frosting	1/8 cake	300	17	220	36	—
Royal						
Cheese Cake Lite No-Bake	1/8 pie	130	3	230	22	—
Cheese Cake Real No-Bake	1/8 pie	160	3	250	29	—

FOOD	PORTION	CAL.	FAT	SOD.	CARB.	FIB.
Wanda's						
Double Chocolate	¼ cup mix per serv (1.4 oz)	170	2	460	35	2

CALABAZA

fresh	½ cup	32	tr	3	8	—

CALZONE

TAKE-OUT

cheese	1 (12 oz)	1020	54	1760	86	8

CANADIAN BACON

unheated	2 slices (1.9 oz)	89	4	799	1	—
Hormel						
Canadian Bacon	2 oz	70	3	610	0	0
Jones						
Slices	1	30	1	160	tr	—
Oscar Mayer						
Canandian Bacon	2 slices (1.6 oz)	50	2	600	0	0

CANDY

(*see also* MARSHMALLOW)

(FAST FACT: Each package of Mars M&M's contains exactly the same percentage of each color: 30% brown, 20% yellow, 20% red, 10% orange, 10% green, 10% blue. In response to consumer input, tan M&M's were replaced by blue.)

boiled sweets	¼ lb	327	0	—	87	0
butterscotch	1 oz	112	1	12	27	—
butterscotch	1 piece (6 g)	24	tr	3	6	—
candied cherries	1 (4 g)	12	tr	—	3	—
candied citron	1 oz	89	tr	82	23	—
candied lemon peel	1 oz	90	tr	14	23	—
candied orange peel	1 oz	90	tr	14	23	—
candied pineapple slice	1 slice (2 oz)	179	tr	—	45	—
candy corn	1 oz	105	0	57	27	—
caramels	1 pkg (2.5 oz)	271	6	174	55	—
caramels	1 piece (8 g)	31	1	20	6	—
caramels chocolate	1 bar (2.3 oz)	231	2	—	56	—
caramels chocolate	1 piece (6 g)	22	tr	—	6	—
carob bar	1 (3.1 oz)	453	28	—	42	—
crisped rice bar almond	1 bar (1 oz)	130	6	66	18	1
crisped rice bar chocolate chip	1 bar (1 oz)	115	4	79	21	1
dark chocolate	1 oz	150	10	5	16	—
fondant chocolate coated	1 sm (0.4 oz)	40	1	3	9	—
fondant chocolate coated	1 lg (1.2 oz)	128	3	9	28	—

FOOD	PORTION	CAL.	FAT	SOD.	CARB.	FIB.
fondant mint	1 oz	105	0	57	27	—
fruit pastilles	1 tube (1.4 oz)	101	0	—	25	—
gumdrops	10 sm (0.4 oz)	135	0	15	35	—
gumdrops	10 lg (3.8 oz)	420	0	48	108	—
hard candy	1 oz	106	0	11	28	—
jelly beans	10 sm (0.4 oz)	40	tr	3	10	—
jelly beans	10 lg (1 oz)	104	tr	7	26	—
lollipop	1 (6 g)	22	0	2	6	—
marzipan	3½ oz	497	25	5	57	—
milk chocolate	1 bar (1.55 oz)	226	14	36	26	—
milk chocolate crisp	1 bar (1.45 oz)	203	11	59	28	—
milk chocolate w/ almonds	1 bar (1.45 oz)	215	14	30	22	—
nougat nut cream	3½ oz	342	31	—	58	—
peanut bar	1 (1.4 oz)	209	14	91	19	—
peanuts chocolate covered	1 cup (5.2 oz)	773	50	61	74	—
peanuts chocolate covered	10 (1.4 oz)	208	13	16	20	—
pretzels chocolate covered	1 (0.4 oz)	50	2	10	8	—
pretzels chocolate covered	1 oz	130	5	—	20	—
sesame crunch	1 oz	146	9	—	14	—
sesame crunch	20 pieces (1.2 oz)	181	12	—	18	—
sweet chocolate	1 oz	143	10	5	17	—
sweet chocolate	1 bar (1.45 oz)	201	14	7	25	—
100 Grand						
Bar	1 bar (1.5 oz)	200	8	75	30	tr
3 Musketeers						
Bar	2 fun size (1.2 oz)	140	4	60	25	0
Bar	1 (2.1 oz)	260	8	110	46	1
5th Avenue						
Bar	1 (2.1 oz)	290	13	140	39	—
After Eight						
Dark Chocolate Wafer Thin Mints	1	35	1	0	6	—
Almond Joy						
Bar	1 (1.76 oz)	250	14	70	28	—
Baby Ruth						
Bar	1 (2.1 oz)	280	12	135	38	2
Fun Size	2 pieces	200	9	95	27	1
Bar None						
Candy	1 (1.5 oz)	240	14	50	23	—
Bit-O-Honey						
Candy	1.7 oz	200	4	125	39	—
Bits O Brickle						
Candy	1 tbsp (0.5 oz)	80	5	85	9	0

FOOD	PORTION	CAL.	FAT	SOD.	CARB.	FIB.
Bonus						
Bar	1 bar (2.1 oz)	290	16	140	34	2
Breath Savers						
Sugar Free Mint Cinnamon	1 piece (2 g)	10	0	0	2	—
Sugar Free Peppermint	1 piece (2 g)	10	0	0	2	—
Sugar Free Spearmint	1 piece (2 g)	10	0	0	2	—
Sugar Free Wintergreen	1 piece (2 g)	10	0	0	2	—
Brock						
Butterscotch Discs	3 pieces (0.6 oz)	70	0	80	17	—
Candy Corn	21 pieces (1.4 oz)	150	0	85	37	—
Candy Rolls	2 rolls (0.5 oz)	50	0	0	12	—
Caramel Dots	3 pieces (1.3 oz)	140	3	50	25	tr
Cinnamon Discs	3 pieces (0.6 oz)	70	0	5	17	—
Circus Peanuts	11 pieces (2.5 oz)	260	0	25	65	—
Coconut Mountains	4 pieces (1.4 oz)	170	6	80	29	—
Fruit Basket	3 pieces (0.6 oz)	60	0	0	15	—
Fruit Kisses	3 pieces (0.6 oz)	70	0	5	17	—
Glitters	2 pieces (0.5 oz)	50	0	15	13	—
Gummy Bears	5 pieces (1.4 oz)	130	0	15	30	—
Gummy Squirms	5 pieces (1.3 oz)	120	0	15	28	—
Jelly Beans	12 pieces (1.4 oz)	140	0	15	36	—
Lemon Drops	3 pieces (0.5 oz)	60	0	5	14	—
Orange Slices	4 pieces (1.5 oz)	140	0	20	36	—
Party Mints	9 pieces (0.5 oz)	60	0	0	15	—
Peanut Butter Crunch	3 pieces (0.6 oz)	80	2	45	15	—
Pops Assorted	2 (0.5 oz)	60	0	5	15	—
Sour Balls	3 pieces (0.6 oz)	70	0	5	17	—
Sour Sharks	23 pieces (2.5 oz)	30	3	45	60	—
Spearmint Starlights	3 pieces (0.6 oz)	60	0	5	16	—
Spice Drops	12 pieces (1.4 oz)	130	0	20	33	—
Starlight Mints	3 pieces (0.6 oz)	60	0	5	16	—
Toffee	6 pieces (1.5 oz)	170	5	45	31	—
Butterfinger						
BB's	1 pkg (1.7 oz)	230	10	90	34	1
Bar	1 (2.1 oz)	280	11	120	41	1
Fun Size	2 bars (1.6 oz)	200	8	85	30	1
Caramello						
Candy	1 (1.6 oz)	220	11	60	28	—
Cellas						
Chocolate Covered Cherries Dark Chocolate	2 pieces (1 oz)	100	4	—	—	—

FOOD	PORTION	CAL.	FAT	SOD.	CARB.	FIB.
Cellas (CONT.)						
Chocolate Covered Cherries Milk Chocolate	2 pieces (1 oz)	110	4	15	18	2
Certs						
Breath Mints	1 piece (1.67 g)	6	0	—	2	—
Mini Sugar Free	1 piece (0.365 g)	1	0	—	tr	—
Sugar Free	1 piece (1.67 g)	7	0	—	2	—
Charleston Chew						
Candy	1 pkg (1.9 oz)	230	7	—	—	—
Chocolate	½ bar	120	3	—	—	—
Strawberry	½ bar	120	3	—	—	—
Vanilla	½ bar	120	3	—	—	—
Charms						
Blow Pop	1 (0.7 oz)	80	0	—	—	—
Pop	1 (0.6 oz)	70	0	—	—	—
Chuckles						
Candy	4 pieces (1.4 oz)	140	0	15	34	—
Chunky						
Bar	1 (1.4 oz)	200	11	20	22	2
Clorets						
Mints	1 piece (1.67 g)	6	0	—	2	—
Crunch						
Fun Size	4 bars (1.5 oz)	200	10	55	25	1
Dove						
Dark Chocolate	1 bar (1.3 oz)	200	12	0	22	2
Dark Chocolate	¼ bar (1.5 oz)	230	14	0	26	3
Dark Chocolate Miniatures	7 (1.5 oz)	220	14	0	26	2
Milk Chocolate	1 bar (1.3 oz)	200	12	25	22	1
Milk Chocolate	¼ bar (1.5 oz)	230	13	30	25	1
Milk Chocolate Miniatures	7 (1.5 oz)	230	13	30	25	1
Truffles	3 (1.2 oz)	200	13	15	19	1
Dream						
Caramel & Nougat In Milk Chocolate	1 bar (1 oz)	90	3	70	21	1
Estee						
Caramels Chocolate & Vanilla No Sugar Added	5 (1.3 oz)	150	5	65	26	0
Dark Chocolate	½ bar (1.4 oz)	200	14	10	23	0
Gum Drops Assorted Fruit Sugar Free	23 (1.4 oz)	140	0	0	36	0

FOOD	PORTION	CAL.	FAT	SOD.	CARB.	FIB.
Estee (CONT.)						
Gum Drops Licorice	23 (1.4 oz)	140	0	0	36	—
Gummy Bears Sugar Free	16 (1.4 oz)	140	0	0	31	—
Hard Candies Assorted Fruit Sugar Free	5 (0.5 oz)	60	0	0	16	0
Hard Candies Assorted Mint Sugar Free	5 (0.5 oz)	60	0	0	16	0
Hard Candies Butterscotch Sugar Free	2 (0.4 oz)	50	0	50	12	—
Hard Candies Peppermint Swirls Sugar Free	3 (0.5 oz)	60	0	0	14	—
Hard Candies Tropical Fruit Sugar Free	5 (0.5 oz)	60	0	0	16	0
Lollipops Assorted Fruit Sugar Free	2 (0.5 oz)	60	0	0	16	—
Milk Chocolate	½ bar (1.4 oz)	230	17	65	17	0
Milk Chocolate With Almonds	½ bar (1.4 oz)	230	17	65	16	0
Milk Chocolate With Crisp Rice	1 bar (2.3 oz)	370	26	110	29	0
Milk Chocolate With Fruit & Nuts	½ bar (1.4 oz)	220	16	65	18	0
Mint Chocolate	½ bar (1.4 oz)	200	14	10	23	0
Peanut Brittle No Sugar Added	⅓ box (1.5 oz)	210	9	115	28	1
Peanut Butter Cups	5 (1.3 oz)	200	12	70	19	1
Peanut Butter Cups	1 (0.3 oz)	40	3	0	3	0
Toffee Sugar Free	5 (0.5 oz)	60	0	0	16	—
Ferrero Rocher						
Candy	2 pieces (0.9 oz)	150	10	24	11	0
Franklin						
Crunch 'N Munch Candied	1.25 oz	170	7	200	28	1
Crunch 'N Munch Caramel	1.25 oz	160	5	130	28	1
Crunch 'N Munch Maple Walnut	1.25 oz	160	6	180	28	1
Crunch 'N Munch Toffee	1.25 oz	160	5	210	28	1
Glenny's						
Brown Rice Treats Carob & Mint With Oat Bran	1 bar (1.75 oz)	180	2	20	37	2

FOOD	PORTION	CAL.	FAT	SOD.	CARB.	FIB.
Glenny's (CONT.)						
Brown Rice Treats Cinnamon & Raisin	1 bar (1.75 oz)	170	1	30	38	—
Brown Rice Treats Peanut & Raisin	1 bar (2 oz)	210	5	29	39	—
Brown Rice Treats Plain & Fancy	1 bar (1.25 oz)	120	1	29	28	—
Brown Rice Treats Raisin Bran	1 bar (1.75 oz)	170	1	17	38	—
Brown Rice Treats Toasted Almond With Oat Bran	1 bar (1.75 oz)	200	5	20	34	2
Fruit Drops Black Cherry	1	6	tr	tr	1	—
Fruit Drops Gentle Mint	1	6	tr	tr	1	—
Fruit Drops Mandarin Orange	1	6	tr	tr	1	—
Fruit Drops Mixed Fruit	1	6	tr	tr	1	—
Fruit Drops Twist Of Lemon	1	6	tr	tr	1	—
Hard Candies Fruit	1	19	tr	tr	4	—
Hard Candies Peppermint	1	19	tr	tr	4	—
Lollipops C Pops	1	35	tr	tr	8	—
Lollipops Fruit	1	21	tr	tr	5	—
Moist & Chewy Coconut Almondine Bar	1 bar (1.5 oz)	190	10	20	22	—
Moist & Chewy Oatmeal Raisin Bar	1 bar (1.5 oz)	160	3	25	30	—
Moist & Chewy Peanut Bar	1 bar (1.5 oz)	180	7	20	24	—
Moist & Chewy Sunflower Bar	1 bar (1.5 oz)	180	7	15	24	—
Snack Bar Fat-Free Apple-Cinnamon	1 (125 oz)	120	1	15	28	—
Snack Bar Fat-Free Caramel	1 (1.25 oz)	120	tr	70	29	—
Snack Bar Fat-Free Chocolate	1 (1.25 oz)	120	tr	10	28	—
Snack Bar Fat-Free Raspberry	1 (1.25 oz)	120	tr	15	29	—
Godiva						
Almond Butter Dome	3 pieces (1.5 oz)	240	17	20	19	0
Bouchee Au Chocolat	1 piece (1.5 oz)	210	11	40	25	0
Bouchee Ivory Raspberry	1 pieces (1 oz)	160	9	25	17	0

FOOD	PORTION	CAL.	FAT	SOD.	CARB.	FIB.
Godiva (CONT.)						
Gold Ballotin	3 pieces (1.5 oz)	210	10	15	27	0
Truffle Amaretto Di Saronno	2 pieces (1.5 oz)	210	12	25	24	0
Truffle Deluxe Liqueur	2 pieces (1.5 oz)	210	13	25	23	0
Golden Almond						
Bar	½ bar	260	17	35	20	—
Golden III						
Bar	½ bar	250	15	40	26	—
Goldenberg's						
Peanut Chews	3 pieces (1.3 oz)	180	9	40	22	1
Goo Goo Supreme						
With Pecans	1 pkg (1.5 oz)	188	5	51	34	4
Goobers						
Peanuts	1 pkg (1.38 oz)	210	13	20	19	3
Good & Fruity						
Candy	1 box (1.8 oz)	140	1	75	35	2
Good & Plenty						
Snacksize	3 boxes (1.5 oz)	140	0	80	34	—
Haviland						
Chocolate Covered Thin Mints	6 (1.5 oz)	170	5	5	33	1
Heath						
Bar	1 (1.4 oz)	210	13	180	25	0
Hershey						
Amazin'Fruit Gummy Candy	2 snack pkg (1.4 oz)	130	0	45	30	—
Bar	1 (1.55 oz)	240	14	40	25	—
Bar With Almonds	1 (1.45 oz)	230	14	55	20	—
Kisses	9 pieces (1.46 oz)	220	13	35	23	—
Special Dark Sweet Chocolate Bar	1 (1.45)	220	12	5	25	—
Jolly Rancher						
Candies	3 pieces (0.6 oz)	60	0	5	14	—
Joyva						
Halvah	1.5 oz	240	16	80	16	2
Halvah Chocolate Covered	1 bar (2 oz)	380	23	95	20	3
Jells Raspberry	3 pieces (1.6 oz)	200	3	15	25	tr
Joys Raspberry	1 (1.6 oz)	200	3	15	25	1
Marshmallow Twists Chocolate Covered	2 (1.5 oz)	190	4	20	21	0
Rings Orange & Raspberry	3 pieces (1.5 oz)	190	3	15	23	tr

FOOD	PORTION	CAL.	FAT	SOD.	CARB.	FIB.
Joyva (CONT.)						
Sesame Crunch	3 pieces (0.5)	80	4	25	7	0
Sticks Orange	3 pieces (1.6 oz)	200	3	15	25	tr
Twists Vanilla & Cherry	2 pieces (1.5 oz)	190	4	20	21	0
Juicefuls						
Candy	3 pieces (0.5 oz)	60	0	0	15	—
Junior Mints						
Candies	1 pkg (1.6 oz)	190	4	—	—	—
Just Born						
Jelly Beans	1 oz	108	tr	—	—	—
Sugar Coated	1½ oz	148	tr	—	—	—
Toasted Coconut	1⅜ oz	140	2	—	—	—
Kit Kat						
Bar	1 (1.625 oz)	250	13	60	29	—
Krackel						
Bar	1 (1.55 oz)	230	13	80	27	—
Laffy Taffy						
Apple Chews	1 oz	110	1	55	26	—
Banana Chews	1 oz	110	1	55	26	—
Grape Chews	1 oz	110	1	60	26	—
Passion Punch Chews	1 oz	110	1	50	26	—
Strawberry Chews	1 oz	110	1	55	26	—
Sweet & Sour Cherry Chews	1 oz	110	1	55	26	—
Watermelon Chews	1 oz	110	1	55	26	—
Lance						
Chocolaty Peanut Bar	1 (57 g)	320	18	40	29	—
Peanut Bar	1 pkg (50 g)	260	14	80	24	—
Popscotch	1 pkg (35 g)	160	6	120	24	—
Lifesavers						
Big Tablet Candy Cane	4 pieces (0.5 oz)	60	0	0	16	—
Cards 'N Candy	4 pieces (0.4 oz)	40	0	0	10	—
Christmas Tin	4 pieces (0.5 oz)	60	0	20	16	—
Egg-Sortment	1 roll (0.4 oz)	40	0	0	10	—
Fruit Juicers Lollipops	1	40	0	0	10	0
Gummi Bunnies	3 pkg (1.6 oz)	140	0	0	34	—
Gummi Savers Five Flavor	1 roll (1.5 oz)	130	0	0	32	—
Gummi Savers Five Flavor	1 pkg (1.8 oz)	160	0	0	38	—
Gummi Savers Mixed Berry	1 roll (1.5 oz)	130	0	0	32	—
Gummi Savers Mixed Berry	1 pkg (1.8 oz)	160	0	0	38	—

FOOD	PORTION	CAL.	FAT	SOD.	CARB.	FIB.
Lifesavers (CONT.)						
Gummi Savers Tangy Fruits	1 roll (1.5 oz)	130	0	0	32	—
Gummi Savers Tangy Fruits	1 pkg (1.8 oz)	160	0	0	38	—
Gummi Savers Variety	2 pkg (1.3 oz)	120	0	0	27	—
Gummi Savers Wacky Frootz	1 roll (1.5 oz)	130	0	0	32	—
Gummi Savers Wacky Frootz	1 pkg (1.8 oz)	160	0	0	38	—
Holes Five Flavor	20 pieces (5 g)	20	0	0	5	—
Holes Island Fruit	20 pieces (5 g)	20	0	0	5	—
Holes Sour 'N Sweet	16 pieces (5 g)	20	0	0	5	—
Holes Sunshine Fruits	20 pieces (0.2 oz)	20	0	0	5	—
Holes Super Tart	20 pieces (5 g)	20	0	0	5	—
Holes Tangerine	1 candy	2	0	0	1	0
Holes Wild Fruits	20 pieces (5 g)	20	0	0	5	—
Lollipops Candy Cane	1 (0.4 oz)	40	0	0	10	—
Lollipops Christmas	1 (0.4 oz)	40	0	0	10	—
Lollipops Easter	1 (0.4 oz)	40	0	0	10	—
Lollipops Fruit Flavors	1 (0.4 oz)	45	0	0	11	0
Lollipops Swirled Flavors	1 (0.4 oz)	40	0	0	10	—
Lollipops Valentine	1 (0.4 oz)	40	0	0	10	—
Roll Butter Rum	2 pieces (5 g)	20	0	20	5	—
Roll Candy Cane	4 pieces (0.4 oz)	40	0	0	10	—
Roll Cryst-O-Mint	2 pieces (5 g)	20	0	0	5	—
Roll Five Flavor	2 pieces (5 g)	20	0	0	5	—
Roll Fruits On Fire	2 pieces (5 g)	20	0	0	5	—
Roll Pep-O-Mint	3 pieces (5 g)	20	0	0	5	—
Roll Spear-O-Mint	3 pieces (5 g)	20	0	0	5	—
Roll Sunshine Fruits	2 pieces (5 g)	20	0	0	5	—
Roll Tangy Fruit Swirl	2 pieces (5 g)	20	0	0	5	—
Roll Tangy Fruit Watermelon	1 pieces (5 g)	20	0	0	5	—
Roll Tangy Fruits	2 pieces (5 g)	20	0	0	5	—
Roll Tropical Fruits	2 pieces (5 g)	20	0	0	5	—
Roll Wild Cherry	1 pieces (5 g)	20	0	0	5	—
Roll Wild Flavors	2 pieces (5 g)	20	0	0	5	—
Roll Wild Sour Berries	2 pieces (5 g)	20	0	0	5	—
Roll Wint-O-Green	3 pieces (5 g)	20	0	0	5	—
Sack'it Butter Rum	4 pieces (0.5 oz)	60	0	65	15	—
Sack'it Five Flavor	4 pieces (0.5 oz)	60	0	0	16	—
Sack'it Holiday Tin	4 pieces (0.5 oz)	60	0	65	16	—

FOOD	PORTION	CAL.	FAT	SOD.	CARB.	FIB.
Lifesavers (CONT.)						
Sack'it Pep-O-Mint	4 pieces (0.5 oz)	60	0	0	16	—
Sack'it Tangy Fruits	4 pieces (0.5 oz)	60	0	0	16	—
Sack'it Wild Cherry	4 pieces (0.5 oz)	60	0	0	16	—
Sack'it Wint-O-Green	4 pieces (0.5 oz)	60	0	0	16	—
Sugar Free Iced Mint	1 pieces (2 g)	10	0	0	2	—
Sugar Free Vanilla Mint	1 pieces (2 g)	10	0	0	2	—
Valentine Book	2 pieces (5 g)	20	0	20	5	—
Lindt						
Truffles	3 pieces (1.3 oz)	220	18	10	14	0
M&M's						
Almond	1.5 oz	220	12	20	24	2
Almond	1 pkg (1.3 oz)	200	11	20	21	2
Mint	1.5 oz	200	9	30	30	1
Mint	1 pkg (1.7 oz)	230	10	35	34	1
Peanut	½ bag king size (1.6 oz)	240	12	25	28	2
Peanut	1 pkg (1.7 oz)	250	13	25	30	2
Peanut	1.5 oz	220	11	20	25	2
Peanut	1 fun size (0.7 oz)	110	5	10	13	1
Peanut Butter	1 fun size (0.7 oz)	110	6	45	12	1
Peanut Butter	1.5 oz	220	12	90	25	2
Peanut Butter	1 pkg (1.6 oz)	240	13	100	27	2
Plain	1 pkg fun size (0.7 oz)	100	4	15	15	0
Plain	1.5 oz	200	9	30	30	1
Plain	1 pkg (1.7 oz)	230	10	35	34	1
Plain	½ pkg king size (1.6 oz)	220	9	30	32	1
Mars						
Almond Bar	2 fun size (1.3 oz)	190	10	55	23	1
Almond Bar	1 bar (1.8 oz)	240	13	70	31	1
Mayfair						
Mints	5 pieces (1.3 oz)	180	9	5	26	tr
Milk Duds						
Pieces	1 box (1.8 oz)	230	8	120	38	0
Snack Size	4 boxes (1.3 oz)	160	5	85	26	0
Milkshake						
Bar	1 bar (1.8 oz)	220	7	120	38	0
Milky Way						
Bar	2 fun size (1.4 oz)	180	7	60	28	0
Bar	1 (2.1 oz)	280	11	90	43	1
Bar	⅓ king size (1.2 oz)	160	6	50	24	0
Dark	1 fun size (0.7 oz)	90	3	35	14	0

FOOD	PORTION	CAL.	FAT	SOD.	CARB.	FIB.
Milky Way (CONT.)						
Dark	1 bar (1.8 oz)	220	8	85	36	1
Miniature	5 (1.5 oz)	190	7	65	30	0
Mounds						
Bar	1 (1.9 oz)	260	14	85	31	—
Mr. Goodbar						
Candy	1 (1.75 oz)	290	19	20	23	—
NECCO						
Mint	1 piece	12	tr	—	—	—
Natural Touch						
Caroby Almond Bar	4 sections (28 g)	150	10	50	12	—
Caroby Milk Bar	4 sections (28 g)	150	9	55	13	—
Caroby Milk Free Bar	4 sections (28 g)	160	11	25	11	—
Caroby Mint Bar	4 sections (28 g)	150	9	55	13	—
Nestle						
Areo Bar	1 bar (1.45 oz)	210	13	20	26	2
Buncha Crunch	1 pkg (1.4 oz)	90	10	95	26	tr
Crunch	1 bar (1.55 oz)	230	12	60	28	1
Milk Chocolate	1 bar (1.45 oz)	220	13	30	23	2
Turtles Pecan Caramel Candy	2 pieces (1.2 oz)	160	9	30	20	1
Newman's Own						
Organics Espresso Sweet Dark Chocolate	1 bar (1.2 oz)	190	12	10	19	0
Nips						
Butter Rum	2 pieces (0.5 oz)	60	2	35	12	—
Caramel	2 pieces (0.5 oz)	60	2	40	12	—
Chocolate Mint	2 pieces (0.5 oz)	60	2	40	11	—
Chocolate Parfait	2 pieces (0.5 oz)	60	2	35	11	—
Peanut Butter Parfait	2 pieces (0.5 oz)	60	2	40	11	—
Ocean Spray						
Fruit Waves Assorted	3 pieces (0.3 oz)	35	0	0	9	—
Oh Henry!						
Bar	1 (1.8 oz)	230	9	125	32	2
PayDay						
Bar	1 (1.85 oz)	240	12	170	28	2
Pearson						
Licorice	2 pieces (0.5 oz)	60	2	40	12	—
Pez						
Candy	1 roll (0.3 oz)	30	0	0	8	—
Sugar Free	1 roll (0.3 oz)	30	0	0	8	0
Planters						
Original Peanut Bar	1 pkg (1.6 oz)	230	14	70	22	2

FOOD	PORTION	CAL.	FAT	SOD.	CARB.	FIB.
Pom Pom						
Candies	1 pkg (1.6 oz)	200	6	—	—	—
Raisinets						
Raisins	1 pkg (1.58 oz)	200	8	15	31	2
Reese's						
Peanut Butter Cups	1 (1.8 oz)	280	17	180	26	—
Pieces	1.85 oz	260	11	90	32	—
Riesen						
Candy	5 pieces (1.4 oz)	180	7	30	29	3
Rolo						
Carmels In Milk Chocolate	8 pieces (1.93 oz)	270	12	110	37	—
Russell Stover						
Assorted Creams	3 pieces (1.4 oz)	180	7	50	29	0
Pecan Roll	1 (2 oz)	300	20	95	26	3
Skittles						
Original	2 pkg fun size (1.6 oz)	180	2	5	41	0
Original	1.5 oz	170	2	5	38	0
Original	½ king size (1.3 oz)	150	2	5	34	0
Original	1 pkg (2.8 oz)	250	3	10	55	0
Tropical	1.5 oz	170	2	5	38	0
Tropical	2 bags fun size (1.4 oz)	160	2	5	36	0
Tropical	1 bag (2.2 oz)	250	3	10	56	0
Wild Berry	2 bags fun size (1.4 oz)	160	2	5	36	0
Wild Berry	1 bag (2.2 oz)	250	3	10	56	0
Wild Berry	1.5 oz	170	2	5	38	0
Skor						
Toffee Bar	1 (1.4 oz)	220	14	125	22	—
Smucker's						
Jelly Beans	1 pkg (0.7 oz)	70	0	10	18	0
Snickers						
Bar	1 bar (2.1 oz)	280	14	150	36	1
Bar	2 bars fun size (1.4 oz)	190	9	100	24	1
Bar	⅓ king size (1.2 oz)	170	8	85	21	1
Miniatures	4 (1.3 oz)	170	8	90	22	1
Munch Bar	1 (1.4 oz)	230	15	150	17	2
Peanut Butter	1 bar (2 oz)	310	20	150	28	1
Sno-Caps						
Candies	1 pkg (2.3 oz)	300	13	0	48	3

FOOD	PORTION	CAL.	FAT	SOD.	CARB.	FIB.
Solitaires						
Candies	½ bag	260	17	25	20	—
Sour Punch						
Candy Straws Sour Apple	6 pieces (1.4 oz)	130	1	10	31	—
Spice Stix						
And Drops	14 pieces (1.6 oz)	140	0	15	35	—
Starburst						
California Fruits	8 pieces (1.4 oz)	160	3	20	33	0
California Fruits	1 stick (2.1 oz)	240	5	35	48	0
Original Fruits	⅓ king size (1.2 oz)	140	3	20	28	0
Original Fruits	8 pieces (1.4 oz)	160	3	20	33	0
Orignal Fruits	1 stick (2.1 oz)	240	5	35	48	0
Strawberry Fruits	8 pieces (1.4 oz)	160	3	20	33	0
Strawberry Fruits	1 stick (2.1 oz)	240	5	35	48	0
Tropical Fruits	1 stick (2.1 oz)	240	5	35	48	0
Tropical Fruits	8 pieces (1.4 oz)	160	3	20	33	0
Sugar Babies						
Candies	1 pkg (1.7 oz)	190	2	—	—	—
Tidbits	1 pkg	180	2	—	—	—
Sugar Daddy						
Candies	1 pkg (1.7 oz)	200	3	—	—	—
Swedish Red Fish						
Candy	19 pieces (1.4 oz)	150	1	20	35	—
Sweet Escapes						
Triple Chocolate Wafer Bars	1 (0.7 oz)	80	3	30	14	—
Switzer						
Cherry Bites	12 pieces (1.6 oz)	50	0	25	11	—
Licorice Bites	12 pieces (1.6 oz)	46	0	56	11	—
Symphony						
Almond Butterchips	1 (1.4 oz)	220	14	40	20	—
Milk Chocolate	1 (1.4 oz)	220	13	35	22	—
Terry's						
Orange Milk Chocolate	5 pieces (1.5 oz)	240	14	40	26	1
Tootsie Roll						
Candy	1 (1 oz)	110	2	—	—	—
Dots	12 (1.5 oz)	160	0	—	—	—
Midgees	6 (1.4 oz)	160	3	—	—	—
Pop	1 (0.6 oz)	60	0	—	—	—
Twix						
Caramel	1 pkg (2 oz)	280	14	115	37	0
Caramel	1 (1 oz)	140	7	60	19	0
Caramel	1 fun size (0.5 oz)	80	4	30	10	0

FOOD	PORTION	CAL.	FAT	SOD.	CARB.	FIB
Twix (CONT.)						
Caramel	1 king size (0.8 oz)	120	6	45	15	1
Peanut Butter	1 (0.9 oz)	130	8	70	13	1
Twizzlers						
Candy	4 pieces (1.4 oz)	130	1	95	30	—
Pull-N-Peel Cherry	1 piece (1.1 oz)	110	0	80	23	—
Velamints						
Cocoamint	1 piece (1.7 g)	5	0	0	2	—
Peppermint	1 piece (1.7 g)	5	0	0	2	—
Spearmint	1 piece (1.7 g)	5	0	0	2	—
Wintergreen	1 piece (1.7 g)	5	0	0	2	—
Very Special						
Chocolate Bottles Liquor Filled	3 pieces (1 oz)	150	6	10	24	2
Whatchamacallit						
Bar	1 (1.8 oz)	260	13	130	30	—
Whitman's						
Assorted	3 pieces (1.4 oz)	190	8	50	27	0
Dark Chocolate	3 pieces (1.4 oz)	200	10	55	25	1
Little Ambassadors	7 pieces (1.4 oz)	190	9	50	26	1
Pecan Delight	1 bar (2 oz)	310	20	75	27	2
Pecan Roll	1 bar (2 oz)	300	20	95	26	1
Sampler	3 pieces (1.4 oz)	200	11	60	25	1
Whoppers						
Candy	1 pkg (1.8 oz)	230	10	130	36	1
Y&S						
Bites Cherry	1 oz	100	1	85	23	—
York						
Peppermint Patty	1 snack size (0.5 oz)	57	1	3	11	—
Peppermint Patty	1 (1.5 oz)	180	4	20	34	—
Zero						
Bar	2 pieces (1.4 oz)	170	6	85	28	0
HOME RECIPE						
divinity	1 recipe 48 pieces (19 oz)	1891	tr	247	486	—
divinity	1 (11 g)	38	0	5	10	—
fondant	1 recipe 60 pieces (32.6 oz)	3327	tr	374	863	—
fondant	1 piece (0.6 oz)	57	0	6	15	—
fudge brown sugar w/ nuts	1 piece (0.5 oz)	56	1	14	11	—
fudge brown sugar w/ nuts	1 recipe 60 pieces (30.7 oz)	3453	88	852	676	—
fudge chocolate	1 piece (0.6 oz)	65	1	10	14	—

FOOD	PORTION	CAL.	FAT	SOD.	CARB.	FIB.
fudge chocolate	1 recipe 48 pieces (29 oz)	3161	70	511	660	—
fudge chocolate marshmallow	1 recipe (43.1 oz)	5182	207	1273	880	—
fudge chocolate marshmallow	1 piece (0.7 oz)	84	3	21	14	—
fudge chocolate marshmallow w/ nuts	1 piece (0.8 oz)	96	4	21	15	—
fudge chocolate marshmallow w/ nuts	1 recipe 60 pieces (43.1 oz)	5182	207	1273	880	—
fudge chocolate marshmallow w/ nuts	1 recipe 60 pieces (46.1 oz)	5742	258	1234	903	—
fudge chocolate w/ nuts	1 piece (0.7 oz)	81	3	11	14	—
fudge chocolate w/ nuts	1 recipe 48 pieces (32.7 oz)	3967	150	562	678	—
fudge peanut butter	1 piece (0.6 oz)	59	1	12	13	—
fudge peanut butter	1 recipe 36 pieces (20.4 oz)	2161	38	424	456	—
fudge vanilla	1 piece (0.6 oz)	59	1	11	13	—
fudge vanilla	1 recipe 48 pieces (27.5 oz)	2893	42	525	644	—
fudge vanilla w/ nuts	1 piece (0.5 oz)	62	2	9	11	—
fudge vanilla w/ nuts	1 recipe 60 pieces (31 oz)	3666	117	538	665	—
peanut brittle	1 recipe (17.6 oz)	2288	95	2269	347	—
peanut brittle	1 oz	128	5	128	20	—
praline	1 piece (1.4 oz)	177	10	24	24	—
praline	1 recipe 23 pieces (31.8 oz)	4116	220	559	562	—
taffy	1 piece (0.5 oz)	56	1	13	14	—
taffy	1 recipe 48 pieces (25 oz)	2677	24	636	651	—
toffee	1 piece (0.4 oz)	65	4	22	8	—
toffee	1 recipe 48 pieces (19.4 oz)	2997	182	1036	356	—
truffles	1 piece (0.4 oz)	59	4	8	5	—
truffles	1 recipe 49 pieces (21.5 oz)	2985	210	433	275	—
CANTALOUPE						
fresh cubed	1 cup	57	tr	14	13	1
fresh half	½	94	1	23	22	2
Big Valley						
Balls frzn	¾ cup (4.9 oz)	40	0	16	10	0

FOOD	PORTION	CAL.	FAT	SOD.	CARB.	FIB.
Chiquita						
Fresh	1 cup	70	0	—	—	—
Dole						
Fresh	¼	50	0	35	11	0
CAPERS						
Progresso						
Capers	1 tsp (5 g)	0	0	105	0	0
Reese						
Capers	1 tsp (5 g)	0	0	105	0	—
CARAWAY						
seed	1 tsp	7	tr	tr	1	—
CARDAMON						
ground	1 tsp	6	tr	tr	1	
CARDOON						
fresh cooked	3½ oz	22	tr	176	5	—
raw shredded	½ cup	36	tr	151	4	—
CARIBOU						
roasted	3 oz	142	4	51	0	
CARISSA						
fresh	1	12	tr	1	3	—
CAROB						
carob mix	3 tsp	45	0	12	11	—
carob mix as prep w/ whole milk	9 oz	195	8	132	23	-
flour	1 tbsp	14	tr	3	7	—
flour	1 cup	185	1	36	92	—
CARP						
fresh cooked	1 fillet (6 oz)	276	12	107	0	
fresh cooked	3 oz	138	6	54	0	—
raw	3 oz	108	5	42	0	-
roe raw	3½ oz	130	2	—	2	—
CARROT JUICE						
canned	6 oz	73	tr	54	17	
Hain						
Juice	6 fl oz	80	0	170	17	
Hollywood						
Juice	6 fl oz	80	0	170	17	2
Odwalla						
Juice	8 fl oz	70	0	200	18	2
CARROTS						
CANNED						
slices	½ cup	17	tr	176	4	

FOOD	PORTION	CAL.	FAT	SOD.	CARB.	FIB.
slices low sodium	½ cup	17	tr	31	4	1
Allen						
Sliced	½ cup (4.5 oz)	35	1	230	8	3
Crest Top						
Sliced	½ cup (4.5 oz)	35	1	230	8	3
Del Monte						
Cut	½ cup (4.3 oz)	35	0	300	8	3
Sliced	½ cup (4.3 oz)	35	0	300	8	3
S&W						
Diced Fancy	½ cup	30	0	240	7	—
Julienne French Style Fancy	½ cup	30	0	240	7	—
Sliced Fancy	½ cup	30	0	240	7	—
Sliced Water Pack	½ cup	30	0	50	7	—
Whole Tiny Fancy	½ cup	30	0	240	7	—
Seneca						
Diced	½ cup	30	0	264	6	2
Sliced	½ cup	30	0	264	6	2
FRESH						
baby raw	1 (½ oz)	6	tr	5	1	—
raw	1 (2.5 oz)	31	tr	25	7	2
raw shredded	½ cup	24	tr	19	6	2
slices cooked	½ cup	35	tr	52	8	—
Dole						
Medium	1	40	1	40	8	1
FROZEN						
slices cooked	½ cup	26	tr	43	6	—
Big Valley						
Carrots	½ cup (3 oz)	35	0	40	8	2
Birds Eye						
Baby Whole Deluxe	½ cup	40	0	45	9	2
Polybag Sliced	¾ cup	35	0	40	8	1
Fresh Like						
Carrots	3.5 oz	42	tr	42	10	—
Green Giant						
Harvest Fresh Baby	½ cup	18	0	75	5	2
Hanover						
Crinkle Sliced	½ cup	35	0	—	—	—

CASABA

cubed	1 cup	45	tr	20	11	—
fresh	1/10	43	tr	20	10	—

CASHEWS

cashew butter w/o salt	1 tbsp	94	8	2	4	—

FOOD	PORTION	CAL.	FAT	SOD.	CARB.	FIB.
dry roasted	1 oz	163	13	4	9	—
dry roasted salted	1 oz	163	13	213	9	—
oil roasted	1 oz	163	14	5	8	—
oil roasted salted	1 oz	163	14	209	8	—
Beer Nuts						
Cashews	1 pkg (1 oz)	170	13	65	8	—
Fisher						
Honey Roasted Halves	1 oz	150	13	—	7	—
Honey Roasted Whole	1 oz	150	13	90	7	—
Oil Roasted Halves	1 oz	170	15	160	8	—
Oil Roasted Whole	1 oz	170	15	140	8	—
Frito Lay						
Cashews	1 oz	170	14	115	9	—
Guy's						
Whole Salted	1 oz	170	14	140	5	—
Hain						
Cashew Butter Raw	2 tbsp	190	15	125	8	—
Cashew Butter Raw Unsalted	2 tbsp	210	19	170	8	—
Cashew Butter Toasted	2 tbsp	210	17	190	7	—
Lance						
Cashews	1 pkg (32 g)	190	15	95	8	—
Planters						
Fancy Oil Roasted	1 oz	170	14	120	8	1
Fancy Oil Roasted	1 pkg (2 oz)	340	29	240	16	3
Halves Lightly Salted Oil Roasted	1 oz	160	13	55	9	2
Halves Oil Roasted	1 oz	170	14	120	8	2
Honey Roasted	1 oz	150	12	120	11	1
Honey Roasted	1 pkg (2 oz)	310	24	240	23	3
Munch'N Go Honey Roasted	1 pkg (2 oz)	310	24	240	23	3
Munch'N Go Singles Oil Roasted	1 pkg (2 oz)	330	28	240	16	3
Oil Roasted	1 pkg (1 oz)	160	14	120	8	1
Oil Roasted	1 pkg (1.5 oz)	250	21	240	12	2

CASSAVA

FOOD	PORTION	CAL.	FAT	SOD.	CARB.	FIB.
raw	3½ oz	120	tr	8	27	—

CATFISH

FOOD	PORTION	CAL.	FAT	SOD.	CARB.	FIB.
channel breaded & fried	3 oz	194	11	238	7	—
channel raw	3 oz	99	4	54	0	—

FOOD	PORTION	CAL.	FAT	SOD.	CARB.	FIB.
CATSUP						
(*see* KETCHUP)						
CAULIFLOWER						
FRESH						
cooked	½ cup (2.2 oz)	14	tr	9	3	1
flowerets cooked	3 (2 oz)	12	tr	8	2	1
flowerets raw	3 (2 oz)	14	tr	17	3	1
green cooked	½ cup (2.2 oz)	20	tr	14	4	—
raw	½ cup (1.8 oz)	13	tr	15	3	1
Dole						
Cauliflower	⅙ med head	18	0	45	3	2
FROZEN						
cooked	½ cup	17	tr	16	3	—
Big Valley						
Florets	¾ cup (3 oz)	25	0	15	4	1
Birds Eye						
Frzn	⅔ cup	25	0	20	5	2
Polybag	½ cup	20	0	15	4	—
With Cheese Sauce	½ pkg	90	5	480	8	1
Fresh Like						
Cauliflower	3.5 oz	26	tr	48	5	1
Green Giant						
Cuts	½ cup	12	0	25	3	1
In Cheese Sauce	½ cup	60	2	500	10	2
One Serve In Cheese Sauce	1 pkg	80	3	690	14	2
Hanover						
Cauliflower	½ cup	20	0	—	—	—
Florets	½ cup	20	0	—	—	—
JARRED						
Vlasic						
Hot & Spicy	1 oz	4	0	435	1	—
Sweet	1 oz	35	0	225	9	—
CAVIAR						
black	1 oz	71	5	420	1	—
black	1 tbsp	40	3	240	1	—
red	1 tbsp	40	3	240	1	—
red	1 oz	71	5	420	1	—
CELERIAC						
fresh cooked	3½ oz	25	tr	61	6	—
raw	½ cup	31	tr	78	7	—

FOOD	PORTION	CAL.	FAT	SOD.	CARB.	FIB.
CELERY						
DRIED						
seed	1 tsp	8	tr	3	1	—
FRESH						
diced cooked	½ cup	13	tr	68	3	—
raw	1 stalk (1.3 oz)	6	tr	35	1	1
raw diced	½ cup	10	tr	52	2	1
Dole						
Stalks	2 med	20	0	140	2	4
FROZEN						
Fresh Like						
Celery	3.5 oz	14	tr	88	3	1
CELTUCE						
raw	3½ oz	22	tr	11	4	—
CEREAL						
all bran	½ cup (1 oz)	76	1	196	21	—
bran flakes	¾ cup (1 oz)	90	1	264	22	—
corn flakes	1¼ cup (1 oz)	110	tr	351	24	—
corn flakes low sodium	1 cup	100	tr	3	22	—
corn grits instant	1 pkg (0.8 oz)	82	tr	344	18	—
corn grits quick	1 cup	146	1	0	31	—
corn grits quick not prep	1 cup	579	2	1	124	—
corn grits quick not prep	1 tbsp	36	tr	0	8	—
corn grits regular	1 cup	146	1	0	31	—
corn grits regular not prep	1 cup	579	2	1	124	—
crispy rice	1 cup	111	tr	205	25	—
farina	¾ cup	87	tr	1	19	3
farina not prep	1 tbsp	40	0	0	9	tr
fortified oat flakes	1 cup	177	1	429	35	—
oatmeal	1 cup	145	2	1	25	—
oatmeal instant cooked w/o salt	1 cup	145	2	2	25	—
oatmeal not prep	1 cup	311	5	3	54	9
oatmeal quick cooked w/o salt	1 cup	145	2	2	25	—
oatmeal regular cooked w/o salt	1 cup	145	2	2	25	—
puffed rice	1 cup	57	tr	0	13	—
puffed wheat	1 cup	44	tr	0	10	—
shredded wheat	1 biscuit	83	tr	0	19	—
sugar-coated corn flakes	¾ cup (1 oz)	110	1	230	26	—
Albers						
Hominy Quick Grits uncooked	¼ cup	140	1	0	31	1

FOOD	PORTION	CAL.	FAT	SOD.	CARB.	FIB.
Arrowhead						
4 Grain + Flax	¼ cup (1.6 oz)	150	2	0	28	6
7 Grain	⅓ cup (1.4 oz)	140	2	0	25	5
Amaranth Flakes	1 cup (1.2 oz)	130	2	0	25	3
Apple Corns	1 cup (1.5 oz)	150	2	110	35	4
Bear Mush	¼ cup (1.6 oz)	160	1	0	33	2
Bran Flakes	1 cup (1 oz)	100	1	80	22	4
Kamut Flakes	1 cup (1.1 oz)	120	1	65	25	3
Maple Corns	1 cup (1.9 oz)	190	3	140	43	6
Multi Grain Flakes	1 cup (1.2 oz)	140	2	130	29	3
Nature O's	1 cup (1.1 oz)	130	2	5	24	3
Oat Bran Flakes	1 cup (1.2 oz)	110	2	60	22	4
Oat Flakes Rolled	⅓ cup (1.2 oz)	130	3	0	23	4
Oat Groats	¼ cup (1.5 oz)	160	3	0	29	4
Oatmeal Instant Original	1 oz	100	0	15	22	—
Puffed Corn	1 cup (0.8 oz)	80	0	0	16	1
Puffed Kamut	1 cup (0.6 oz)	50	0	0	11	2
Puffed Millet	1 cup (0.9 oz)	90	1	0	19	1
Puffed Rice	1 cup (0.8 oz)	90	0	0	19	1
Puffed Wheat	1 cup (0.9)	90	1	0	20	2
Rice & Shine	¼ cup (1.5 oz)	150	1	0	32	2
Spelt Flakes	1 cup (1.1 oz)	100	1	60	22	3
Wheat Flakes Rolled	⅓ cup (1.2 oz)	110	1	0	24	5
Aunt Jemima						
Enriched White Hominy Grits Regular	3 tbsp	101	tr	1	22	1
Betty Crocker						
Dutch Apple	1 cup (1.9 oz)	220	2	330	47	1
Streusel	¾ cup (1 oz)	120	2	170	25	1
Cap'n Crunch						
Crunchberries	¾ cup	113	2	247	24	1
Original	¾ cup	113	2	241	24	1
Peanut Butter Crunch	¾ cup	119	3	281	22	1
Erewhon						
Aztec	1 oz	100	0	85	24	1
Barley Plus	1 oz	110	1	0	22	1
Brown Rice Cream	1 oz	110	1	20	23	—
Crispy Brown Rice	1 oz	110	1	185	24	4
Fruit 'n Wheat	1 oz	100	1	75	21	3
Oat Bran With Toasted Wheat Germ	1 oz	115	2	15	18	3
Oatmeal Instant Apple Cinnamon	1.25 oz	145	3	100	25	—
Oatmeal Instant Apple Raisin	1.3 oz	150	3	100	27	—

FOOD	PORTION	CAL.	FAT	SOD.	CARB.	FIB.
Erewhon (CONT.)						
Oatmeal Instant Dates & Walnuts	1.2 oz	130	3	60	24	3
Oatmeal Instant Maple Spice	1.2 oz	140	3	100	24	—
Oatmeal Instant With Added Oat Bran	1.25 oz	125	3	0	23	4
Raisin Bran	1 oz	100	0	80	22	3
Super-O's	1 oz	110	0	5	24	4
Wheat Flakes	1 oz	100	0	75	22	4
Estee						
Corn Flakes	1 pkg (1 oz)	90	0	310	24	4
Raisin Bran	1 pkg (1 oz)	90	1	100	21	3
General Mills						
Apple Cinnamon Cheerios	¾ cup (1 oz)	120	2	160	25	1
Basic 4	1 cup (1.9 oz)	200	2	320	43	3
Berry Berry Kix	¾ cup (1 oz)	120	2	180	26	0
Body Buddies Natural Fruit	1 cup (1 oz)	120	2	290	26	0
Booberry	1 cup (1 oz)	120	1	220	27	0
Cheerios	1 cup (1 oz)	110	2	280	22	3
Cinnamon Grahams	¾ cup (1 oz)	120	1	240	26	1
Cinnamon Toast Crunch	¾ cup (1 oz)	130	4	210	24	1
Cocoa Puffs	1 cup (1 oz)	120	1	190	27	0
Cookie Crisp	1 cup (1 oz)	120	2	115	25	0
Corn Chex	1 cup (1 oz)	110	0	300	26	0
Count Chocula	1 cup (1 oz)	120	1	180	26	0
Country Corn Flakes	1 cup (1 oz)	120	1	290	26	0
Crispy Wheaties 'n Raisins	1 cup (1.9 oz)	190	1	270	44	4
Fiber One	½ cup (1 oz)	60	1	135	24	13
Frankenberry	1 cup (1 oz)	120	1	210	27	0
French Toast Crunch	¾ cup (1 oz)	120	2	170	26	0
Frosted Cheerios	1 cup (1 oz)	120	1	210	25	1
Golden Grahams	¾ cup (1 oz)	120	1	280	25	1
Honey Frosted Wheaties	¾ cup (1 oz)	110	1	200	27	0
Honey Nut Cheerios	1 cup (1 oz)	120	2	270	24	2
Honey Nut Clusters	1 cup (1.9 oz)	210	3	270	46	3
Jurassic Park Crunch	1 cup (1 oz)	120	1	200	26	1
Kaboom	1¼ cup (1 oz)	120	2	280	24	1
Kix	1 ⅓ cup (1 oz)	120	1	270	26	1
Lucky Charms	1 cup (1 oz)	120	1	210	25	1
Multi-Bran Chex	1 cup (2 oz)	200	2	360	49	7

FOOD	PORTION	CAL.	FAT	SOD.	CARB.	FIB.
General Mills (CONT.)						
Multi-Grain Cheerios	1 cup (1 oz)	110	1	210	24	3
Oatmeal Crisp Almond	1 cup (1.9 oz)	220	5	250	42	4
Oatmeal Crisp Apple Cinnamon	1 cup (1.9 oz)	210	2	280	46	4
Oatmeal Crisp Raisin	1 cup (1.9 oz)	210	3	210	44	3
Raisin Nut Bran	¾ cup (1.9 oz)	200	4	250	41	5
Reese's Peanut Butter Puffs	¾ cup (1 oz)	130	3	210	24	0
Rice Chex	1¼ cup (1.1 oz)	120	0	280	27	0
S'Mores Grahams	¾ cup (1 oz)	120	1	370	26	0
Sun Crunchers	1 cup (1.9 oz)	220	3	370	45	2
Team Cheerios	1 cup (1 oz)	120	1	220	25	1
Total Corn Flakes	1 ⅓ cup (1 oz)	110	1	210	25	0
Total Raisin Bran	1 cup (1.9 oz)	180	1	240	43	5
Total Whole Grain	¾ cup (1 oz)	110	1	200	24	3
Trix	1 cup (1 oz)	120	2	200	26	1
Wheat Chex	1 cup (1.9 oz)	180	1	420	41	5
Wheat Hearts not prep	¼ cup (1.3 oz)	130	1	0	26	2
Wheaties	1 cup (1 oz)	110	1	220	24	3
Glenny's						
Maple Frosted Corn	1 oz	109	tr	50	20	—
Oat Mini Puffs	1 oz	108	tr	30	22	—
Oat Mini Puffs No Salt No Sugar	1 oz	108	tr	7	22	—
Rice Mini Puffs	1 oz	109	tr	30	20	—
Good Shepherd						
Millet Rice Flakes Wheat Free	1 oz	95	1	30	19	1
Spelt	1 oz	90	tr	0	20	3
Spelt Flakes	1 oz	100	6	80	21	2
Grist Mill						
Apple Cinnamon Natural	½ cup (1.9 oz)	260	10	20	36	3
Bran	½ cup (1.9 oz)	250	8	40	37	11
Oat & Honey Natural	½ cup (1.9 oz)	270	12	10	34	4
Oat Honey & Raisin Natural	½ cup (1.9 oz)	260	10	10	35	4
H-O						
Farina Instant	1 pkg	110	0	235	22	3
Farina not prep	3 tbsp	120	0	0	26	3
Oatmeal Instant	½ cup	130	2	<5	22	3
Oatmeal Instant	1 pkg	110	2	230	18	3
Oatmeal Instant Apple Cinnamon	1 pkg	130	2	220	26	3

FOOD	PORTION	CAL.	FAT	SOD.	CARB.	FIB.
H-O (CONT.)						
Oatmeal Instant Maple Brown Sugar	1 pkg	160	2	285	32	3
Oatmeal Instant Raisin & Spice	1 pkg	150	2	140	32	3
Oatmeal Instant Sweet 'n Mellow	1 pkg	150	2	270	30	3
Oats 'n Fiber	⅓ cup	100	2	5	15	3
Oats 'n Fiber	1 pkg	110	2	140	18	3
Oats 'n Fiber Apple & Bran	1 pkg	130	2	140	26	3
Oats 'n Fiber Raisin & Bran	1 pkg	150	2	140	32	3
Oats Gourmet	⅓ cup	100	2	0	18	3
Oats Quick	½ cup	130	2	<5	22	3
Health Valley						
100% Natural Bran With Apples & Cinnamon	¼ cup (1 oz)	100	1	10	22	5
Blue Corn Flakes 100% Organic	½ cup (1 oz)	90	tr	10	19	3
Bran Cereal With Dates 100% Organic	¼ cup (1 oz)	100	1	5	20	5
Bran Cereal With Raisins 100% Organic	¼ cup (1 oz)	100	1	5	20	5
Fiber 7 Flakes 100% Organic	½ cup (1 oz)	90	tr	0	20	5
Fiber 7 Flakes With Raisins 100% Organic	½ cup (1 oz)	90	tr	0	20	5
Fruit & Fitness	1 cup (2 oz)	220	4	5	37	11
Fruit Lites Corn	½ cup (0.5 oz)	45	0	2	10	tr
Fruit Lites Rice	½ cup (0.5 oz)	45	1	2	11	tr
Fruit Lites Wheat	½ cup (0.5 oz)	45	1	2	11	2
Healthy Crunch Almond Date	¼ cup (1 oz)	110	3	5	18	4
Healthy Crunch Apple Cinnamon	¼ cup (1 oz)	110	3	10	18	4
Healthy O's 100% Organic	¾ cup (1 oz)	90	1	1	18	3
Lites Puffed Corn	½ cup (1 oz)	50	0	0	11	tr
Lites Puffed Rice	½ cup (1 oz)	50	0	0	12	tr
Lites Puffed Wheat	½ cup (1 oz)	50	0	0	11	1
Oat Bran Flakes 100% Organic	½ cup (1 oz)	100	tr	0	20	4

FOOD	PORTION	CAL.	FAT	SOD.	CARB.	FIB.
Health Valley (CONT.)						
Oat Bran Flakes Almonds/Dates 100% Organic	½ cup (1 oz)	100	tr	0	20	4
Oat Bran Flakes With Raisins 100% Organic	½ cup (1 oz)	100	tr	0	20	4
Oat Bran Natural Apples & Cinnamon	¼ cup (1 oz)	100	tr	10	19	4
Oat Bran Natural Raisins & Spice	¼ cup	100	tr	10	19	4
Oat Bran O's 100% Organic	½ cup (1 oz)	110	tr	0	20	3
Oat Bran O's Fruit & Nuts	½ cup (1 oz)	110	3	0	19	3
Orangeola Almonds & Dates	¼ cup	110	3	5	18	4
Orangeola Bananas & Hawaiian Fruit	¼ cup (1 oz)	120	4	10	20	4
Raisin Bran Flakes 100% Organic	½ cup (1 oz)	100	tr	5	21	6
Real Oat Bran Almond Crunch	¼ cup (1 oz)	110	3	2	17	4
Real Oat Bran Hawaiian Fruit	¼ cup (1 oz)	130	3	2	22	5
Real Oat Bran Raisin Nut	¼ cup (1 oz)	130	3	2	21	5
Rice Bran O's	½ cup	110	1	5	22	2
Rice Bran With Almonds & Dates	½ cup (1 oz)	110	3	2	19	2
Sprouts 7 Bananas & Hawaiian Fruit	¼ cup (1 oz)	90	1	5	16	4
Sprouts 7 Raisin	¼ cup	90	1	5	16	5
Swiss Breakfast Raisin Nut	¼ cup (1 oz)	100	3	10	19	3
Swiss Breakfast Tropical Fruit	¼ cup (1 oz)	100	3	10	19	3
Healthy Choice						
Multi-Grain Flakes	1 cup (1.1 oz)	100	0	210	26	3
Multi-Grain Raisins & Almonds	1¼ cup (2 oz)	200	2	240	44	4
Multi-Grain Squares	1¼ cup (2 oz)	190	1	0	45	6
Heartland						
Coconut	1 oz	130	5	80	18	2
Plain	1 oz	130	4	80	18	2
Raisin	1 oz	130	4	80	18	2

FOOD	PORTION	CAL.	FAT	SOD.	CARB.	FIB.
Kashi						
5-Bran	2½ oz	281	6	13	47	16
Brittles Sesame/Maple	3½ oz	473	19	85	65	—
Cereal	2 oz	177	1	5	38	5
Puffed	¾ oz	74	1	2	16	2
Kellogg's						
All-Bran	½ cup (1 oz)	80	1	280	22	10
All-Bran With Extra Fiber	½ cup (1 oz)	50	1	150	22	15
Apple Cinnamon Rice Krispies	¾ cup (1 oz)	110	0	220	27	1
Apple Cinnamon Squares	¾ cup (1.9 oz)	180	1	15	44	0
Apple Jacks	1 cup (1 oz)	110	0	135	26	1
Apple Raisin Crisp	1 cup (1.9 oz)	180	0	340	46	4
Blueberry Squares	¾ cup (1.9 oz)	180	1	15	44	5
Bran Buds	⅓ cup (1 oz)	70	1	210	24	11
Cinnamon Mini Buns	¾ cup (1 oz)	120	1	210	27	1
Cocoa Krispies	¾ cup (1 oz)	120	1	190	27	0
Common Sense Oat Bran	¾ cup (1 oz)	110	1	270	23	4
Complete Bran Flakes	¾ cup (1 oz)	100	1	230	25	5
Corn Flakes	1 cup (1 oz)	110	0	330	26	1
Corn Pops	1 cup (1 oz)	110	0	95	27	1
Cracklin' Oat Bran	¾ cup (1.9 oz)	230	8	180	40	6
Crispix	1 cup (1 oz)	110	0	230	26	1
Double Dip Crunch	¾ cup (1 oz)	110	0	160	27	0
Froot Loops	1 cup (1 oz)	120	1	150	26	1
Frosted Bran	¾ cup (1 oz)	100	0	200	26	3
Frosted Flakes	¾ cup (1 oz)	120	0	200	28	0
Frosted Krispies	¾ cup (1 oz)	110	0	230	27	0
Frosted Mini-Wheats	1 cup (1.9 oz)	190	1	0	45	6
Frosted Mini-Wheats Bite Size	1 cup (1.9 oz)	190	1	0	45	6
Fruitful Bran	1¼ cup (1.9 oz)	170	1	330	44	6
Fruity Marshmallow Krispies	¾ cups (1 oz)	110	0	180	27	0
Just Right Crunchy Nuggets	1 cup (1.9 oz)	200	2	340	46	3
Just Right Fruit & Nut	1 cup (1.9 oz)	210	2	260	46	3
Mueslix Golden Crunch	¾ cup (1.9 oz)	210	5	280	40	6
Nut & Honey Crunch	1¼ cup (1.9 oz)	220	4	370	45	1
Oatbake Raisin Nut	⅓ cup (1 oz)	110	3	190	21	3
Pop-Tart Crunch Frosted Brown Sugar Cinnamon	¾ cup (1 oz)	120	1	160	26	0

FOOD	PORTION	CAL.	FAT	SOD.	CARB.	FIB.
Kellogg's (CONT.)						
Pop-Tart Crunch Frosted Strawberry	¾ cup (1 oz)	120	1	125	27	0
Product 19	1 cup (1 oz)	110	0	280	25	1
Raisin Bran	1 cup (1.9 oz)	170	1	310	43	7
Raisin Squares	¾ cup (1.9 oz)	180	1	0	44	5
Rice Krispies	1¼ cup (1 oz)	110	0	320	26	1
Special K	1 cup (1 oz)	110	0	250	21	1
Strawberry Squares	¾ cup (1.9 oz)	180	1	10	44	5
Temptations French Vanilla Almond	¾ cup (1 oz)	120	2	210	24	1
Temptations Honey Roasted Pecan	1 cup (1 oz)	120	3	240	24	0
Kolln						
Crispy Oats	1 cup (1.8 oz)	190	3	210	40	2
Oat Bran Crunch	⅔ cup (2.1 oz)	220	5	0	41	9
Oat Muesli Fruit	¾ cup (2 oz)	200	5	15	39	4
LaLoma						
Ruskets Biscuits	2 biscuits (30 g)	110	0	95	22	—
Life						
Cinnamon	⅔ cup	101	2	182	19	3
Original	⅔ cup	101	2	186	19	3
Little Crow						
Coco Wheat	3 tbsp (36 g)	130	1	12	28	4
Maltex						
Cereal	1 oz	105	1	0	21	3
Maypo						
30 Second	1 oz	100	1	0	19	2
Vermont Style	1 oz	105	1	0	20	2
With Oat Bran	1 oz	130	2	1	26	4
McCann's						
Irish Oatmeal	1 oz	110	2	0	20	3
Morning Traditions						
Banana Nut Crunch	1 cup (2 oz)	250	6	240	43	4
Blueberry Morning	1¼ cup (1.9 oz)	220	3	250	43	2
Cranberry Almond Crunch	1 cup (1.9 oz)	220	3	200	44	3
Great Grains Crunchy Pecan	⅔ cup (1.9 oz)	220	6	190	38	4
Great Grains Raisins Dates & Pecans	⅔ cup (1.9 oz)	210	5	160	39	4
Mother's						
Oatmeal Instant	½ cup (1.4 oz)	150	3	0	27	4
Whole Wheat Natural	½ cup (1.4 oz)	130	1	0	30	4

FOOD	PORTION	CAL.	FAT	SOD.	CARB.	FIB.
Mueslix						
Crispy Blend	⅔ cup (1.9 oz)	200	2	190	42	4
Nabisco						
100% Bran	⅓ cup (1 oz)	80	1	120	23	8
Cream Of Rice	1 oz	100	0	0	23	—
Cream Of Wheat Instant as prep	1 cup	120	0	0	25	1
Cream Of Wheat Quick as prep	1 cup	120	0	—	25	1
Cream Of Wheat Regular as prep	1 cup	120	0	0	25	1
Frosted Shredded Wheat Bite Size	1 cup (1.8 oz)	190	1	10	44	5
Honey Nut Shredded Wheat Bite Size	1 cup (1.8 oz)	200	2	40	43	4
Mix'n Eat Cream Of Wheat Apple & Cinnamon	1 pkg (1¼ oz)	130	0	250	29	1
Mix'n Eat Cream Of Wheat Brown Sugar Cinnamon	1 pkg (1¼ oz)	130	0	230	29	1
Mix'n Eat Cream Of Wheat Maple Brown Sugar	1 pkg (1¼ oz)	130	0	180	29	1
Mix'n Eat Cream Of Wheat Our Original	1 pkg (1¼ oz)	100	0	170	21	1
Original Shredded Wheat	2 biscuits (1.6 oz)	160	1	0	38	5
Original Shredded Wheat 'N Bran	1¼ cup (2.1 oz)	200	1	0	47	8
Original Shredded Wheat Spoon Size	1 cup (1.7 oz)	170	1	0	41	5
Nut & Honey						
Crunch O's	¾ cup (1 oz)	120	3	200	23	2
Nutri-Grain						
Almond Raisin	1¼ cup (2 oz)	200	3	200	43	4
Golden Wheat	¾ cup (1.1 oz)	100	1	220	24	4
Golden Wheat & Raisin	1¼ cup (2 oz)	180	1	280	45	6
Pillsbury						
Farina	⅔ cup	80	tr	170	17	—
Post						
Alpha-Bits	1 cup (1 oz)	130	2	210	27	1
Bran Flakes	¾ cup (1 oz)	100	1	220	24	5
Cocoa Pebbles	¾ cup (1 oz)	120	1	160	26	0
Fruit & Fibre Dates Raisins & Walnuts	1 cup (1.9 oz)	210	3	250	42	5

FOOD	PORTION	CAL.	FAT	SOD.	CARB.	FIB.
Post (CONT.)						
Fruit & Fibre Peaches Raisins & Almonds	1 cup (1.9 oz)	210	3	260	42	5
Fruity Pebbles	¾ cup (1 oz)	110	1	160	24	0
Golden Crisp	¾ cup (1 oz)	110	0	40	25	0
Grape-Nuts	½ cup (2 oz)	200	1	350	47	5
Grape-Nuts	¼ cup (1 oz)	100	1	140	24	3
Honey Bunches Of Oats	¾ cup (1 oz)	120	2	190	25	1
Honey Bunches Of Oats With Almonds	¾ cup (1.1 oz)	130	3	180	24	1
Honeycomb	1⅓ cups (1 oz)	110	1	220	26	tr
Marshmallow Alpha-Bits	1 cup (1 oz)	120	1	160	25	0
Post Toasties	1 cup (1 oz)	100	0	270	24	1
Raisin Bran	1 cup (2 oz)	190	1	300	47	8
Waffle Crisp	1 cup (1 oz)	130	3	120	24	0
Pritikin						
Apple Raisin Spice	1 pkg (1.6 oz)	170	3	5	34	—
Multigrain	1 pkg	160	2	0	33	—
Quaker						
100% Natural	¼ cup	127	6	14	18	2
100% Natural Apples & Cinnamon	¼ cup	126	5	13	19	2
100% Natural Raisin & Date	¼ cup	123	5	14	18	2
Crunchy Bran	⅔ cup	89	1	316	23	5
Crunchy Nut Oh!s	1 cup	127	4	164	22	1
Enriched White Hominy Grits Quick	3 tbsp	101	tr	1	22	1
Enriched Yellow Hominy Quick Grits	3 tbsp	101	tr	1	22	1
Honey Graham Oh!s	1 cup	122	3	217	23	1
Instant Grits White Hominy	1 pkg	79	tr	440	18	1
Instant Grits With Imitation Bacon Bits	1 pkg	101	tr	590	22	2
Instant Grits With Imitation Ham Bits	1 pkg	99	tr	800	21	2
Instant Grits With Real Cheddar Cheese	1 pkg	104	1	497	22	1
King Vitaman	1½ cup	110	1	280	23	1
Multigrain	½ cup	130	2	10	29	5
Oat Squares	½ cup	105	2	159	21	2
Oatmeal Instant	1 pkg (1.2 oz)	130	3	95	22	3

FOOD	PORTION	CAL.	FAT	SOD.	CARB.	FIB.
Quaker (CONT.)						
Oatmeal Instant Apples & Cinnamon	1 pkg (1.2 oz)	130	2	105	26	3
Oatmeal Instant Cinnamon Graham Cookie	1 pkg (1.4 oz)	150	3	170	30	3
Oatmeal Instant Cinnamon Spice	1 pkg (1.6 oz)	170	2	290	36	3
Oatmeal Instant Cinnamon Toast	1 pkg (1.2 oz)	130	2	160	27	2
Oatmeal Instant Fruit & Cream Blueberry	1 pkg (1.2 oz)	130	3	140	27	2
Oatmeal Instant Honey Nut	1 pkg (1.2 oz)	130	3	210	25	2
Oatmeal Instant Kids Choice Radical Raspberry	1 pkg (1.4 oz)	150	3	170	29	3
Oatmeal Instant Maple Brown Sugar	1 pkg (1.5 oz)	160	2	240	33	3
Oatmeal Instant Peaches & Cream	1 pkg (1.2 oz)	130	2	150	27	2
Oatmeal Instant Raisin & Walnut	1 pkg (1.3 oz)	140	3	160	27	3
Oatmeal Instant Raisin Date Walnut	1 pkg (1.3 oz)	130	3	240	27	3
Oatmeal Instant Raisin Spice	1 pkg (1.5 oz)	160	2	250	32	3
Oatmeal Instant Strawberries & Cream	1 pkg (1.2 oz)	130	2	160	27	2
Oatmeal Instant Strawberries 'N Stuff	1 pkg (1.4 oz)	150	2	170	30	3
Oats Old Fashion	½ cup	150	3	0	27	4
Oats Quick	½ cup	150	3	0	27	4
Popeye Sweet Crunch	1 cup	113	2	254	24	1
Puffed Rice	1 cup	54	tr	1	13	tr
Puffed Wheat	1 cup	50	tr	1	11	1
Shredded Wheat	2 biscuits	132	1	1	32	4
Ralston						
Almond Delight	1 cup (1.8 oz)	210	3	410	41	4
Bran Flakes	¾ cup (1.1 oz)	110	1	220	24	5
Chex Multi-Bran	1¼ cup (2 oz)	220	2	320	46	7
Cocoa Crispy Rice	1 cup (1.8 oz)	200	1	340	45	tr
Cocoa Crunchies	¾ cup (1.1 oz)	120	1	170	26	0
Cookie Crisp	1 cup (1 oz)	120	2	110	25	0

FOOD	PORTION	CAL.	FAT	SOD.	CARB.	FIB.
Ralston (CONT.)						
Corn Flakes	1¼ cup (1.1 oz)	120	0	280	27	1
Crisp Crunch	¾ cup (1.1 oz)	120	1	240	26	tr
Crisp Rice	1¼ cup (1.2 oz)	130	0	330	28	0
Frosted Flakes	¾ cup (1.1 oz)	120	0	180	28	1
Fruit Rings	¾ cup (0.9 oz)	100	1	115	23	0
Magic Stair	¾ cup (1.1 oz)	120	1	160	26	tr
Muesli Blueberry	1 cup (1.9 oz)	200	3	170	41	4
Muesli Cranberry	¾ cup (1.9 oz)	200	3	180	40	4
Muesli Peach	¾ cup (1.9 oz)	200	3	170	39	4
Muesli Raspberry	¾ cup (2 oz)	220	3	170	44	4
Muesli Strawberry	1 cup (1.9 oz)	210	3	170	41	4
Multi Vitamin Whole Grain Flakes	1 cup (1.1 oz)	120	1	300	25	3
Nutty Nuggets	½ cup (1.7 oz)	180	2	220	38	5
Raisin Bran	¾ cup (1.9 oz)	190	1	290	41	6
Tasteeos	1¼ cup (1.1 oz)	130	3	260	22	3
Tasteeos Apple Cinnamon	1 cup (1.2 oz)	130	2	150	27	1
Tasteeos Honey Nut	1 cup (1.2 oz)	130	2	250	28	1
Rice Krispies						
Treats	¾ cup (1 oz)	120	1	170	25	0
Roman Meal						
Apple Cinnamon	1.2 oz	105	2	6	18	6
Cream Of Rye	1.3 oz	111	1	2	20	5
Oats Wheat Dates Raisins Almonds	1.3 oz	129	2	3	24	3
Oats Wheat Honey Coconuts Almonds	1.3 oz	155	5	8	22	3
Original	1 oz	83	1	tr	15	5
Original With Oats	1.2 oz	108	1	1	19	5
Smacks						
Cereal	¾ cup (1 oz)	110	1	75	26	1
Stone-Buhr						
4 Grain	⅓ cup (1.6 oz)	140	2	0	31	5
7 Grain	⅓ cup (1.6 oz)	140	2	0	31	7
Bran Flakes	¼ cup (0.6 oz)	64	0	160	14	2
Cracked Wheat	¼ cup (2.4 oz)	210	1	0	48	6
Manna Golden	6 tsp (1.6 oz)	160	0	0	35	1
Rolled Oats Old Fashion	6 tsp (1.6 oz)	150	3	0	28	5
Scotch Oats	¼ cup (1.6 oz)	150	4	0	28	4
Sunbelt						
Muesli	1.9 oz	210	2	70	44	3

FOOD	PORTION	CAL.	FAT	SOD.	CARB.	FIB.
US Mills						
Poppets	1 oz	110	1	10	24	1
Uncle Sam	1 oz	110	1	65	20	7
Uncle Roy's						
Muesli Swiss Style	½ cup (1.6 oz)	170	5	20	32	3
Weetabix						
Cereal	2 (1.3 oz)	142	1	—	31	3
Wheatena						
Cereal	⅓ cup (1.4 oz)	150	1	0	32	5

CEREAL BARS
(*see also* GRANOLA BARS, NUTRITIONAL SUPPLEMENTS)

FOOD	PORTION	CAL.	FAT	SOD.	CARB.	FIB.
Cap'n Crunch						
Bar	1 (0.8 oz)	90	2	105	17	—
Berries Bar	1 (0.8 oz)	90	2	110	17	—
Rice Krispies						
Treats	1 bar (0.8 oz)	90	2	105	17	0
Treats Chocolate Chip	1 (1 oz)	120	4	60	20	[illegible]

CHAMPAGNE

FOOD	PORTION	CAL.	FAT	SOD.	CARB.	FIB.
sekt german champagne	3.5 fl oz	84	0	—	5	–
Andre						
Blush	1 fl oz	22	0	1	1	—
Brut	1 fl oz	21	0	1	1	—
Cold Duck	1 fl oz	25	0	1	2	—
Extra Dry	1 fl oz	23	0	1	1	—
Ballatore						
Spumante	1 fl oz	23	0	2	2	—
Eden Roc						
Brut	1 fl oz	21	0	1	1	—
Brut Rosé	1 fl oz	22	0	1	2	—
Extra Dry	1 fl oz	21	0	1	1	—
Tott's						
Blanc de Noir	1 fl oz	22	0	1	2	—
Brut	1 fl oz	20	0	1	tr	—
Extra Dry	1 fl oz	21	0	1	1	—

CHAYOTE

FOOD	PORTION	CAL.	FAT	SOD.	CARB.	FIB.
fresh cooked	1 cup	38	1	1	8	—
raw	1 (7 oz)	49	1	8	11	—
raw cut up	1 cup	32	tr	198	7	—

CHEESE
(*see also* CHEESE DISHES, CHEESE SUBSTITUTES, COTTAGE CHEESE, CREAM CHEESE)

FOOD	PORTION	CAL.	FAT	SOD.	CARB.	FIB.
american	1 oz	93	7	337	2	—

FOOD	PORTION	CAL.	FAT	SOD.	CARB.	FIB.
american cheese food	1 pkg (8 oz)	745	56	2700	17	—
american cheese spread	1 jar (5 oz)	412	30	1910	12	—
american cold pack	1 pkg (8 oz)	752	56	2193	19	—
american cheese spread	1 oz	82	6	381	2	—
bel paese	3½ oz	391	30	—	0	—
blue	1 oz	100	8	396	1	—
blue crumbled	1 cup (4.7 oz)	477	39	1884	3	—
brick	1 oz	105	8	159	1	—
brie	1 oz	95	8	178	tr	—
cacio di roma sheep's milk cheese	1 oz	130	10	170	0	—
caerphilly	1.4 oz	150	13	—	0	0
camembert	1 oz	85	7	239	tr	—
camembert	1 wedge (1 ⅓ oz)	114	9	320	tr	—
caraway	1 oz	107	8	196	1	—
cheddar	1 oz	114	9	176	tr	—
cheddar low fat	1 oz	49	2	174	1	—
cheddar low sodium	1 oz	113	9	6	1	—
cheddar reduced fat	1.4 oz	104	6	—	0	0
cheddar shredded	1 cup	455	37	701	1	—
cheshire	1 oz	110	9	198	1	—
cheshire reduced fat	1.4 oz	108	6	—	tr	0
colby	1 oz	112	9	171	1	—
colby low fat	1 oz	49	2	174	1	—
colby low sodium	1 oz	113	9	6	1	—
derby	1.4 oz	161	14	—	0	0
edam	1 oz	101	8	274	tr	—
edam reduced fat	1.4 oz	92	4	—	tr	0
emmentaler	3½ oz	403	30	450	tr	—
feta	1 oz	75	6	316	1	—
fontina	1 oz	110	9	—	tr	—
fromage frais	1.6 oz	51	3	—	3	0
gjetost	1 oz	132	8	170	12	—
gloucester double	1.4 oz	162	14	—	0	0
goat hard	1 oz	128	10	98	1	—
goat semisoft	1 oz	103	8	146	1	—
goat soft	1 oz	76	6	104	tr	—
gorgonzola	3½ oz	376	31	—	1	—
gouda	1 oz	101	8	232	1	—
gruyere	1 oz	117	9	95	tr	—
lancashire	1.4 oz	149	12	—	0	0
leicester	1.4 oz	160	14	—	0	0
limburger	1 oz	93	8	227	tr	—
lymeswold	1.4 oz	170	16	—	tr	0

FOOD	PORTION	CAL.	FAT	SOD.	CARB.	FIB.
monterey	1 oz	106	9	152	tr	—
mozzarella	1 oz	80	6	106	1	—
mozzarella	1 lb	1276	98	1692	10	—
mozzarella low moisture	1 oz	90	7	118	1	—
mozzarella low moisture part skim	1 oz	79	5	150	1	—
mozzarella part skim	1 oz	72	5	132	1	—
muenster	1 oz	104	9	178	tr	—
parmesan grated	1 tbsp (5 g)	23	2	93	tr	—
parmesan grated	1 oz	129	9	528	1	—
parmesan hard	1 oz	111	7	454	1	—
pimento	1 oz	106	9	405	tr	—
port du salut	1 oz	100	8	151	tr	—
provolone	1 oz	100	8	248	1	—
quark 20% fat	3½ oz	116	5	35	3	—
quark 40% fat	3½ oz	167	11	34	3	—
quark made w/ skim milk	3½ oz	78	tr	40	4	—
queso anego	1 oz	106	9	321	1	—
queso asadero	1 oz	101	8	186	1	—
queso chichuahua	1 oz	106	8	175	2	—
ricotta part skim	1 cup (8.6 oz)	340	19	307	13	—
ricotta part skim	½ cup (4.4 oz)	171	10	155	6	—
ricotta whole milk	½ cup (4.4 oz)	216	16	104	4	—
ricotta whole milk	1 cup (8.6 oz)	428	32	207	7	—
romadur 40% fat	3½ oz	289	20	—	tr	—
romano	1 oz	110	8	340	1	—
roquefort	1 oz	105	9	513	1	—
stilton blue	1.4 oz	164	14	—	0	0
stilton white	1.4 oz	145	13	—	0	0
swiss	1 oz	107	8	74	1	—
swiss cheese food	1 pkg (8 oz)	734	55	3523	10	—
swiss processed	1 oz	95	7	388	1	—
tilsit	1 oz	96	7	213	1	—
wensleydale	1.4 oz	151	13	—	0	0
whey cheese	3.5 oz	440	27	511	33	0
yogurt cheese	1 oz	20	0	—	—	—
Alouette						
Brie Baby	1 oz	110	9	180	2	0
Brie Baby With Herbs	1 oz	110	9	180	2	0
French Onion	2 tbsp (0.8 oz)	70	7	160	1	0
Garlic	2 tbsp (0.8 oz)	70	7	135	1	0
Light Dill	2 tbsp (0.8 oz)	50	4	120	2	0
Light Garlic	2 tbsp (0.8 oz)	50	4	120	1	1
Light Herb	2 tbsp (0.8 oz)	50	4	125	2	0

FOOD	PORTION	CAL.	FAT	SOD.	CARB.	FIB.
Alouette (CONT.)						
Light Herbs & Garlic	2 tbsp (0.8 oz)	50	4	120	1	0
Light Spring Vegetable	2 tbsp (0.8 oz)	50	4	110	1	0
Salmon	2 tbsp (0.8 oz)	60	5	95	1	0
Scallions	2 tbsp (0.8 oz)	70	7	120	1	0
Spinach	2 tbsp (0.8 oz)	60	6	85	1	0
Alpine Lace						
American	1 slice (0.66 oz)	50	3	260	1	0
American Fat Free	1 piece (1 oz)	45	tr	280	2	0
American Hot Pepper Less Fat Less Sodium	1 piece (1 oz)	80	20	260	2	0
American Less Fat Less Sodium	1 piece (1 oz)	80	6	200	2	0
Cheddar Fat Free	1 piece (1 oz)	45	tr	280	2	0
Cheddar Reduced Fat	1 piece (1 oz)	80	5	135	1	0
Colby Reduced Fat	1 piece (1 oz)	80	5	115	1	0
Fat Free For Parmesan Lovers	2 tsp (5 g)	10	0	65	0	0
Fat Free Mexican Macho	2 tbsp (1 oz)	30	tr	165	1	0
Fat Free Singles	1 slice (0.66 oz)	25	0	280	tr	0
Feta Reduced Fat	1 piece (1 oz)	60	4	370	1	0
Goat	1 oz	40	3	130	tr	—
Mozzarella Fat Free	1 piece (1 oz)	45	tr	280	2	0
Mozzarella Reduced Sodium Part Skim	1 piece (1 oz)	70	5	75	1	0
Muenster Reduced Sodium	1 piece (1 oz)	100	9	85	1	0
Provolone Smoked Reduced Fat	1 piece (1 oz)	70	5	120	1	0
Swiss Reduced Fat	1 piece (1 oz)	90	6	35	1	0
Armour						
Cheddar	1 oz	110	9	—	—	—
Cheddar Lower Salt	1 oz	110	9	106	—	—
Colby Lower Salt	1 oz	110	9	—	—	—
Monterey Jack	1 oz	110	9	—	—	—
Monterey Jack Lower Salt	1 oz	110	9	111	—	—
BabyBel						
Mini Light	1 (0.7 oz)	45	3	180	0	0
Bongrain						
Chavrie	2 tbsp (0.8 oz)	40	3	110	1	0
Montrachet	1 oz	70	6	135	tr	0
Montrachet Chive	1 oz	70	6	135	tr	0
Montrachet Classic	1 oz	70	6	130	tr	0

FOOD	PORTION	CAL.	FAT	SOD.	CARB.	FIB.
Bongrain (CONT.)						
Montrachet Classic Herb	1 oz	70	6	150	tr	0
Montrachet Herbs & Garlic	1 oz	70	6	150	tr	0
Montrachet In Oil drained	1 oz	70	6	130	tr	0
Montrachet With Ash	1 oz	70	6	125	tr	0
Borden						
American Slices	1 oz	110	9	490	1	—
American Very Sharp	1 oz	110	9	490	1	—
Lite Line Mozzarella	1 oz	50	2	—	—	—
Lite Line Sharp Cheddar	1 oz	50	2	—	—	—
Lite Line Swiss	1 oz	50	2	—	—	—
Swiss Slices	1 oz	100	8	380	1	—
Breakstone's						
Ricotta	¼ cup (2.2 oz)	110	8	90	3	0
Bresse						
Brie	1 oz	110	9	180	2	0
Brie Light	1 oz	70	4	160	1	tr
Brie With Herbs	1 oz	110	9	180	2	0
Creme De Brie	2 tbsp (1 oz)	90	8	220	tr	0
Creme De Brie Herb	2 tbsp (1 oz)	90	8	220	tr	0
Brier Run						
Chevre	1 oz	61	5	70	—	—
Quark	1 oz	34	3	15	—	—
Bristol Gold						
Cheddar Light	1 oz	70	4	150	3	—
French Onion Light	1 oz	70	4	150	3	—
Garlic & Herb Light	1 oz	70	4	150	3	—
Horseradish Light	1 oz	70	4	150	3	—
Smoke Light	1 oz	70	4	150	3	—
Wine Light	1 oz	70	4	150	3	—
Cabot						
Cheddar	1 oz	110	9	175	0	—
Mediterranean Cheddar		110	9	180	1	0
Monterey Jack	1 oz	80	5	200	1	—
Vermont Cheddar 50% Light	1 oz	70	5	170	1	0
Vitalait	1 oz	70	4	170	1	—
Vitalait Jalapeno	1 oz	70	4	170	1	—
Cheez Whiz						
Light	2 tbsp (1.2 oz)	80	3	540	6	0
Churney						
Diet Snack Cheddar Flavored	1 oz	70	3	—	—	—

FOOD	PORTION	CAL.	FAT	SOD.	CARB.	FIB.
Churney (CONT.)						
Diet Snack Port Wine Flavored	1 oz	70	3	—	—	—
Feta	1 oz	80	6	320	tr	0
Cracker Barrel						
Baby Swiss	1 oz	110	9	110	0	0
Cheddar Extra Sharp	1 oz	120	10	180	0	0
Cheddar Marbled Sharp	1 oz	110	9	180	tr	0
Cheddar New York Aged	1 oz	120	10	180	0	0
Cheddar Sharp	1 oz	120	10	180	0	0
Cheddar Vermont Sharp	1 oz	110	9	180	tr	0
Reduced Fat Cheddar Extra Sharp	1 oz	90	6	240	tr	0
Reduced Fat Cheddar Sharp	1 oz	90	6	240	tr	0
Reduced Fat Cheddar Vermont Sharp	1 oz	90	6	240	tr	0
Whipped Spreadable Cream Cheese & Extra Sharp Cheddar	2 tbsp (0.9 oz)	80	8	180	tr	0
Whipped Spreadable Cream Cheese & Sharp Cheddar	2 tbsp (0.9 oz)	80	8	180	tr	0
Whipped Spreadable Cream Cheese & Sharp Cheddar w/ Herbs	2 tbsp (0.9 oz)	80	8	180	tr	0
Delice De France						
Cheese	1 oz	110	9	180	2	0
With Herbs	1 oz	110	9	180	2	0
Delico						
Alouette Cajun	2 tbsp (0.8 oz)	70	7	120	1	0
Alouette French Onion	2 tbsp (0.8 oz)	70	7	160	1	0
Alouette Garden Vegetable	2 tbsp (0.8 oz)	60	6	130	1	0
Alouette Garlic	2 tbsp (0.8 oz)	70	7	135	1	0
Alouette Horseradish & Chive	2 tbsp (0.8 oz)	60	7	100	1	0
Alouette Spinach	2 tbsp (0.8 oz)	60	6	85	1	0
Di Giorno						
Parmesan Grated	2 tsp (5 g)	25	2	85	0	0
Parmesan Shredded	2 tsp (5 g)	20	2	75	0	0
Parmesan Shredded	2 tsp (5 g)	20	2	75	0	0
Romano Grated	2 tsp (5 g)	25	2	90	0	0

FOOD	PORTION	CAL.	FAT	SOD.	CARB.	FIB.
Di Giorno (CONT.)						
Romano Shredded	2 tsp (5 g)	20	2	70	0	0
Dorman						
Cheda-Jack Reduced Fat Low Sodium	1 oz	80	5	140	1	—
Cheddar	1 oz	110	9	200	1	—
Cheddar Reduced Fat Low Sodium	1 oz	80	5	140	1	—
Colby	1 oz	110	9	190	1	—
Edam	1 oz	100	8	200	1	—
Gouda	1 oz	100	8	210	1	—
Lo-Chol Cheddar	1 oz	100	7	140	1	—
Lo-Chol Colby	1 oz	100	7	140	1	—
Lo-Chol Mozzarella	1 oz	90	6	140	1	—
Lo-Chol Muenster	1 oz	100	7	140	1	—
Lo-Chol Swiss	1 oz	100	7	140	1	—
Monterey Reduced Fat Low Sodium	1 oz	80	5	140	1	—
Monterey Jack	1 oz	100	8	180	1	—
Mozzarella Park Skim	1 oz	90	7	190	1	—
Mozzarella Reduced Fat Low Sodium	1 oz	80	4	140	1	—
Muenster	1 oz	110	9	190	0	—
Muenster Low Sodium	1 oz	110	9	95	0	—
Muenster Reduced Fat Low Sodium	1 oz	80	5	140	tr	—
Parmesan	1 oz	110	7	350	1	—
Provolone	1 oz	90	7	290	1	—
Provolone Reduced Fat Low Sodium	1 oz	80	4	140	1	—
Romano	1 oz	100	7	350	1	—
Swiss	1 oz	100	8	80	0	—
Swiss No Salt Added	1 oz	100	8	10	tr	—
Swiss Reduced Fat Low Sodium	1 oz	90	5	60	tr	—
Easy Cheese						
Spread American	2 tbsp (1.2 oz)	100	7	400	2	0
Spread Cheddar	2 tbsp (1.2 oz)	100	7	410	3	0
Spread Cheddar'n Bacon	2 tbsp (1.2 oz)	100	7	410	3	0
Spread Nacho	2 tbsp (1.2 oz)	100	7	390	3	0
Spread Sharp Cheddar	2 tbsp (1.2 oz)	100	7	440	3	0
Father Time						
Cheddar Extra-Sharp Premium	1 oz	110	9	180	1	0

FOOD	PORTION	CAL.	FAT	SOD.	CARB.	FIB.
Formagg						
Formaggio D'Oro	1 oz	70	5	450	1	0
Friendship						
Farmer	2 tbsp (1 oz)	50	3	120	0	0
Farmer No Salt Added	2 tbsp (1 oz)	50	3	10	0	0
Hoop	2 tbsp (1 oz)	20	0	10	0	0
Frigo						
Asiago	1 oz	110	9	400	1	—
Blue	1 oz	100	8	400	1	—
Cheddar	1 oz	110	9	200	1	—
Cheddar Lite	1 oz	80	5	190	1	—
Feta	1 oz	100	8	400	1	—
Impastata	1 oz	60	5	50	1	—
Mozzarella Part Skim Low Moisture	1 oz	80	5	190	1	—
Mozzarella Whole Milk Low Moisture	1 oz	90	7	190	1	—
Mozzarella Lite Whole Milk Low Moisture	1 oz	60	2	140	1	—
Parmazest	1 oz	120	7	410	5	—
Parmesan & Romano Dry Grated	1 oz	130	9	510	1	—
Parmesan & Romano Grated	1 oz	110	7	350	1	—
Parmesan Dry Grated	1 oz	130	9	510	1	—
Parmesan Grated	1 oz	110	7	350	1	—
Parmesan Whole	1 oz	110	7	350	1	—
Pizza Shredded	1 oz	65	3	150	1	—
Provolone	1 oz	100	7	230	1	—
Provolone Lite	1 oz	70	4	205	1	—
Ricotta Low Fat Low Salt	1 oz	30	1	10	1	—
Ricotta Part Skim	1 oz	40	3	30	1	—
Ricotta Whole Milk	1 oz	60	5	40	1	—
Romano Dry Grated	1 oz	130	9	510	1	—
Romano Grated	1 oz	110	8	350	1	—
Romano Whole	1 oz	110	8	350	1	—
String	1 oz	80	5	190	1	—
String Lite	1 oz	60	2	140	1	—
Swiss	1 oz	110	8	80	1	—
Taco Shredded	1 oz	110	9	200	1	—
Gerard						
Brie	1 oz	90	7	180	2	0
Handi-Snacks						
Cheez'n Breadsticks	1 pkg (1.1 oz)	120	6	320	12	0

FOOD	PORTION	CAL.	FAT	SOD.	CARB.	FIB.
Handi-Snacks (CONT.)						
Cheez'n Breadsticks	1 pkg (1.1 oz)	130	7	340	11	0
Cheez'n Crackers	1 pkg (1.1 oz)	110	7	300	9	0
Cheez'n Pretzels	1 pkg (1 oz)	100	5	410	11	tr
Mozzarella String Cheese	1 piece (1 oz)	80	6	240	0	0
Nacho Stix'n Cheez	1 pkg (1.1 oz)	110	6	320	11	0
Healthy Choice						
American Singles White	1 slice (0.7 oz)	30	0	290	2	—
American Singles Yellow	1 slice (0.7 oz)	30	0	290	2	—
Cheddar Fancy Shreds	¼ cup (1 oz)	45	0	200	2	—
Cheddar Shreds	¼ cup (1 oz)	45	0	200	2	—
Loaf	1 in cube (1 oz)	35	0	390	3	—
Mexican Shreds	¼ cup (1 oz)	45	0	200	2	—
Mozzarella	1 oz	45	0	200	1	—
Mozzarella Fancy Shreds	¼ cup (1 oz)	45	0	200	2	—
Mozzarella Shreds	¼ cup (1 oz)	45	0	200	2	—
Mozzarella String Cheese	1 stick (1 oz)	45	0	200	1	—
Pizza Fancy Shreds	¼ cup (1 oz)	45	0	200	2	—
Pizza String	1 stick (1 oz)	45	0	200	1	—
Heluva Good Cheese						
American	1 slice (0.7)	45	5	390	2	0
Cheddar Curds Snack	1 oz	113	9	179	1	0
Cheddar Extra-Sharp	1 oz	110	9	180	1	0
Cheddar Mild	1 oz	110	9	180	1	0
Cheddar Mild Reduced Fat	1 oz	80	6	200	1	0
Cheddar Mild White	1 oz	110	9	180	1	0
Cheddar Sharp	1 oz	110	9	180	1	0
Cheddar Sharp White	1 oz	110	9	180	1	0
Cheddar Shredded	¼ cup (1 oz)	110	9	180	1	0
Cheddar Very Low Sodium	1 oz	110	9	140	0	0
Cheddar White Extra-Sharp	1 oz	110	9	180	1	0
Cheddar White Very Low Sodium	1 oz	110	9	140	0	0
Cheddar White Shredded	¼ cup (1 oz)	110	9	180	1	0
Colby	1 oz	117	9	186	0	0
Colby-Jack	1 oz	110	9	200	0	0
Cold Pack Cheddar Sharp	2 tbsp (1 oz)	90	7	210	3	0
Cold Pack Cheddar Sharp With Bacon	2 tbsp (1 oz)	90	7	210	3	0

FOOD	PORTION	CAL.	FAT	SOD.	CARB.	FIB.
Heluva Good Cheese (CONT.)						
Cold Pack Cheddar Sharp With Horseradish	2 tbsp (1 oz)	90	7	210	3	0
Cold Pack Cheddar Sharp With Jalapenos	2 tbsp (1 oz)	90	7	210	3	0
Cold Pack Cheddar Sharp With Port Wine	2 tbsp (1 oz)	90	7	210	3	0
Monterey Jack	1 oz	100	8	180	0	0
Monterey Jack Shredded	¼ cup (1 oz)	100	8	170	1	0
Monterey Jack With Jalapenos	1 oz	100	8	180	0	0
Mozzarella Part Skim Low Moisture Shredded	¼ cup (1 oz)	80	5	170	1	0
Mozzarella Whole Milk	1 oz	80	6	220	tr	0
Muenster	1 oz	100	8	180	0	0
Swiss	1 oz	112	8	62	0	0
Washed Curd Cheese	1 oz	110	9	170	1	0
Hoffman						
American Yellow	1 oz	110	9	400	1	0
Hot Pepper	1 oz	90	7	460	2	0
Super Sharp	1 oz	110	9	380	1	0
Holland Farm						
Edam	1 oz	97	8	—	—	—
Farmer	1 oz	102	8	—	—	—
Gouda	1 oz	103	8	—	—	—
Monterey Jack	1 oz	102	9	—	—	—
Muenster	1 oz	102	9	—	—	—
Hollow Road Farms						
Sheep's Milk	1 oz	45	3	65	1	—
Keller's						
Chub	2 tbsp (1 oz)	100	10	120	1	0
Kraft						
Cheddar Extra Sharp	1 oz	120	10	180	0	0
Cheddar Medium	1 oz	110	9	180	tr	0
Cheddar Mild	1 oz	110	9	180	tr	0
Cheddar Sharp	1 oz	120	10	180	0	0
Cheddary Melts Medium Cheddar	1 oz	110	9	390	2	0
Cheddary Melts Mild Cheddar	1 oz	110	9	390	2	0
Cheddary Melts Shreds Medium Cheddar	¼ cup (1.1 oz)	120	9	420	2	0

FOOD	PORTION	CAL.	FAT	SOD.	CARB.	FIB.
Kraft (CONT.)						
Cheddary Melts Shreds Mild Cheddar	¼ cup (1.1 oz)	120	9	420	2	0
Cheese Food w/ Garlic	1 oz	90	7	370	2	0
Cheese Food w/ Jalapeno Peppers	1 oz	90	7	370	2	0
Colby	1 oz	110	9	180	tr	0
Colby Monterey Jack	1 oz	110	9	180	0	0
Deluxe American	1 oz	100	9	430	tr	0
Deluxe American White	1 oz	100	9	430	tr	0
Deluxe Singles American	1 (1 oz)	110	9	460	tr	0
Deluxe Singles American	1 (0.7 oz)	70	6	310	tr	0
Deluxe Singles Pimento	1 (1 oz)	100	8	430	tr	0
Deluxe Singles Swiss	1 (1 oz)	90	7	410	0	0
Deluxe Singles Swiss	1 slice (0.7 oz)	70	5	310	0	0
Free Grated	2 tsp (5 g)	15	0	75	3	0
Free Shredded Cheddar	¼ cup (0.9 oz)	40	0	270	1	0
Free Shredded Mozzarella	¼ cup (1 oz)	45	0	340	2	tr
Free Singles White	1 slice (0.7 oz)	30	0	320	3	0
Grated Parm Plus! Garlic Herb	2 tsp (5 g)	15	0	110	2	0
Grated Parm Plus! Zesty Red Pepper	2 tsp (5 g)	15	0	110	2	0
Grated Parmesan	2 tsp (5 g)	20	2	85	0	0
Grated Romano	2 tsp (5 g)	20	2	70	0	0
Marbled Cheddar Mild	1 oz	110	9	180	tr	0
Marbled Cheddar & Monterey Jack	1 oz	110	9	190	tr	0
Marbled Cheddar & Whole Milk Mozzarella	1 oz	100	8	190	tr	0
Marbled Colby Monterey Jack	1 oz	110	9	180	0	0
Monterey Jack	1 oz	110	9	190	0	0
Monterey Jack w/ Jalapeno Peppers	1 oz	110	9	190	tr	0
Mozzarella Part Skim Low Moisture	1 oz	80	5	200	tr	0
Mozzarella String Cheese Low Moisture Part Skim	1 piece (1 oz)	80	6	240	0	0
Pizza Shredded Four Cheese	¼ cup (0.9 oz)	90	7	220	tr	0
Pizza Shredded Mozzarella & Cheddar	⅓ cup (1.1 oz)	120	9	220	1	0

FOOD	PORTION	CAL.	FAT	SOD.	CARB.	FIB.
Kraft (CONT.)						
Pizza Shredded Mozzarella & Provolone w/ Smoke Flavor	¼ cup (0.9 oz)	90	7	200	tr	0
Reduced Fat Cheddar Mild	1 oz	90	6	240	tr	0
Reduced Fat Cheddar Sharp	1 oz	90	6	240	tr	0
Reduced Fat Colby	1 oz	80	6	220	0	0
Reduced Fat Monterey Jack	1 oz	80	6	240	tr	0
Shredded Cheddar Medium	¼ cup (0.9 oz)	100	8	170	tr	0
Shredded Cheddar Mild	¼ cup (0.9 oz)	100	8	170	tr	0
Shredded Cheddar Sharp	1 oz (0.9 oz)	110	9	170	tr	0
Shredded Cheddar & Monterey Jack	¼ cup (0.9 oz)	100	8	170	tr	0
Shredded Colby & Monterey Jack	¼ cup (0.9 oz)	100	8	170	tr	0
Shredded Hearty Italian	⅓ cup (1.1 oz)	100	8	230	2	0
Shredded Italian Style Classic Garlic	⅓ cup (1.1 oz)	100	8	240	2	tr
Shredded Italian Style Mozzarelle & Parmesan	⅓ cup (1.1 oz)	100	8	240	1	0
Shredded Lower Fat Cheddar Mild	¼ cup (0.9 oz)	80	6	220	tr	0
Shredded Lower Fat Cheddar Sharp	¼ cup (0.9 oz)	80	6	220	tr	0
Shredded Lower Fat Colby & Monterey Jack	¼ cup (0.9 oz)	80	5	210	tr	0
Shredded Lower Fat Mozzarella	⅓ cup (1.1 oz)	80	5	210	tr	0
Shredded Lower Fat Pizza Cheese	⅓ cup (1.1 oz)	90	6	240	1	0
Shredded Mexican Style Cheddar & Monterey Jack	⅓ cup (1.1 oz)	120	10	200	tr	0
Shredded Mexican Style Cheddar & Monterey Jack w/ Jalapeno Peppers	⅓ cup (1.1 oz)	120	10	200	tr	0

FOOD	PORTION	CAL.	FAT	SOD.	CARB.	FIB.
Kraft (CONT.)						
Shredded Mexican Style Four Cheese	⅓ cup (1.1 oz)	120	10	210	tr	0
Shredded Mexican Style Taco Cheese	⅓ cup (1.1 oz)	120	10	240	1	0
Shredded Monterey Jack	¼ cup (0.9 oz)	100	8	170	tr	0
Shredded Parmesan	2 tsp (5 g)	20	2	75	0	0
Shredded Part Skim Mozzarella	¼ cup (1.1 oz)	90	6	220	tr	0
Shredded Swiss	¼ cup (0.9 oz)	100	8	25	tr	0
Shredded Whole Milk Mozzarella	¼ cup (1.1 oz)	100	8	220	1	0
Shredded Finely Cheddar Mild	¼ cup (1.1 oz)	120	10	190	tr	0
Shredded Finely Cheddar Sharp	¼ cup (1.1 oz)	120	10	190	tr	0
Shredded Finely Colby & Monterey Jack	¼ cup (1 oz)	110	9	190	tr	0
Shredded Finely Lower Fat Cheddar Milk	⅓ cup (1.1 oz)	100	7	260	1	0
Shredded Finely Lower Fat Cheddar Sharp	⅓ cup (1.1 oz)	100	7	260	1	0
Shredded Finely Part Skim Mozzarella	¼ cup (1.1 oz)	90	6	220	tr	0
Shredded Finely Swiss	¼ cup (0.9 oz)	110	8	45	tr	0
Singles American	1 (0.7 oz)	60	5	260	2	0
Singles American	1 (0.6 oz)	60	5	260	2	0
Singles American	1 (1.2 oz)	110	8	460	3	0
Singles Mild Mexican	1 (0.7 oz)	70	5	280	2	0
Singles Monterey	1 slice (0.7 oz)	70	5	290	2	0
Singles Pimento	1 (0.7 oz)	60	5	260	1	0
Singles Reduced Fat American	1 (0.7 oz)	50	3	320	2	0
Singles Reduced Fat American White	1 (0.7 oz)	50	3	320	2	0
Singles Sharp	1 slice (0.7 oz)	70	6	300	tr	0
Singles Swiss	1 slice (0.7 oz)	70	5	320	1	0
Singles Nonfat American	1 (0.7 oz)	30	0	270	3	0
Singles Nonfat Sharp Cheddar	1 (0.7 oz)	35	0	300	3	0
Singles Nonfat Swiss	1 slice (0.7 oz)	30	0	270	3	0
Slices Cheddar Mild	1 (1 oz)	110	9	180	tr	0
Slices Colby	1 (1.6 oz)	180	14	290	tr	0
Slices Part Skim Mozzarella	1 (1.5 oz)	120	8	310	tr	0

FOOD	PORTION	CAL.	FAT	SOD.	CARB.	FIB.
Kraft (CONT.)						
Slices Part Skim Mozzarella	1 (1.6 oz)	130	8	320	tr	0
Slices Provolone Smoke Flavor	1 (1.5 oz)	150	11	370	tr	0
Slices Swiss	1 (1.3 oz)	150	12	65	tr	0
Slices Swiss	1 (0.8 oz)	90	7	40	0	0
Slices Swiss	1 (1.5 oz)	170	13	45	tr	0
Slices Swiss	1 (1.6 oz)	180	14	45	tr	0
Slices Swiss Aged	1 (1.5 oz)	170	13	75	tr	0
Slices Deli-Thin Part Skim Mozzarella	1 (1 oz)	80	5	200	tr	0
Slices Deli-Thin Swiss	1 (0.8 oz)	90	7	40	0	0
Slices Deli-Thin Swiss Aged	1 (0.8 oz)	90	7	40	0	0
Slices Reduced Fat Swiss	1 (1.3 oz)	130	9	90	tr	0
Spread Bacon	2 tbsp (1.1 oz)	90	8	570	tr	0
Spread Jalapeno Pepper	1 oz	80	6	470	2	0
Spread Olive & Pimento	2 tbsp (1.1 oz)	70	6	220	3	0
Spread Pimento	2 tbsp (1.1 oz)	80	6	170	3	0
Spread Pineapple	2 tbsp (1.1 oz)	70	5	120	4	0
Spread Pineapple	2 tbsp (1.1 oz)	70	5	115	4	0
Spread Roka Brand Blue	2 tbsp (1.1 oz)	90	8	520	tr	0
Swiss	1 oz	110	9	50	0	0
Lactaid						
American	3.5 oz	328	25	1189	7	0
Land O'Lakes						
American	1 slice (0.75 oz)	80	6	340	tr	0
American	2 slices (1 oz)	100	9	460	1	0
American	1 oz	110	9	430	tr	0
American Less Salt	1 oz	110	9	270	tr	0
American Light	1 oz	70	5	400	2	0
American Sharp	1 oz	110	9	360	tr	0
American & Swiss	1 oz	100	8	380	0	0
Baby Swiss	1 oz	110	8	125	0	0
Brick	1 oz	100	8	160	tr	0
Chedarella	1 oz	100	8	200	0	0
Cheddar Light	1 oz	70	4	230	tr	0
Gouda	1 oz	110	8	230	1	—
Jalapeno Light	1 oz	70	4	400	1	0
Monterey Jack	1 oz	110	9	160	tr	0
Mozzarella	1 oz	80	6	190	tr	0
Muenster	1 oz	100	8	220	0	0

FOOD	PORTION	CAL.	FAT	SOD.	CARB.	FIB.
Land O'Lakes (CONT.)						
Provolone	1 oz	100	8	240	tr	0
Swiss	1 oz	110	8	75	tr	0
Swiss Light	1 oz	80	4	60	tr	0
Laughing Cow						
Assorted Wedge	1 (1 oz)	70	6	370	1	0
Babybel	1 oz	90	7	230	0	0
Babybel Mini	1 (0.7 oz)	70	6	170	0	0
Bonbel	1 oz	100	8	230	0	0
Bonbel Mini	1 (0.7 oz)	70	6	170	0	0
Cheesebits	6 pieces (1 oz)	70	6	370	1	0
Gouda Mini	1 (0.7 oz)	80	6	170	0	0
Original Wedge	1 (1 oz)	70	6	370	1	0
Wedge Light	1 (1 oz)	50	3	370	1	0
Lifetime						
Cheddar Fat Free	1 oz	40	0	220	1	0
Cheddar Fat Free Lactose Free	1 oz	40	0	220	1	0
Garden Vegetable Fat Free	1 oz	40	0	220	1	0
Jalapeno Jack Fat Free	1 oz	40	0	220	1	0
Jalapeno Jack Fat Free Lactose Free	1 oz	40	0	220	1	0
Mild Mexican Fat Free	1 oz	40	0	220	1	0
Monterey Jack Fat Free	1 oz	40	0	220	1	0
Mozzarella Fat Free	1 oz	40	0	220	1	0
Mozzarella Fat Free Lactose Free	1 oz	40	0	220	1	0
Onions & Chives Fat Free	1 oz	40	0	220	1	0
Sharp Cheddar Fat Free	1 oz	40	0	220	1	0
Smoked Cheddar Fat Free	1 oz	40	0	220	1	0
Swiss Fat Free	1 oz	40	0	220	1	0
Light N'Lively						
Singles American	1 (0.7 oz)	45	3	280	2	0
Marin French Cheese						
Breakfast	1 oz	86	7	—	1	—
Brie	1 oz	86	7	—	1	—
Camembert	1 oz	86	7	—	1	—
Schloss	1 oz	86	7	—	1	—
MayBud						
Edam	1 oz	100	8	210	1	0
Gouda	1 oz	100	8	210	1	0
Gouda Round	1 oz	100	8	210	1	0

FOOD	PORTION	CAL.	FAT	SOD.	CARB.	FIB.
New Holland						
Cheese	1 oz	90	7	105	0	0
Garlic	1 oz	90	7	105	tr	0
Havarti Lower Fat Garden Vegetable	1 oz	80	6	145	0	0
Jalapeno	1 oz	80	6	140	tr	0
Natural Vegetable	1 oz	80	6	110	0	0
Northfield						
Naturally Slender	1 oz	90	7	—	—	—
Old English						
American Sharp	1 slice (1 oz)	100	9	460	tr	0
Polly-O						
Mozzarella Free	1 oz	35	0	220	tr	—
Mozzarella Lite	1 oz	60	3	230	tr	—
Mozzarella Part Skim	1 oz	70	5	220	tr	—
Mozzarella Part Skim Shredded	¼ cup	80	5	200	tr	—
Mozzarella Shredded Free	¼ cup	45	0	270	1	—
Mozzarella Shredded Lite	¼ cup	60	3	220	1	—
Mozzarella Whole Milk	1 oz	80	6	220	tr	—
Mozzarella Whole Milk Shredded	¼ cup	90	7	200	tr	—
Ricotta Free	¼ cup	50	0	80	2	—
Ricotta Lite	¼ cup	70	3	80	3	—
Ricotta Part Skim	¼ cup	90	6	65	2	—
Ricotta Whole Milk	¼ cup	110	8	60	2	—
String	1 oz	80	6	200	1	—
String Lite	1 piece (1 oz)	60	3	230	tr	0
President						
Feta Fat Free	1 oz	30	0	450	2	0
Price's						
Cheese & Bacon Spread	2 tbsp (1.1 oz)	90	7	340	2	0
Jalapeno Nacho Dip Hot	2 tbsp (1.1 oz)	80	7	370	2	0
Jalapeno Nacho Dip Mild	2 tbsp (1.1 oz)	80	7	370	2	0
Pimento Cheese Spread	2 tbsp (1.1 oz)	80	7	320	2	0
Pimento Cheese Spread Light	2 tbsp (1.1 oz)	60	4	260	3	0
Vegetable Garden	2 tbsp (1.1 oz)	70	5	290	3	0
Quaker						
Chub	2 tbsp (1 oz)	100	10	120	1	0
Rondele						
Light Soft Spreadable Garlic & Herb	2 tbsp (0.9 oz)	60	4	190	2	0

FOOD	PORTION	CAL.	FAT	SOD.	CARB.	FIB.
Rondele (CONT.)						
Soft Spreadable Garlic & Herbs	2 tbsp (1 oz)	100	9	180	1	0
Sargento						
4 Cheese Mexican Recipe Blend Shredded	¼ cup (1 oz)	110	9	200	tr	0
6 Cheese Italian Recipe Blend Shredded	¼ cup (1 oz)	90	7	180	0	0
Blue Crumbled	¼ cup (1 oz)	100	8	350	1	0
Cheddar	1 slice (1 oz)	110	9	160	1	0
Cheddar Mild Shredded Classic Supreme	¼ cup (1 oz)	110	9	160	1	0
Cheddar Mild Shredded Fancy Supreme	¼ cup (1 oz)	110	9	160	1	0
Cheddar Mild Shredded Preferred Light	¼ cup (1 oz)	70	5	200	tr	0
Cheddar Mild White Shredded Classic Supreme	¼ cup (1 oz)	110	9	160	1	0
Cheddar New York Sharp Shredded Classic Supreme	¼ cup (1 oz)	110	9	160	1	0
Cheddar Sharp Shredded Classic Supreme	¼ cup (1 oz)	110	9	160	1	0
Cheddar Sharp Shredded Fancy Supreme	¼ cup (1 oz)	110	9	160	1	0
Cheese For Nachos & Tacos Shredded	¼ cup (1 oz)	110	9	240	1	0
Cheese For Pizza Shredded	¼ cup (1 oz)	90	6	210	0	0
Cheese For Tacos Shredded	¼ cup (1 oz)	110	9	220	1	0
Cheese For Tacos Shredded Preferred Light	¼ cup (1 oz)	70	5	240	tr	0
Colby	1 slice (1 oz)	110	9	190	0	0
Colby-Jack Shredded Fancy Supreme	¼ cup (1 oz)	110	9	190	tr	0
Gourmet Parm	1 tbsp	20	1	95	tr	—
Jarlsberg	1 slice (1.2 oz)	120	9	50	1	0
Monterey Jack	1 slice (1 oz)	100	9	190	0	0

FOOD	PORTION	CAL.	FAT	SOD.	CARB.	FIB.
Sargento (CONT.)						
MooTown Snackers Cheddar	1 piece (0.8 oz)	100	8	130	1	0
MooTown Snackers Cheddar Mild Light	1 piece (0.8 oz)	60	4	170	tr	0
MooTown Snackers Cheese & Pretzels	1 pkg (1 oz)	90	3	320	12	0
MooTown Snackers Cheese & Sticks	1 pkg (1 oz)	100	4	260	13	0
MooTown Snackers Colby-Jack	1 piece (0.8 oz)	90	8	160	tr	0
MooTown Snackers Pizza Cheese & Sticks	1 pkg (1 oz)	100	4	260	13	0
MooTown Snackers String	1 piece (0.8 oz)	70	5	170	tr	0
MooTown Snackers String Light	1 piece (0.8 oz)	60	3	200	tr	0
Mozzarella	1 slice (1.5 oz)	130	9	230	2	0
Mozzarella Preferred Light	1 slice (1.5 oz)	100	5	210	0	0
Mozzarella Shredded Classic Supreme	¼ cup (1 oz)	80	6	150	1	0
Mozzarella Shredded Fancy Supreme	¼ cup (1 oz)	80	6	150	1	0
Mozzarella Shredded Preferred Light	¼ cup (1 oz)	70	3	140	tr	0
Muenster	1 slice (1 oz)	100	9	200	tr	0
Parmesan Fresh	1 oz	111	7	454	1	—
Parmesan Shredded	¼ cup (1 oz)	110	7	300	1	0
Parmesan & Romano Shredded	¼ cup (1 oz)	110	7	340	1	0
Pizza Double Cheese Shredded	¼ cup (1 oz)	90	6	150	1	0
Provolone	1 slice (1 oz)	100	8	190	0	0
Ricotta Light	¼ cup (2.2 oz)	60	3	55	3	0
Ricotta Old Fashioned	¼ cup (2.2 oz)	90	6	75	3	0
Ricotta Part Skim	¼ cup (2.2 oz)	80	5	75	2	0
Swiss	1 slice (0.7 oz)	80	6	30	0	0
Swiss Preferred Light	1 slice (1 oz)	80	4	50	tr	0
Swiss Shredded Fancy Supreme	¼ cup (1 oz)	110	8	40	0	0
Swiss Wafer Thin	2 slices (1 oz)	110	9	40	0	0
Smart Beat						
American Fat Free	1 slice (0.6 oz)	25	0	180	3	—

FOOD	PORTION	CAL.	FAT	SOD.	CARB.	FIB.
Smart Beat (CONT.)						
Lactose Free Fat Free	1 slice (0.6 oz)	25	0	180	3	—
Mellow Cheddar Fat Free	1 slice (0.6 oz)	25	0	180	3	—
Sharp Cheddar Fat Free	1 slice (0.6 oz)	25	0	220	3	—
Treasure Cave						
Blue Crumbled	1 oz	110	9	400	tr	0
Feta Crumbled	1 oz	80	6	370	tr	0
Tree Of Life						
Cheddar 33% Reduced Fat Organic Milk	1 oz	90	6	135	1	—
Cheddar Low Sodium Raw Milk	1 oz	110	9	110	0	—
Cheddar Mild Organic Milk	1 oz	110	9	190	1	—
Cheddar Mild Raw Milk	1 oz	110	9	180	0	—
Cheddar Razor Sharp Raw Milk	1 oz	110	9	180	0	—
Cheddar Sharp Organic Milk	1 oz	110	9	190	0	—
Cheddar Sharp Raw Milk	1 oz	110	9	180	0	—
Colby Organic Milk	1 oz	120	10	190	1	—
Colby Raw Milk	1 oz	110	9	170	1	—
Farmer Part-Skim Organic Milk	1 oz	90	6	110	1	—
Jalapeno Jack Organic Milk	1 oz	110	9	190	1	—
Jalapeno Jack Semi-Soft Organic Milk	1 oz	110	9	150	0	—
Monterey Jack 35% Reduced Fat Organic Milk	1 oz	80	5	190	1	—
Monterey Jack Organic Milk	1 oz	100	8	185	1	—
Monterey Jack Semi-Soft Raw Milk	1 oz	110	9	150	0	—
Mozzarella Low Moisture Part Skim	1 oz	80	5	150	1	—
Mozzarella Low Moisture Part Skim Organic Milk	1 oz	80	5	170	1	—
Muenster Organic Milk	1 oz	100	8	185	1	—
Muenster Semi-Soft Raw Milk	1 oz	100	9	180	0	—
Provolone	1 oz	100	8	250	1	—

FOOD	PORTION	CAL.	FAT	SOD.	CARB.	FIB.
Tree Of Life (CONT.)						
Swiss Raw Milk	1 oz	110	8	75	1	—
Velveeta						
Cheese	1 slice (0.7 oz)	60	5	300	2	0
Cheese	1 slice (1.2 oz)	100	7	480	3	0
Cheese	1 slice (0.8 oz)	70	5	310	2	0
Light	1 oz	60	3	440	3	0
Shredded	¼ cup (1.3 oz)	130	9	500	3	0
Shredded Mild Mexican w/ Jalapeno Pepper	¼ cup (1.3 oz)	120	9	520	3	0
Spread	1 oz	90	6	420	3	0
Spread Hot Mexican	1 oz	90	6	420	3	0
Spread Italiana	1 oz	60	6	430	2	0
Spread Mild Mexican	1 oz	90	6	420	3	0
Weight Watchers						
Cheddar Mild Yellow	1 oz	80	5	180	1	0
Cheddar Sharp Yellow	1 oz	80	5	180	1	0
Fat Free Grated Italian Topping	1 tbsp	20	0	60	2	0
Fat Free Reduced Sodium American Yellow	2 slices (0.75 oz)	30	0	160	3	0
Fat Free Sharp Cheddar	2 slices (0.75 oz)	30	0	320	3	0
Fat Free Swiss	2 slices (0.75 oz)	30	0	320	2	0
Fat Free White	2 slices (0.75 oz)	30	0	320	3	0
Fat Free Yellow	2 slices (0.75 oz)	30	0	320	3	0
Low Sodium Cheddar Mild	1 oz	80	5	70	1	0
Monterey Jack	1 oz	80	5	180	1	0
Reduced Sodium American White	2 slices (0.75 oz)	30	0	150	2	0
White Clover						
Cheddar Light With Simplesse	1 oz	80	4	160	tr	—
Colby Light With Simplesse	1 oz	80	4	180	tr	—
Monterey Jack Light With Simplesse	1 oz	70	4	190	tr	—
Muenster Light With Simplesse	1 oz	70	4	190	tr	—
WisPride						
Chunk	1 oz	110	8	180	4	0
Garlic & Herb Cup	2 tbsp (1.1 oz)	100	7	270	4	0
Hickory Smoked Cup	2 tbsp (1.1 oz)	100	7	230	4	0

FOOD	PORTION	CAL.	FAT	SOD.	CARB.	FIB.
WisPride (CONT.)						
Port Wine Ball	2 tbsp (1.1 oz)	100	8	190	4	0
Port Wine Cup	2 tbsp (1.1 oz)	100	7	230	4	0
Port Wine Light Cup	2 tbsp (1.1 oz)	80	3	200	5	0
Sharp Ball	2 tbsp (1.1 oz)	100	8	190	4	0
Sharp Cheddar Ball	2 tbsp (1.1 oz)	100	8	190	4	0
Sharp Cup	2 tbsp (1.1 oz)	100	7	230	4	0
Sharp Light Cup	2 tbsp (1.1 oz)	80	3	200	5	0
Swiss Ball	2 tbsp (1.1 oz)	110	8	125	5	0

CHEESE DISHES

FOOD	PORTION	CAL.	FAT	SOD.	CARB.	FIB.
FROZEN						
Stouffer's						
Welsh Rarebit	¼ cup (1.1 oz)	120	9	280	5	—
HOME RECIPE						
welsh rarebit as prep w/ 1 white toast	1 slice	228	16	—	14	1
TAKE-OUT						
cheese omelette as prep w/ 2 eggs	1 (6.8 oz)	519	44	—	tr	0
fondue	1 cup (7.5 oz)	492	29	283	8	—
fondue	½ cup (3.8 oz)	247	15	142	4	—

CHEESE SUBSTITUTES

FOOD	PORTION	CAL.	FAT	SOD.	CARB.	FIB.
mozzarella	1 oz	70	3	194	7	—
Borden						
Cheese Two	1 oz	90	7	360	2	—
Taco-Mate	1 oz	100	7	360	2	—
Formagg						
American White	1 slice (0.66 oz)	60	4	260	tr	0
American Yellow	1 slice (0.66 oz)	60	4	260	tr	0
Caesar's Italian Garden American	1 oz	60	3	240	1	0
Cheddar	1 slice (0.66 oz)	60	4	260	tr	0
Cheddar Shredded	1 oz	60	3	190	1	0
Classic American	1 oz	60	3	290	1	0
Macaroni And Cheese Sauce	⅔ cup (5 oz)	190	2	470	35	0
Mozzarella Shredded	1 oz	60	3	140	1	0
Old World Mozzarella	1 oz	60	3	140	1	0
Parmesan Grated	2 tsp (5 g)	15	1	80	tr	tr
Swiss	1 oz	60	3	240	1	0
Swiss White	1 slice (0.66 oz)	60	4	260	tr	0
Vintage Provolone	1 oz	60	3	190	1	0
Zesty Jalapeno American	1 oz	60	3	290	1	0

FOOD	PORTION	CAL.	FAT	SOD.	CARB.	FIB.
Frigo						
Imitation Cheddar	1 oz	90	7	280	1	—
Imitation Mozzeralla	1 oz	90	7	240	1	—
Georgio's						
Imitation Cheddar Shredded	¼ cup (1 oz)	90	7	450	1	0
Imitation Mozzarella Shredded	¼ cup (1 oz)	90	7	350	1	0
Sargento						
Classic Supreme Cheddar Shredded	¼ cup (1 oz)	90	6	470	2	0
Classic Supreme Mozzarella Shredded	¼ cup (1 oz)	80	6	320	tr	0
Fancy Supreme Cheddar Shredded	¼ cup (1 oz)	90	6	470	2	0
White Wave						
Soy A Melt Cheddar	1 oz	80	5	170	1	—
Soy A Melt Fat Free Cheddar	1 oz	40	tr	370	3	—
Soy A Melt Fat Free Mozzarella	1 oz	40	tr	370	3	—
Soy A Melt Garlic Herb	1 oz	80	5	170	1	—
Soy A Melt Jalapeno Jack	1 oz	80	5	170	1	—
Soy A Melt Monterey Jack	1 oz	80	5	170	1	—
Soy A Melt Mozzarella	1 oz	80	5	170	1	—
Soy A Melt Singles American	1 slice (¾ oz)	60	4	280	1	—
Soy A Melt Singles Mozzarella	1 slice (¾ oz)	60	4	280	1	—

CHERIMOYA

fresh	1	515	2	—	131	—

CHERRIES

CANNED

sour in heavy syrup	½ cup	232	tr	18	60	—
sour in light syrup	½ cup	189	tr	18	49	—
sour water packed	1 cup	87	tr	17	22	—
sweet in heavy syrup	½ cup	107	tr	3	27	—
sweet in light syrup	½ cup	85	tr	3	22	—
sweet juice pack	½ cup	68	tr	3	17	—
sweet water pack	½ cup	57	tr	2	15	—

FOOD	PORTION	CAL.	FAT	SOD.	CARB.	FIB.
Del Monte						
Dark Pitted In Heavy Syrup	½ cup (4.2 oz)	120	0	10	24	tr
Sweet Dark Whole Unpitted In Heavy Syrup	½ cup (4.2 oz)	120	0	10	24	tr
DRIED						
Chukar						
Bing	2 oz	160	1	3	35	—
Rainer	2 oz	160	1	3	35	—
Tart	2 oz	170	0	10	43	—
Tart 'n Sweet	2 oz	180	0	10	43	—
Sonoma						
Pitted	¼ cup (1.4 oz)	140	0	0	34	2
FRESH						
sour	1 cup	51	tr	3	13	—
sweet	10	49	1	0	11	—
Dole						
Cherries	1 cup	90	1	0	19	3
FROZEN						
sour unsweetened	1 cup	72	1	1	17	—
sweet sweetened	1 cup	232	tr	3	58	—
Big Valley						
Dark Sweet	¾ cup (4.9 oz)	90	0	0	20	3

CHERRY JUICE

FOOD	PORTION	CAL.	FAT	SOD.	CARB.	FIB.
After The Fall						
Black Cherry	1 can (12 oz)	170	0	20	42	0
Capri Sun						
Wild Cherry Drink	1 pkg (7 oz)	100	0	20	30	0
Hi-C						
Box	8.45 fl oz	140	0	30	35	—
Drink	8 fl oz	130	0	30	33	—
Juice Works						
Drink	6 oz	100	0	—	—	—
Juicy Juice						
Drink	1 bottle (6 fl oz)	90	0	10	23	—
Drink	1 box (8.45 fl oz)	130	0	10	30	—
Kool-Aid						
Black Cherry Drink as prep w/ sugar	1 serv (8 oz)	100	0	15	25	0
Bursts Cherry Drink	1 (7 oz)	100	0	30	25	0
Drink as prep w/ sugar	1 serv (8 oz)	100	0	5	25	0
Splash Drink	1 serv (8 oz)	110	0	35	29	0

FOOD	PORTION	CAL.	FAT	SOD.	CARB.	FIB.
Kool-Aid (CONT.)						
Sugar Free Drink Mix as prep	1 serv (8 oz)	5	0	5	0	0
Sipps						
Wild Cherry	8.45 oz	130	0	—	—	—
Smucker's						
Black Cherry	8 oz	130	0	10	31	—
Black Cherry Sparkler	10 oz	120	tr	5	30	—
Tree Of Life						
Concentrate	8 tsp (1.4 oz)	110	0	0	28	—
CHERVIL						
seed	1 tsp	1	tr	tr	tr	—
CHESTNUTS						
chinese cooked	1 oz	44	tr	1	10	—
chinese dried	1 oz	103	tr	2	23	—
chinese raw	1 oz	64	tr	1	14	—
chinese roasted	1 oz	68	tr	1	15	—
cooked	1 oz	37	tr	8	8	—
dried peeled	1 oz	105	1	11	22	—
japanese cooked	1 oz	16	tr	1	4	—
japanese dried	1 oz	102	tr	10	23	—
japanese raw	1 oz	44	tr	4	10	—
japanese roasted	1 oz	57	tr	—	13	—
raw peeled	1 oz	56	tr	1	13	—
roasted	2 to 3 (1 oz)	70	1	1	15	—
roasted	1 cup	350	3	3	76	—
CHEWING GUM						
bubble gum	1 block (8 g)	27	0	0	8	—
stick	1 (3 g)	10	0	0	3	—
Bazooka						
Fruit Chunk	1 piece (6 g)	25	0	0	5	—
Fruit Soft	1 piece (6 g)	25	0	0	5	—
Gum	1 piece (4 g)	15	0	0	4	—
Gum	1 piece (6 g)	25	0	0	5	—
Beech-Nut						
Peppermint	1 stick (3 g)	10	0	0	2	0
Spearmint	1 stick (3 g)	10	0	0	2	0
Big Red						
Stick	1	10	tr	0	2	—
Brock						
Bubble Gum	1 piece (0.2 oz)	20	0	0	4	—
Bubble Yum						
Bananaberry Split	1 piece (0.3 oz)	25	0	0	6	—

FOOD	PORTION	CAL.	FAT	SOD.	CARB.	FIB.
Bubble Yum (CONT.)						
Cotton Candy	1 piece (0.3 oz)	25	0	0	6	—
Grape	1 piece (0.3 oz)	25	0	0	6	—
Luscious Lime	1 piece (0.3 oz)	25	0	0	6	—
Regular	1 piece (0.3 oz)	25	0	0	6	0
Sour Apple	1 piece (0.3 oz)	25	0	0	6	1
Sour Cherry	1 piece (0.3 oz)	25	0	0	6	0
Sugarless	1 piece (0.2 oz)	15	0	0	3	—
Sugarless Grape	1 piece (0.2 oz)	15	0	0	3	—
Sugarless Peppermint	1 piece (0.2 oz)	15	0	0	3	—
Sugarless Strawberry	1 piece (0.2 oz)	15	0	0	3	—
Sugarless Variety	1 piece (0.2 oz)	15	0	0	3	—
Variety Pack	1 piece (0.3 oz)	25	0	0	6	0
Watermelon	1 piece (0.3 oz)	25	0	0	6	0
Wild Strawberry	1 piece (0.3 oz)	25	0	0	6	0
Bubblicious						
Gum	1 piece (7.9 g)	25	0	—	6	—
*Care*Free*						
Sugarless Bubble Gum	1 stick (3 g)	10	0	0	2	—
Sugarless Cinnamon	1 piece (3 g)	5	0	0	2	—
Sugarless Peppermint	1 piece (3 g)	5	0	0	2	—
Sugarless Spearmint	1 piece (3 g)	5	0	0	2	—
Sugarless Wild Cherry	1 stick (3 g)	10	0	0	2	—
Chiclets						
Original	1 piece (1.59 g)	6	0	—	2	—
Tiny Size	8 pieces (0.13 g)	tr	0	—	tr	—
Clorets	1 piece (1.59 g)	6	0	—	2	—
Dentyne						
Cinn-A-Burst	1 piece (3.2 g)	9	0	—	2	—
Gum	1 piece (1.88 g)	6	0	—	1	—
Sugar Free	1 piece (1.88 g)	5	0	—	1	—
Doublemint						
Chewing Gum	1 piece	10	tr	0	2	—
Extra Sugar Free						
Cinnamon	1 piece	8	tr	0	tr	—
Spearmint & Peppermint	1 stick	8	tr	0	tr	—
Winter Fresh	1 piece	8	tr	0	tr	—
Freedent						
Spearmint Peppermint & Cinnamon	1 stick	10	tr	0	3	—
Freshen-Up						
Gum	1 piece (4.2 g)	13	0	—	3	—
Fruit Stripe						
Bubble Gum Jumbo Pack	1 stick (3 g)	10	0	0	2	0

FOOD	PORTION	CAL.	FAT	SOD.	CARB.	FIB.
Fruit Stripe (CONT.)						
Variety Pack Chewing & Bubble Gum	1 stick (3 g)	10	0	0	2	0
Hubba Bubba						
Bubble Gum Cola	1 piece	23	tr	0	6	—
Bubble Gum Sugarfree Grape	1 piece	13	tr	0	tr	—
Bubble Gum Sugarfree Original	1 piece	14	tr	0	tr	—
Original	1 piece	23	tr	0	6	—
Strawberry Grape Raspberry	1 piece	23	tr	0	6	—
Juicy Fruit						
Stick	1	10	tr	0	2	—
Rain-Blo						
Bubble Gum Balls	1 piece (2 g)	5	0	0	2	—
*Stick*Free*						
Sugarless Peppermint	1 stick (3 g)	10	0	0	2	—
Sugarless Spearmint	1 stick (3 g)	10	0	0	2	—
Swell						
Bubble Gum	1 piece (3 g)	10	0	0	2	—
Trident						
Gum	1 piece (1.88 g)	5	0	—	1	—
Soft Bubble Gum	1 piece (3.3 g)	9	0	—	2	—
Wrigley's						
Spearmint	1 stick	10	tr	0	2	—
CHIA SEEDS						
dried	1 oz	134	7	—	14	—
CHICKEN						
(*see also* CHICKEN DISHES, CHICKEN SUBSTITUTES, DINNER, HOT DOGS)						
CANNED						
chicken spread	1 oz	55	3	—	2	—
chicken spread	1 tbsp	25	2	—	1	—
chicken spread barbeque flavored	1 oz	55	3	—	2	—
w/ broth	1 can (5 oz)	234	11	714	0	—
w/ broth	½ can (2.5 oz)	117	6	357	0	—
Hormel						
Chunk	2 oz	70	3	200	0	0
Chunk Breast	2 oz	60	2	100	0	0
No Salt Chunk Breast	2 oz	60	2	20	0	0
Swanson						
Chunk Style Mixin' Chicken	2½ oz	130	8	230	1	—

FOOD	PORTION	CAL.	FAT	SOD.	CARB.	FIB.
Swanson (CONT.)						
White	2½ oz	100	4	235	0	—
White & Dark	2½ oz	100	4	240	0	—
Underwood						
Chunky	2.08 oz	150	9	440	2	—
Chunky Light	2.08 oz	80	3	330	2	—
Smoky	2.08 oz	150	8	290	10	—
FRESH						
broiler/fryer back w/ skin batter dipped & fried	½ back (2.5 oz)	238	16	228	7	—
broiler/fryer back w/ skin floured & fried	1.5 oz	146	9	40	3	—
broiler/fryer back w/ skin roasted	1 oz	96	7	28	0	—
broiler/fryer back w/ skin stewed	½ back (2.1 oz)	158	11	39	0	—
broiler/fryer back w/o skin fried	½ back (2 oz)	167	9	58	3	—
broiler/fryer breast w/ skin batter dipped & fried	½ breast (4.9 oz)	364	18	385	13	—
broiler/fryer breast w/ skin batter dipped & fried	2.9 oz	218	11	231	8	—
broiler/fryer breast w/ skin roasted	½ breast (3.4 oz)	193	8	69	0	—
broiler/fryer breast w/ skin roasted	2 oz	115	5	41	0	—
broiler/fryer breast w/ skin stewed	½ breast (3.9 oz)	202	8	68	0	—
broiler/fryer breast w/o skin fried	½ breast (3 oz)	161	4	68	tr	—
broiler/fryer breast w/o skin roasted	½ breast (3 oz)	142	3	63	0	—
broiler/fryer breast w/o skin stewed	2 oz	86	2	36	0	—
broiler/fryer dark meat w/ skin batter dipped & fried	5.9 oz	497	31	493	16	—
broiler/fryer dark meat w/ skin floured & fried	3.9 oz	313	19	98	4	—
broiler/fryer dark meat w/ skin roasted	3.5 oz	256	16	88	0	—
broiler/fryer dark meat w/ skin stewed	3.9 oz	256	16	77	0	—
broiler/fryer dark meat w/o skin fried	1 cup (5 oz)	334	16	136	4	—

FOOD	PORTION	CAL.	FAT	SOD.	CARB.	FIB.
broiler/fryer dark meat w/o skin roasted	1 cup (5 oz)	286	14	130	0	—
broiler/fryer dark meat w/o skin stewed	1 cup (5 oz)	269	13	104	0	—
broiler/fryer dark meat w/o skin stewed	3 oz	165	8	64	0	—
broiler/fryer drumstick w/ skin batter dipped & fried	1 (2.6 oz)	193	11	194	6	—
broiler/fryer drumstick w/ skin floured & fried	1 (1.7 oz)	120	7	44	1	—
broiler/fryer drumstick w/ skin roasted	1 (1.8 oz)	112	6	47	0	—
broiler/fryer drumstick w/ skin stewed	1 (2 oz)	116	6	43	0	—
broiler/fryer drumstick w/o skin fried	1 (1.5 oz)	82	3	40	0	—
broiler/fryer drumstick w/o skin roasted	1 (1.5 oz)	76	2	42	0	—
broiler/fryer drumstick w/o skin stewed	1 (1.6 oz)	78	3	37	0	—
broiler/fryer leg w/ skin batter dipped & fried	1 (5.5 oz)	431	26	442	14	—
broiler/fryer leg w/ skin floured & fried	1 (3.9 oz)	285	16	99	3	—
broiler/fryer leg w/ skin roasted	1 (4 oz)	265	15	99	0	—
broiler/fryer leg w/ skin stewed	1 (4.4 oz)	275	16	92	0	—
broiler/fryer leg w/o skin fried	1 (3.3 oz)	195	9	90	1	—
broiler/fryer leg w/o skin roasted	1 (3.3 oz)	182	8	87	0	—
broiler/fryer leg w/o skin stewed	1 (3.5 oz)	187	8	78	0	—
broiler/fryer light meat w/ skin batter dipped & fried	4 oz	312	17	324	11	—
broiler/fryer light meat w/ skin floured & fried	2.7 oz	192	9	60	1	—
broiler/fryer light meat w/ skin roasted	2.8 oz	175	9	59	0	—
broiler/fryer light meat w/ skin stewed	3.2 oz	181	9	57	0	—

FOOD	PORTION	CAL.	FAT	SOD.	CARB.	FIB.
broiler/fryer light meat w/o skin fried	1 cup (5 oz)	268	8	114	1	—
broiler/fryer light meat w/o skin roasted	1 cup (5 oz)	242	6	108	0	—
broiler/fryer light meat w/o skin stewed	1 cup (5 oz)	223	6	91	0	—
broiler/fryer neck w/ skin stewed	1 (1.3 oz)	94	7	20	0	—
broiler/fryer neck w/o skin stewed	1 (.6 oz)	32	1	12	0	—
broiler/fryer skin batter dipped & fried	4 oz	449	33	663	26	—
broiler/fryer skin batter dipped & fried	from ½ chicken (6.7 oz)	748	55	1105	44	—
broiler/fryer skin floured & fried	1 oz	166	14	18	3	—
broiler/fryer skin floured & fried	from ½ chicken (2 oz)	281	24	30	5	—
broiler/fryer skin roasted	from ½ chicken (2 oz)	254	23	36	0	—
broiler/fryer skin stewed	from ½ chicken (2.5 oz)	261	24	40	0	—
broiler/fryer thigh w/ skin batter dipped & fried	1 (3 oz)	238	14	248	8	—
broiler/fryer thigh w/ skin floured & fried	1 (2.2 oz)	162	9	55	2	—
broiler/fryer thigh w/ skin roasted	1 (2.2 oz)	153	10	52	0	—
broiler/fryer thigh w/ skin stewed	1 (2.4 oz)	158	10	49	0	—
broiler/fryer thigh w/o skin fried	1 (1.8 oz)	113	5	49	1	—
broiler/fryer thigh w/o skin roasted	1 (1.8 oz)	109	6	46	0	—
broiler/fryer thigh w/o skin stewed	1 (1.9 oz)	107	5	41	0	—
broiler/fryer w/ skin floured & fried	½ chicken (11 oz)	844	47	264	10	—
broiler/fryer w/ skin floured & fried	½ breast (3.4 oz)	218	9	75	2	—
broiler/fryer w/ skin fried	½ chicken (16.4 oz)	1347	81	1360	44	—
broiler/fryer w/ skin roasted	½ chicken (10.5 oz)	715	41	244	0	—
broiler/fryer w/ skin stewed	½ chicken (11.7 oz)	730	42	224	0	—

FOOD	PORTION	CAL.	FAT	SOD.	CARB.	FIB.
broiler/fryer w/ skin neck & giblets batter dipped & fried	1 chicken (2.3 lbs)	2987	180	2921	93	—
broiler/fryer w/ skin neck & giblets roasted	1 chicken (1.5 lbs)	1598	90	536	tr	—
broiler/fryer w/ skin neck & giblets stewed	1 chicken (1.6 lbs)	1625	93	494	tr	—
broiler/fryer w/o skin fried	1 cup	307	13	127	2	—
broiler/fryer w/o skin roasted	1 cup (5 oz)	266	10	120	0	—
broiler/fryer w/o skin stewed	1 cup (5 oz)	248	9	98	0	—
broiler/fryer w/o skin stewed	1 oz	54	3	18	0	—
broiler/fryer wing w/ skin batter dipped & fried	1 (1.7 oz)	159	11	157	5	—
broiler/fryer wing w/ skin floured & fried	1 (1.1 oz)	103	7	25	1	—
broiler/fryer wing w/ skin roasted	1 (1.2 oz)	99	7	28	0	—
broiler/fryer wing w/ skin stewed	1 (1.4 oz)	100	7	27	0	—
capon w/ skin neck & giblets roasted	1 chicken (3.1 lbs)	3211	165	704	1	—
cornish hen w/ skin roasted	1 hen (8 oz)	595	42	146	0	—
cornish hen w/o skin & bone roasted	1 hen (3.8 oz)	144	4	67	0	—
cornish hen w/o skin & bone roasted	½ hen (2 oz)	72	2	34	0	—
cornish hen w/skin roasted	½ hen (4 oz)	296	21	73	0	—
roaster dark meat w/o skin roasted	1 cup (5 oz)	250	12	133	0	—
roaster light meat w/o skin roasted	1 cup (5 oz)	214	6	71	0	—
roaster w/ skin neck & giblets roasted	1 chicken (2.4 lbs)	2363	140	760	1	—
roaster w/ skin roasted	½ chicken (1.1 lbs)	1071	64	349	0	—
roaster w/o skin roasted	1 cup (5 oz)	469	28	105	0	—
stewing dark meat w/o skin stewed	1 cup (5 oz)	361	21	133	0	—
stewing w/ skin neck & giblets stewed	1 chicken (1.3 lbs)	1636	107	419	tr	—
stewing w/ skin stewed	6.2 oz	507	34	130	0	—
stewing w/ skin stewed	½ chicken (9.2 oz)	744	49	190	0	—

FOOD	PORTION	CAL.	FAT	SOD.	CARB.	FIB.
Perdue						
Boneless Breasts Cooked	3 oz	120	2	10	0	—
Boneless Breast Tenderloins Cooked	3 oz	100	1	25	0	—
Boneless Thighs Roasted	2 (3.5 oz)	200	11	60	0	—
Breast Quarters Cooked	3 oz	180	10	35	0	—
Burger Cooked	1 (3 oz)	170	11	35	0	—
Chicken Breast Seasoned Barbecue Cooked	3 oz	110	1	420	5	—
Chicken Breast Seasoned Italian Cooked	3 oz	100	1	520	2	—
Chicken Breast Seasoned Lemon Pepper Cooked	3 oz	90	1	520	2	—
Chicken Breast Seasoned Oriental Cooked	3 oz	100	1	550	3	—
Cornish Hen Split Dark Meat Roasted	1 half (6.5 oz)	210	15	45	0	0
Cornish Hen White Meat Cooked	3 oz	170	9	40	0	—
Drumsticks Roasted	1 (2 oz)	110	6	50	0	—
Drumsticks Skinless Roasted	2 (3.5 oz)	150	6	85	0	—
Ground Cooked	3 oz	180	12	55	0	—
Jumbo Drumsticks Roasted	1 (2 oz)	110	6	50	0	—
Jumbo Split Breast Roasted	1 (7 oz)	370	20	80	0	—
Jumbo Thighs Roasted	1 (3 oz)	240	18	60	0	—
Jumbo Whole Leg Roasted	2 (5.5 oz)	360	25	110	0	—
Jumbo Wings Roasted	2 (3 oz)	210	15	75	0	—
Leg Quarters Cooked	3 oz	210	16	55	0	—
Oven Stuffer Boneless Breast Cooked	3 oz	120	2	25	0	—
Oven Stuffer Boneless Breast Thin Sliced Cooked	1 slice (2 oz)	80	1	10	0	—
Oven Stuffer Boneless Thighs Roasted	1 (3.5 oz)	170	8	40	0	—

FOOD	PORTION	CAL.	FAT	SOD.	CARB.	FIB.
Perdue (CONT.)						
Oven Stuffer Dark Meat Roasted	3 oz	200	14	50	0	—
Oven Stuffer Drumbstick Roasted	1 (3.5 oz)	190	11	80	0	—
Oven Stuffer White Meat Roasted	3 oz	160	8	45	0	—
Oven Stuffer Whole Breast Cooked	3 oz	150	7	35	0	—
Oven Stuffer Wing Drummettes Roasted	2 (2.5 oz)	170	11	45	0	—
Split Breast Skinless Roasted	1 (6 oz)	250	8	55	0	—
Split Breasts Roasted	1 (7 oz)	370	20	80	0	—
Thighs Roasted	1 (3 oz)	240	18	60	0	—
Thighs Skinless Roasted	1 (2.5 oz)	160	9	55	0	—
Whole White Meat Cooked	3 oz	160	9	40	0	0
Whole Leg Roasted	1 (5.5 oz)	360	25	110	0	—
Wingettes Roasted	3 (3 oz)	200	14	65	0	0
Wings Roasted	2 (3 oz)	210	15	75	0	—
Tyson						
Breast	3 oz	116	2	63	0	—
Cornish Hen	3.5 oz	250	15	80	1	—
Drumstick	3 oz	131	4	81	0	—
Thigh	3 oz	152	7	75	0	—
Whole	3 oz	134	4	73	0	—
Wing	3 oz	147	6	78	0	—
Wampler Longacre						
Ground raw	1 oz	50	4	20	0	—
FROZEN						
Banquet						
Country Fried	1 serv (3 oz)	270	18	620	13	1
Drum Snackers	2.25 oz	190	13	460	12	1
Fried Breast	1 piece (4.45 oz)	240	26	600	18	4
Fried Hot & Spicy	1 serv (3 oz)	260	18	590	13	1
Fried Original	1 serv (3 oz)	270	18	620	13	1
Fried Thigh & Drumsticks	1 serv (3 oz)	260	18	540	10	2
Hot & Spicy Nuggets	2.5 oz	230	17	320	11	1
Hot Popcorn Chicken	1 pkg (3 oz)	290	19	790	18	2
Nuggets	3 oz	240	15	540	12	1
Nuggets Chicken & Cheddar	2.7 oz	280	19	560	13	1

FOOD	PORTION	CAL.	FAT	SOD.	CARB.	FIB.
Banquet (CONT.)						
Nuggets Chicken & Mozzarella	6 (2.8 oz)	210	11	1060	20	2
Nuggets Southern Fried	6 (4.5 oz)	340	20	840	22	2
Nuggets Sweet & Sour	6 (4.5 oz)	320	18	670	25	2
Patties	1 (2.5 oz)	180	11	360	10	tr
Patties Southern Fried	1 (2.5 oz)	190	12	480	12	tr
Skinless Fried	1 serv (3 oz)	210	13	480	7	2
Skinless Fried Honey BBQ	1 serv (3 oz)	210	13	480	7	2
Southern Fried	1 serv (3 oz)	270	18	590	13	1
Tenders	3 pieces (3 oz)	260	16	490	16	2
Tenders Southern Fried	3 pieces (3 oz)	260	16	480	16	1
Wings Hot & Spicy	4 pieces (5 oz)	230	16	280	5	1
Country Skillet						
Chicken Chunks	5 (3.1 oz)	270	17	720	18	1
Chicken Nuggets	10 (3.3 oz)	280	18	620	16	1
Chicken Patties	2.5 oz	190	12	500	12	1
Southern Fried Chicken Chunks	5 (3.1 oz)	250	15	550	16	1
Southern Fried Chicken Patties	1 (2.5 oz)	190	12	450	12	1
Empire						
Nuggets	5 (3 oz)	180	9	370	12	1
Stix	4 (3.1 oz)	180	9	420	6	2
Ozark Valley						
Nuggets	4 (2.9 oz)	210	10	590	16	2
Patties	1 (3 oz)	210	11	550	14	1
Sensible Chef						
Fried Breast	1 (3 oz)	200	10	310	8	2
Swanson						
Chicken Nibbles	3¼ oz	300	19	690	19	—
Chicken Nuggets	3 oz	230	14	360	14	—
Fried Chicken Breast Portion	4½ oz	360	20	800	21	—
Pre-Fried Chicken Parts	3¼ oz	270	16	650	16	—
Thighs & Drumsticks	3¼ oz	290	18	610	17	—
Tyson						
BBQ Breast Fillets	3 oz	110	2	200	13	—
Boneless Breasts	3.5 oz	210	12	50	0	—
Boneless Skinless Breast	3.5 oz	130	2	50	0	—
Boneless Skinless Thighs	3.5 oz	200	10	70	0	—
Breaded Patties	3 oz	300	20	—	15	—

FOOD	PORTION	CAL.	FAT	SOD.	CARB.	FIB.
Tyson (CONT.)						
Breast Chunks	3 oz	240	17	430	10	—
Breast Fillets	3 oz	190	9	400	15	—
Breast Patties	2.6 oz	220	15	640	11	—
Breast Tenders	3 oz	220	12	500	13	—
Chick'n Cheddar	2.6 oz	220	15	310	11	—
Chick'n Chunks	2.6 oz	220	15	500	11	—
Cordon Blue Mini	1	90	4	210	5	—
Diced	3 oz	130	3	40	1	—
Drums & Thighs	3.5 oz	270	17	110	0	—
Grilled Sandwich	3.5 oz	200	5	470	25	—
Hors D'Oeuvres Mesquite Chunks	3.5 oz	100	1	600	1	—
Hot BBQ Breast Tenders	2.75 oz	110	3	580	4	—
Mesquite Breast Fillets	2.75 oz	100	2	250	3	—
Mesquite Breast Strips	2.75 oz	100	2	240	2	—
Mesquite Breast Tenders	2.75 oz	110	2	290	2	—
Microwave Chunks	3.5 oz	220	15	—	11	—
Microwave Chunks BBQ Sandwich	4 oz	230	6	600	27	—
Microwave Tenders	3.5 oz	230	11	600	19	—
Roasted Breast Fillets	1 oz	50	2	160	—	—
Roasted Breasts	1 oz	50	3	160	—	—
Roasted Drumsticks	1 oz	50	3	190	—	—
Roasted Half Chicken	1 oz	60	4	150	—	—
Roasted Thighs	1 oz	70	5	180	—	—
Roasted Whole Chicken	1 oz	60	4	150	—	—
Skinless Breast Tenders	3.5 oz	120	1	55	0	—
Southern Fried Breast Fillets	3 oz	220	11	630	15	—
Southern Fried Breast Patties	2.6 oz	220	15	460	9	—
Southern Fried Chick'n Chunks	2.6 oz	220	15	540	11	—
Thick & Crispy Patties	2.6 oz	220	14	490	13	—
Weaver						
Batter Dipped Breast	4.4 oz	310	20	220	13	—
Batter Dipped Drums & Thighs	3 oz	210	14	220	11	—
Batter Dipped Wings	4 oz	400	28	520	20	—
Breast Fillets	4.5 oz	270	13	520	18	—
Breast Fillets Strips	3.3 oz	200	10	500	14	—
Breast Patties	3 oz	205	11	640	14	—
Chicken Nuggets	2.6 oz	190	12	450	10	—

FOOD	PORTION	CAL.	FAT	SOD.	CARB.	FIB.
Weaver (CONT.)						
Crispy Dutch Frye Assorted	3.6 oz	290	18	550	16	—
Crispy Dutch Frye Breasts	4.5 oz	350	22	520	17	—
Crispy Dutch Frye Drums & Thighs	3.5 oz	290	19	640	14	—
Crispy Dutch Frye Wings	4 oz	400	28	520	20	—
Crispy Light Skinless	2.9 oz	170	9	320	9	—
Croquettes	2 pieces	280	16	780	22	—
Croquettes With Gravy	2 pieces + ½ cup gravy	282	18	1040	26	—
Honey Batter Tenders	3 oz	220	12	500	14	—
Hot Wings	2.7 oz	170	11	670	1	—
Mini Drums Crispy	3 oz	210	12	480	13	—
Mini Drums Herbs & Spice	3 oz	200	11	320	13	—
Premium Tenders	3 oz	170	9	500	11	—
Rondelets Cheese	1 (2.6 oz)	190	11	520	12	—
Rondelets Italian	1 (2.6 oz)	190	11	560	11	—
Rondelets Original	1 (3 oz)	190	10	610	13	—
READY-TO-EAT						
chicken roll light meat	2 oz	90	4	331	1	—
chicken roll light meat	1 pkg (6 oz)	271	13	992	4	—
poultry salad sandwich spread	1 oz	238	4	107	2	—
poultry salad sandwich spread	1 tbsp (13 g)	109	2	49	1	—
Banquet						
Breast Tenders Fat Free	3 (3.2 oz)	130	0	480	20	2
Carl Buddig						
Chicken	1 oz	50	3	320	1	0
Chicken By George						
Cajun	1 breast (4 oz)	120	4	650	2	0
Caribbean Grill	1 breast (4 oz)	150	4	550	8	0
Garlic & Herb	1 breast (4 oz)	120	3	800	3	0
Italian Bleu Cheese	1 breast (4 oz)	130	5	790	2	0
Lemon Herb	1 breast (4 oz)	120	3	800	3	0
Lemon Oregano	1 breast (4 oz)	130	4	600	3	0
Mesquite Barbecue	1 breast (4 oz)	120	2	800	5	0
Mustard Dill	1 breast (4 oz)	140	5	650	2	0
Roasted	1 breast (4 oz)	110	3	500	1	0
Teriyaki	1 breast (4 oz)	130	3	650	6	0
Tomato Herb With Basil	1 breast (4 oz)	140	5	630	5	0

FOOD	PORTION	CAL.	FAT	SOD.	CARB.	FIB.
Empire						
Barbarcue Whole	5 oz	280	17	460	1	0
Battered & Breaded Cutlets	1 (3.3 oz)	200	9	320	11	2
Battered & Breaded Fried Breasts	3 oz	170	8	440	3	tr
Battered & Breaded Nuggets	5 (3 oz)	200	13	650	9	1
Bologna	3 slices (1.8 oz)	200	7	360	2	0
Fried Drum & Thigh	3 oz	240	16	260	7	2
Falls						
BBQ	3 oz	150	8	310	—	—
Healthy Choice						
Deli-Thin Oven Roasted Breast	6 slices (2 oz)	45	0	410	0	0
Deli-Thin Smoked Breast	6 slices (2 oz)	60	2	420	1	0
Fresh-Trak Oven Roasted Breast	1 slice (1 oz)	30	1	290	0	0
Oven Roasted Breast	1 slice (1 oz)	25	0	220	0	0
Smoked Breast	1 slice (1 oz)	35	1	220	0	0
Hebrew National						
Deli Thin Oven Roasted	1.8 oz	45	1	460	—	—
Hillshire						
Deli Select Oven Roasted Breast	1 slice	10	tr	115	tr	—
Deli Select Smoked Breast	1 slice	10	tr	95	tr	—
Flavor Pack 90-99% Fat Free Smoked Breast	1 slice (0.75 oz)	20	tr	220	tr	—
Lunch 'N Munch Smoked Chicken/ Monterey Jack	1 pkg (4.5 oz)	350	20	1260	19	—
Lunch 'N Munch Smoked Chicken/ Monterey/ Snickers	1 pkg (4.25 oz)	400	23	1080	31	—
Louis Rich						
Deli-Thin Oven Roasted Breast	4 slices (1.8 oz)	60	2	620	1	0
Deluxe Oven Roasted Breast	1 slice (1 oz)	40	1	330	1	0
Hickory Smoked Breast	1 slice (1 oz)	30	1	360	1	0
Oven Roasted Breast	1 slice (1 oz)	40	3	350	1	0
Mr. Turkey						
Deli Cuts Hardwood Smoked	3 slices	30	tr	305	2	—

FOOD	PORTION	CAL.	FAT	SOD.	CARB.	FIB.
Mr. Turkey (CONT.)						
Deli Cuts Oven Roasted	3 slices	25	0	220	2	—
Oscar Mayer						
Deli-Thin Honey Glazed Breast	4 slices (1.8 oz)	60	1	740	2	0
Free Oven Roasted Breast	4 slices (1.8 oz)	45	0	650	1	—
Healthy Favorites Oven Roasted Breast	4 slices (1.8 oz)	40	0	620	1	0
Lunchables Chicken/ Monterey Jack	1 pkg (4.5 oz)	350	21	1690	20	1
Lunchables Deluxe Chicken/Turkey	1 pkg (5.1 oz)	380	22	1840	24	1
Lunchables Dessert Chocolate Pudding/ Chicken/ Jack	1 pkg (6.2 oz)	370	18	1490	33	0
Smoked Breast	1 slice (1 oz)	25	tr	397	tr	—
Perdue						
Cornish Hen Dark Meat Cooked	3 oz	200	15	45	0	—
Cornish Hen Split White Meat Roasted	½ hen (6.5 oz)	200	11	45	0	0
Nuggets Chicken & Cheese	5 (3 oz)	220	15	550	11	2
Nuggets Chik-Tac-Toe Cooked	5 (3 oz)	200	12	390	15	2
Nuggets Football Basketball Baseball	4 (3 oz)	230	15	500	14	—
Nuggets Original	5 (3 oz)	200	12	390	15	2
Nuggets Star & Drumstick	4 (3 oz)	200	12	390	15	2
Original Tenderloins Cooked	3 oz	160	7	320	7	2
Original Cutlets Cooked	1 (3.5 oz)	230	13	450	18	2
Oven Roasted Breast	1 (5 oz)	190	6	540	0	0
Oven Roasted Drumsticks	2 (2.5 oz)	100	4	350	0	0
Oven Roasted Half Dark Meat	3 oz	170	11	320	0	0
Oven Roasted Half White Meat	3 oz	140	7	320	0	0
Oven Roasted Thighs	1 (3 oz)	170	12	360	0	0
Oven Roasted Whole Chicken Dark Meat	3 oz	170	11	320	0	0

FOOD	PORTION	CAL.	FAT	SOD.	CARB.	FIB.
Perdue (CONT.)						
Oven Roasted Whole Chicken White Meat	3 oz	140	7	320	0	0
Perdue Done It! Nuggets Original	1 (.67 oz)	48	3	85	3	—
Short Cuts Italian	3 oz	110	2	540	1	0
Short Cuts Lemon Pepper	½ cup (2.5 oz)	90	2	530	2	—
Short Cuts Mesquite	3 oz	110	2	510	2	0
Short Cuts Oven Roasted	3 oz	110	2	765	2	0
Wings Barbecued	3 oz	200	13	600	3	1
Wings Hot & Spicy	3 oz	190	13	610	2	1
Tyson						
Bologna	1 slice	44	1	185	4	—
Hickory Smoked Breast	1 slice	25	1	195	1	—
Honey Flavored Breast	1 slice	25	1	—	1	—
Oven Roasted Breast	1 slice	25	1	185	1	—
Oven Roasted Mesquite Breast	1 slice	25	1	—	1	—
Roasted Drumsticks w/ Skin	2 (3.8 oz)	220	12	580	1	—
Roll	1 slice	26	1	153	1	—
Wings Barbecue	6-7 (3.5 oz)	218	14	400	0	—
Wings Hot & Spicy	6-7 (3.5 oz)	218	14	400	0	—
Wings Roasted	6-7 (3.5 oz)	218	14	400	0	—
Wings Teriyaki	6-7 (3.5 oz)	218	14	400	0	—
Wampler Longacre						
Breast	1 oz	35	1	200	1	—
Chef's Select Breast	1 oz	35	1	320	tr	—
Premium Oven Roasted Breast	1 oz	50	3	350	2	—
Roll	1 oz	65	5	240	tr	—
Roll Sliced	1 slice (0.8 oz)	50	4	170	1	—
Weaver						
Roasted Wings	1 oz	70	5	180	—	—
Weight Watchers						
Roasted & Smoked Breast	2 slices (¾ oz)	25	1	220	tr	—
Roasted Ham	2 slices (¾ oz)	25	1	210	tr	—
TAKE-OUT						
boneless breaded & fried w/ barbecue sauce	6 pieces (4.6 oz)	330	18	830	25	—
boneless breaded & fried w/ honey	6 pieces (4 oz)	339	18	537	27	—

boneless breaded & fried w/ mustard sauce	6 pieces (4.6 oz)	323	17	791	21	—
boneless breaded & fried w/ sweet & sour sauce	6 pieces (4.6 oz)	346	18	791	29	—
breast & wing breaded & fried	2 pieces (5.7 oz)	494	30	975	20	—
drumstick breaded & fried	2 pieces (5.2 oz)	430	27	756	16	—
oven roasted breast of chicken	2 oz	60	1	470	0	—
thigh breaded & fried	2 pieces (5.2 oz)	430	27	756	16	—

CHICKEN DISHES

(*see also* CHICKEN SUBSTITUTES, DINNER)

CANNED						
Dinty Moore						
Microwave Cup Chicken & Dumpling	1 cup (7.5 oz)	200	6	890	21	1
Stew	1 cup (8.5 oz)	220	11	980	16	2
Swanson						
Chicken & Dumplings	7½ oz	220	11	980	19	—
Chicken Ala King	5¼ oz	190	12	690	9	—
Chicken Stew	7⅝ oz	160	7	990	15	—
FROZEN						
Croissant Pocket						
Stuffed Sandwich Chicken Broccoli & Cheddar	1 piece (4.5 oz)	300	11	640	37	5
Hot Pocket						
Stuffed Sandwich Chicken & Cheddar With Broccoli	1 (4.5 oz)	300	12	620	37	tr
Jimmy Dean						
Grilled Breast Sandwich	1 (5.5 oz)	330	11	730	27	1
Lean Pockets						
Stuffed Sandwich Chicken Fajita	1 (4.5 oz)	260	8	770	36	3
Stuffed Sandwich Chicken Parmesan	1 (4.5 oz)	260	8	630	34	1
Stuffed Sandwich Glazed Chicken Supreme	1 (4.5 oz)	240	7	600	34	1
Luigino's						
Chicken A La King With Noodles	1 pkg (8 oz)	240	7	660	28	2
Noodles With Chicken Peas & Carrots	1 pkg (8 oz)	300	11	640	38	2

FOOD	PORTION	CAL.	FAT	SOD.	CARB.	FIB.
Luigino's (CONT.)						
Noodles With Chicken Peas & Carrots	1 cup (6.3 oz)	260	10	560	33	2
Sweet & Sour Chicken With Rice	1 pkg (8 oz)	300	6	480	50	2
MicroMagic						
Chicken Sandwich	1 pkg (4.5 oz)	390	16	650	42	—
Ovenstuffs						
Chicken Turnover	1 (4.75 oz)	350	16	690	36	—
Tyson						
Microwave Breast Sandwich	4.25 oz	328	14	520	33	—
White Castle						
Grilled Chicken Sandwich	2 (4 oz)	250	9	490	24	5
Grilled Chicken Sandwich w/ Sauce	2 (4.8 oz)	290	9	600	33	5
MIX						
Chicken Skillet Helper						
Stir-Fried Chicken as prep	1 cup	270	9	810	30	1
Hamburger Helper						
Cheddar Spirals Reduced Sodium Chicken Recipe as prep	1 cup	240	6	630	27	1
Italian Herb Reduced Sodium Chicken Recipe as prep	1 cup	200	2	630	29	2
Southwestern Beef Reduced Sodium Chicken Recipe as prep	1 cup	220	3	630	32	2
READY-TO-EAT						
Spreadables						
Chicken Salad	¼ can	100	6	—	—	—
Wampler Longacre						
Cacciatore	1 serv (4 oz)	118	3	267	5	—
Salad	1 oz	70	3	125	3	—
Salad Lite	1 oz	45	2	95	3	—
Smokey Barbecue	1 serv (4 oz)	175	7	460	11	—
Sweet N Sour	1 serv (4 oz)	106	tr	231	16	—

FOOD	PORTION	CAL.	FAT	SOD.	CARB.	FIB.
Wampler Longacre (CONT.)						
Szechwan With Peanuts	1 serv (4 oz)	112	4	560	6	—
SHELF-STABLE						
Dinty Moore						
Stew	1 cup (7.5 oz)	180	8	920	18	2
Lunch Bucket						
Dumplings'n Chicken	1 pkg (7.5 oz)	140	2	880	25	—
Light'n Healthy Chicken Fiesta	1 pkg (7.5 oz)	170	3	600	28	—
Top Shelf						
Chicken Cacciatore	1 bowl (10 oz)	210	3	850	26	3
Chicken Acapulco Fiesta Chicken	1 bowl (10 oz)	420	16	1070	45	2
Chicken Ala King	1 bowl (10 oz)	380	12	960	47	2
Glazed Breast Of Chicken	1 bowl (10 oz)	200	5	910	17	2
TAKE-OUT						
chicken & dumplings	¾ cup	256	12	1283	12	tr
chicken & noodles	1 cup	365	18	600	26	—
chicken a la king	1 cup	470	34	760	12	—
chicken cacciatore	¾ cup	394	24	671	9	2
chicken paprikash	1½ cups	296	10	—	—	—
chicken pie w/ top crust	1 slice (5.6 oz)	472	31	—	32	1
fillet sandwich plain	1	515	29	957	39	—
fillet sandwich w/ cheese lettuce mayonnaise & tomato	1	632	39	1238	42	—

CHICKEN SUBSTITUTES

FOOD	PORTION	CAL.	FAT	SOD.	CARB.	FIB.
Harvest Direct						
TVP Poultry Chunks	3.5 oz	280	1	15	32	18
TVP Poultry Ground	3.5 oz	280	1	15	32	18
Jaclyn's						
Salsa Chicken Style Dinner	11.5 oz	325	9	290	35	—
Sesame Chicken Style Dinner	11.5 oz	345	8	635	40	—
Knox Mountain Farm						
Chick'N Wheat Mix	1 serv (1/9 pkg)	110	1	220	3	2
LaLoma						
Chicken Supreme not prep	¼ cup (16 g)	50	0	450	4	—
Chik Nuggets	5 nuggets (85 g)	270	20	530	8	—
Fried Chicken	1 piece (57 g)	180	14	570	2	—
Fried Chicken w/ Gravy	2 piece (85 g)	140	10	340	4	—

FOOD	PORTION	CAL.	FAT	SOD.	CARB.	FIB.
Soy Is Us						
Chicken Not!	½ cup (1.75 oz)	140	2	5	15	9
White Wave						
Meatless Sandwich Slices	2 slices (1.6 oz)	80	0	260	8	0
Worthington						
Chick-ketts	½ cup (84 g)	160	7	640	6	—
ChickStiks	1 (47 g)	110	7	380	4	—
Chicken Sliced	2 slices (57 g)	130	9	460	3	—
CrispyChik	1 patty (71 g)	220	15	620	13	—
CrispyChik	6 nuggets (85 g)	280	19	500	17	—
Cutlets	1.5 slices (92 g)	100	2	270	4	—
Diced Chik	¼ cup (60 g)	90	8	330	2	—
FriChik	2 pieces (90 g)	180	13	610	13	—
Golden Croquettes	5 pieces (106 g)	280	14	890	20	—
Savory Slices	2 slices (60 g)	90	8	330	2	—
Vegetarian Chicken Pie	1 (227 g)	380	20	1200	43	—

CHICKPEAS

CANNED

FOOD	PORTION	CAL.	FAT	SOD.	CARB.	FIB.
chickpeas	1 cup	285	3	718	54	—
Allen						
Garbanzo	½ cup (4.4 oz)	120	3	330	19	8
East Texas Fair						
Garbanzo	½ cup (4.4 oz)	120	3	330	19	8
Eden						
Organic	½ cup (4.1 oz)	110	2	10	17	4
Goya						
Spanish Style	7.5 oz	150	2	890	32	9
Green Giant						
Garbanzo	½ cup	90	2	320	18	5
Hanover						
Chickpeas	½ cup	100	1	—	—	—
Old El Paso						
Garbanzo	½ cup (4.6 oz)	120	3	280	20	7
Progresso						
Chick Peas	½ cup (4.6 oz)	120	3	280	20	7
S&W						
Garbanzo Lite 50% Less Salt	½ cup	110	0	295	21	—
Garbanzo Premium Large	½ cup	110	1	470	20	—
Garbanzo Water Pack	½ cup	105	1	5	19	—

DRIED

FOOD	PORTION	CAL.	FAT	SOD.	CARB.	FIB.
cooked	1 cup	269	4	11	45	—

FOOD	PORTION	CAL.	FAT	SOD.	CARB.	FIB.
Bean Cuisine						
Garbanzo	½ cup	115	1	5	—	5
CHICORY						
greens raw chopped	½ cup	21	tr	41	4	—
root raw	1 (2.1 oz)	44	tr	30	11	—
roots raw cut up	½ cup (1.6 oz)	33	tr	23	8	—
witloof head raw	1 (1.9 oz)	9	tr	1	2	—
witloof raw	½ cup (1.6 oz)	8	tr	1	2	—
CHILI						
CANNED						
chili w/ beans	1 cup	286	14	1330	30	—
Allen						
Mexican Chili Beans	½ cup (4.5 oz)	120	1	300	22	8
Armour						
Chili No Beans	1 cup (8.7 oz)	470	38	1200	18	—
Chili With Beans	1 cup (8.9 oz)	440	28	1270	34	—
Chili With Beans Hot	1 cup (8.9 oz)	440	28	1270	34	—
Chili With Beans Western Style	1 cup (8.8 oz)	460	32	1130	29	—
Brown Beauty						
Mexican Chili Beans	½ cup (4.5 oz)	120	1	300	22	8
Chi-Chi's						
San Antonio	1 cup (8.5 oz)	240	19	900	23	6
Del Monte						
Sauce	1 tbsp (0.6 oz)	20	0	480	0	0
Dennison's						
Chili Beans In Chili Gravy	7.5 oz	180	1	—	—	—
Chili Con Carne w/ Beans	7.5 oz	310	15	—	—	—
Chili Con Carne w/ Beans	7.5 oz	300	19	—	—	—
Chunky Chili w/ Beans	7.5 oz	310	14	—	—	—
Cook-off Chili w/ Beans	7.5 oz	340	19	—	—	—
Hot Chili Con Carne w/ Beans	7.5 oz	310	16	—	—	—
Gebhardt						
Hot With Beans	1 cup	470	27	1000	47	6
Plain	1 cup	530	43	990	20	1
With Beans	1 cup	495	28	1010	47	6
Hain						
Spicy Tempeh	7½ oz	160	4	1350	24	—
Spicy Vegetarian	7½ oz	160	1	1060	29	—
Spicy Vegetarian Reduced Sodium	7½ oz	170	1	200	31	—
Spicy With Chicken	7½ oz	130	2	1030	19	—

FOOD	PORTION	CAL.	FAT	SOD.	CARB.	FIB.
Health Valley						
Mild Vegetarian With Beans	5 oz	160	3	290	21	12
Mild Vegetarian With Beans No Salt Added	5 oz	160	3	30	21	12
Mild Vegetarian With Lentils	5 oz	140	4	290	15	7
Mild Vegetarian With Lentils No Salt Added	5 oz	140	4	50	15	7
Spicy Vegetarian With Beans	5 oz	160	4	280	21	12
Hormel						
Chunky With Beans	1 cup (8.7 oz)	270	7	1240	34	7
Hot No Beans	1 cup (8.2 oz)	210	9	910	17	3
Hot With Beans	1 cup (8.7 oz)	270	7	1240	33	7
No Beans	1 cup (8.2 oz)	210	9	910	17	3
Turkey With Beans	1 cup (8.7 oz)	210	3	1180	30	5
Turkey No Beans	1 cup (8.2 oz)	190	3	1250	17	3
Vegetarian	1 cup (8.7 oz)	200	1	780	38	7
With Beans	1 cup (8.7 oz)	270	7	1240	33	7
Hunt's						
Chili Beans	½ cup (4.5 oz)	87	1	597	17	6
Just Rite						
Hot With Beans	4 oz	195	10	495	16	1
With Beans	4 oz	200	11	500	16	1
Without Beans	4 oz	180	11	515	9	tr
Luck's						
Hot Chili Beans	7.5 oz	200	2	—	—	—
Natural Touch						
Vegetarian	⅔ cup (190 g)	230	12	890	19	—
Old El Paso						
Chili With Beans	1 cup (8 oz)	200	7	420	15	6
S&W						
Chili Beans	½ cup	130	1	520	23	—
Chili Makin's Original	½ cup	100	1	782	20	—
Van Camp's						
Chilee Beanee Weenee	1 can (8 oz)	240	12	1090	27	9
Chili With Beans	1 cup (8.9 oz)	350	21	1020	28	7
Wolf Brand						
Chili-Mac	7.5 oz	317	20	854	23	—
Extra Spicy With Beans	7.5 oz	324	21	926	21	—
Extra Spicy Without Beans	7.5 oz	363	25	962	15	—
Plain	7.5 oz	330	22	1165	10	—

FOOD	PORTION	CAL.	FAT	SOD.	CARB.	FIB.
Wolf Brand (CONT.)						
With Beans	7.5 oz	345	22	1013	22	—
Without Beans	1 cup	387	27	1042	16	—
Worthington						
Chili	⅔ cup (141 g)	190	10	550	15	—
DRIED						
powder	1 tsp	8	tr	26	1	—
Gebhardt						
Chili Powder	1 tsp	15	tr	0	3	tr
Chili Quik Seasoning	1 tsp	10	tr	165	2	tr
Hain						
Hot Chili	¼ pkg	30	1	370	5	—
Medium Chili	¼ pkg	30	1	300	5	—
Mild Chili	¼ pkg	30	1	330	5	—
Nile Spice						
Chili'n Beans Original	1 pkg	150	2	670	25	6
Chili'n Beans Spicy	1 pkg	150	2	720	25	6
Old El Paso						
Chili Seasoning Mix	1 tbsp (0.3 oz)	25	1	770	4	1
Watkins						
Chili Seasoning	1¼ tsp (4 g)	15	0	110	2	0
Powder	¼ tsp (0.5 g)	0	0	10	0	0
FROZEN						
Lean Cuisine						
Three Bean w/ Rice	1 pkg (10 oz)	250	6	590	38	9
Lightlife						
Chili	4.3 oz	110	3	360	14	—
Luigino's						
Chili-Mac	1 pkg (8 oz)	230	7	770	29	3
Stouffer's						
With Beans	1 pkg (8.75 oz)	270	10	1130	29	8
Swanson						
Homestyle Chili Con Carne	8¼ oz	270	10	740	26	—
Tabatchnick						
Vegetarian	7.5 oz	210	6	530	28	10
Tyson						
Chicken Chili	3.5 oz	105	3	420	11	—
SHELF-STABLE						
Lunch Bucket						
Chili With Beans	1 pkg (7.5 oz)	300	14	1120	26	—
Micro Cup Meals						
Chili Mac	1 cup (7.5 oz)	200	9	980	17	2
Chili No Beans	1 cup (7.5 oz)	290	17	830	15	3

FOOD	PORTION	CAL.	FAT	SOD.	CARB.	FIB.
Micro Cup Meals (CONT.)						
Chili With Beans	1 cup (7.5 oz)	250	11	980	23	6
Chili With Beans	1 cup (10.4 oz)	410	17	1430	41	12
Hot Chili With Beans	1 cup (7.5 oz)	250	11	980	23	6
Wampler Longacre						
Turkey	1 serv (4 oz)	118	3	850	10	—
TAKE-OUT						
con carne w/ beans	8.9 oz	254	8	1008	22	—

CHINESE CABBAGE

(*see* CABBAGE

CHINESE FOOD

(*see* ASIAN FOOD)

CHINESE PRESERVING MELON

cooked	½ cup	11	tr	93	3	—

CHIPS

(*see also* POPCORN, PRETZELS, SNACKS)

CORN						
barbecue	1 bag (7 oz)	1036	65	1511	111	10
barbecue	1 oz	148	9	216	16	1
cones nacho	1 oz	152	9	270	17	—
cones plain	1 oz	145	8	290	18	—
onion	1 oz	142	6	278	19	—
plain	1 oz	153	10	179	16	1
plain	1 bag (7 oz)	1067	66	1248	113	9
puffs cheese	1 oz	157	10	298	15	tr
puffs cheese	1 bag (8 oz)	1256	78	2383	122	2
twists cheese	1 oz	157	10	298	15	tr
twists cheese	1 bag (8 oz)	1256	78	2383	122	2
Energy Food Factory						
Corn Pops Fat Free	½ oz	50	0	110	11	1
Corn Pops Nacho	½ oz	50	1	150	12	1
Corn Pops Original	½ oz	50	1	110	11	1
Fritos						
Chili Cheese	34 pieces (1 oz)	160	10	300	15	1
Crisp 'N Thin	18 pieces (1 oz)	160	10	240	16	1
Dip Size	13 pieces (1 oz)	150	10	240	16	1
Non-Stop Nacho Cheese	34 pieces (1 oz)	150	9	220	16	1
Rowdy Rustlers Bar-B-Q	34 pieces (1 oz)	150	9	300	17	1
Wild 'N Mild	32 pieces (1 oz)	160	9	240	16	1
Health Valley						
Chips	1 oz	160	11	90	13	1
No Salt Added	1 oz	160	11	1	13	1

FOOD	PORTION	CAL.	FAT	SOD.	CARB.	FIB.
Health Valley (CONT.)						
With Cheddar Cheese	1 oz	160	10	120	15	1
Lance						
BBQ	1 pkg (50 g)	260	16	360	25	—
Chips	1 pkg (50 g)	270	17	350	26	—
Planters						
Corn Chips	34 chips (1 oz)	170	10	180	17	2
King Size	17 chips (1 oz)	160	10	180	16	2
Snacks To Go	1 pkg (1.5 oz)	240	15	260	23	3
Snyder's						
BBQ	1 oz	160	11	200	14	2
Chips	1 oz	160	11	150	14	2
Wise						
Corn Crunchies	1 oz	160	10	180	15	—
Crispy Corn	1 oz	160	10	125	15	—
Crispy Corn Nacho Cheese	1 oz	160	10	190	16	—
Dipsy Doodles	1 pkg (1.5 oz)	240	15	270	24	1
MULTIGRAIN						
Sunchips						
Chips	12 pieces (1 oz)	150	8	100	18	—
French Onion	12 pieces (1 oz)	140	7	120	18	—
POTATO						
barbecue	1 bag (7 oz)	971	64	1486	105	—
barbecue	1 oz	139	9	213	15	—
cheese	1 bag (6 oz)	842	46	1348	98	—
cheese	1 oz	140	8	225	16	—
light	1 bag (6 oz)	801	35	836	114	—
light	1 oz	134	6	139	19	—
potato	1 oz	152	10	168	15	—
potato	1 bag (8 oz)	1217	79	1347	120	—
sour cream & onion	1 oz	150	10	177	15	—
sour cream & onion	1 bag (7 oz)	1051	67	1237	102	—
sticks	1 oz	148	10	71	15	1
sticks	½ cup (0.6 oz)	94	6	45	10	1
sticks	1 pkg (1 oz)	148	10	71	15	—
Barrel O' Fun						
Barbeque	1 oz	145	9	250	16	0
Chips	1 oz	150	9	160	15	0
Sour Cream & Onion	1 oz	150	9	230	15	0
Butterfield						
Sticks	⅔ cup (1 oz)	150	9	90	16	2
Sticks	1 pkg (1.7 oz)	250	15	150	26	3

FOOD	PORTION	CAL.	FAT	SOD.	CARB.	FIB.
Cape Cod						
Chips	19 chips (1 oz)	150	8	110	17	1
Cottage Fries						
No Salt Added	1 oz	160	11	5	14	—
Energy Food Factory						
Potato Pops Au Gratin	½ oz	60	2	110	12	1
Potato Pops Fat Free	½ oz	50	0	110	13	1
Potato Pops Herb & Garlic	½ oz	50	1	110	11	1
Potato Pops Mesquite	½ oz	50	1	110	12	1
Potato Pops Original	½ oz	50	1	110	11	1
Potato Pops Salt N' Vinegar	½ oz	50	1	110	11	1
Health Valley						
Country Ripple	1 oz	160	10	60	15	1
Country Ripple No Salt Added	1 oz	160	10	1	15	1
Dip Chips	1 oz	160	10	60	15	1
Dip Chips No Salt Added	1 oz	160	10	1	15	1
Natural	1 oz	160	10	60	15	1
Natural No Salt Added	1 oz	160	10	1	15	1
Herr's						
Potato	1 oz	140	8	180	16	1
Kelly's						
Bar-B-Q	1 oz	150	9	230	15	1
Chips	1 oz	150	9	160	14	2
Crunchy	1 oz	150	9	140	17	2
Rippled	1 oz	150	9	160	14	2
Sour Cream n' Onion	1 oz	150	9	170	15	1
Unsalted	1 oz	150	10	5	14	—
Lance						
BBQ	1 pkg (32 g)	190	12	270	18	—
Cajun Style	1 pkg (32 g)	160	11	250	16	—
Chips	1 pkg (32 g)	190	15	220	12	—
Hot Fries	1 pkg (28 g)	160	10	220	14	—
Ripple	1 pkg (32 g)	190	15	220	12	—
Sour Cream & Onion	1 pkg (32 g)	190	12	390	18	—
Lay's						
Baked KC Masterpiece	11 pieces (1 oz)	110	2	200	23	2
Baked Original	12 chips (1 oz)	110	2	150	23	2
Baked Sour Cream & Onion	12 chips (1 oz)	110	2	170	23	2
Bar-B-Q	17 pieces (1 oz)	150	9	270	15	1
Cheddar Cheese	17 pieces (1 oz)	150	10	300	14	1

FOOD	PORTION	CAL.	FAT	SOD.	CARB.	FIB.
Lay's (CONT.)						
Crunch Tators	16 pieces (1 oz)	150	8	120	17	1
Crunch Tators Amazin' Cajun	16 pieces (1 oz)	150	8	150	17	—
Crunch Tators Hoppin' Jalapeno	16 pieces (1 oz)	140	7	200	18	1
Crunch Tators Mighty Mesquite	16 pieces (1 oz)	150	8	135	17	—
Crunch Tators Supreme Sour Cream	16 pieces (1 oz)	150	8	180	16	—
Flamin' Hot	17 pieces (1 oz)	150	9	190	15	1
Reduced Fat Original	21 chips (1 oz)	150	8	160	18	1
Salt & Vinegar	17 pieces (1 oz)	150	10	390	14	1
Tangy Ranch	17 pieces (1 oz)	160	10	210	15	1
Unsalted	17 pieces (1 oz)	150	10	10	15	1
Wow Original	25 chips (1 oz)	80	0	180	19	1
Wow Original	1 pkg (0.75 oz)	55	0	130	13	1
Louise's						
"1g" Mesquite BBQ	1 oz	110	1	180	24	2
"1g" Original	1 oz	110	1	180	24	2
70% Less Fat Mesquite BBQ	1 oz	110	3	180	21	2
70% Less Fat Original	1 oz	110	3	200	21	2
Fat-Free Maui Onion	1 oz	110	0	180	23	2
Fat-Free Mesquite BBQ	1 oz	110	0	180	23	2
Fat-Free No Salt	1 oz	110	0	10	24	2
Fat-Free Original	1 oz	110	0	180	23	2
Fat-Free Vinegar & Salt	1 oz	110	0	300	23	2
Mr. Phipps						
Tater Crisps Bar-B-Que	21 (1 oz)	130	4	270	21	1
Tater Crisps Original	23 (1 oz)	120	7	220	20	1
Tater Crisps Sour Cream 'n Onion	22 (1 oz)	130	4	210	21	1
New York Deli						
Chips	1 oz	160	11	120	14	—
Old Dutch Foods						
Augratin	1 oz	150	8	220	15	—
BBQ	1 oz	140	8	360	16	—
Chips	1 oz	150	9	160	16	—
Dill Flavored	1 oz	150	8	340	16	—
Onion & Garlic	1 oz	150	9	420	15	—
Ripple	1 oz	150	9	150	16	—
Sour Cream & Onion	1 oz	150	10	220	15	—

FOOD	PORTION	CAL.	FAT	SOD.	CARB.	FIB.
Pringles						
BBQ	14 chips (1 oz)	150	6	200	15	—
Cheez-ums	14 chips (1 oz)	150	10	190	—	—
Original	14 chips (1 oz)	160	11	170	—	—
Ranch	14 chips (1 oz)	150	10	130	—	—
Ridges Cheddar & Sour Cream	12 chips (1 oz)	150	10	200	—	—
Ridges Mesquite BBQ	12 chips (1 oz)	150	10	220	—	—
Ridges Original	12 chips (1 oz)	150	10	150	—	—
Right BBQ	16 chips (1 oz)	140	7	160	18	—
Right Original	16 chips (1 oz)	140	7	135	—	—
Right Ranch	16 chips (1 oz)	140	7	120	18	—
Right Sour Cream 'N Onion	16 chips (1 oz)	140	7	120	18	—
Rippled Original	10 chips (1 oz)	160	11	150	15	—
Sour Cream N'Onion	14 chips (1 oz)	160	10	135	15	—
Ruffles						
Cheddar Cheese & Sour Cream	18 chips (1 oz)	160	10	250	15	1
Chips	18 chips (1 oz)	150	10	135	15	1
Mesquite Grille B-B-Q	18 chips (1 oz)	160	10	270	15	1
Monterey Jack Cheese Attack	18 chips (1 oz)	160	10	200	15	1
Ranch	18 chips (1 oz)	160	10	220	15	1
Reduced Fat	16 chips (1 oz)	140	7	130	18	1
Sour Cream & Onion	18 chips (1 oz)	160	10	220	15	1
Snyder's						
BBQ	1 oz	150	10	370	13	1
Cheddar Bacon	1 oz	150	10	260	13	1
Chips	1 oz	150	10	130	13	1
Coney Island	1 oz	150	10	280	13	1
Grilled Steak & Onion	1 oz	150	10	260	13	1
Hot Buffalo Wings	1 oz	150	10	200	13	1
Kosher Dill	1 oz	150	10	400	13	1
No Salt	1 oz	150	10	0	13	1
Salt & Vinegar	1 oz	150	10	200	13	1
Sausage Pizza	1 oz	150	10	230	13	1
Sour Cream & Onion	1 oz	150	10	190	13	1
Sour Cream & Onion Unsalted	1 oz	150	10	10	13	1
State Line						
Chips	1 pkg (0.5 oz)	80	5	70	7	tr
Suprimos						
Cheddar & Jack	1 oz	140	6	180	17	—

FOOD	PORTION	CAL.	FAT	SOD.	CARB.	FIB.
Suprimos (CONT.)						
Cool Onion	1 oz	140	6	170	17	—
Weight Watchers						
Barbecue Curls	1 pkg (0.5 oz)	60	3	110	11	1
Wise						
Natural	1 oz	160	11	190	14	—
Ridgies Barbecue	1 oz	150	10	240	14	—
TORTILLA						
nacho	1 oz	141	7	201	18	2
nacho	1 bag (8 oz)	1131	58	1606	142	12
nacho light	1 oz	126	4	284	20	—
nacho light	1 bag (6 oz)	757	26	1705	122	—
plain	1 oz	142	7	150	18	2
plain	1 bag (7.5 oz)	1067	56	1124	134	14
ranch	1 bag (7 oz)	969	47	1212	128	—
ranch	1 oz	139	7	174	18	—
taco	1 oz	136	7	223	18	—
taco	1 bag (8 oz)	1089	55	1788	143	—
Barrel O' Fun						
Nacho	1 oz	140	6	160	19	1
Tostada Yellow	1 oz	140	6	40	19	0
White	1 oz	140	6	50	20	0
Doritos						
Reduced Fat Cooler Ranch	13 chips (1 oz)	130	5	200	20	1
Reduced Fat Nacho Cheesier	13 chips (1 oz)	130	5	210	19	1
Wow Nacho Cheese	11 chips (1 oz)	97	1	260	21	1
Wow Nacho Cheesier	1 pkg (0.75 oz)	70	1	180	13	1
Frito Lay						
Salsa 'N Cheese	16 (1 oz)	150	8	180	17	2
Guiltless Gourmet						
Baked	22-26 chips (1 oz)	110	1	119	21	1
Hain						
Sesame	1 oz	140	7	190	19	—
Sesame Cheese	1 oz	160	8	270	20	—
Sesame No Salt Added	1 oz	140	7	<5	19	—
Taco Style	1 oz	160	11	320	15	—
Herr's						
Restaurant Style White Corn	10 chips (1 oz)	140	6	90	18	2
La FAMOUS						
No Salt Added	1 oz	140	7	5	18	—

FOOD	PORTION	CAL.	FAT	SOD.	CARB.	FIB.
La FAMOUS (CONT.)						
Tortilla	1 oz	140	7	180	18	—
Lance						
Jalapeno Cheese	1 pkg (1⅛ oz)	160	8	—	—	—
Nacho	1 pkg (32 g)	160	8	240	19	—
Louise's						
95% Fat-Free	1 oz	120	2	170	23	1
Mr. Phipps						
Nacho	28 (1 oz)	130	4	150	20	3
Original	28 (1 oz)	130	4	130	21	3
Old El Paso						
NACHIPS	9 chips (1 oz)	150	8	85	17	2
White Corn	11 chips (1 oz)	140	8	60	18	1
Santitas						
Cantina Style	1 oz	140	6	75	19	2
Cantina Style Fajita	1 oz	140	7	95	19	2
Chips	1 oz	140	7	50	19	2
Strips	1 oz	140	7	65	19	2
Snyder's						
Chips	1 oz	140	7	130	18	2
Enchilada	1 oz	140	7	220	18	2
Nacho Cheese	1 oz	140	7	130	18	2
No Salt	1 oz	140	7	0	18	2
Ranch	1 oz	140	7	150	18	2
Tostitos						
Baked Cool Ranch	11 chips (1 oz)	120	3	170	21	1
Baked Original	9 chips (1 oz)	110	tr	200	24	2
Baked Unsalted	13 chips (1 oz)	110	1	10	24	2
Bite Size	16 pieces (1 oz)	150	8	110	18	2
Chips	11 pieces (1 oz)	140	8	160	18	2
Restaurant Style Lime 'N Chili	7 pieces (1 oz)	150	7	190	18	2
Restaurant Style White Corn	7 pieces (1 oz)	150	6	75	20	2
Tyson						
Nacho Cheese	1 oz	140	7	145	17	—
Ranch Flavor	1 oz	140	2	—	17	—
Traditional	1 oz	140	7	95	17	—
Unsalted	1 oz	140	7	7	17	—
Wise						
Bravos	1 oz	150	8	180	18	—
VEGETABLE						
taro	10 (0.8 oz)	115	6	79	16	—
taro	1 oz	141	7	97	19	—

FOOD	PORTION	CAL.	FAT	SOD.	CARB.	FIB.
Eden						
Vegetable Chips	50 (1 oz)	130	4	260	24	0
Wasabi Chip Hot & Spicy	50 (1 oz)	130	4	260	24	0
Hain						
Carrot Chips	1 oz	150	9	160	16	0
Carrot Chips Barbecue	1 oz	140	8	160	16	0
Carrot Chips No Salt Added	1 oz	150	7	30	16	0
Health Valley						
Carrot Lites	0.5 oz	75	4	5	9	tr
Terra Chips						
Sweet Potato	1 oz	140	7	10	18	1
Sweet Potato Spiced	1 oz	140	7	105	16	3
Taro Spiced	1 oz	130	5	170	20	2
Vegetable	1 oz	140	7	70	18	3
Top Banana						
Plantain Chips	1 oz	150	8	85	17	—

CHITTERLINGS

FOOD	PORTION	CAL.	FAT	SOD.	CARB.	FIB.
pork simmered	3 oz	258	24	33	0	—

CHIVES

FOOD	PORTION	CAL.	FAT	SOD.	CARB.	FIB.
freeze-dried	1 tbsp	1	tr	—	tr	—
fresh chopped	1 tbsp	1	tr	0	tr	—
fresh chopped	1 tsp	0	tr	0	tr	—

CHOCOLATE

(*see also* CANDY, CAROB, COCOA, ICE CREAM TOPPINGS, MILK DRINKS)

FOOD	PORTION	CAL.	FAT	SOD.	CARB.	FIB.
BAKING						
baking	1 oz	145	15	1	8	—
grated unsweetened	1 cup (4.6 oz)	690	73	18	37	18
liquid unsweetened	1 oz	134	14	3	10	—
squares unsweetened	1 square (1 oz)	148	16	4	8	4
Baker's						
Bittersweet	½ square (0.5 oz)	70	6	0	7	1
German's Sweet	2 squares (0.5 oz)	60	4	0	8	tr
Semi-Sweet	½ square (0.5 oz)	70	5	0	8	1
Unsweetened	½ square (0.5 oz)	70	7	0	4	2
White	½ square (0.5 oz)	80	5	15	8	0
Hershey						
Premium Semi-Sweet	1 oz	140	8	—	16	—
Premium Unsweetened	1 oz	190	16	5	7	—
Nestle						
Choco Bake	½ oz	80	8	0	5	3

FOOD	PORTION	CAL.	FAT	SOD.	CARB.	FIB.
Nestle (CONT.)						
Premier White	½ oz	80	5	15	8	—
Semi-Sweet	½ oz	70	4	0	9	2
Unsweetened	½ oz	80	7	0	5	3
CHIPS						
milk chocolate	1 cup (6 oz)	862	52	138	100	—
semisweet	60 pieces (1 oz)	136	9	3	18	—
semisweet	1 cup (6 oz)	804	50	19	106	—
Baker's						
Chips	1 oz	143	8	25	18	—
Real Milk Chocolate	½ oz	70	4	10	9	0
Real Semi-Sweet	½ oz	60	4	0	9	1
Semi-Sweet	½ oz	70	4	15	10	0
Hershey						
Chunks Milk Chocolate	1 oz	160	9	25	16	—
Chunks Semi-Sweet	1 oz	140	8	—	15	—
Milk Chocolate	1 oz	150	12	55	27	—
Mint Chocolate	¼ cup	230	12	—	28	—
Semi-Sweet	¼ cup (1.5 oz)	220	12	5	26	—
Semi-Sweet Miniature	¼ cup (1.5 oz)	220	12	5	26	—
M&M's						
Baking Bits Milk Chocolate	0.5 oz	70	3	0	10	0
Baking Bits Semi-Sweet	0.5 oz	70	4	0	9	1
Nestle						
Morsels Milk Chocolate	1 tbsp	70	4	0	10	—
Morsels Mint Chocolate	1 tbsp	70	4	0	9	2
Morsels Rainbow	1 tbsp	70	3	0	10	1
Morsels Mini Semi-Sweet	1 tbsp	70	4	0	9	2
Semi-Sweet Morsels	1 tbsp	40	4	0	9	2
MIX						
powder	2-3 heaping tsp	75	1	45	20	—
powder as prep w/ whole milk	9 oz	226	9	165	31	—
Hershey						
Chocolate Milk Mix	3 tbsp	90	4	40	22	—

CHOCOLATE MILK

(*see* CHOCOLATE, COCOA, MILK DRINKS, MILKSHAKE)

CHOCOLATE SYRUP

FOOD	PORTION	CAL.	FAT	SOD.	CARB.	FIB.
chocolate fudge	1 cup (11.9 oz)	1176	46	442	200	—
chocolate fudge	1 tbsp (0.7 oz)	73	3	27	12	—
syrup	1 cup	653	3	287	177	—

FOOD	PORTION	CAL.	FAT	SOD.	CARB.	FIB.
syrup	2 tbsp	82	tr	36	22	—
syrup as prep w/ whole milk	9 oz	232	9	156	34	—
Estee						
Choco-Syp	2 tbsp (1.2 oz)	50	0	15	11	—
Hershey						
Syrup	2 tbsp	80	1	20	17	—
Marzetti						
Syrup	2 tbsp	40	4	50	21	0
Quik						
Chocolate	1 ⅔ tbsp	100	1	45	22	—
Chocolate	2½ tsp (0.75 oz)	90	1	25	20	—
Sugar Free Chocolate	1 heaping tsp (5.8 g)	18	tr	35	3	—
Red Wing						
Syrup	2 tbsp (1.4 oz)	110	1	10	25	0
CHUTNEY						
apple	1.2 oz	68	0	—	18	1
apple cranberry	1 tbsp	16	0	1	4	—
coconut	¼ cup	74	7	5	4	2
tomato	1.2 oz	54	0	—	14	1
Sonoma						
Dried Tomato	1 tbsp (0.7 g)	35	0	0	9	0
CILANTRO						
fresh	¼ cup	1	tr	1	tr	—
Watkins						
Dried	¼ tsp (0.5 oz)	0	0	0	0	0
CINNAMON						
ground	1 tsp	6	tr	1	2	—
sticks	0.5 oz	39	tr	4	8	3
Watkins						
Ground	¼ tsp (0.5 g)	0	0	0	0	0
CISCO						
raw	3 oz	84	2	47	0	—
smoked	1 oz	50	3	135	0	—
smoked	3 oz	151	10	409	0	—
CLAM JUICE						
Doxsee						
Canned	3 fl oz	4	0	110	0	—
CLAMS						
CANNED						
liquid only	3 oz	2	tr	183	tr	—

FOOD	PORTION	CAL.	FAT	SOD.	CARB.	FIB.
liquid only	1 cup	6	tr	516	tr	—
meat only	1 cup	236	3	179	8	—
meat only	3 oz	126	2	95	4	—
Doxsee						
Chopped	6.5 oz	90	tr	1020	6	—
Empress						
Whole Baby	4 oz	60	1	540	2	—
Gorton's						
Minced & Chopped	½ can	70	1	640	4	—
Progresso						
Creamy Clam	½ cup (4.2 oz)	100	6	560	8	0
Minced	¼ cup (2 oz)	25	0	250	2	0
Red Clam	½ cup (4.4 oz)	80	3	620	8	1
White Clam Sauce	½ cup (4.4 oz)	120	9	310	1	0
S&W						
Fancy Chopped	2 oz	28	0	280	2	—
Fancy Minced	2 oz	28	0	280	2	—
Whole Baby Chowder Clams	2 oz	33	0	—	1	—
Snow's						
Minced	6.5 oz	90	tr	1020	6	—
FRESH						
cooked	3 oz	126	2	95	4	—
cooked	20 sm	133	2	100	5	—
raw	3 oz	63	1	47	2	—
raw	9 lg (180 g)	133	2	100	5	—
raw	20 sm (180 g)	133	2	100	5	—
FROZEN						
Gorton's						
Microwave Crunchy Clam Strips	3.5 oz	330	22	430	24	—
Mrs. Paul's						
Fried	2½ oz	200	9	450	21	—
Microwave Fried Clams	2.5 oz	260	15	410	23	—
HOME RECIPE						
breaded & fried	20 sm	379	21	684	19	—
breaded & fried	3 oz	171	9	309	9	—
TAKE-OUT						
breaded & fried	¾ cup	451	26	833	39	—

CLOVES

ground	1 tsp	7	tr	5	1	—

COCOA

(*see also* CHOCOLATE)

hot cocoa	1 cup	218	9	123	26	—

FOOD	PORTION	CAL.	FAT	SOD.	CARB.	FIB.
mix as prep w/ water	7 oz	103	1	149	23	—
mix w/ Equal as prep w/ water	7 oz	48	tr	173	9	—
powder unsweetened	1 tbsp (5 g)	11	1	1	3	2
powder unsweetened	1 cup (3 oz)	197	12	18	47	29
Carnation						
Hot Cocoa 70 Calorie	3 tsp (21 g)	70	tr	—	—	—
Hot Cocoa Milk Chocolate	1 pkg or 4 heaping tsp (1 oz)	110	1	—	—	—
Hot Cocoa Natural Mint	1 pkg or 4 heaping tsp (1 oz)	110	1	—	—	—
Hot Cocoa Rich Chocolate	1 pkg or 4 heaping tsp (1 oz)	110	1	—	—	—
Hot Cocoa Rich Chocolate w/ Marshmallows	1 pkg or 4 heaping tsp (1 oz)	110	1	—	—	—
Hot Cocoa Sugar Free Mint	1 pkg or 4 heaping tsp (15 g)	50	tr	—	—	—
Hot Cocoa Sugar Free Rich Chocolate	1 pkg or 4 heaping tsp (15 g)	50	tr	—	—	—
Hershey						
Cocoa	⅓ cup (1 oz)	120	4	10	13	—
European Cocoa	1 oz	90	3	15	8	—
Hills Bros.						
Hot Cocoa	6 oz	110	2	—	—	—
Hot Cocoa Sugar Free	6 oz	60	2	—	—	—
Nestle						
Cocoa	1 tbsp	15	1	0	3	2
Hot Cocoa Mix	1 oz	110	1	100	23	—
Hot Cocoa Mix With Marshmallows	1 oz	120	1	115	23	—
Hot Cocoa Mix With Marshmallows as prep w/ 2% milk	6 oz	220	5	190	32	—
Hot Cocoa Mix With Marshmallows as prep w/ skim milk	6 oz	190	1	200	32	—
Hot Cocoa Mix With Marshmallows as prep w/ whole milk	6 oz	240	8	240	32	—
Hot Cocoa Mix as prep w/ 2% milk	6 oz	210	5	190	32	—
Hot Cocoa Mix as prep w/ skim milk	6 oz	180	1	200	32	—

FOOD	PORTION	CAL.	FAT	SOD.	CARB.	FIB.
Nestle (CONT.)						
Hot Cocoa Mix as prep w/ whole milk	6 oz	230	8	240	32	—
Swiss Miss						
Cocoa Diet	6 oz	20	tr	180	3	0
Hot Cocoa Bavarian Chocolate	6 oz	110	3	170	20	0
Hot Cocoa Double Rich	6 oz	110	1	150	22	0
Hot Cocoa Milk Chocolate	6 oz	110	1	125	24	0
Hot Cocoa Milk Chocolate	1 serv	110	1	139	24	1
Hot Cocoa Mini-Marshmallow	1 serv	109	1	149	24	1
Hot Cocoa Rich Chocolate	1 serv	110	1	166	24	1
Hot Cocoa Sugar Free	1 serv	67	tr	242	13	1
Hot Cocoa Sugar Free Milk Chocolate	1 serv	49	tr	179	10	1
Hot Cocoa Sugar Free Mini-Marshmallow	1 serv	51	1	159	11	1
Hot Cocoa White Chocolate	1 serv	109	1	128	21	tr
Hot Cocoa With Mini Marshmallows	6 oz	110	1	170	23	0
Hot Cocoa Lite	1 serv	74	tr	197	17	2
Lite as prep	6 oz	70	tr	160	17	0
Sugar Free With Sugar Free Marshmallows as prep	6 oz	50	tr	120	9	0
Sugar Free as prep	6 oz	60	tr	125	10	0
Ultra Slim-Fast						
Hot Cocoa as prep w/ water	8 oz	190	tr	140	35	5
Weight Watchers						
Hot Cocoa Mix as prep	1 pkg	70	0	160	7	1
COCONUT						
coconut water	1 cup	46	tr	252	9	—
coconut water	1 tbsp	3	tr	16	1	—
cream canned	1 cup	568	52	149	25	—
cream canned	1 tbsp	36	3	10	2	—
dried sweetened flaked	7 oz pkg	944	64	509	95	—
dried sweetened flaked	1 cup	351	24	189	35	—

FOOD	PORTION	CAL.	FAT	SOD.	CARB.	FIB.
dried sweetened flaked canned	1 cup	341	24	15	32	—
dried sweetened shredded	7 oz pkg	997	71	522	95	—
dried sweetened shredded	1 cup	466	33	244	44	—
dried toasted	1 oz	168	13	11	13	—
dried unsweetened	1 oz	187	18	11	7	—
fresh	1 piece (1.5 oz)	159	15	9	7	4
fresh shredded	1 cup	283	27	16	12	7
milk canned	1 tbsp	30	3	2	tr	—
milk canned	1 cup	445	48	29	6	—
milk frozen	1 tbsp	30	3	2	1	—
milk frozen	1 cup	486	50	29	13	—
Baker's						
Angel Flake	1 tbsp (0.5 oz)	70	5	45	6	1
Angel Flake (canned)	2 tbsp (0.5 oz)	70	6	0	6	1
Premium Shred	2 tbsp (0.5 oz)	70	5	45	6	1
Coco Lopez						
Cream Of Coconut	2 tbsp	120	5	10	20	—
COD						
CANNED						
atlantic	1 can (11 oz)	327	3	680	0	—
atlantic	3 oz	89	1	185	0	—
roe	3.5 oz	118	3	—	tr	—
DRIED						
atlantic	3 oz	246	2	5973	0	—
FRESH						
atlantic cooked	1 fillet (6.3 oz)	189	2	141	0	—
atlantic cooked	3 oz	89	1	66	0	—
atlantic raw	3 oz	70	1	46	0	—
pacific baked	3 oz	95	1	82	0	—
roe baked w/ butter & lemon juice	3.5 oz	126	3	73	2	—
roe raw	3½ oz	130	2	—	2	—
FROZEN						
Gorton's						
Fishmarket Fresh	5 oz	110	1	90	0	—
Mrs. Paul's						
Light Fillets	1 fillet	240	11	430	22	—
Van De Kamp's						
Lightly Breaded Fillets	1 (4 oz)	220	10	410	19	0
COFFEE						
(*see also* COFFEE BEVERAGES, COFFEE SUBSTITUTES)						
INSTANT						
cappuccino mix as prep	7 oz	62	2	104	11	—

FOOD	PORTION	CAL.	FAT	SOD.	CARB.	FIB.
decaffeinated	1 rounded tsp (1.8 g)	4	0	0	1	—
decaffeinated as prep	6 oz	4	0	6	1	—
french mix as prep	7 oz	57	3	—	7	—
mocha mix as prep	7 oz	51	2	36	8	—
regular	1 rounded tsp	4	0	1	1	—
regular as prep	6 oz	4	0	6	1	—
regular w/ chicory	1 rounded tsp	6	0	5	1	—
regular w/ chicory as prep	6 oz	6	0	10	1	—
REGULAR						
brewed	6 oz	4	0	4	1	—
Folgers						
Colombian Supreme	1 tbsp	16	tr	tr	3	—
Custom Roast	1 tbsp	16	tr	tr	3	—
Decaffeinated	1 tbsp	17	tr	tr	3	—
French Roast	1 tbsp	16	tr	tr	3	—
Gourmet Supreme	1 tbsp	16	tr	tr	3	—
Instant	1 tsp	8	tr	1	1	—
Instant Decaffeinated	1 tsp	8	tr	2	2	—
Singles	1 bag	21	tr	1	4	—
Singles Decaffeinated	1 bag	21	tr	2	4	—
Special Roast	1 tbsp	16	tr	tr	3	—
Vacuum Pack	1 tbsp	16	tr	tr	3	—
Maryland Club						
Ground	1 tbsp	16	tr	tr	3	—
TAKE-OUT						
cafe au lait	1 cup (8 fl oz)	77	4	62	6	—
cafe brulot	1 cup (4.8 fl oz)	48	0	2	3	—
cappuccino	1 cup (8 fl oz)	77	4	62	6	—
coffee con leche	1 cup (8 fl oz)	77	4	62	6	—
espresso	1 cup (3 fl oz)	2	0	2	tr	—
irish coffee	1 serv (9 fl oz)	107	3	25	3	—
mocha	1 mug (9.6 fl oz)	202	15	28	17	—

COFFEE BEVERAGES

(*see also* COFFEE SUBSTITUTES)

FOOD	PORTION	CAL.	FAT	SOD.	CARB.	FIB.
Chock o'ccino						
Cinnamon	8 oz	120	2	55	25	—
Coffee	8 oz	120	2	55	25	—
Mocha	8 oz	120	2	55	25	—
General Foods						
International Coffee Sugar Free Cafe Vienna as prep	1 serv (8 oz)	30	2	75	3	0

FOOD	PORTION	CAL.	FAT	SOD.	CARB.	FIB.
General Foods (CONT.)						
International Coffee Sugar Free Fat Free Suisse Mocha as prep	1 serv (8 oz)	25	0	35	5	tr
International Coffees Cafe Francais as prep	1 serv (8 oz)	60	4	95	7	0
International Coffees Cafe Vienna as prep	1 serv (8 oz)	70	3	110	11	tr
International Coffees Decaffeinated French Vanilla Cafe as prep	1 serv (8 oz)	60	3	55	10	0
International Coffees Decaffeinated Suisse Mocha as prep	1 serv (8 oz)	60	2	35	9	0
International Coffees French Vanilla Cafe as prep	1 serv (8 oz)	60	3	55	10	0
International Coffees Hazelnut Belgian Cafe as prep	1 serv (8 oz)	70	2	60	12	0
International Coffees Irish Creme Cafe as prep	1 serv (8 oz)	60	2	45	10	0
International Coffees Italian Cappuccino as prep	1 serv (8 oz)	60	2	50	10	0
International Coffees Kahlua Cafe as prep	1 serv (8 oz)	60	2	55	10	0
International Coffees Orange Cappuccino as prep	1 serv (8 oz)	70	2	100	11	tr
International Coffees Suisse Mocha as prep	1 serv (8 oz)	60	2	35	8	0
International Coffees Viennese Chocolate Cafe as prep	1 serv (8 oz)	50	2	30	10	0
International Coffees Sugar Free Fat Free Decaffeinated French Vanilla	1 serv (8 oz)	25	0	65	5	0
International Coffees Sugar Free Fat Free Decaffeinated Suisse Mocha	1 serv (8 oz)	25	0	35	5	tr

FOOD	PORTION	CAL.	FAT	SOD.	CARB.	FIB.
General Foods (CONT.)						
International Coffees Sugar Free Fat Free French Vanilla Cafe as prep	1 serv (8 oz)	25	0	65	5	0
Maxwell House						
Cafe Cappuccino Amaretto as prep	1 serv (8 oz)	90	1	65	19	0
Cafe Cappuccino Decaffeinated Mocha as prep	1 serv (8 oz)	100	3	70	17	0
Cafe Cappuccino Decaffeinated Vanilla as prep	1 serv (8 oz)	90	1	65	19	0
Cafe Cappuccino Irish Cream as prep	1 serv (8 oz)	90	1	65	19	0
Cafe Cappuccino Mocha as prep	1 serv (8 oz)	100	3	65	17	0
Cafe Cappuccino Sugar Free Mocha as prep	1 serv (8 oz)	60	3	80	7	tr
Cafe Cappuccino Sugar Free Vanilla as prep	1 serv (8 oz)	60	3	85	7	0
Cafe Cappuccino Vanilla as prep	1 serv (8 oz)	90	1	65	19	0
Iced Cappuccino as prep w/ 2% milk	1 serv (8 oz)	180	5	125	27	tr
Starbucks						
Frappuccino	1 bottle (9.5 fl oz)	190	3	110	39	0
COFFEE SUBSTITUTES						
powder	1 tsp	9	tr	2	2	—
powder as prep	6 oz	9	tr	7	2	—
powder as prep w/ milk	6 oz	121	6	91	10	—
Kava						
Instant	1 tsp	2	0	<5	1	—
Natural Touch						
Kaffree Roma	1 tsp	6	0	—	1	—
Pero						
Instant Grain Beverage	1 tsp (1.5 g)	5	0	0	1	—
Postum						
Instant Coffee Flavor as prep	1 serv (8 oz)	10	0	0	3	0
Instant as prep	1 serv (8 oz)	10	0	0	3	0
COFFEE WHITENERS (*see also* MILK SUBSTITUTES)						
liquid nondairy frzn	1 tbsp (0.5 oz)	20	2	12	2	—

FOOD	PORTION	CAL.	FAT	SOD.	CARB.	FIB.
powder nondairy	1 tsp	11	tr	4	1	—
Coffee-Mate						
Liquid	1 tbsp (0.5 fl oz)	16	1	5	2	—
Powder	1 tsp (2 g)	10	1	5	1	—
Cremora						
Whitener	1 tsp	12	1	5	1	—
Hood						
Non Dairy	1 tbsp (0.5 oz)	20	2	0	2	0
International Delight						
Amaretto	1 tbsp (0.6 fl oz)	45	2	5	7	0
Cinnamon Hazelnut	1 tbsp (0.6 fl oz)	45	2	5	7	0
Irish Creme	1 tbsp (0.6 fl oz)	45	2	5	7	0
No Fat Amaretto	1 tbsp (0.5 fl oz)	30	0	5	7	0
No Fat French Vanilla Royale	1 tbsp (0.5 fl oz)	30	0	5	7	0
No Fat Hawaiian Macadamia	1 tbsp (0.5 fl oz)	30	0	5	7	0
No Fat Irish Creme	1 tbsp (0.5 fl oz)	30	0	5	7	0
Suisse Chocolate Mocha	1 tbsp (0.6 fl oz)	45	2	10	7	0
Mocha Mix						
Fat-Free	1 tbsp (0.5 fl oz)	10	0	0	1	0
Lite	1 tbsp (0.5 fl oz)	10	tr	0	tr	0
Lite	4 fl oz	80	7	24	3	0
Original	1 tbsp (0.5 fl oz)	20	2	5	1	0
Signature Flavors French Vanilla	1 tbsp (0.5 fl oz)	35	0	5	8	—
Signature Flavors Irish Creme	1 tbsp (0.5 fl oz)	35	0	5	8	—
Signature Flavors Kahlua	1 tbsp (0.5 fl oz)	35	0	5	8	—
Signature Flavors Mauna Loa Macadamia Nut	1 tbsp (0.5 fl oz)	35	0	5	8	—
N-Rich Creamer						
Whitener	1 tsp	10	tr	0	1	0

COLESLAW

TAKE-OUT

FOOD	PORTION	CAL.	FAT	SOD.	CARB.	FIB.
coleslaw w/ dressing	½ cup	42	2	14	7	—

COLLARDS

CANNED

FOOD	PORTION	CAL.	FAT	SOD.	CARB.	FIB.
Allen						
Collards	½ cup (4.1 oz)	30	1	20	5	3
Sunshine						
Collards	½ cup (4.1 oz)	30	1	20	5	3

FOOD	PORTION	CAL.	FAT	SOD.	CARB.	FIB.
FRESH						
cooked	½ cup	17	tr	10	4	—
raw chopped	½ cup	6	tr	4	1	—
FROZEN						
chopped cooked	½ cup	31	tr	42	6	—

COOKIES

(*see also* BROWNIE, CAKE, DOUGHNUT, PIE)

FOOD	PORTION	CAL.	FAT	SOD.	CARB.	FIB.
HOME RECIPE						
chocolate chip as prep w/ butter	1 (0.42 oz)	78	5	55	9	—
chocolate chip as prep w/ margarine	1 (0.56 oz)	78	5	58	9	—
macaroons	1 (0.8 oz)	97	3	59	17	—
oatmeal	1 (0.5 oz)	67	3	90	10	—
oatmeal w/ raisins	1 (0.52 oz)	65	2	81	10	—
peanut butter	1 (0.7 oz)	95	5	104	12	—
shortbread as prep w/ butter	1 (0.38 oz)	60	4	51	6	—
shortbread as prep w/ margarine	1 (0.38 oz)	60	4	56	6	—
sugar as prep w/ butter	1 (0.49 oz)	66	3	64	8	—
sugar as prep w/ margarine	1 (0.49 oz)	66	3	69	8	—
MIX						
chocolate chip	1 (0.56 oz)	79	4	47	10	—
oatmeal	1 (0.6 oz)	74	3	75	10	tr
oatmeal raisin	1 (0.6 oz)	74	3	75	10	tr
Betty Crocker						
Chocolate Chip Big Batch	2	120	6	100	16	—
Date Bar Classic Dessert	1	60	2	35	9	—
Estee						
Chocolate Chip	3	130	7	120	17	0
READY-TO-EAT						
animal	11 crackers (1 oz)	126	4	112	21	—
animal crackers	1 box (2.4 oz)	299	9	274	51	—
animal crackers	1 (2.5 g)	11	tr	10	2	—
butter	1 (5 g)	23	1	18	3	tr
chocolate chip	1 (0.4 oz)	48	2	32	7	tr
chocolate chip	1 box (1.9 oz)	233	12	188	36	—
chocolate chip low fat	1 (0.25 oz)	45	2	38	7	—
chocolate chip low sugar low sodium	1 (0.24 oz)	31	1	1	5	—
chocolate chip soft-type	1 (0.5 oz)	69	4	49	9	tr

FOOD	PORTION	CAL.	FAT	SOD.	CARB.	FIB.
chocolate w/ creme filling	1 (0.35 oz)	47	2	36	7	tr
chocolate w/ creme filling chocolate coated	1 (0.60 oz)	82	5	55	11	—
chocolate w/ creme filling sugar free low sodium	1 (0.35 oz)	46	2	24	7	—
chocolate w/ extra creme filling	1 (0.46 oz)	65	3	64	9	—
chocolate wafer	1 (0.2 oz)	26	1	35	4	—
chocolate wafer cookie crumbs	½ cup (5.9 oz)	728	25	980	120	—
digestive biscuits plain	2	141	7	—	21	1
fig bars	1 (0.56 oz)	56	1	56	11	1
fortune	1 (0.28 oz)	30	tr	22	7	tr
fudge	1 (0.73 oz)	73	1	40	17	tr
gingersnaps	1 (0.24 oz)	29	1	48	5	—
graham	1 squares (0.24 oz)	30	1	42	5	—
graham chocolate covered	1 (0.49 oz)	68	3	41	9	—
graham honey	1 (0.24 oz)	30	1	42	5	tr
ladyfingers	1 (0.38 oz)	40	1	16	7	—
marshmallow chocolate coated	1 (0.46 oz)	55	2	22	9	—
marshmallow pie chocolate coated	1 (1.4 oz)	165	7	66	26	—
molasses	1 (0.5 oz)	65	2	69	11	—
oatmeal	1 (0.6 oz)	81	3	69	12	1
oatmeal	1 (0.52 oz)	71	4	62	9	tr
oatmeal soft-type	1 (0.5 oz)	61	2	52	10	tr
oatmeal raisin	1 (0.6 oz)	81	3	69	12	1
oatmeal raisin low sugar no sodium	1 (0.24 oz)	31	1	1	5	—
oatmeal raisin soft-type	1 (0.5 oz)	61	2	52	10	tr
peanut butter sandwich	1 (0.5 oz)	67	3	52	9	—
peanut butter sandwich sugar free low sodium	1 (0.35 oz)	54	3	41	5	—
peanut butter soft-type	1 (0.5 oz)	69	4	50	9	tr
raisin soft-type	1 (0.5 oz)	60	2	51	10	—
shortbread	1 (0.28 oz)	40	2	36	5	—
shortbread pecan	1 (0.49 oz)	79	5	39	8	tr
sugar	1 (0.52 oz)	72	3	53	10	—
sugar low sugar sodium free	1 (0.24 oz)	30	1	0	5	—
sugar wafers w/ creme filling	1 (0.12 oz)	18	1	5	3	—

FOOD	PORTION	CAL.	FAT	SOD.	CARB.	FIB.
sugar wafers w/ creme filling sugar free sodium free	1 (0.14 oz)	20	1	0	3	—
vanilla sandwich	1 (0.35 oz)	48	2	35	7	tr
vanilla wafers	1 (0.21 oz)	28	1	18	4	—
Archway						
Almond Crescents	2 (0.8 oz)	100	4	75	17	tr
Apple N'Raisin	1 (1.1 oz)	130	52	105	20	1
Apricot Filled	1 (1 oz)	110	4	90	18	tr
Bells And Stars	3 (1 oz)	150	7	100	19	tr
Blueberry Filled	1 (1 oz)	110	4	115	19	tr
Carrot Cake	1 (1 oz)	120	5	180	18	0
Cherry Filled	1 (1 oz)	110	4	100	19	tr
Cherry Nougat	3 (1 oz)	150	9	40	18	0
Chocolate Chip	1 (1 oz)	130	6	150	19	0
Chocolate Chip & Toffee	1 (1 oz)	140	7	120	19	tr
Chocolate Chip Bag	3 (0.9 oz)	130	7	70	17	0
Chocolate Chip Drop	1 (1 oz)	140	10	105	11	tr
Chocolate Chip Ice Box	1 (1 oz)	140	7	80	19	0
Chocolate Chip Mini	12 (1.1 oz)	150	7	95	20	0
Cinnamon Snaps	12 (1.1 oz)	150	7	115	19	0
Coconut Macaroon	1 (0.8 oz)	90	5	55	14	2
Cookie Jar Hermits	1 (1 oz)	110	3	160	19	tr
Dark Chocolate	1 (1 oz)	110	4	150	20	tr
Dutch Chocolate	1 (1 oz)	120	4	110	19	0
Fig Bars Low Fat	2 (1.1 oz)	100	1	105	23	1
Frosty Lemon	1 (1 oz)	120	5	110	19	0
Frosty Orange	1 (1 oz)	120	4	140	19	1
Fruit And Honey Bar	1 (1 oz)	110	4	120	18	tr
Fruit Bar No Fat	1 (1 oz)	90	0	95	21	0
Fruit Cake	1 (1.1 oz)	140	7	100	20	2
Fudge Nut Bar	1 (1 oz)	110	5	120	17	tr
Fun Chip Mini	12 (1.1 oz)	140	6	100	21	0
Gingersnaps	5 (1.1 oz)	130	5	110	22	0
Granola No Fat	1 (0.5 oz)	50	0	60	11	tr
Holiday Pak	3 (1.1 oz)	150	8	95	19	tr
Iced Gingerbread	3 (1.1 oz)	140	5	130	23	0
Iced Molasses	1 (1 oz)	110	5	170	19	tr
Iced Oatmeal	1 (1 oz)	120	5	85	19	1
Lemon Snaps	12 (1.1 oz)	150	7	120	19	0
New Orleans Cake	1 (1 oz)	110	4	105	18	tr
Nutty Nougat	3 (1.1 oz)	160	10	60	18	0
Oatmeal	1 (0.9 oz)	110	3	95	19	tr
Oatmeal Apple Filled	1 (1 oz)	110	3	105	18	0

FOOD	PORTION	CAL.	FAT	SOD.	CARB.	FIB.
Archway (CONT.)						
Oatmeal Date Filled	1 (1 oz)	110	4	120	18	tr
Oatmeal Mini	12 (1.1 oz)	150	8	130	19	1
Oatmeal Pecan	1 (1 oz)	120	5	100	18	1
Oatmeal Raisin	1 (1 oz)	110	4	115	19	tr
Oatmeal Raisin Bran	1 (1 oz)	110	4	100	19	tr
Old Fashioned Molasses	1 (1 oz)	120	3	150	20	0
Old Fashioned Windmill	1 (0.7 oz)	100	4	95	15	0
Party Treats	3 (1.1 oz)	140	7	105	20	0
Peanut Butter	1 (1 oz)	140	7	125	16	tr
Peanut Butter & Chip	3 (0.9 oz)	130	7	125	16	0
Peanut Butter N' Chips	1 (1 oz)	140	7	115	16	tr
Peanut Butter Nougat	3 (1.1 oz)	160	9	140	18	1
Pecan Crunch	6 (1.1 oz)	150	8	120	18	0
Pecan Ice Box	1 (1 oz)	140	7	100	18	0
Pecan Malted Nougat	3 (1.1 oz)	160	10	60	17	2
Pfeffernusse	2 (1.3 oz)	140	1	100	32	tr
Pineapple Filled	1 (0.9 oz)	100	4	75	16	1
Raisin Oatmeal	1 (1 oz)	130	5	40	19	1
Raisin Oatmeal Bag	3 (1 oz)	130	6	55	19	1
Raspberry Filled	1 (1 oz)	110	4	90	18	tr
Rocky Road	1 (1 oz)	130	6	85	18	tr
Ruth's Golden Oatmeal	1 (1 oz)	120	5	135	19	tr
Select Assortment	3 (0.9 oz)	130	6	80	18	0
Soft Molasses Drop	1 (1 oz)	110	4	160	18	1
Soft Sugar	1 (1 oz)	110	4	110	18	0
Strawberry Filled	1 (1 oz)	110	4	90	18	tr
Sugar	1 (1 oz)	120	4	190	20	0
Vanilla Wafer	5 (1.1 oz)	130	4	130	22	0
Wedding Cakes	3 (1.1 oz)	160	8	45	20	0
Bakery Wagon						
Apple Walnut Raisin	1	100	4	130	16	1
Cobbler Apple Cranberry Fat Free	1	70	0	60	16	1
Cobbler Apple Fat Free	1	70	0	55	17	1
Cobbler Mixed Fruit Fat Free	1	70	0	65	16	1
Cobbler Raspberry Fat Free	1	70	0	60	17	1
Ginger Snaps	5	160	7	140	22	1
Honey Fruit Bars	1	100	3	80	17	1
Iced Molasses	1	100	3	120	18	1
Iced Molasses Mini	3	130	3	170	18	1
Oatmeal Apple Filled	1	90	3	65	14	1

FOOD	PORTION	CAL.	FAT	SOD.	CARB.	FIB.
Bakery Wagon (CONT.)						
Oatmeal Chocolate Chunk	1	100	3	75	16	1
Oatmeal Date Filled	1	90	3	90	17	1
Oatmeal Raspberry Filled	1	100	3	105	16	1
Oatmeal Soft	1	100	4	90	16	1
Oatmeal Walnut Raisin	1	100	4	125	17	1
Vanilla Wafers Cholesterol Free	6	130	6	140	22	1
Baking On The Lite Side						
Oatmeal Crunchy	2 (0.6 oz)	60	0	20	13	0
Raspberry Linzer	1 (0.6 oz)	55	0	20	12	0
Barnum's						
Animal Crackers	12 (1.1 oz)	140	4	160	23	1
Biscos						
Sugar Wafers	8 (1 oz)	140	6	40	21	tr
Waffle Cremes	4 (1.2 oz)	180	9	35	24	tr
Cadbury						
Fingers	3	85	4	30	11	tr
Chip-A-Roos						
Cookies	3 (1.3 oz)	190	10	150	23	1
Chips Ahoy!						
Bit Size Chocolate Chip	14 (1.1 oz)	170	7	105	21	tr
Chewy Chocolate Chip	3 (1.3 oz)	170	8	125	23	tr
Chunky Chocolate Chip	1 (0.5 oz)	80	4	60	11	tr
Real Chocolate Chip	3 (1.1 oz)	160	8	105	21	1
Reduced Fat	3 (1.1 oz)	150	6	150	23	1
Sprinkled Real Chocolate Chip	3 (1.3 oz)	170	8	120	24	tr
Striped Chocolate Chip	1 (0.5 oz)	80	4	45	10	tr
Chortles						
Cookies	½ pkg. (1 oz)	125	3	109	23	1
Cookie Lover's						
Blue Ribbon Brownies	1 (0.8 oz)	90	3	75	14	0
Classic Shortbread	1 (0.8 oz)	110	7	75	12	0
Dutch Chocolate Chip	1 (0.8 oz)	90	4	65	12	0
Fancy Peanut Butter	1 (0.8 oz)	100	6	90	10	0
Grahams Cinnamon Honey	2 (1 oz)	110	1	130	24	1
Grahams Honey	2 (1 oz)	100	2	130	22	1
Old-Time Raisin	1 (0.8 oz)	90	3	60	14	0
Delacre						
Cookie Assortment	4 (1.1 oz)	130	<5	35	18	1

FOOD	PORTION	CAL.	FAT	SOD.	CARB.	FIB.
Drake's						
Chocolate Chip	2 (1 oz)	140	6	110	18	—
Chocolate- Chocolate Chip	2 (1 oz)	130	5	85	19	—
Coconut	2 (1 oz)	130	5	95	20	—
Coconut Macaroon	1 (1 oz)	135	7	80	17	—
Hermit	1 (2 oz)	230	7	280	38	—
Oatmeal	2 (1 oz)	120	5	50	19	—
Oatmeal Creme	1 (2 oz)	240	9	250	9	—
Peanut Butter Wafers	1 (2.25 oz)	324	16	135	43	—
Dutch Mill						
Chocolate Chip	3 (1.1 oz)	160	10	85	18	1
Coconut Macaroons	3 (1 oz)	120	7	115	14	0
Oatmeal Raisin	3 (1 oz)	130	6	75	18	1
Entenmann's						
Chocolate Chip	3 (0.9 oz)	140	7	85	19	—
Estee						
Chocolate Chip	4 (1.1 oz)	150	7	30	21	tr
Coconut	4 (1 oz)	140	6	25	19	tr
Creme Wafers Chocolate	7 (1.1 oz)	160	8	0	21	tr
Creme Wafers Lemon	5 (1.2 oz)	170	8	10	23	0
Creme Wafers Peanut Butter	5 (1.2 oz)	170	9	85	21	0
Creme Wafers Triple Decker Banana Split	3 (0.9 oz)	140	7	0	18	0
Creme Wafers Triple Decker Chocolate Caramel & Peanut Butter	3 (0.9 oz)	140	7	45	17	0
Creme Wafers Vanilla	7 (1.1 oz)	160	7	0	22	0
Creme Wafers Vanilla & Strawberry	5 (1.2 oz)	170	8	0	23	0
Fig Bars Apple Low Fat	2 (1 oz)	100	1	25	22	3
Fig Bars Cranberry Low Fat	2 (1 oz)	100	1	20	22	3
Fig Bars Low Fat	2 (1 oz)	100	0	20	23	3
Fudge	4 (1 oz)	150	7	45	19	1
Lemon	4 (1 oz)	140	6	25	19	tr
Oatmeal Raisin	4 (1 oz)	130	5	25	19	1
Sandwich Chocolate	3 (1.2 oz)	160	6	60	24	1
Sandwich Original	3 (1.2 oz)	160	6	45	24	1
Sandwich Peanut Butter	3 (1.2 oz)	160	7	55	22	1
Sandwich Vanilla	3 (1.2 oz)	160	5	35	25	tr
Shortbread Reduced Fat	4 (1 oz)	130	4	150	22	tr

FOOD	PORTION	CAL.	FAT	SOD.	CARB.	FIB.
Estee (CONT.)						
Vanilla	4 (1 oz)	140	6	25	19	tr
FFV						
Animal Crackers	9	110	3	—	—	—
Caramel Patties	2	150	7	—	—	—
Fig Bars Vanilla	1	60	1	—	—	—
Fig Bars Whole Wheat	1	60	1	—	—	—
Ginger Boys Calcium Enriched	6	120	3	—	—	—
Jelly Tarts	2	110	4	—	—	—
Mint Sandwich	2	160	7	—	—	—
Oatmeal Calcium Enriched	5	130	5	—	—	—
Peanut Butter Sandwich	2	170	8	—	—	—
Regal Grahams	2	140	7	—	—	—
Royal Dainty	2	120	6	—	—	—
T.C. Rounds	2	160	8	—	—	—
Tango	2	160	5	—	—	—
Trolley Cakes Devilsfood	2	120	2	—	—	—
Vanilla Wafers	8	120	5	—	—	—
Famous Amos						
Chocolate Chip	3 (1 oz)	140	6	100	20	—
Chocolate Chip Pecan	3 (1 oz)	150	8	98	18	—
Oatmeal Raisin	3 (1 oz)	134	6	137	19	—
Freihofer's						
Chocolate Chip	2 (0.9 oz)	120	6	75	16	1
Frito Lay						
Peanut Butter Bar	1.75 oz	270	16	65	30	—
Frookie						
7-Grain Oatmeal	1	45	2	35	7	—
Animal Frackers	6	60	2	25	9	—
Apple Cinnamon Oat Bran	1	45	2	35	7	—
Apple Cinnamon Oat Bran	1 lg	120	4	100	18	—
Apple Fruitins	1	60	1	25	12	—
Chocolate Chip	1	45	2	35	7	—
Chocolate Chip	1 lg	120	4	100	18	—
Chocolate Chip Mint	1	45	2	35	7	—
Fig Fruitins	1	60	1	25	12	—
Ginger Spice	1	45	2	35	7	—
Mandarin Chocolate Chip	1	45	2	35	7	—
Oat Bran Muffin	1 lg	120	4	100	18	—

FOOD	PORTION	CAL.	FAT	SOD.	CARB.	FIB.
Frookie (CONT.)						
Oat Bran Muffin	1	45	2	35	7	—
Oatmeal Raisin	1	45	2	35	7	—
Oatmeal Raisin	1 lg	120	4	100	18	—
General Mills						
Dunkaroos	1 pkg (1 oz)	130	5	70	19	—
FundaMiddles Vanilla Creme In Chocolate Graham Shells	1 pkg (0.8 oz)	110	4	120	18	—
Girl Scout						
Chalet Cremes Sugar Free	4 (1 oz)	150	6	55	22	1
Do-si-dos	3 (1.2 oz)	170	8	105	22	1
Samoas	2 (1 oz)	160	9	45	17	2
Snaps	7 (1.1 oz)	130	2	210	26	1
Striped Chocolate Chip	3 (1.2 oz)	180	10	100	20	1
Tagalongs	2 (0.9 oz)	150	10	85	13	2
Thin Mints	4 (1 oz)	140	8	80	18	1
Trefoils	5 (1.1 oz)	160	8	90	20	1
Glenny's						
Noah'N Friends Animal Peanut Butter	0.5 oz	65	3	35	9	—
Noah'N Friends Animal Vanilla	0.5 oz	65	2	35	10	—
Noah'N Friends Animal Wheat-Free Oatmeal	0.5 oz	65	2	20	10	—
Nookie Bar	1 (1.15 oz)	138	3	—	18	—
Sesame Nookie	1 (0.5 oz)	60	4	8	6	—
Sesame Nookie	1 pkg (1.5 oz)	180	12	24	18	—
Golden Fruit						
Apple	1 (0.7 oz)	80	2	55	15	tr
Cranberry	1 (0.7 oz)	70	1	55	15	tr
Cranberry Low Fat	1 (0.7 oz)	70	1	55	15	tr
Raisin	1 (0.7 oz)	80	2	40	15	tr
Grandma's						
Animal Cookies Candied	5 (1 oz)	140	6	80	20	—
Chocolate Chip	2 (2.75 oz)	370	17	270	50	—
Chocolate Chip Rich'N Chewy	3 (1 oz)	140	6	80	20	—
Fudge Chocolate Chip	2 (2.75 oz)	350	13	380	54	—
Grab Cookie Bits Chocolate	8 (1 oz)	140	6	180	19	—
Grab Cookie Bits Peanut Butter	8 (1 oz)	140	6	125	19	—

FOOD	PORTION	CAL.	FAT	SOD.	CARB.	FIB.
Grandma's (CONT.)						
Grab Cookie Bits Vanilla	8 (1 oz)	140	6	75	20	—
Oatmeal Apple Spice	2 (2.75 oz)	330	12	570	51	—
Old Time Molasses	2 (2.75 oz)	320	9	520	58	—
Peanut Butter	2 (2.75 oz)	410	30	410	43	—
Raisin Soft	2 (2.75 oz)	320	10	280	54	—
Handi-Snack						
Cookie Jammers Cookies & Fruit Spread	1 pkg (1.3 oz)	130	3	125	26	tr
Health Valley						
Amaranth Cookies	1	70	3	30	12	2
Fancy Fruit Chunks Apricot Almond	2	90	4	45	12	2
Fancy Fruit Chunks Date Pecan	2	90	4	45	13	2
Fancy Fruit Chunks Raisin Oat Bran	2	70	2	95	13	2
Fancy Fruit Chunks Tropical Fruit	2	90	3	45	15	2
Fancy Peanut Chunks	2	90	3	55	12	2
Fat Free Apple Spice	3	75	tr	40	17	3
Fat Free Apricot Delight	3	75	tr	40	16	3
Fat Free Date Delight	3	75	tr	40	17	3
Fat Free Hawaiian Fruit	3	75	tr	40	16	3
Fat Free Jumbos Apple Raisin	1	70	tr	35	16	3
Fat Free Jumbos Raisin	1	70	tr	35	16	3
Fat Free Jumbos Raspberry	1	70	tr	35	16	3
Fat Free Raisin Oatmeal	3	75	tr	40	17	3
Fiber Jumbos Blueberry Nut	1	100	3	45	14	3
Fiber Jumbos Chunky Pecan	1	100	3	45	14	3
Fiber Jumbos Raisin Nut	1	100	3	45	14	3
Fruit & Fitness	5	200	6	115	34	6
Fruit Jumbos Almond Date	1	70	3	30	10	1
Fruit Jumbos Oat Bran	1	70	2	35	12	2
Fruit Jumbos Raisin Nut	1	70	3	35	10	1
Fruit Jumbos Tropical Fruit	1	70	3	35	10	2
Graham Amaranth	7	110	3	110	25	3

FOOD	PORTION	CAL.	FAT	SOD.	CARB.	FIB.
Health Valley (CONT.)						
Graham Honey	7	100	4	125	18	2
Graham Oat Bran	7	120	3	45	20	5
Honey Jumbos Crisp Cinnamon	1	70	4	35	9	1
Honey Jumbos Crisp Peanut Butter	1	70	2	35	11	1
Honey Jumbos Fancy Oat Bran	2	130	4	50	20	4
Oat Bran Animal Cookies	7	110	4	50	17	3
Oat Bran Fruit & Nut	2	110	4	70	17	3
The Great Tofu	2	90	3	30	14	4
The Great Wheat Free	2	80	3	35	14	3
Heyday						
Caramel & Peanut	1 (0.8 oz)	110	5	40	13	tr
Fudge	1 (0.8 oz)	110	5	40	13	tr
Honey Maid						
Cinnamon Grahams	10 (1.1 oz)	140	3	210	26	1
Honey Grahams	8 (1 oz)	120	3	180	22	1
Hydrox						
Original	3	150	7	125	21	1
Reduced Fat	3 (1.1 oz)	130	4	140	24	1
Keebler						
Buttercup	3	70	3	110	11	—
Chocolate Fudge Sandwich	1	80	4	70	12	—
Commodore	1	60	2	65	10	—
Cookies Mates	2	50	2	55	8	—
French Vanilla Creme	1	80	4	80	12	—
Graham Honey Fiber Enriched	2	90	2	110	16	—
Graham Kitchen Rich	2	60	2	55	9	—
Homeplate	1	60	2	130	10	—
Keebies	1	80	3	80	12	—
Krisp Kreem Wafers	2	50	3	20	7	—
Old Fashion Chocolate Chip	1	80	4	75	11	—
Old Fashion Double Fudge	1	80	4	65	11	—
Old Fashion Oatmeal	1	80	4	110	13	—
Old Fashion Peanut Butter	1	80	4	100	10	—
Old Fashion Sugar	1	80	3	70	13	—
Pitter Patter	1	90	4	115	12	—

FOOD	PORTION	CAL.	FAT	SOD.	CARB.	FIB.
Keebler (CONT.)						
Vanilla Wafers	4	80	4	60	10	—
LU						
Chocolatiers	4 (1.1 oz)	170	8	35	20	2
Chocolatiers Dipped	3 (1 oz)	170	11	15	17	1
Le Petit Ecolier Dark Chocolate	2 (0.9 oz)	130	6	55	17	1
Little Schoolboy Milk Chocolate	2 (0.9 oz)	130	7	85	15	0
Marie Lu	3 (1.2 oz)	170	6	170	25	1
Truffle Lu	4 (1.2 oz)	180	11	410	18	1
La Choy						
Fortune	1	15	tr	1	4	tr
Lance						
Choc-O-Lunch	1 pkg (37 g)	180	7	150	26	—
Choc-O-Mint	1 pkg (35 g)	180	10	90	22	—
Chocolate Chip Fudge	1 (28 g)	130	5	130	20	—
Chocolate Chip Soft	1 (28 g)	130	5	100	19	—
Coated Graham	1 pkg (50 g)	200	10	60	24	—
Fig Bar	1 pkg (42 g)	150	2	85	30	—
Lem-O-Lunch	1 pkg (48 g)	240	11	190	32	—
Lemon Nekot	1 pkg (42 g)	220	11	100	28	—
Malt	1 pkg (35 g)	190	11	125	16	—
Nut-O-Lunch	1 oz	140	5	—	—	—
Oatmeal	1 (57 G)	130	5	70	20	—
Peanut Butter Creme Filled Wafer	1 pkg (50 g)	240	10	80	34	—
Van-O-Lunch	1 pkg (37 g)	180	7	150	26	—
Little Debbie						
Animal	1 pkg (1.5 oz)	190	5	110	33	0
Caramel Cookie Bars	1 pkg (1.2 oz)	160	8	90	23	1
Chocolate Chip Chewy	1 pkg (2 oz)	370	19	280	47	1
Chocolate Chip Crisp	1 pkg (1.5 oz)	210	12	150	26	1
Cookie Wreaths	1 pkg (0.6 oz)	90	5	45	11	0
Creme Filled Chocolate	1 pkg (1.2 oz)	180	8	115	24	1
Creme Filled Chocolate	1 pkg (1.8 oz)	260	11	230	36	1
Easter Puffs	1 pkg (1.2 oz)	140	5	65	25	0
Figaroos	1 pkg (1.5 oz)	160	4	115	31	3
Figaroos	1 pkg (2 oz)	200	5	160	40	2
Fudge Macaroons	1 pkg (1 oz)	140	8	65	18	1
Ginger	1 pkg (0.7 oz)	90	3	55	14	1
Oatmeal Crisp	1 pkg (1.5 oz)	210	11	230	27	1
Oatmeal Lights	1 pkg (1.3 oz)	140	4	190	28	1
Oatmeal Raisin	1 pkg (2.7 oz)	320	13	330	50	2

FOOD	PORTION	CAL.	FAT	SOD.	CARB.	FIB.
Little Debbie (CONT.)						
Peanut Butter	1 pkg (1.5 oz)	210	10	230	27	1
Peanut Butter & Jelly Sandwich	1 pkg (1.1 oz)	130	5	100	22	1
Peanut Butter Bars	1 pkg (1.9 oz)	270	15	190	33	1
Peanut Clusters	1 pkg (1.4 oz)	190	11	125	23	1
Pecan Spinwheels	1 pkg (1 oz)	110	4	100	16	1
Pecan Shortbread	1 pkg (1.5 oz)	220	13	170	26	0
Lorna Doone						
Cookies	4 (1 oz)	140	7	130	19	tr
Mallomars						
Cookies	2 (0.9 oz)	120	5	35	17	1
Mallopuffs						
Cookies	1 (0.6 oz)	70	2	35	12	tr
Manischewitz						
Macaroons Chocolate	2 (0.9 oz)	90	4	80	15	4
Mother's						
Almond Shortbread	3	180	11	115	19	1
Butter	5	140	6	95	21	—
Checkerboard Wafers	8	150	8	40	20	1
Chocolate Chip	2	160	8	105	20	0
Chocolate Chip Angel	3	180	9	70	21	1
Chocolate Chip Bag	4	140	5	85	23	1
Chocolate Chip Parade	4	130	5	100	19	1
Circus Animals	6	140	6	55	20	0
Cocadas	5	150	7	140	20	2
Cookie Parade	4	140	7	95	18	2
Dinosaur Grrrahams	2	130	3	130	24	—
Double Fudge	3	170	8	100	22	2
Duplex Creme	3	170	8	130	23	1
English Tea	2	180	7	100	26	1
Fig Bar	2	130	4	105	24	0
Fig Bar Fat Free	1	70	0	65	16	1
Fig Bar Whole Wheat	2	130	5	140	20	3
Fig Bar Whole Wheat Fat Free	1	70	0	60	17	1
Flaky Flix Fudge	2	140	7	50	17	2
Flaky Flix Vanilla	2	140	8	40	17	1
Frosted Holiday	4	130	6	50	19	0
Fudge Bowl Crowns	2	140	6	55	21	1
Fudge Bowl Nuggets	2	140	6	70	21	1
Gaucho Peanut Butter	2	190	10	200	22	2
Gingerbread Man	6	140	6	160	21	1
Iced Oatmeal	2	120	4	150	20	1

FOOD	PORTION	CAL.	FAT	SOD.	CARB.	FIB.
SnackWell's (CONT.)						
Reduced Fat Vanilla Sandwich	2 (0.9 oz)	110	3	95	21	1
Social Tea						
Cookies	6 (1 oz)	120	4	105	20	tr
Stella D'Oro						
Almond Toast Mandel	1	60	1	43	10	—
Angel Bars	1	80	5	15	7	—
Angel Wings	1	70	5	40	7	—
Angelica Goodies	1	110	4	45	16	—
Anginetti	1	30	1	3	5	—
Anisette Sponge	1	50	1	40	10	—
Anisette Toast	1	50	1	50	9	—
Anisette Toast Jumbo	1	110	1	65	23	—
Apple Pastry Low Sodium	1	80	3	5	14	—
Biscottini Cashews	1	110	6	50	14	—
Breakfast Treats	1	100	4	80	15	—
Castelets Chocolate	1	60	3	33	9	—
Chinese Dessert Cookies	1	170	9	90	19	—
Como Delight	1	150	7	60	18	—
Deep Night Fudge	1	65	4	33	8	—
Dutch Apple Bars	1	110	3	35	19	—
Egg Biscuits Low Sodium	3	120	3	15	20	—
Egg Biscuits Sugared	1	80	1	45	14	—
Egg Jumbo	1	50	1	30	9	—
Fruit Delight Apple Cinnamon Fat Free	1	70	0	50	17	—
Fruit Delight Peach Apricot Fat Free	1	70	0	35	17	—
Fruit Delight Raspberry Fat Free	1	70	0	40	17	—
Fruit Slices	1	60	2	45	9	—
Fruit Slices Fat Free	1	50	0	60	12	—
Golden Bars	1	110	4	65	16	—
Holiday Rings & Stars	1	47	1	12	7	—
Holiday Trinkets	1	40	2	31	5	—
Hostess Assortment	1	40	2	20	6	—
Indulgente Cashew Biscottini	1 (1.1 oz)	150	8	70	19	tr
Kichel Low Sodium	21	150	9	25	13	—
Lady Stella Assortment	1	40	2	22	6	—
Margherite Chocolate	1	70	3	40	10	—

FOOD	PORTION	CAL.	FAT	SOD.	CARB.	FIB.
Stella D'Oro (CONT.)						
Margherite Vanilla	1	70	3	45	11	—
Peach Apricot Pastry Sodium Free	1	80	3	0	13	—
Pfeffernusse Spice Drops	1	40	1	18	7	—
Prune Pastry Dietetic	1	90	3	0	14	—
Roman Egg Biscuits	1	140	5	125	20	—
Royal Nuggets	1	2	tr	—	tr	—
Sesame Regina	1	50	2	28	6	—
Swiss Fudge	1	70	3	33	9	—
Sunshine						
Almond Crescents	4 (1.1 oz)	150	6	105	22	tr
Animal Crackers	1 box (2 oz)	260	7	230	43	1
Animal Crackers	14 (1.1 oz)	140	4	125	24	tr
Classics Chocolate Chip With Pecans	1 (0.7 oz)	110	7	45	11	tr
Classics Chocolate Chip With Walnuts	1 (0.7 oz)	100	6	70	11	1
Classics Premier Chocolate Chip	1 (0.7 oz)	100	5	75	13	tr
Dixie Vanilla	2 (0.9 oz)	120	5	105	19	tr
Fig Bars	2 (1 oz)	110	3	60	20	1
Fudge Family Bears Vanilla	2 (1 oz)	140	6	115	20	tr
Fudge Mint Patties	2 (0.8 oz)	130	7	60	16	tr
Fudge Striped Shortbread	3 (1.1 oz)	160	8	85	20	1
Ginger Snaps	7 (1 oz)	130	5	150	22	tr
Grahams Cinnamon	2 (1.1 oz)	140	6	150	22	tr
Grahams Fudge Dipped	4 (1.2 oz)	170	9	75	21	1
Grahams Honey	2 (1 oz)	120	4	130	20	1
Grahamy Bears	1 pkg (2 oz)	260	10	230	41	2
Grahamy Bears	10 (1.1 oz)	140	5	125	22	1
Iced Gingerbread	5 (1 oz)	130	6	135	19	tr
Iced Oatmeal	2 (0.9 oz)	120	5	90	18	tr
Jingles	6 (1.1 oz)	150	5	115	22	tr
Lemon Coolers	5 (1 oz)	140	6	100	21	tr
Mini Chocolate Chip Cookies	5 (1.1 oz)	160	8	120	20	tr
Mini Fudge Royals	15 (1.1 oz)	160	8	90	20	1
Oatmeal Chocolate Chip	3 (1.3 oz)	170	8	130	23	2
Oatmeal Country Style	3 (1.2 oz)	170	7	160	24	1
School House Cookies	20 (1.1 oz)	140	5	115	23	tr

FOOD	PORTION	CAL.	FAT	SOD.	CARB.	FIB.
Sunshine (CONT.)						
Sugar Wafers Chocolate	3 (0.9 oz)	130	7	30	17	tr
Sugar Wafers Peanut Butter	4 (1.1 oz)	170	9	75	19	1
Sugar Wafers Vanilla	3 (0.9 oz)	130	6	20	18	tr
Tru Blu Chocolate	1 (0.6 oz)	80	3	64	11	tr
Tru Blu Lemon	1 (0.6 oz)	80	3	65	11	tr
Tru Blu Vanilla	1 (0.5 oz)	80	3	65	11	tr
Vanilla Wafers	7 (1.1 oz)	150	7	110	20	tr
Vienna Fingers	2 (1 oz)	140	6	105	21	tr
Tastykake						
Chocolate Chip Bar	1 (43 g)	190	8	95	28	1
Chocolate Chunk Macadamia Nut	1 pkg (56 g)	310	14	180	42	2
Fudge Bar	1 (50 g)	200	7	160	35	1
Oatmeal Raisin Bar	1 (50 g)	210	8	250	32	1
Soft'N Chewy Chocolate Chip	1 (39 g)	170	7	170	25	1
Soft'n Chewy Chocolate Chocolate Chip	1 (32 g)	170	7	110	26	1
Soft'n Chewy Oatmeal Raisin	1 (39 g)	160	5	160	27	1
Vanilla Sugar Wafer	1 (6 g)	36	2	10	4	0
Teddy Grahams						
Chocolate	24 (1 oz)	140	5	150	22	1
Cinnamon	24 (1 oz)	140	4	150	23	1
Honey	24 (1 oz)	140	4	150	22	1
Tree Of Life						
Creme Supremes	2 (0.9 oz)	120	5	90	18	1
Creme Supremes Mint	2 (0.9 oz)	120	5	90	18	1
Fat Free Classic Carrot Cake	1 (0.8 oz)	60	0	50	14	1
Fat Free Devil's Food Chocolate	1 (0.8 oz)	70	0	80	15	1
Fat Free Golden Oatmeal Raisin	1 (0.8 oz)	70	0	40	16	1
Fat Free Harvest Fruit & Nut	1 (0.8 oz)	70	0	45	16	1
Fat Free Toasted Almond Butter	1 (0.8 oz)	70	0	35	16	1
Fruit Bars Apple Spice	2 (1.3 oz)	120	3	120	22	2
Fruit Bars Fat Free Fig	1 (0.8 oz)	70	0	100	16	2
Fruit Bars Fat Free Peach Apricot	1 (0.8 oz)	70	0	110	17	1

FOOD	PORTION	CAL.	FAT	SOD.	CARB.	FIB.
Tree Of Life (CONT.)						
Fruit Bars Fat Free Wildberry	1 (0.8 oz)	70	0	170	16	2
Fruit Bars Fig	2 (1.3 oz)	120	3	100	21	3
Fruit Bars Peach Apricot	2 (1.3 oz)	120	3	105	22	2
Honey-Sweet Colossal Carrot Cake	1 (0.8 oz)	110	5	105	16	1
Honey-Sweet Lemon Burst	1 (0.8 oz)	110	5	25	15	1
Honey-Sweet Oh-So-Oatmeal	1 (0.8 oz)	110	5	140	14	1
Honey-Sweet Pecans-A-Plenty	1 (0.8 oz)	125	7	30	14	1
Monster Fat Free Carrot Cake	¼ cookie (0.9 oz)	60	0	30	15	1
Monster Fat Free Devil's Food Chocolate	¼ cookie (0.9 oz)	80	0	45	20	2
Monster Fat Free Gingerbread	¼ cookie (0.9 oz)	80	0	50	19	2
Monster Fat Free Maple Pecan	¼ cookie (0.9 oz)	90	0	50	20	2
Royal Vanilla	2 (0.9 oz)	120	5	115	17	0
Small World Animal Grahams	7 (1 oz)	120	3	60	21	3
Small World Chocolate Chip	7 (1 oz)	120	4	60	20	3
Soft-Bake Chocolate Chip	1 (0.8 oz)	125	7	15	15	1
Soft-Bake Double Fudge	1 (0.8 oz)	110	5	20	16	2
Soft-Bake Maui Macaroon	1 (0.8 oz)	135	10	0	12	2
Soft-Bake Oatmeal	1 (0.8 oz)	115	5	20	16	2
Soft-Bake Peanut Butter	1 (0.8 oz)	125	7	60	13	1
Wheat-Free American Oatmeal	1 (0.8 oz)	90	5	25	11	1
Wheat-Free California Carob	1 (0.8 oz)	105	5	75	14	6
Wheat-Free Georgia Peanut Butter	1 (0.8 oz)	95	6	110	8	1
Wheat-Free Mountain Maple Walnut	1 (0.8 oz)	100	6	50	9	6
Vienna Fingers						
Low Fat	2 (1 oz)	130	4	95	23	tr

FOOD	PORTION	CAL.	FAT	SOD.	CARB.	FIB.
Weight Watchers						
Apple Raisin Bar	1 (0.75 oz)	70	2	60	14	2
Chocolate Chip	2 (1.06 oz)	140	5	90	22	1
Chocolate Sandwich	2 (1.06)	140	4	160	23	1
Fruit Filled Fig	1 (0.7 oz)	70	0	50	16	0
Fruit Filled Raspberry	1 (0.7 oz)	70	0	45	16	0
Oatmeal Raisin	2 (1.06 oz)	120	2	90	22	1
Vanilla Sandwich	2 (1.06 oz)	140	3	80	25	1
REFRIGERATED						
chocolate chip	1 (0.42 oz)	59	3	28	8	—
chocolate chip unbaked	1 oz	126	6	59	17	—
oatmeal	1 (0.4 oz)	56	3	39	8	—
oatmeal raisin	1 (0.4 oz)	56	3	39	8	—
peanut butter	1 (0.4 oz)	60	3	52	7	—
peanut butter dough	1 oz	130	7	112	15	—
sugar	1 (0.42 oz)	58	3	56	8	—
sugar dough	1 oz	124	6	120	17	—
Pillsbury						
Chocolate Chip	1	70	3	55	9	—
Oatmeal Raisin	1	60	2	55	10	—
Peanut Butter	1	70	3	75	9	—
Sugar	1	70	3	70	9	—
TAKE-OUT						
biscotti with nuts chocolate dipped	1 (1.3 oz)	117	6	33	16	1

CORIANDER

leaf dried	1 tsp	2	tr	1	tr	—
leaf fresh	¼ cup	1	tr	1	tr	—
seed	1 tsp	5	tr	1	1	—

CORN

(*see also* BRAN, CEREAL, CORNMEAL)

CANNED						
cream style	½ cup	93	1	365	23	—
w/ red & green peppers	½ cup	86	1	396	21	—
white	½ cup	66	1	—	15	—
yellow	½ cup	66	1	—	15	1
Del Monte						
Cream Style Golden	½ cup (4.4 oz)	90	1	360	20	2
Cream Style Golden 50% Less Salt	½ cup (4.4 oz)	90	1	180	20	2
Cream Style Golden No Salt Added	½ cup (4.4 oz)	90	1	10	20	2
Cream Style Supersweet Golden	½ cup (4.4 oz)	60	1	360	14	2

FOOD	PORTION	CAL.	FAT	SOD.	CARB.	FIB.
Del Monte (CONT.)						
Cream Style White	½ cup (4.4 oz)	100	0	360	21	2
Whole Kernel Golden	½ cup (4.4 oz)	90	0	360	18	3
Whole Kernel Golden Supersweet 50% Less Salt	½ cup (4.4 oz)	60	1	130	11	3
Whole Kernel Golden Supersweet No Salt Added	½ cup (4.4 oz)	60	1	10	11	3
Whole Kernel Golden Supersweet No Sugar	½ cup (4.4 oz)	60	0	360	11	3
Whole Kernel Golden Supersweet Vacuum Packed	½ cup (3.7 oz)	70	1	270	13	3
Whole Kernel Golden Supersweet Vacuum Packed No Salt Added	½ cup (3.7 oz)	70	1	10	13	3
Whole Kernel White Sweet	½ cup (4.4 oz)	80	0	360	17	2
Green Giant						
50% Less Salt No Sugar Added	½ cup	50	1	140	11	2
Corn	½ cup	70	0	350	10	2
Cream Style	½ cup	100	tr	390	24	2
Deli Corn	½ cup	80	tr	350	19	2
Golden Kernel 50% Less Salt	½ cup	70	tr	175	16	2
Golden Vacuum Packed	½ cup	80	0	330	20	2
Mexi Corn	½ cup	80	tr	450	19	2
No Salt No Sugar	½ cup	80	tr	0	18	2
Sweet Select	½ cup	60	1	280	12	2
White Vacuum Packed	½ cup	80	0	290	20	2
Ka-Me						
Baby	½ cup (4.5 oz)	20	0	10	3	2
Stir Fry	½ cup (4.5 oz)	20	0	10	3	2
Owatonna						
Cream Style	½ cup	100	1	—	—	—
Whole Kernel In Brine	½ cup	90	1	—	—	—
Whole Kernel Vacuum Pack	½ cup	100	1	—	—	—
S&W						
Cream Style Diet	½ cup	100	1	0	21	—
Cream Style Premium Homestyle	½ cup	105	1	435	25	—

FOOD	PORTION	CAL.	FAT	SOD.	CARB.	FIB.
S&W (CONT.)						
Sweet 'N Natural	½ cup	90	1	180	20	—
Whole Kernel Tender Young	½ cup	90	1	295	20	—
Whole Kernel Water Pack	½ cup	80	1	0	15	—
Seneca						
Cream Style	½ cup	80	0	288	18	1
Whole Kernel	½ cup	90	0	288	21	2
Whole Kernel Natural Pack	½ cup	80	1	0	18	2
DRIED						
Goya						
Giant White	⅓ cup (1.6 oz)	160	2	10	35	4
FRESH						
on-the-cob w/ butter cooked	1 ear	155	3	30	32	—
white cooked	½ cup	89	1	14	21	—
white raw	½ cup	66	1	12	15	—
yellow cooked	1 ear (2.7 oz)	83	1	13	19	—
yellow cooked	½ cup	89	1	14	21	—
yellow raw	1 ear (3 oz)	77	1	14	17	—
yellow raw	½ cup	66	1	12	15	—
FROZEN						
cooked	½ cup	67	tr	4	17	—
on-the-cob cooked	1 ear (2.2 oz)	59	tr	3	14	—
Birds Eye						
Big Ears	1 ear	160	1	0	37	—
In Butter Sauce	½ cup	90	2	170	19	2
Little Ears	2 ears	130	1	0	30	—
On The Cob	1 ear	120	1	0	29	—
Polybag Cut	½ cup	80	1	0	19	2
Polybag Deluxe Tender Sweet	½ cup	80	1	0	20	2
Sweet	½ cup	80	1	0	20	2
Fresh Like						
Cob Corn	1 ear (3 in)	96	1	4	24	1
Cob Corn	1 ear (5 in)	96	1	4	23	1
Cut	3.5 oz	85	1	5	21	1
Green Giant						
Cream Style	½ cup	110	1	370	25	3
Harvest Fresh Niblets	½ cup	80	1	40	17	2
Harvest Fresh White Shoepeg	½ cup	90	1	60	19	2

FOOD	PORTION	CAL.	FAT	SOD.	CARB.	FIB.
Green Giant (CONT.)						
In Butter Sauce	½ cup	100	2	310	19	—
Nibblers Corn On The Cob	2 ears	120	1	10	27	2
Niblet Ears	1 ear	120	1	10	27	2
Niblets	½ cup	90	tr	5	19	2
One Serve Niblets In Butter Sauce	1 pkg	120	2	350	24	3
One Serve On The Cob	1 pkg	120	1	10	26	2
Super Sweet Nibblers Corn On The Cob	2 ears	90	2	10	19	2
Super Sweet Niblet Ears	1 ear	90	2	10	19	2
Super Sweet Niblet Select	½ cup	60	1	5	13	2
White In Butter Sauce	½ cup	100	2	280	20	2
White Select	½ cup	90	1	5	19	2
Hanover						
White Shoepeg	½ cup	80	0	—	—	—
White Sweet	½ cup	80	0	—	—	—
Yellow Sweet	½ cup	80	0	—	—	—
Mrs. Paul's						
Fritters	2	240	9	560	35	—
Ore Ida						
Cob Corn	1 ear (6.1 oz)	180	3	5	33	4
Cob Corn Mini-Gold	1 ear (3.1 oz)	90	1	0	16	2
Stouffer's						
Souffle	½ cup (2.4 oz)	170	7	490	21	1
Tree Of Life						
Corn	⅔ cup (3.2 oz)	80	1	10	19	1
SHELF-STABLE						
Pantry Express						
Golden Whole Kernel	½ cup	60	tr	210	18	1
TAKE-OUT						
fritters	1 (1 oz)	62	2	126	9	1
scalloped	½ cup	258	7	246	43	—

CORN CHIPS

(*see* CHIPS)

CORNISH HENS

(*see* CHICKEN)

CORNMEAL

FOOD	PORTION	CAL.	FAT	SOD.	CARB.	FIB.
corn grits cooked	1 cup	146	tr	0	31	—
corn grits uncooked	1 cup	579	2	1	124	—

FOOD	PORTION	CAL.	FAT	SOD.	CARB.	FIB.
degermed	1 cup	506	2	5	107	7
self-rising degermed	1 cup	489	2	1860	103	—
whole grain	1 cup	442	4	43	94	13
Albers						
White	3 tbsp	110	0	0	34	tr
Yellow	3 tbsp	110	0	0	34	tr
Arrowhead						
Yellow	¼ cup (1.2 oz)	120	1	0	27	3
Aunt Jemima						
White	3 tbsp	102	1	1	22	1
Yellow	3 tbsp	102	1	1	22	1
Quaker						
White	3 tbsp	102	1	1	22	1
Yellow	3 tbsp	102	1	1	22	1
MIX						
Arrowhead						
Corn Bread	¼ cup (1.2 oz)	120	1	270	24	4
Aunt Jemima						
Bolded White Mix	3 tbsp	99	1	337	21	—
Buttermilk Self Rising White Mix	3 tbsp	101	1	439	21	—
Self Rising White Mix	3 tbsp	98	1	381	21	1
Self Rising Yellow Mix	3 tbsp	100	1	490	21	—
Golden Dipt						
Corny Dog Batter Mix	1 oz	100	0	490	22	—
Hush Puppy Deluxe Mix	1¼ oz	120	0	520	26	—
Hush Puppy Jalapeno Mix	1¼ oz	120	0	570	27	—
Hush Puppy With Onion	1¼ oz	120	0	520	27	—
Hodgson Mill						
Yellow	¼ cup (1 oz)	100	1	0	22	3
Yellow Self Rising	¼ cup (1 oz)	90	1	260	21	3
Kentucky Kernal						
White Corn Meal Mix	¼ cup (1 oz)	100	1	210	22	2
Miracle Maize						
Complete as prep	1 piece (1.5 oz)	193	3	193	34	2
Country Style as prep	1 piece 2 in x 2 in (1.8 oz)	230	5	406	38	2
Sweet as prep	1 piece 2 in x 2 in (1.8 oz)	236	5	260	41	1
Stone-Buhr						
Yellow Corn Meal	¼ cup (1 oz)	100	0	0	23	1
READY-TO-EAT						
Aurora						
Polenta	½ cup (5 oz)	110	0	470	24	1

FOOD	PORTION	CAL.	FAT	SOD.	CARB.	FIB.
TAKE-OUT						
hush puppies	5 (2.7 oz)	256	12	965	35	4
hush puppies	1 (0.75 oz)	74	3	147	10	1
CORNSALAD						
raw	1 cup	12	tr	—	2	—
CORNSTARCH						
cornstarch	⅓ cup	164	tr	4	39	tr
Argo						
Cornstarch	1 tbsp (8 g)	30	0	0	7	—
Cornstarch	1 cup (128 g)	460	tr	tr	115	—
Hodgson Mill						
Cornstarch	2 tsp (0.4 oz)	35	0	0	9	—
Kingsford's						
Cornstarch	1 cup (128 g)	460	tr	tr	115	—
Cornstarch	1 tbsp (8 g)	30	tr	0	7	—
COTTAGE CHEESE						
creamed	4 oz	117	5	457	3	—
creamed	1 cup (7.4 oz)	217	9	850	6	—
creamed w/ fruit	4 oz	140	4	457	15	—
dry curd	1 cup (5.1 oz)	123	1	19	3	—
dry curd	4 oz	96	tr	14	2	—
lowfat 1%	1 cup (7.9 oz)	164	2	918	6	—
lowfat 1%	4 oz	82	1	459	3	—
lowfat 2%	4 oz	101	2	459	4	—
lowfat 2%	1 cup (7.9 oz)	203	4	918	8	—
Axelrod						
Nonfat	½ cup (4.4 oz)	90	0	500	7	0
Borden						
4%	½ cup	120	5	400	4	—
Dry Curd 0.5%	½ cup	80	1	20	3	—
Unsalted 4%	½ cup	120	5	40	4	—
Breakstone's						
2% Fat Large Curd	½ cup (4.2 oz)	90	3	390	4	0
2% Fat Small Curd	½ cup (4.2 oz)	90	3	390	4	0
4% Fat Large Curd	½ cup (4.2 oz)	120	5	400	5	0
4% Fat Small Curd	½ cup (4.2 oz)	120	5	400	5	0
Dry Curd	¼ cup (1.9 oz)	45	0	30	3	0
Free	½ cup (4.4 oz)	80	0	440	6	0
Snack 2% Fat Small Curd	1 pkg (4 oz)	90	2	370	4	0
Snack 4% Fat Small Curd	1 pkg (4 oz)	110	5	380	4	0

FOOD	PORTION	CAL.	FAT	SOD.	CARB.	FIB.
Breakstone's (CONT.)						
Snack Free	1 pkg (4 oz)	70	0	400	6	0
Cabot						
Cottage Cheese	4 oz	120	5	455	3	—
Light	4 oz	90	1	360	3	—
Friendship						
California Style	½ cup (4 oz)	115	5	380	4	0
Lowfat No Salt Added	½ cup (4 oz)	90	1	40	4	0
Lowfat Pineapple	½ cup (4 oz)	120	1	300	17	0
Lowfat 1%	½ cup (4 oz)	90	1	360	4	0
Nonfat	½ cup (4 oz)	80	0	380	5	0
Nonfat Plus Peach	½ cup (4 oz)	110	0	300	15	0
Pot Style	½ cup (4 oz)	90	3	430	3	0
With Pineapple	½ cup (4 oz)	140	4	310	15	0
Hood						
1% Fat	½ cup (4 oz)	90	2	390	6	0
1% Fat Chive & Onion	½ cup (4 oz)	90	2	390	6	0
1% Fat No Salt Added	½ cup (4 oz)	90	2	65	6	0
1% Fat Pepper & Herb	½ cup (4 oz)	90	2	450	6	0
1% Fat Pineapple Cherry	½ cup (4 oz)	110	1	290	15	0
4% Fat	½ cup (4 oz)	120	4	390	5	0
4% Fat Chive	½ cup (4 oz)	130	4	380	5	0
4% Fat Pineapple	½ cup (4 oz)	130	4	290	15	0
Nonfat	½ cup (4 oz)	80	0	330	6	0
Nonfat Pineapple	½ cup (4 oz)	110	0	250	16	0
Knudsen						
1.5% Fat Small Curd Pineapple	½ cup (4.6 oz)	120	2	330	14	0
2% Fat Small Curd	½ cup (4.2 oz)	100	3	400	5	0
4% Fat Large Curd	½ cup (4.5 oz)	130	5	330	4	0
4% Fat Small Curd	½ cup (4.3 oz)	120	5	400	4	0
Free	½ cup (4.2 oz)	80	0	380	4	0
On The Go! 1.5% Fat Peach	1 pkg (4 oz)	110	2	300	13	0
On The Go! 1.5% Fat Pineapple	1 pkg (4 oz)	110	2	300	13	0
On The Go! 1.5% Fat Strawberry	1 pkg (4 oz)	110	2	290	13	0
On The Go! 1.5% Fat Tropical Fruit	1 pkg (4 oz)	110	2	300	13	0
On The Go! 2% Fat	1 pkg (4 oz)	90	2	370	5	0
On The Go! Free	1 pkg (4 oz)	70	0	350	4	0
Lactaid						
1%	4 oz	72	1	406	3	—

FOOD	PORTION	CAL.	FAT	SOD.	CARB.	FIB.
Light N'Lively						
1% Fat	½ cup (4 oz)	80	1	370	5	0
1% Fat Garden Salad	½ cup (4.2 oz)	80	2	390	5	0
1% Fat Peach & Pineapple	½ cup (4.3 oz)	110	1	340	15	0
Fat Free	½ cup (4.4 oz)	80	0	440	6	0
Lite Line						
Lowfat 1 ½%	½ cup	90	2	400	4	—
Viva						
Nonfat	½ cup	70	0	430	5	—
Weight Watchers						
1%	½ cup	90	1	460	4	0
2%	½ cup	90	2	460	4	0
COTTONSEED						
kernels roasted	1 tbsp	51	4	3	2	—
COUGH DROPS						
Halls						
Cough Drops	1 (3.8 g)	15	0	—	4	—
Plus	1 (4.7 g)	18	0	—	5	—
With Vitamin C	1 (3.8 g)	14	0	—	4	—
Lifesavers						
Menthol	2 (0.5 oz)	60	0	0	14	—
COUSCOUS						
cooked	½ cup	101	tr	4	21	—
dry	½ cup	346	tr	9	71	—
Casbah						
Almond Chicken Vegetarian	1 pkg (1.5 oz)	160	2	470	29	tr
Asparagus Au Gratin Organic	1 pkg (1.5 oz)	150	2	400	28	1
Cheddar Broccoli	1 pkg (1.3 oz)	130	2	470	23	tr
Hearty Harvest Zestful Organic as prep	1 pkg (10 fl oz)	180	1	460	36	2
Moroccan Stew	1 pkg (2 oz)	180	1	430	36	1
Pilaf as prep	1 cup	200	tr	480	40	tr
Tomato Parmesan	1 pkg (1.8 oz)	170	2	460	34	2
Kitchen Del Sol						
Aegean Citrus as prep	½ cup (1.1 oz)	110	3	290	20	1
Moroccan Ginger as prep	½ cup (1.1 oz)	120	3	290	21	1
Spicy Vegetable as prep	½ cup (1.1 oz)	120	3	290	20	1
Tomato & Olive	½ cup (1 oz)	120	4	290	19	1

FOOD	PORTION	CAL.	FAT	SOD.	CARB.	FIB.
Kitchen Del Sol (CONT.)						
Tomato & Olive	½ cup (1.1 oz)	120	4	290	19	1
Near East						
As Prep	1¼ cup	260	6	65	46	2
COWPEAS						
catjang dried cooked	1 cup	200	1	32	35	—
common canned	1 cup	184	1	718	33	—
frozen cooked	½ cup	112	tr	5	20	—
leafy tips chopped cooked	1 cup	12	tr	3	1	—
leafy tips raw chopped	1 cup	10	tr	2	2	—
CRAB						
CANNED						
blue	3 oz	84	1	283	0	—
blue	1 cup	133	2	5	0	—
S&W						
Dungeness Crab	3.25 oz	81	2	920	1	—
FRESH						
alaska king cooked	1 leg (4.7 oz)	129	2	1436	0	—
alaska king cooked	3 oz	82	1	911	0	—
alaska king raw	3 oz	71	1	711	0	—
alaska king raw	1 leg (6 oz)	144	1	1438	0	—
blue cooked	1 cup	138	2	376	0	—
blue cooked	3 oz	87	2	237	0	—
blue raw	1 crab (7 oz)	18	tr	62	tr	—
blue raw	3 oz	74	1	249	tr	—
dungeness raw	1 crab (5.7 oz)	140	2	481	1	—
dungeness raw	3 oz	73	1	251	1	—
queen steamed	3 oz	98	1	587	0	—
FROZEN						
Mrs. Paul's						
Deviled Crab	1 cake	180	9	480	18	—
Deviled Crab Miniatures	3½ oz	240	12	540	25	—
TAKE-OUT						
baked	1 (3.8 oz)	160	2	550	4	—
cake	1 (2 oz)	160	10	492	5	—
crab cakes	1 (2.1 oz)	93	5	198	tr	—
soft-shell fried	1 (4.4 oz)	334	18	1118	31	—
CRACKER CRUMBS						
cracker meal	1 cup (4 oz)	440	2	32	93	—
graham cracker crumbs	½ cup (4.4 oz)	540	13	756	97	3
Golden Dipt						
Cracker Meal	1 oz	100	0	0	22	—

FOOD	PORTION	CAL.	FAT	SOD.	CARB.	FIB.
Honey Maid						
Graham Cracker	0.5 oz	70	2	90	13	tr
Keebler						
Cracker Meal	1 cup	100	3	5	23	—
Graham Crumbs	1 cup	520	14	630	90	—
Zesty Meal	1 cup	85	10	100	61	—
Kellogg's						
Corn Flake Crumbs	2 tbsp (0.4 oz)	40	0	120	9	0
Lance						
Cracker Meal	1 oz	100	1	1	21	—
Nabisco						
Nilla Cookie Crumbs	2 tbsp (0.5 oz)	70	3	55	13	tr
Oreo						
Cookie Crumbs	2 tbsp (0.5 oz)	80	3	140	13	1
Premium						
Fat Free Cracker Crumbs	¼ cup (1 oz)	100	0	0	23	1
Ritz						
Cracker Crumbs	⅓ cup (1 oz)	140	7	270	17	1
Sunshine						
Graham	3 tbsp (0.6 oz)	80	2	150	13	tr

CRACKERS

(*see also* CRACKER CRUMBS)

FOOD	PORTION	CAL.	FAT	SOD.	CARB.	FIB.
cheese	14 (½ oz)	71	4	141	8	—
cheese	1 (1 in sq) (1 g)	5	tr	10	1	—
cheese low sodium	14 (½ oz)	71	4	68	8	—
cheese low sodium	1 (1 in sq) (1 g)	5	tr	5	1	—
cheese w/ peanut butter filling	1 (0.24 oz)	34	2	69	4	tr
crispbread	3	61	2	—	9	1
crispbread rye	1 (0.35 oz)	37	tr	26	8	2
crispbread rye	3	77	1	—	17	3
melba toast plain	1 (5 g)	19	tr	41	4	tr
melba toast pumpernickel	1 (5 g)	19	tr	45	4	tr
melba toast rye	1 (5 g)	19	tr	45	4	tr
melba toast wheat	1 (5 g)	19	tr	42	4	tr
milk	1 (0.42 oz)	55	2	71	8	—
oyster cracker	1 (1 g)	4	tr	13	1	tr
peanut butter sandwich	1 (7 g)	34	2	66	4	—
rusk toast	1 (0.35 oz)	41	1	25	7	—
rye w/ cheese filling	1 (0.24 oz)	34	2	73	4	—
rye wafers plain	1 (0.9 oz)	84	tr	199	20	—
rye wafers seasoned	1 (0.8 oz)	84	2	195	16	—
saltines	1 (3 g)	13	tr	38	2	tr

FOOD	PORTION	CAL.	FAT	SOD.	CARB.	FIB.
saltines fat free low sodium	6 (1 oz)	118	tr	191	25	—
saltines fat free low sodium	3 (0.5 oz)	59	tr	95	12	—
saltines low salt	1 (3 g)	13	tr	19	2	tr
snack cracker	1 (3 g)	15	1	25	2	tr
snack cracker low salt	1 (3 g)	15	1	11	2	tr
snack cracker w/ cheese filling	1 (7 g)	33	2	98	4	—
soup cracker	1 (1 g)	4	tr	13	1	tr
water biscuits	3	92	3	—	16	1
wheat w/ cheese filling	1 (0.24 oz)	35	2	64	4	—
wheat w/ peanut butter filling	1 (0.24 oz)	35	2	57	4	—
wheat thins	1 (2 g)	9	tr	16	1	—
wheat thins	7 (0.5 oz)	67	3	113	9	1
wheat thins low salt	7 (0.5 oz)	67	3	40	9	1
whole wheat	1 (4 g)	18	1	26	3	—
whole wheat low salt	1 (4 g)	18	1	10	3	—
zwieback	3½ oz	374	4	263	73	4
Adrienne's						
Gourmet Flatbread Caraway & Rye	2	20	tr	45	4	—
Gourmet Flatbread Classic Island	2	20	tr	45	3	—
Gourmet Flatbread Slightly Onion	2	20	tr	45	3	—
Gourmet Flatbread Ten Grain	2	20	tr	45	3	1
Ak-mak						
100% Whole Wheat	5 (1 oz)	116	2	214	19	4
American Heritage						
Sesame	9 (1.1 oz)	160	9	300	17	1
Wheat & Bran	9 (1 oz)	140	7	280	17	2
Better Cheddars						
Crackers	22 (1 oz)	70	8	290	17	tr
Low Sodium	22 (1 oz)	150	7	75	18	tr
Reduced Fat	24 (1 oz)	140	6	350	19	tr
Burns & Ricker						
Bagel Crisps Garlic	5 (1 oz)	100	0	280	22	1
Cheez-It						
Crackers	27 (1 oz)	160	8	240	16	tr
Crackers	1 pkg (1.5 oz)	220	12	340	23	1
Crackers	1 pkg (2 oz)	290	16	450	31	2
Hot & Spicy	26 (1 oz)	160	8	220	17	1
Hot & Spicy	1 pkg (1.5 oz)	220	12	310	25	1

FOOD	PORTION	CAL.	FAT	SOD.	CARB.	FIB.
Cheez-It (CONT.)						
Low Sodium	27 (1 oz)	160	8	70	16	tr
Party Mix	½ cup (1 oz)	140	5	270	19	1
Reduced Fat	30 (1 oz)	130	5	280	19	tr
White Cheddar	1 pkg (1.5 oz)	220	12	400	24	tr
White Cheddar	26 (1 oz)	160	9	280	17	tr
Crown Pilot						
Crackers	1 (0.5 oz)	70	2	85	13	tr
Devonsheer						
Melba Rounds Garlic	½ oz	56	1	132	9	1
Melba Rounds Honey Bran	½ oz	52	1	98	9	1
Melba Rounds Onion	½ oz	51	1	120	10	1
Melba Rounds Plain	½ oz	53	1	111	10	1
Melba Rounds Plain Unsalted	½ oz	52	1	<5	10	1
Melba Rounds Rye	½ oz	53	1	130	10	1
Melba Rounds Sesame	½ oz	57	2	131	8	1
Eden						
Brown Rice	5 (1 oz)	120	2	230	22	2
Escort						
Crackers	3 (0.5 oz)	70	4	115	9	—
Estee						
Unsalted	1 (0.5 oz)	70	2	0	10	0
FFV						
Ham & Cheese Crispy Wafers	7	70	2	—	—	—
Frito Lay						
Cheese Filled	6 (1.5 oz)	210	10	470	24	—
Cracker Snacks Cheddar	13-16 (1 oz)	70	4	150	8	—
Cracker Snacks Zesty Italian	13-16 (1 oz)	70	3	115	9	—
Peanut Butter Filled	6 (1.5 oz)	210	10	450	24	—
Goya						
Butter Crackers	1	40	1	60	6	—
Crackers	1	30	0	45	5	—
Hain						
Cheese	1 oz	130	6	180	17	—
Onion	1 oz	130	6	160	17	—
Onion No Salt Added	1 oz	130	6	5	17	—
Rich	1 oz	130	5	160	18	—
Rich No Salt Added	1 oz	130	5	15	18	—
Rye	1 oz	120	4	200	19	—
Rye No Salt Added	1 oz	120	4	10	19	—

FOOD	PORTION	CAL.	FAT	SOD.	CARB.	FIB.
Hain (CONT.)						
Sesame	1 oz	140	7	210	16	—
Sesame No Salt Added	1 oz	140	7	5	16	—
Sour Cream & Chive	1 oz	130	6	150	15	—
Sour Cream & Chive No Salt Added	1 oz	130	6	25	15	—
Sourdough	½ oz	65	3	100	9	—
Sourdough Low Salt	1 oz	130	5	10	18	—
Vegetable	1 oz	130	5	180	10	—
Vegetable No Salt Added	1 oz	130	5	50	10	—
Harvest Crisps						
5 Grain	13 (1.1 oz)	130	4	300	23	1
Oat	13 (1.1 oz)	140	5	300	22	1
Health Valley						
Herb Stoned Wheat	13	55	2	80	9	2
Herb Stoned Wheat No Salt	13	55	2	30	9	2
Rice Bran	7	130	4	65	19	2
Sesame Stoned Wheat	13	55	2	80	9	2
Sesame Stoned Wheat No Salt Added	13	55	2	30	9	2
Seven Grain Vegetable Stoned Wheat	13	55	2	80	9	2
Seven Grain Vegetable Stoned Wheat No Salt Added	13	55	2	30	9	2
Stoned Wheat	13	55	2	80	9	2
Stoned Wheat No Salt Added	13	55	2	30	9	2
Healthy Choice						
Bread Crisps Garlic Herb	11 (1 oz)	110	2	115	22	2
Hi Ho						
Butter Flavored	9 (1.1 oz)	160	9	280	19	tr
Cracked Pepper	9 (1.1 oz)	160	9	280	18	tr
Crackers	9	160	9	280	18	tr
Low Salt	9 (1.1 oz)	160	9	135	18	tr
Multi Grain	9 (1.1 oz)	160	9	370	18	1
Reduced Fat	10 (1.1 oz)	140	5	280	21	tr
Whole Wheat	9 (1.1 oz)	150	8	280	18	2
J.J. Flats						
Breadflats Caraway	1	52	1	126	10	1
Breadflats Caraway And Salt	1	51	1	213	9	1
Breadflats Cinnamon	1	53	1	126	10	1

FOOD	PORTION	CAL.	FAT	SOD.	CARB.	FIB.
J.J. Flats (CONT.)						
Breadflats Flavorall	1	52	1	139	10	1
Breadflats Garlic	1	52	1	127	10	1
Breadflats Oat Bran	1	49	1	141	8	2
Breadflats Onion	1	53	1	140	10	1
Breadflats Plain	1	53	1	143	10	1
Breadflats Poppy	1	53	1	126	9	1
Breadflats Sesame	1	55	2	124	9	1
Kavli						
Crackers	1 piece	40	tr	40	10	2
Keebler						
Club	2	30	2	75	4	—
Melba Toast Garlic	2	25	tr	35	4	—
Melba Toast Long	2	30	tr	10	7	—
Melba Toast Onion	2	25	tr	35	4	—
Melba Toast Plain	2	25	tr	35	4	—
Melba Toast Sesame	2	25	tr	35	4	—
Oyster Crackers Large	26	80	2	175	13	—
Oyster Crackers Small	50	80	2	175	13	—
Snack Crackers Toasted Rye	2	30	2	70	4	—
Snack Crackers Toasted Sesame	2	30	2	65	4	—
Snack Crackers Toasted Wheat	2	30	2	60	4	—
Toasted Snack Bacon	2	30	2	65	4	—
Toasted Snack Onion	2	30	2	70	4	—
Toasted Snack Pumpernickel	2	30	2	55	4	—
Wholegrain Wheat	2	30	1	70	5	—
Krispy						
Cracked Pepper	5 (0.5 oz)	60	2	180	10	tr
Fat Free	5 (0.5 oz)	60	0	135	12	tr
Mild Cheddar	5 (0.5 oz)	60	2	180	10	tr
Original	5 (0.5 oz)	60	2	180	10	tr
Soup & Oyster Crackers	17 (0.5 oz)	60	2	200	11	tr
Unsalted Tops	5 (0.5 oz)	60	2	120	10	tr
Whole Wheat	5 (0.5 oz)	60	2	130	10	tr
Lance						
Bonnie	1 pkg (34 g)	160	7	170	24	—
Captain Wafers	2	30	1	60	5	—
Captain Wafers Very Low Sodium	2	30	1	25	5	—
Captain Wafers w/ Cream Cheese & Chives	1 pkg (37 g)	170	9	260	23	—

FOOD	PORTION	CAL.	FAT	SOD.	CARB.	FIB.
Lance (CONT.)						
Cheese-On-Wheat	1 pkg (37 g)	180	9	260	22	—
Lanchee	1 pkg (35 g)	180	11	110	19	—
Melba Toast Oblong	2	30	0	50	7	—
Melba Toast Plain	2	20	0	30	4	—
Melba Toast Round Garlic	2	20	0	35	4	—
Melba Toast Round Onion	2	20	0	30	4	—
Melba Toast Sesame	2	25	0	35	4	—
Nekot	1 pkg (42 g)	210	10	95	24	—
Nip-Chee	1 pkg (37 g)	180	8	320	21	—
Oyster Crackers	1 pkg (14 g)	70	2	170	10	—
Peanut Butter Wheat	1 pkg (37 g)	190	11	210	18	—
Rye Twins	2	30	1	65	5	—
Rye-Chee	1 pkg (41 g)	190	9	320	22	—
Saltines	2	25	1	65	4	—
Saltines Slug Pack	4 crackers	50	1	130	8	—
Sesame Twins	2	40	1	65	6	—
Toastchee	1 pkg (39 g)	190	11	310	19	—
Toasty	1 pkg (35 g)	180	10	160	17	—
Wheat Twins	2	30	1	70	5	—
Wheatswafer	2	30	1	50	4	—
Lavash						
Bread Crisp Original	2 (0.5 oz)	60	1	90	11	—
Bread Crisp Sesame	2 (0.5 oz)	60	1	70	10	—
Little Debbie						
Cheese Crackers With Peanut Butter	1 pkg (0.9 oz)	140	7	290	16	1
Cheese Crackers With Peanut Butter	1 pkg (1.4 oz)	210	10	430	23	1
Toasty Crackers With Peanut Butter	1 pkg (0.9 oz)	140	7	290	16	1
Toasty Crackers With Peanut Butter	1 pkg (1.4 oz)	200	10	350	20	1
Wheat Crackers With Cheddar Cheese	1 pkg (0.9 oz)	140	7	270	16	0
Manischewitz						
Tam Tams	10	147	8	171	17	—
Tam Tams No Salt	10	138	7	—	18	—
Tams Garlic	10	153	8	165	19	—
Tams Onion	10	150	8	157	18	—
Tams Wheat	10	150	8	180	18	—

FOOD	PORTION	CAL.	FAT	SOD.	CARB.	FIB.
McCrackens						
Cracker Crisp Country Butter	1 oz	140	8	170	18	—
Cracker Crisp Sour Cream & Chives	1 oz	140	8	170	18	—
Cracker Crisp Tangy Cheddar	1 oz	140	8	170	18	—
Cracker Crisp Toasted Wheat	1 oz	140	8	170	18	—
NABS						
Cheese Peanut Butter Sandwich	6 (1.4 oz)	190	10	390	24	1
Peanut Butter Toast Sandwich	6 (1.4 oz)	190	10	380	24	1
Nabisco						
Bacon Flavored	15 (1.1 oz)	160	8	460	19	tr
Chicken In A Biskit	14 (1 oz)	160	9	270	17	tr
Garden Crisps	15 (1 oz)	130	4	290	22	1
Oat Thins	18 (1 oz)	140	1	190	20	2
Royal Lunch	1 (0.4 oz)	50	2	65	8	0
Swiss	15 (1 oz)	140	7	350	18	tr
Tid-Bit Cheese	32 (1 oz)	150	8	420	17	tr
Vegetable Thins	14 (1.1 oz)	160	9	310	19	1
Wheat Thins Original	16 (1 oz)	140	6	170	19	2
Wheat Thins Reduced Fat	18 (1 oz)	120	4	220	21	2
Zings!	1 pkg (1.8 oz)	240	11	420	34	2
Nips						
Cheese	29 (1 oz)	150	6	310	18	tr
Old London						
Melba Toast Pumpernickel	½ oz	54	1	156	10	1
Melba Toast Rye	½ oz	52	1	132	10	—
Melba Toast Sesame	½ oz	55	2	148	8	1
Melba Toast Sesame Unsalted	½ oz	55	2	5	8	1
Melba Toast Wheat	½ oz	51	1	121	10	1
Melba Toast White	½ oz	51	1	111	10	1
Melba Toast White Unsalted	½ oz	51	1	4	10	1
Melba Toast Whole Grain	½ oz	52	1	116	9	1
Melba Toast Whole Grain Unsalted	½ oz	53	1	4	10	1
Rounds Bacon	½ oz	53	1	126	9	1

FOOD	PORTION	CAL.	FAT	SOD.	CARB.	FIB.
Old London (CONT.)						
Rounds Garlic	½ oz	56	1	132	9	1
Rounds Onion	½ oz	52	1	121	10	1
Rounds Rye	½ oz	52	1	132	10	—
Rounds Sesame	½ oz	56	2	149	8	1
Rounds White	½ oz	48	1	111	9	1
Rounds Whole Grain	½ oz	54	1	102	9	1
Oysterettes						
Crackers	19 (0.5 oz)	60	3	150	10	tr
Partners						
Walla Walla Sweet Onion Preservative Free	0.5 oz	65	3	60	8	tr
Pepperidge Farm						
Butter Thins	4	70	3	115	10	0
Cracked Wheat	3	100	4	180	14	1
Crispy Graham	4	70	2	115	13	—
English Water Biscuits	4	70	1	100	13	0
Flutters Garden Herb	¾ oz	100	4	190	14	—
Flutters Golden Sesame	¾ oz	110	5	150	13	—
Flutters Original Butter	¾ oz	100	4	150	15	—
Flutters Toasted Wheat	¾ oz	110	5	170	13	—
Garden Vegetable	5	60	2	125	10	—
Goldfish Cheddar Cheese	1 pkg (1½ oz)	190	6	340	28	1
Goldfish Cheddar Cheese	1 oz	120	4	230	19	1
Goldfish Cheese Thins	4	50	2	160	—	0
Goldfish Original	1 oz	130	5	190	18	1
Goldfish Parmesan Cheese	1 oz	120	4	330	19	1
Goldfish Pizza Flavored	1 oz	130	5	220	19	[illegible]
Goldfish Pretzel	1 oz	110	3	160	20	1
Hearty Wheat	4	100	5	140	13	1
Multi Grain	4	70	2	115	12	—
Sesame	4	80	4	140	12	2
Snack Mix Classic	1 oz	140	8	360	14	1
Snack Mix Lightly Smoked	1 oz	150	9	350	13	1
Snack Sticks Cheese	8	130	5	400	19	1
Snack Sticks Pretzel	8	120	3	430	23	1
Snack Sticks Pumpernickel	8	140	6	330	20	1
Snack Sticks Sesame	8	140	5	280	19	1
Spicy Lightly Smoked	1 oz	140	8	340	14	1

FOOD	PORTION	CAL.	FAT	SOD.	CARB.	FIB.
Pepperidge Farm (CONT.)						
Toasted Rice	4	60	2	140	10	—
Toasted Wheat With Onion	4	80	3	140	12	0
Planters						
Cheese Peanut Butter Sandwiches	1 pkg (1.4 oz)	190	10	390	24	1
Toast Peanut Butter Sandwiches	1 pkg (1.4 oz)	190	10	380	24	1
Premium						
Saltine Bits	34 (1 oz)	150	7	340	19	tr
Saltine Fat Free	5 (0.5 oz)	50	0	130	11	0
Saltine Low Sodium	5 (0.5 oz)	60	1	35	10	tr
Saltine Original	5 (0.5 oz)	60	2	180	10	tr
Saltine Unsalted Tops	5 (0.5 oz)	60	2	135	10	tr
Soup & Oyster	23 (0.5 oz)	60	2	230	11	tr
Ralston						
Oat Bran Krisp	2	60	3	140	6	3
Ritz						
Bits	48 (1 oz)	160	9	250	18	1
Bits Sandwiches With Peanut Butter	13 (1 oz)	150	8	130	17	1
Bits Sandwiches With Real Cheese	14 (1.1 oz)	160	10	300	17	1
Crackers	5 (0.5 oz)	80	4	135	10	tr
Low Sodium	5 (0.5 oz)	80	4	35	10	tr
Sandwiches With Real Cheese	1 pkg (1.4 oz)	210	12	450	21	1
Rykrisp						
Natural	2	40	0	75	7	4
Seasoned	2	45	1	105	8	3
Seasoned Twindividuals	2	45	1	105	8	3
Sesame	2	50	2	105	7	3
Ryvita						
Crisp Bread Dark Finn Crisp	2	38	tr	—	—	—
Crisp Bread Dark Rye	1	26	tr	—	—	—
Crisp Bread Dark w/ Caraway Seeds Finn Crisp	2	38	tr	—	—	—
Crisp Bread High Fiber	1	23	tr	—	—	—
Crisp Bread Light Rye	1	26	tr	—	—	—
Crisp Bread Toasted Sesame Rye	1	31	tr	—	—	—

FOOD	PORTION	CAL.	FAT	SOD.	CARB.	FIB.
Ryvita (CONT.)						
Snackbread High Fiber	1	14	tr	—	—	—
Snackbread Original Wheat	1	20	tr	—	—	—
Savory Thins						
Toasted Onion & Garlic	15 (1 oz)	110	1	90	23	2
Sesmark						
Brown Rice	15 (1 oz)	120	2	85	25	tr
Cheese Thins	15 (1 oz)	130	3	110	26	tr
Rice Thins Original	15 (1 oz)	130	3	150	24	tr
Rice Thins Teriyaki Flavored	13 (1 oz)	130	3	170	24	tr
Savory Thins Original	15 (1 oz)	125	2	125	25	1
Sesame Thins Cheddar	9 (1 oz)	150	8	400	15	3
Sesame Thins Garlic	9 (1 oz)	150	8	340	16	3
Sesame Thins Original	9 (1 oz)	150	8	380	16	2
Sesame Thins Unsalted	11 (1 oz)	150	8	1	17	3
SnackWell's						
Cracked Pepper	7 (0.5 oz)	60	0	150	13	tr
Fat Free Wheat	5 (0.5 oz)	60	0	170	12	1
Reduced Fat Cheese	38 (1 oz)	130	2	340	23	1
Reduced Fat Classic Golden	6 (0.5 oz)	60	1	140	11	0
Salsa Cheddar	32 (1 oz)	120	2	340	23	1
Snorkles						
Cheddar	56 (1 oz)	140	5	200	19	1
Sociables						
Crackers	7 (0.5 oz)	80	4	150	9	tr
Sunshine						
Saltines Cracked Pepper	5 (0.5 oz)	60	2	180	10	tr
Town House						
Crackers	2	35	2	60	4	—
Tree Of Life						
Bite Size Fat Free Corn & Salsa	12	60	0	90	12	0
Bite Size Fat Free Cracked Pepper	12	55	0	80	12	0
Bite Size Fat Free Garden Vegetable	12	55	0	80	12	0
Bite Size Fat Free Garlic & Herb	12	55	0	80	12	0
Bite Size Fat Free Soya Nut	12	60	0	80	12	0
Bite Size Fat Free Toasted Onion	12	60	0	80	12	0

FOOD	PORTION	CAL.	FAT	SOD.	CARB.	FIB.
Tree Of Life (CONT.)						
Bite Size Fat Free Whole Wheat	12	60	0	85	12	2
Fat Free Oyster	40 (0.5 oz)	60	0	130	13	0
Saltine Cracked Pepper Fat Free	4 (0.5 oz)	60	0	130	13	1
Saltine Fat Free	4 (0.5 oz)	50	0	140	11	0
Triscuit						
Crackers	7 (1.1 oz)	140	5	170	21	4
Deli-Style Rye	7 (1.1 oz)	140	5	180	22	4
Garden Herb	6 (1 oz)	130	5	120	20	3
Low Sodium	7 (1.1 oz)	150	6	50	21	3
Reduced Fat	8 (1.1 oz)	130	3	180	24	4
Wheat 'n Bran	7 (1.1 oz)	140	5	170	22	4
Tuscany						
Pita Crisps	1 oz	90	1	—	—	—
Pita Crisps Sesame	1 oz	96	2	—	—	—
Toast	1 oz	95	2	—	—	—
Toast Pepato	1 oz	93	2	—	—	—
Toast Pesto	1 oz	96	2	—	—	—
Toast Tomato	1 oz	95	2	—	—	—
Twigs						
Sesame & Cheese Sticks	15 (1 oz)	150	7	300	17	tr
Uneeda Biscuit						
Unsalted Tops	2 (0.5 oz)	60	2	110	11	tr
Venus						
Armenian Thin Bread	2 (0.9 oz)	100	1	165	19	—
Bran Wafers Salt Free	5 (0.5 oz)	60	1	0	11	2
Corn Crackers Salt Free	5 (0.5 oz)	60	1	0	10	2
Cracked Wheat Wafers Salt Free	5 (0.5 oz)	60	1	0	11	—
Cracker Bread	5 (0.5 oz)	60	1	90	11	—
Hors D'oeuvre	3 (0.5 oz)	60	2	20	11	—
Oat Bran Wafers	5 (0.5 oz)	60	1	105	11	2
Oat Bran Wafers Salt Free	5 (0.5 oz)	60	1	0	11	1
Old Brussels Cheddar Waferettes	5 (0.5 oz)	80	5	160	7	—
Old Brussels Jalapeno Waferettes	5 (0.5 oz)	80	5	160	7	1
Rye Wafers Low Salt	5 (0.5 oz)	60	1	110	11	—
Stoned Wheat Wafers Bite Size	7 (0.5 oz)	60	1	180	11	—
Water Crackers Fat Free	5 (0.5 oz)	55	0	70	11	—

FOOD	PORTION	CAL.	FAT	SOD.	CARB.	FIB.
Venus (CONT.)						
Wheat Wafers Low Salt	5 (0.5 oz)	60	2	110	10	1
Waldorf						
Sodium Free	2	30	1	0	5	—
Wasa						
Crisp	3 (0.5 oz)	50	0	100	11	2
Crisp'N Light Sourdough Rye	3 (0.6 oz)	60	0	120	12	1
Crisp'N Light Wheat	2 (0.5 oz)	50	0	100	10	1
Crispbread Cinnamon Toast	1 (0.6 oz)	60	1	65	11	1
Crispbread Fiber Rye	1 (0.4 oz)	30	1	60	4	2
Crispbread Gluten & Wheat Free Corn	1 (0.4 oz)	40	1	90	7	0
Crispbread Hearty Rye	1 (0.5 oz)	45	0	40	9	2
Crispbread Light Rye	1 (0.3 oz)	25	0	40	5	1
Crispbread Multi Grain	1 (0.5 oz)	45	0	85	8	2
Crispbread Organic Rye	1 (0.3 oz)	25	0	50	7	1
Crispbread Sodium Free Rye	1 (0.3 oz)	30	0	0	7	2
Crispbread Sourdough Rye	1 (0.4 oz)	35	0	55	7	1
Crispbread Toasted Wheat	1 (0.5 oz)	50	2	85	8	1
Crispbread Whole Wheat	1 (0.5 oz)	50	1	55	11	1
Waverly						
Crackers	5 (0.5 oz)	70	4	135	10	0
Wheat Thins						
Low Salt	16 (1 oz)	140	6	75	20	2
Multi-Grain	17 (1 oz)	130	4	290	21	2
Wheatworth						
Stone Ground	5 (0.5 oz)	80	4	170	10	1
Zesta						
Saltine	2	25	1	75	4	—
Saltine Unsalted Top	2	25	1	35	4	—
Zwieback						
Crackers	1 (8 g)	35	1	10	5	tr

CRANBERRIES

CANNED

FOOD	PORTION	CAL.	FAT	SOD.	CARB.	FIB.
cranberry sauce sweetened	½ cup	209	tr	40	54	—
Ocean Spray						
CranFruit Cranberry Orange Sauce	2 oz	100	0	10	23	—

FOOD	PORTION	CAL.	FAT	SOD.	CARB.	FIB.
Ocean Spray (CONT.)						
CranFruit Cranberry Raspberry Sauce	2 oz	100	0	10	23	—
CranFruit Cranberry Strawberry Sauce	2 oz	100	0	10	23	—
Cranberry Sauce Jellied	2 oz	90	0	10	22	—
Whole Berry Sauce	2 oz	90	0	10	23	—
S&W						
Cranberry Sauce Jellied Old Fashioned	½ cup	90	0	20	22	—
Cranberry Sauce Whole Berry Old Fashioned	½ cup	90	0	20	22	—
DRIED						
Ocean Spray						
Craisins	⅓ cup (1.4 oz)	130	0	0	33	2
FRESH						
chopped	1 cup	54	tr	1	14	—
Ocean Spray						
Fresh	½ cup	25	0	0	6	—

CRANBERRY BEANS

FOOD	PORTION	CAL.	FAT	SOD.	CARB.	FIB.
CANNED						
cranberry beans	1 cup	216	1	863	39	—
DRIED						
cooked	1 cup	240	1	1	43	—
Bean Cuisine						
Dried	½ cup	115	1	5	—	5

CRANBERRY JUICE

FOOD	PORTION	CAL.	FAT	SOD.	CARB.	FIB.
cocktail	1 cup	147	tr	10	38	—
cranberry juice cocktail	6 oz	108	tr	4	27	—
cranberry juice cocktail low calorie	6 oz	33	0	6	9	—
cranberry juice cocktail frzn	12 oz can	821	0	13	210	—
cranberry juice cocktail frzn as prep	6 oz	102	0	6	26	—
After The Fall						
Cape Cod Cranberry	1 bottle (10 oz)	130	0	25	30	—
Cranberry Ginger Ale	1 can (12 oz)	140	0	65	35	0
Apple & Eve						
Juice	6 fl oz	100	0	10	25	—
Crystal Light						
Cranberry Breeze Drink	1 serv (8 oz)	5	0	20	0	0
Cranberry Breeze Drink Mix as prep	1 serv (8 oz)	5	0	0	0	0

FOOD	PORTION	CAL.	FAT	SOD.	CARB.	FIB.
Everfresh						
Cranberry Cocktail	1 can (8 oz)	140	0	0	36	0
Ocean Spray						
Cocktail	8 fl oz	140	0	35	34	0
Cocktail Reduced Calorie	8 fl oz	50	0	35	13	0
Lightstyle Low Calorie Cranberry Juice Cocktail	8 fl oz	40	0	35	10	0
Seneca						
Cocktail frzn as prep	8 fl oz	140	0	0	36	0
Smucker's						
Juice Sparkler	10 oz	140	tr	5	34	—
Snapple						
Cranberry Royal	10 fl oz	150	0	25	37	—
Tree Of Life						
Concentrate	8 tsp (1.4 oz)	110	0	0	28	—
Tropicana						
Twister Ruby Red	1 bottle (10 fl oz)	150	0	30	37	—
Twister Ruby Red	8 fl oz	120	0	25	30	—
Veryfine						
Drink	8 oz	160	0	<10	40	—
CRAYFISH						
(*see also* LOBSTER)						
cooked	3 oz	97	1	58	0	—
raw	3 oz	76	1	45	0	—
raw	8	24	tr	14	0	—
CREAM						
(*see also* SOUR CREAM, SOUR CREAM SUBSTITUTES, WHIPPED TOPPINGS)						
LIQUID						
half & half	1 tbsp (0.5 oz)	20	2	6	1	—
half & half	1 cup (8.5 oz)	315	28	98	10	—
heavy whipping	1 tbsp (0.5 oz)	52	6	6	tr	—
light coffee	1 tbsp (0.5 oz)	29	3	6	1	—
light coffee	1 cup (8.4 oz)	496	46	95	9	—
light whipping	1 tbsp (0.5 oz)	44	5	5	tr	—
Farmland						
Half & Half	2 tbsp	40	3	15	2	0
Light Cream	2 tbsp	30	3	10	1	0
Hood						
Half & Half	2 tbsp (1 oz)	40	4	15	1	0
Heavy	1 tbsp (0.5 oz)	50	5	0	0	0
Light	1 tbsp (0.5 oz)	30	3	10	tr	0
Whipping Cream	1 tbsp (0.5 oz)	45	5	5	tr	0

FOOD	PORTION	CAL.	FAT	SOD.	CARB.	FIB.
Parmalat						
Half & Half	2 tbsp (1 oz)	40	3	20	2	0
WHIPPED						
heavy whipping	1 cup (4.1 oz)	411	44	89	7	—
light whipping	1 cup (4.2 oz)	345	37	82	7	—

CREAM CHEESE

FOOD	PORTION	CAL.	FAT	SOD.	CARB.	FIB.
cream cheese	1 oz	99	10	84	1	—
cream cheese	1 pkg (3 oz)	297	30	251	2	—
Alpine Lace						
Fat Free Garden Vegetable	2 tbsp (1 oz)	30	tr	165	1	0
Fat Free Garlic & Herbs	2 tbsp (1 oz)	30	tr	165	1	0
Breakstone's						
Temp-Tee Whipped	2 tbsp (0.8 oz)	80	8	70	tr	0
Fleur De Lait						
Bermuda Onion & Chives	2 tbsp (0.9 oz)	90	8	130	2	0
Cinnamon Raisin	2 tbsp (0.9 oz)	90	8	90	6	0
Date Nut Rum	2 tbsp (0.9 oz)	90	8	90	4	0
Fresh Cut Garden Vegetable	2 tbsp (0.9 oz)	80	8	200	1	0
Garden Vegetable	2 tbsp (0.9 oz)	80	8	200	1	0
Garlic & Spice	2 tbsp (0.9 oz)	90	9	160	1	0
Herb & Spice	2 tbsp (0.9 oz)	90	9	190	2	0
Irish Creme	2 tbsp (0.9 oz)	100	9	95	2	0
Lemon	2 tbsp (0.9 oz)	90	7	90	5	0
Lox	2 tbsp (0.9 oz)	90	8	125	1	0
Mandarin Orange	2 tbsp (0.9 oz)	90	7	90	3	0
Peach	2 tbsp (0.9 oz)	90	7	90	3	0
Pineapple	2 tbsp (0.9 oz)	90	8	95	3	0
Plain	2 tbsp (1 oz)	100	10	60	1	0
Strawberry	2 tbsp (0.9 oz)	90	8	90	3	0
Toasted Onion	2 tbsp (0.9 oz)	90	9	190	2	0
Wildberry	2 tbsp (0.9 oz)	90	7	90	4	0
Fresh Cut						
Bac'n & Horseradish	2 tbsp (0.9 oz)	90	9	135	1	0
Bermuda Onion & Chives	2 tbsp (0.9 oz)	90	8	130	2	0
Date Nut & Rum	2 tbsp (0.9 oz)	90	8	90	4	0
Garlic & Spice	2 tbsp (0.9 oz)	90	9	160	1	0
Herb & Spice	2 tbsp (0.9 oz)	90	9	190	2	0
Lox	2 tbsp (0.9 oz)	90	8	125	1	0
Peaches & Cream	2 tbsp (0.9 oz)	90	7	90	3	0

FOOD	PORTION	CAL.	FAT	SOD.	CARB.	FIB.
Fresh Cut (CONT.)						
Strawberry	2 tbsp (0.9 oz)	90	8	90	3	0
Friendship						
NY Style Reduced Fat	2 tbsp (1 oz)	50	3	120	0	0
Healthy Choice						
Herbs & Garlic	2 tbsp (1 oz)	25	0	200	2	—
Plain	2 tbsp (1 oz)	25	0	200	2	—
Strawberry	2 tbsp (1 oz)	30	0	200	5	—
Heluva Good Cheese						
Cream Cheese	1 tbsp (1 oz)	100	10	85	1	0
Philadelphia						
Free	1 oz	30	0	140	2	0
Regular	1 oz	100	10	90	tr	0
Soft	2 tbsp (1 oz)	100	10	100	1	0
Soft Apple Cinnamon	2 tbsp (1.1 oz)	100	8	100	5	0
Soft Chives & Onions	2 tbsp (1.1 oz)	110	10	135	2	0
Soft Pineapple	2 tbsp (1.1 oz)	100	9	100	4	0
Soft Salmon	3 tbsp (1.1 oz)	100	9	200	2	0
Soft Strawberry	2 tbsp (1.1 oz)	100	9	100	5	0
Soft Free	2 tbsp (1.2 oz)	30	0	200	2	0
Soft Free Garden Vegetable	2 tbsp (1.2 oz)	30	0	220	2	0
Soft Free Strawberries	2 tbsp (1.2 oz)	45	0	180	6	0
Soft Light	2 tbsp (1.1 oz)	70	5	150	2	0
Soft Light Jalapeno	2 tbsp (1.1 oz)	60	5	210	2	0
Soft Light Raspberry	2 tbsp (1.1 oz)	70	5	125	6	0
Soft Light Roasted Garlic	2 tbsp (1.1 oz)	70	5	180	2	0
Whipped	2 tbsp (0.7 oz)	70	7	85	tr	0
Whipped Chives	2 tbsp (0.7 oz)	70	6	130	tr	0
Whipped Smoked Salmon	2 tbsp (0.7 oz)	70	6	140	1	0
With Chives	1 oz	90	9	135	tr	0
Ultra Delight						
Cheddar Cream Cheese	2 tbsp (0.9 oz)	60	4	150	2	1
Chive	2 tbsp (0.9 oz)	60	4	130	2	1
Garlic	2 tbsp (0.9 oz)	60	4	130	2	1
Mixed Berry	2 tbsp (0.9 oz)	70	4	70	5	1
Nacho	2 tbsp (0.9 oz)	60	4	190	2	1
Salsa	2 tbsp (0.9 oz)	60	4	140	2	1
Shrimp	2 tbsp (0.9 oz)	60	4	130	2	1
Strawberry	2 tbsp (0.9 oz)	60	4	80	4	1
Vegetable	2 tbsp (0.9 oz)	50	4	150	2	1

FOOD	PORTION	CAL.	FAT	SOD.	CARB.	FIB.
Weight Watchers						
Light	2 tbsp	40	3	105	1	0
CREAM CHEESE SUBSTITUTES						
Tofutti						
Better Than Cream Cheese French Onion	1 oz	80	8	135	1	—
Better Than Cream Cheese Herb & Chive	1 oz	80	8	135	1	—
Better Than Cream Cheese Plain	1 oz	80	8	135	1	—
CREAM OF TARTAR						
cream of tartar	1 tsp	8	0	2	2	—
CREPES						
basic crepe unfilled	1	75	2	—	—	—
CRESS (*see also* WATERCRESS)						
garden cooked	½ cup	16	tr	5	3	—
garden raw	½ cup	8	tr	4	1	—
CROAKER						
atlantic breaded & fried	3 oz	188	11	296	6	—
atlantic raw	3 oz	89	3	47	0	—
CROISSANT						
apple	1 (2 oz)	145	5	156	21	1
cheese	1 (2 oz)	236	12	316	27	2
plain	1 (2 oz)	232	12	424	26	2
plain	1 mini (1 oz)	115	6	211	13	1
Pepperidge Farm						
Croissant Sandwich Quartet	1	170	7	250	22	tr
Petite All Butter	1	120	6	170	13	—
Rudy's Farm						
Ham & Swiss Sandwich	1 (3.4 oz)	310	18	830	27	1
Sara Lee						
All Butter	1	170	9	240	19	—
All Butter Petite Size	1	120	6	160	13	—
TAKE-OUT						
w/ egg & cheese	1	369	25	551	24	—
w/ egg cheese & bacon	1	413	28	889	24	—
w/ egg cheese & ham	1	475	34	1080	24	—
w/ egg cheese & sausage	1	524	38	1115	25	—

FOOD	PORTION	CAL.	FAT	SOD.	CARB.	FIB.
CROUTONS						
plain	1 cup (1 oz)	122	2	209	22	2
seasoned	1 cup (1.4 oz)	186	7	495	25	2
Arnold						
Crispy Cheddar Romano	½ oz	64	3	154	8	tr
Crispy Cheese Garlic	½ oz	60	2	130	9	tr
Crispy Fine Herbs	½ oz	50	1	150	10	1
Crispy Italian	½ oz	60	3	150	8	tr
Crispy Onion & Garlic	½	60	2	190	9	—
Crispy Seasoned	½ oz	60	3	160	8	—
Brownberry						
Ceasar Salad	½ oz	62	3	165	8	1
Cheddar Cheese	½ oz	63	3	155	8	tr
Onion & Garlic	½ oz	60	2	190	9	tr
Seasoned	½ oz	59	2	155	8	1
Toasted	½ oz	56	1	145	10	tr
Pepperidge Farm						
Cheddar & Romano Cheese	½ oz	60	2	200	10	—
Cheese & Garlic	½ oz	70	3	180	9	—
Onion & Garlic	½ oz	70	3	160	9	—
Seasoned	½ oz	70	3	180	9	—
Sour Cream & Chive	½ oz	70	3	170	9	—
CUCUMBER						
FRESH						
raw	1 (11 oz)	38	tr	6	8	3
raw sliced	½ cup (1.8 oz)	7	tr	1	1	1
JARRED						
Rosoff's						
Salad	3 slices (1 oz)	12	0	220	3	—
Schorr's						
Cucumber Garden Salad	3 slices (1 oz)	12	0	220	3	—
TAKE-OUT						
cucumber salad	3.5 oz	50	tr	480	11	—
CUMIN						
seed	1 tsp	8	tr	4	1	—
CURRANT JUICE						
black currant nectar	3½ oz	55	0	5	13	—
red currant nectar	3½ oz	54	tr	tr	13	—
CURRANTS						
black fresh	½ cup	36	tr	1	9	—
zante dried	½ cup	204	tr	6	53	—

FOOD	PORTION	CAL.	FAT	SOD.	CARB.	FIB.
CUSK						
fillet baked	3 oz	106	1	38	0	—
CUSTARD						
HOME RECIPE						
baked	1 recipe 4 serv (19.8 oz)	549	26	436	60	—
flan	1 recipe 10 serv (53.7 oz)	2206	63	864	349	—
MIX						
as prep w/ 2% milk	½ cup (4.7 oz)	148	4	200	24	—
as prep w/ 2% milk	1 recipe 4 serv (18.7 oz)	595	15	801	95	—
as prep w/ whole milk	1 recipe 4 serv (18.7 oz)	652	22	—	94	—
as prep w/ whole milk	½ cup (4.7 oz)	163	5	—	23	—
flan as prep w/ 2% milk	1 recipe 4 serv (18.7 oz)	542	9	265	102	—
flan as prep w/ 2% milk	½ cup (4.7 oz)	135	2	68	26	—
flan as prep w/ whole milk	½ cup (4.7 oz)	150	4	65	25	—
flan as prep w/ whole milk	1 recipe 4 serv (18.7 oz)	600	16	291	102	—
Jell-O						
Americana Custard Dessert as prep w/ 2% milk	½ cup (5 oz)	140	3	190	25	0
Flan as prep w/ 2% milk	½ cup (5.1 oz)	140	3	65	26	0
Royal						
Custard	mix for 1 serv	60	0	75	16	—
Flan Caramel Custard	mix for 1 serv	60	0	55	15	—
READY-TO-EAT						
Kozy Shack						
Flan	1 pkg (4 oz)	150	4	90	25	0
TAKE-OUT						
baked	½ cup (5 oz)	148	7	109	15	—
flan	½ cup (5.4 oz)	220	6	86	35	—
zabaione	½ cup (57.2 g)	135	5	9	13	0
CUTTLEFISH						
steamed	3 oz	134	1	632	1	—
DANDELION GREENS						
fresh cooked	½ cup	17	tr	23	3	—
raw chopped	½ cup	13	tr	21	3	—

FOOD	PORTION	CAL.	FAT	SOD.	CARB.	FIB.
DANISH PASTRY						
FROZEN						
Morton						
Honey Buns	1 (2.28 oz)	250	10	160	35	2
Honey Buns Mini	1 (1.23 oz)	160	8	100	19	tr
Pepperidge Farm						
Apple	1	220	8	130	35	—
Cheese	1	240	14	230	25	—
Cinnamon Raisin	1	250	11	170	35	—
Raspberry	1	220	9	140	31	—
Sara Lee						
Apple	1	120	6	120	15	—
Apple Danish Twist	1 slice (1.9 oz)	190	10	200	22	—
Apple Free & Light	1 slice (2 oz)	130	0	120	30	—
Cheese	1	130	8	130	13	—
Cheese Danish Twist	1 slice (1.9 oz)	200	12	270	21	—
Cinnamon Raisin	1	150	8	140	17	—
Raspberry Danish Twist	1 slice (1.9 oz)	200	9	220	25	—
READY-TO-EAT						
plain ring	1 (12 oz)	1305	71	1302	152	—
Hostess						
Apple	1 (3.8 oz)	400	22	340	47	2
Apple Fruit Roll	1 (2 oz)	180	4	170	33	1
Coffee Cake Raspberry	1 (1.2 oz)	110	3	110	21	tr
REFRIGERATED						
Pillsbury						
Caramel Danish w/ Nuts	1	160	8	240	19	—
Cinnamon Raisin Danish w/ Icing	1	150	7	230	20	—
Orange Danish w/ Icing	1	150	7	250	19	—
TAKE-OUT						
almond	1 (4¼ in) (2.3 oz)	280	16	236	30	2
apple	1 (4¼ in) (2.5 oz)	264	13	251	34	1
cheese	1 (3 oz)	353	25	320	29	—
cheese	1 (4¼ in) (2.5 oz)	266	16	319	26	—
cinnamon	1 (3 oz)	349	17	326	47	—
cinnamon	1 (4¼ in) (2.3 oz)	262	15	241	29	1
cinnamon nut	1 (4¼ in) (2.3 oz)	280	16	236	30	2
fruit	1 (3.3 oz)	335	16	333	45	—
lemon	1 (4¼ in) (2.5 oz)	264	13	251	34	1
raisin	1 (4¼ in) (2.5 oz)	264	13	251	34	1
raisin nut	1 (4¼ in) (2.3 oz)	280	16	236	30	2
raspberry	1 (4¼ in) (2.5 oz)	264	13	251	34	1
strawberry	1 (4¼ in) (2.5 oz)	264	13	251	34	1

FOOD	PORTION	CAL.	FAT	SOD.	CARB.	FIB.
DATES						
DRIED						
chopped	1 cup	489	1	5	131	—
deglet noor	10	240	0	—	—	—
whole	10	228	tr	2	61	—
Bordo						
Diced	2 oz	203	1	5	48	—
Dole						
Chopped	½ cup	230	0	5	56	—
Pitted	½ cup	280	0	0	62	—
Dromedary						
Chopped	¼ cup	130	0	0	31	—
Pitted	5	100	0	0	23	—
Sonoma						
Dried	5-6 (1.4 oz)	110	0	15	30	5
DEER						
(*see* VENISON)						
DELI MEATS/COLD CUTS						
(*see also* CHICKEN, HAM, MEAT SUBSTITUTES, TURKEY)						
barbecue loaf pork & beef	1 oz	49	3	378	2	—
beerwurst beef	1 slice (2¾ in x 1/16 in)	20	2	62	tr	—
beerwurst beef	1 slice (4 in x ⅛ in)	75	7	214	tr	—
beerwurst pork	1 slice (2¾in x 1/16 in)	14	1	74	tr	—
beerwurst pork	1 slice (4 in x ⅛ in)	55	4	285	tr	—
berliner pork & beef	1 oz	65	4	368	1	—
blood sausage	1 oz	95	9	—	tr	—
bologna beef	1 oz	88	8	278	tr	—
bologna beef & pork	1 oz	89	8	289	1	—
bologna pork	1 oz	70	6	336	tr	—
braunschweiger pork	1 oz	102	9	324	1	—
braunschweiger pork	1 slice (2½ in x ¼ in)	65	6	206	1	—
corned beef loaf	1 oz	43	2	270	0	—
dried beef	5 slices (21 g)	35	tr	—	tr	—
dried beef	1 oz	47	1	—	tr	—
dutch brand loaf pork & beef	1 oz	68	5	354	2	—
headcheese pork	1 oz	60	5	356	tr	—
honey loaf pork & beef	1 oz	36	1	374	2	—
honey roll sausage beef	1 oz	42	2	304	1	—
lebanon bologna beef	1 oz	60	4	379	1	—

FOOD	PORTION	CAL.	FAT	SOD.	CARB.	FIB.
liver cheese pork	1 oz	86	7	347	1	—
liverwurst pork	1 oz	92	8	—	1	—
luncheon meat beef	1 oz	87	7	377	1	—
luncheon meat pork & beef	1 oz	100	9	367	1	—
luncheon meat pork canned	1 oz	95	9	365	1	—
luncheon sausage pork & beef	1 oz	74	6	335	tr	—
luxury loaf pork	1 oz	40	1	347	1	—
mortadella beef & pork	1 oz	88	7	353	1	—
mother's loaf pork	1 oz	80	6	320	2	—
new england sausage pork & beef	1 oz	46	2	346	1	—
olive loaf pork	1 oz	67	5	421	3	—
peppered loaf pork & beef	1 oz	42	2	432	1	—
pepperoni pork & beef	1 slice (0.2 oz)	27	2	112	tr	—
pepperoni pork & beef	1 (9 oz)	1248	110	5120	7	—
pickle & pimiento loaf pork	1 oz	74	6	394	2	—
picnic loaf pork & beef	1 oz	66	5	330	1	–
salami cooked beef & pork	1 oz	71	6	302	1	—
salami hard pork	1 slice (⅓ oz)	41	4	226	3	—
salami hard pork	1 pkg (4 oz)	460	38	2554	2	—
salami hard pork & beef	1 slice (⅓ oz)	42	3	186	tr	—
salami hard pork & beef	1 pkg (4 oz)	472	39	2101	3	—
sandwich spread pork & beef	1 tbsp	35	3	152	2	—
sandwich spread pork & beef	1 oz	67	5	287	3	—
summer sausage thuringer cervelat	1 oz	98	8	412	1	—
Armour						
Beef Bologna Lower Salt	1 oz	90	8	—	—	—
Bologna Lower Salt	1 oz	90	8	—	—	—
Salami Lower Salt	1 oz	80	7	—	—	—
Carl Buddig						
Beef	1 oz	40	2	430	1	0
Corned Beef	1 oz	40	2	380	1	0
Pastrami	1 oz	40	2	320	1	0
DiLusso						
Genoa	1 oz	100	8	500	0	0
Hansel n'Gretel						
Healthy Deli Bologna Beef & Pork	1 oz	41	2	200	1	—
Healthy Deli Cooked Corn Beef	1 oz	35	1	210	1	—

FOOD	PORTION	CAL.	FAT	SOD.	CARB.	FIB.
Hansel n'Gretel (CONT.)						
Healthy Deli Italian Roast Beef	1 oz	31	1	140	tr	—
Healthy Deli Pastrami Round	1 oz	34	1	195	1	—
Healthy Deli Regular Roast Beef	1 oz	30	tr	130	tr	—
Healthy Deli St Paddy's Corned Beef	1 oz	24	tr	290	1	—
Healthy Choice						
Bologna	1 slice (1 oz)	30	1	290	1	0
Bologna Beef	1 slice (1 oz)	35	1	280	3	0
Deli-Thin Bologna	4 slices (1.8 oz)	60	2	560	3	0
Well-Pack Bologna	1 slice (1 oz)	30	1	290	1	0
Hebrew National						
Bologna Beef	2 oz	180	16	440	—	—
Bologna Beef Reduced Fat	2 oz	130	12	320	—	—
Bologna Lean Chub	2 oz	90	6	430	—	—
Bologna Midget	2 oz	180	16	440	—	—
Deli Pastrami	2 oz	80	3	510	—	—
Deli Express Corned Beef	2 oz	80	3	450	—	—
Deli Express Tongue Sliced	2 oz	120	9	330	—	—
Salami Beef	2 oz	170	14	420	—	—
Salami Beef Reduced Fat	2 oz	110	8	380	—	—
Salami Sean Chub	2 oz	90	6	340	—	—
Salami Midget	2 oz	170	14	420	—	—
Hillshire						
Bologna Large	1 oz	90	8	260	tr	—
Bologna Ring	1 oz	90	8	230	tr	—
Brunschweiger	1 oz	95	8	270	2	—
Deli Select Corned Beef	1 slice	10	tr	100	tr	—
Deli Select Light Bologna	1 slice	12	1	85	tr	—
Deli Select Oven Roasted Cured Beef	1 slice	10	tr	95	tr	—
Deli Select Pastrami	1 slice	10	tr	100	tr	—
Deli Select Roast Beef	1 slice	10	tr	135	tr	—
Deli Select Smoked Beef	1 slice	10	tr	100	tr	—
Flavor Pack 90-99% Fat Free Light Bologna	1 slice (0.73 oz)	30	2	190	1	—
Flavor Pack 90-99% Fat Free Pastrami	1 slice (0.6 oz)	18	tr	180	tr	—

FOOD	PORTION	CAL.	FAT	SOD.	CARB.	FIB.
Hillshire (CONT.)						
Lunch 'N Munch Bologna/ American/ Snickers	1 pkg (4.25 oz)	490	34	1110	31	—
Lunch 'N Munch Bologna/American/ Snickers/Hi-C	1 pkg (4.25 oz + 6 fl oz)	590	34	1130	55	—
Lunch 'N Munch Bologna/American	1 pkg (4.5 oz)	480	37	1390	20	—
Lunch 'N Munch Cotto Salami/Monterey Jack	1 pkg (4.5 oz)	440	32	1270	21	—
Lunch 'N Munch Pepperoni/ American	1 pkg (4.5 oz)	570	46	1670	20	—
Pepperoni	1 oz	110	10	450	0	—
Salami Hard	1 oz	100	9	450	0	—
Salami Hard	1 oz	90	7	470	1	—
Summer Sausage	2 oz	180	16	670	1	—
Summer Sausage Beef	2 oz	190	17	612	1	—
Summer Sausage Light	2 oz	150	12	630	1	—
Summer Sausage w/ Cheddar Cheese	2 oz	200	18	605	1	—
Homeland						
Hard Salami	1 oz	110	10	450	0	0
Hormel						
Liverwurst Spread	4 tbsp (2 oz)	130	10	650	2	0
Pepperoni Chunk	1 oz	140	13	470	0	0
Pepperoni Sliced	15 slices (1 oz)	140	13	470	0	0
Pepperoni Twin	1 oz	140	13	470	0	0
Pillow Pack Genoa Salami	4 slices (1.1 oz)	120	10	540	0	0
Pillow Pack Pepperoni	16 slices (1 oz)	140	13	470	0	0
Pillow Pack Pepperoni	1 oz	140	13	470	0	0
Jones						
Liver Sausage	1 slice	80	7	180	tr	—
Liver Sausage Chub	1 slice	80	7	230	tr	—
Jordan's						
Healthy Trim 95% Fat Free Macaroni & Cheese Loaf	2 slices (1.6 oz)	50	2	290	3	0
Healthy Trim 95% Fat Free Olive Loaf	2 slices (1.6 oz)	50	2	290	2	0
Healthy Trim 95% Fat Free Pickle & Pepper Loaf	2 slices (1.6 oz)	50	2	290	2	0

FOOD	PORTION	CAL.	FAT	SOD.	CARB.	FIB.
Jordan's (CONT.)						
Healthy Trim 97% Fat Free Corned Beef	2 slices (1.6 oz)	45	2	290	0	0
Healthy Trim Low Fat Cooked Salami	3 slices (2 oz)	70	3	360	2	0
Healthy Trim Low Fat German Brand Bologna	3 slices (2 oz)	70	3	360	3	0
Oscar Mayer						
Bologna Beef	1 slice (1 oz)	90	8	300	1	0
Bologna Garlic	1 slice (1.4 oz)	110	12	400	1	0
Bologna Light	1 slice (1 oz)	60	4	310	2	0
Bologna Light Beef	1 slice (1 oz)	60	4	310	2	0
Bologna Pork & Chicken & Beef	1 slice (1 oz)	90	8	270	0	0
Bologna Wisconsin Made Ring	2 oz	140	16	470	1	0
Braunschweiger	1 slice (1 oz)	100	9	320	1	0
Braunschweiger	2 oz	190	17	610	2	0
Braunschweiger German Brand	2 oz	200	18	650	1	0
Cotto Salami	2 slices (1.6 oz)	100	8	520	1	0
Cotto Salami Beef	2 slices (1.6 oz)	90	7	590	0	0
Free Bologna	2 slices (1.6 oz)	35	0	480	2	—
Genoa Salami	3 slices (1 oz)	100	9	490	0	0
Hard Salami	3 slices (1 oz)	100	9	510	0	0
Head Cheese	1 slice (1 oz)	50	4	360	0	0
Healthy Favorites Bologna	2 slices (1.6 oz)	45	1	510	2	0
Honey Loaf	1 slice (1 oz)	35	1	380	1	0
Liver Cheese	1 slice (1.3 oz)	120	10	420	1	0
Lunchables Bologna/American	1 pkg (4.5 oz)	450	34	1620	19	0
Lunchables Deluxe Turkey/Ham	1 pkg (5.1 oz)	360	19	1930	23	1
Lunchables Dessert Jello/Honey Turkey/Cheddar	1 pkg (5.7 oz)	320	16	1360	27	tr
Lunchables Fun Pack Bologna/Wild Cherry	1 pkg (11.2 oz)	530	29	1120	58	tr
Lunchables Fun Pack Ham/Fruit Punch	1 pkg (11.2 oz)	450	20	1260	53	tr
Lunchables Ham/Swiss	1 pkg (4.5 oz)	320	17	1770	19	0
Lunchables Pepperoni/American	1 pkg (4.5 oz)	480	36	1840	19	0

FOOD	PORTION	CAL.	FAT	SOD.	CARB.	FIB.
Oscar Mayer (CONT.)						
Lunchables Salami/ American	1 pkg (4.5 oz)	430	32	1740	18	0
Luncheon Loaf Spiced	1 slice (1 oz)	70	5	340	2	0
New England Brand Sausage	2 slices (1.6 oz)	60	3	570	1	0
Old Fashioned Loaf	1 slice (1 oz)	60	5	340	2	0
Olive Loaf	1 slice (1 oz)	70	5	370	2	0
Peppered Loaf	1 slice (1 oz)	39	2	367	1	—
Pickle And Pimiento Loaf	1 slice (1 oz)	70	6	360	2	0
Salami For Beer	1 slices (1.6 oz)	110	9	580	1	0
Salami Machaich Brand Beef	2 slices (1.6 oz)	120	10	510	1	0
Sandwich Spread	2 oz	140	10	530	9	0
Summer Sausage	2 slices (1.6 oz)	140	13	650	0	0
Summer Sausage Beef	2 slices (1.6 oz)	140	12	640	1	0
Russer						
Bologna	2 oz	180	15	540	3	—
Bologna Jalapeno Pepper	2 oz	170	14	600	3	—
Bologna Wunderbar German Brand	2 oz	190	16	600	5	—
Bologna Beef	2 oz	180	15	600	3	—
Bologna Garlic	2 oz	180	16	520	3	—
Bologna Italian Brand Sweet Red Pepper	2 oz	180	15	540	3	—
Braunschweiger	2 oz	170	14	600	3	—
Cooked Salami	2 oz	120	8	600	3	—
Dutch Brand	2 oz	130	8	600	6	—
Hot Cooked Salami	2 oz	110	7	600	3	—
Italian Brand Loaf	2 oz	130	8	600	5	—
Jalapeno Loaf With Monterey Jack Cheese	2 oz	160	13	650	4	—
Kielbasa Loaf	2 oz	120	8	600	5	—
Light Bologna	2 oz	120	8	400	3	—
Light Bologna Beef	2 oz	120	8	400	3	—
Light Braunschweiger	2 oz	120	8	400	3	—
Light Old Fashioned Loaf	2 oz	90	4	430	4	—
Light P&P Loaf	2 oz	100	6	430	4	—
Light Salami Cooked	2 oz	90	5	400	4	—
Olive Loaf	2 oz	160	13	600	4	—
P&P Loaf	2 oz	160	13	600	4	—
Pepper Loaf	2 oz	90	3	600	6	—
Polish Loaf	2 oz	140	10	600	7	—

FOOD	PORTION	CAL.	FAT	SOD.	CARB.	FIB.
Sara Lee						
Pastrami Beef	2 oz	100	6	540	1	1
Peppered Beef	2 oz	70	2	200	1	—
Shofar						
Salami Beef	2 oz	160	15	410	0	0
Spam						
Less Salt	2 oz	170	16	560	0	0
Lite	2 oz	110	8	560	0	0
Original	2 oz	170	16	750	0	0
Underwood						
Liverwurst	2.08 oz	180	15	470	4	—
Weight Watchers						
Bologna	2 slices (¾ oz)	35	2	220	1	—
TAKE-OUT						
corned beef	2 oz	70	2	390	0	—
corned beef brisket	2 oz	90	5	370	0	—

DIETING AIDS

(*see* NUTRITIONAL SUPPLEMENTS)

DILL

FOOD	PORTION	CAL.	FAT	SOD.	CARB.	FIB.
seed	1 tsp	6	tr	tr	1	—
sprigs fresh	5	0	tr	1	tr	—
sprigs fresh	1 cup	4	tr	5	1	—
weed dry	1 tsp	3	tr	2	1	—
Watkins						
Liquid Spice	1 tbsp (0.5 oz)	120	14	0	0	0

DINNER

(*see also* ASIAN FOOD, PASTA DISHES, POT PIES, SPANISH FOOD)

(FAST FACT: Frozen dinners have come a long way since they were introduced as TV dinners in 1954. In fact, the name TV dinner is no longer used on the package and the packaging now is microwaveable instead of the original sectioned aluminum tray.)

FOOD	PORTION	CAL.	FAT	SOD.	CARB.	FIB.
FROZEN						
Armour						
Classics Chicken Parmigiana	1 meal (10.75 oz)	360	18	1020	25	7
Classics Chicken & Noodles	1 meal (11 oz)	280	9	550	30	6
Classics Chicken Mesquite	1 meal (9.5 oz)	280	13	630	39	5
Classics Chicken w/ Wine & Mushroom	1 meal (10 oz)	260	11	540	20	4
Classics Glazed Chicken	1 meal (10.75 oz)	280	14	740	20	4

FOOD	PORTION	CAL.	FAT	SOD.	CARB.	FIB.
Armour (CONT.)						
Classics Meatloaf	1 meal (11.25 oz)	300	10	600	33	7
Classics Salisbury Steak	1 meal (11.25 oz)	330	18	1310	20	4
Classics Swedish Meatballs	1 meal (10 oz)	300	17	940	20	4
Classics Turkey and Dressing	1 meal (11.25 oz)	270	7	1020	34	5
Classics Veal Parmigiana	1 meal (11.25 oz)	400	22	1050	35	5
Classics Lite Beef Pepper	1 meal (11 oz)	210	4	870	29	5
Classics Lite Chicken Burgundy	1 meal (10 oz)	210	5	760	20	4
Classics Lite Salisbury Steak	1 meal (11.5 oz)	260	7	860	26	6
Classics Lite Shrimp Creole	1 meal (10 oz)	220	1	720	49	16
Classics Lite Sweet & Sour Chicken	1 meal (11 oz)	220	1	520	38	4
Banquet						
BBQ Style Chicken	1 meal (9 oz)	320	12	800	36	3
Beef	1 meal (9 oz)	240	7	660	19	12
Chicken Parmigiana	1 pkg (9.5 oz)	290	15	900	27	3
Chicken & Dumplings	1 meal (10 oz)	260	8	780	35	16
Chicken Fried Steak	1 pkg (10 oz)	400	20	1180	39	4
Chicken Nuggets	1 pkg (6.75 oz)	410	21	650	38	11
Extra Helping All White Chicken	1 meal (18 oz)	820	41	1890	72	8
Extra Helping Chicken Parmigiana	1 meal (19 oz)	650	33	1770	64	9
Extra Helping Chicken Fried Steak	1 meal (18.5 oz)	800	44	2050	73	6
Extra Helping Fried Chicken	1 meal (18 oz)	790	39	1820	72	8
Extra Helping Meatloaf	1 meal (19 oz)	650	38	2140	49	10
Extra Helping Mexican Style	1 meal (22 oz)	820	34	2060	100	20
Extra Helping Salisbury Steak	1 meal (19 oz)	740	46	1860	52	11
Extra Helping Southern Fried Chicken	1 meal (17.5 oz)	750	37	2140	67	9
Extra Helping Turkey Dinner	1 meal (18.8 oz)	560	20	1910	63	7
Family Entree Beef Stew	1 serv (8.13 oz)	160	4	1120	17	4
Family Entree Chicken Parmigiana	1 serv (4.67 oz)	240	13	690	18	2

FOOD	PORTION	CAL.	FAT	SOD.	CARB.	FIB.
Banquet (CONT.)						
Family Entree Chicken & Dumplings	1 serv (7.47 oz)	290	14	1270	30	2
Family Entree Gravy & Sliced Turkey	1 serv (4.8 oz)	100	5	590	5	tr
Family Entree Gravy w/ Charbroiled Beef	1 serv (4.67 oz)	180	13	640	7	2
Family Entree Onion Gravy w/ Beef	1 serv (4.67 oz)	180	14	630	7	2
Family Entree Salisbury Steak	1 serv (4.67 oz)	200	14	610	7	2
Family Entree Veal Parmigiana	1 serv (4.67 oz)	230	14	740	19	2
Family Entrees Dumplings & Chicken	7 oz	280	14	—	28	—
Family Entrees Gravy & Sliced Beef	1 serv (5.6 oz)	100	3	850	7	tr
Family Entrees Gravy & Sliced Turkey	6 oz	120	6	—	6	—
Fried Chicken	1 meal (9 oz)	470	27	980	35	6
Gravy w/ Beef Patty	1 pkg (9.5 oz)	300	20	1060	21	2
Hot Sandwich Toppers Chicken Ala King	1 pkg (4.5 oz)	100	4	480	7	1
Hot Sandwich Toppers Creamed Chipped Beef	1 pkg (4 oz)	100	3	700	8	0
Hot Sandwich Toppers Gravy & Sliced Beef	1 pkg (4 oz)	70	2	440	5	tr
Hot Sandwich Toppers Gravy & Sliced Turkey	1 pkg (5 oz)	90	4	670	7	tr
Hot Sandwich Toppers Salisbury Steak	1 pkg (5 oz)	220	16	790	8	2
Hot Sandwich Toppers Sloppy Joe	1 meal (4 oz)	140	7	530	12	1
Meatloaf	1 meal (9.5 oz)	280	17	1100	23	2
Mexican Style Combo Meal	1 pkg (11 oz)	380	11	1370	55	9
Mexican Style Meal	1 pkg (11 oz)	340	13	1520	56	10
Oriental Style Chicken	1 pkg (9 oz)	260	9	610	34	4
Salisbury Steak	1 meal (9.5 oz)	310	16	910	28	2
Southern Fried Chicken Meal	1 pkg (8.75 oz)	260	30	1610	44	4
Turkey	1 meal (9.25 oz)	270	10	1100	31	3
Veal Parmagiana	1 pkg (9 oz)	530	14	960	35	7

FOOD	PORTION	CAL.	FAT	SOD.	CARB.	FIB.
Banquet (CONT.)						
Western Style Meal	1 meal (9.5 oz)	210	20	1400	28	5
White Meat Chicken Meal	1 pkg (8.75 oz)	470	28	1100	33	2
Birds Eye						
Easy Recipe Beef Burgundy not prep	½ pkg	120	5	670	17	4
Easy Recipe Beef Fajitas not prep	½ pkg	80	3	390	14	3
Budget Gourmet						
Beef Cantonese	1 meal (9.1 oz)	270	9	880	31	—
Beef Stroganoff	1 meal (8.75 oz)	260	10	840	27	—
Chicken And Egg Noodles	1 meal (10 oz)	440	26	880	28	—
Chicken Au Gratin	1 meal (9.1 oz)	230	8	820	23	—
Chicken Breast Parmigiana	1 pkg (11 oz)	270	9	530	30	—
Chicken Marsala	1 meal (9 oz)	260	8	730	31	—
Chicken With Fettucini	1 meal (10 oz)	400	21	700	29	—
Chinese Style Vegetables & Chicken	1 meal (10 oz)	280	7	590	47	—
French Recipe Chicken	1 meal (10 oz)	220	9	870	21	—
Glazed Turkey	1 meal (9 oz)	260	5	710	38	—
Ham & Asparagus Au Gratin	1 meal (8.7 oz)	300	14	860	26	—
Herbed Chicken Breast With Fettucini	1 pkg (11 oz)	240	6	430	30	—
Italian Style Vegetables & Chicken	1 meal (10.25 oz)	310	8	690	50	—
Mandarin Chicken	1 meal (10 oz)	240	5	710	38	—
Mesquite Chicken Breast	1 pkg (11 oz)	250	6	550	33	—
Orange Glazed Chicken	1 meal (9 oz)	270	3	870	46	—
Oriental Beef	1 meal (10 oz)	290	8	840	36	—
Oriental Chicken With Vegetables	1 meal (9 oz)	280	6	690	44	—
Pepper Steak With Rice	1 meal (10 oz)	300	8	720	40	—
Pot Roast Beef	1 meal (10.5 oz)	230	7	510	19	—
Roast Chicken With Homestyle Gravy	1 meal (11 oz)	280	8	560	36	—
Roast Sirloin Supreme	1 meal (9 oz)	320	15	630	28	—
Sirloin Salisbury Steak	1 meal (11 oz)	280	9	530	30	—
Sirloin Salisbury Steak	1 meal (9 oz)	220	8	730	24	—
Sirloin Cheddar Melt	1 meal (9.4 oz)	380	21	950	29	—
Sirloin Of Beef In Herb Sauce	1 meal (9.5 oz)	250	9	860	21	—

FOOD	PORTION	CAL.	FAT	SOD.	CARB.	FIB.
Budget Gourmet (CONT.)						
Sirloin Of Beef In Wine Sauce	1 pkg (11 oz)	280	8	560	36	—
Sirloin Tips And Country Vegetables	1 meal (10 oz)	290	17	810	19	—
Special Recipe Sirloin Of Beef	1 meal (11 oz)	250	9	560	29	—
Stuffed Turkey Breast	1 pkg (11 oz)	250	6	570	31	—
Swedish Meatballs With Noodles	1 meal (10 oz)	590	38	920	37	—
Sweet And Sour Chicken	1 meal (10 oz)	340	5	620	55	—
Teriyaki Beef	1 pkg (10.75 oz)	260	7	530	37	—
Teriyaki Chicken Breast	1 meal (11 oz)	300	8	480	41	—
Healthy Choice						
Beef & Peppers Cantonese	1 meal (11.5 oz)	270	5	560	40	5
Beef Pepper Steak Oriental	1 meal (9.5 oz)	250	4	470	34	3
Beef Tips Francais	1 meal (9.5 oz)	280	5	520	40	4
Beef Tips With Sauce	1 meal (11 oz)	290	6	270	40	5
Chicken Cantonese	1 meal (11.25)	210	1	360	31	5
Chicken Parmigiana	1 meal (11.5 oz)	300	2	490	47	6
Chicken & Vegetables Marsala	1 meal (11.5 oz)	220	1	440	32	3
Chicken Bangkok	1 meal (9.5 oz)	270	4	390	35	5
Chicken Dijon	1 meal (11 oz)	280	4	410	41	9
Chicken Imperial	1 meal (9 oz)	230	4	470	31	3
Chicken Picante	1 meal (11.25 oz)	220	2	330	30	6
Chicken Teriyaki	1 meal (12.25 oz)	270	2	420	42	5
Classics Beef Broccoli Beijing	1 meal (12 oz)	330	3	500	55	5
Classics Cacciatore Chicken	1 meal (12.5 oz)	260	3	510	36	6
Classics Chicken Fransesca	1 meal (12.5 oz)	360	5	500	51	5
Classics Country Inn Roast Turkey	1 meal (10 oz)	250	4	530	29	6
Classics Ginger Chicken Hunan	1 meal (12.6 oz)	350	3	430	59	5
Classics Mesquite Beef Barbecue	1 meal (11 oz)	310	4	490	45	6
Classics Salisbury Steak	1 meal (11 oz)	260	6	500	32	5
Classics Sesame Chicken Shanghai	1 meal (12 oz)	310	5	460	42	5

FOOD	PORTION	CAL.	FAT	SOD.	CARB.	FIB.
Healthy Choice (CONT.)						
Classics Shrimp & Vegetables Maria	1 meal (12.5 oz)	260	2	540	46	5
Country Glazed Chicken	1 meal (8.5 oz)	200	2	480	30	3
Country Herb Chicken	1 meal (11.5 oz)	270	4	340	40	6
Country Roast Turkey With Mushroom	1 meal (8.5 oz)	220	4	440	28	3
Country Turkey & Pasta	1 meal (12.6 oz)	300	4	450	42	6
Homestyle Turkey With Vegetables	1 meal (9.5 oz)	260	2	490	34	3
Honey Mustard Chicken	1 meal (9.5 oz)	260	2	550	40	4
Lemon Pepper Fish	1 meal (10.7 oz)	290	5	360	47	7
Mandarin Chicken	1 meal (10 oz)	280	3	520	44	4
Mesquite Chicken Barbecue	1 meal (10.5 oz)	320	2	290	55	6
Shrimp Marinara	1 meal (10.5 oz)	220	1	220	44	5
Smoky Chicken Barbecue	1 meal (12.75 oz)	380	5	450	57	7
Southwestern Glazed Chicken	1 meal (12.5 oz)	300	3	430	48	6
Sweet & Sour Chicken	1 meal (11.5 oz)	310	5	250	42	5
Traditional Breast Of Turkey	1 meal (10.5 oz)	280	3	460	40	7
Traditional Meat Loaf	1 meal (12 oz)	320	8	460	46	7
Traditional Beef Tips	1 meal (11.25 oz)	260	5	390	32	6
Tradtional Salisbury Steak	1 meal (11.5 oz)	320	6	470	48	7
Yankee Pot Roast	1 meal (11 oz)	280	5	460	38	5
Kid Cuisine						
Chicken Sandwich	1 pkg (9.43 oz)	480	15	770	71	4
Chicken Nuggets	1 pkg (9.1 oz)	440	16	1070	54	5
Fish Sticks	1 pkg (8.25 oz)	370	12	550	55	4
Fried Chicken	1 pkg (10.1 oz)	440	19	940	49	5
Hot Dogs w/ Buns	6.7 oz	450	19	880	57	—
Macaroni & Beef	1 pkg (9.6 oz)	370	9	900	58	5
Le Menu						
Beef Sirloin Tips	11½ oz	400	18	760	29	—
Beef Stroganoff	10 oz	430	24	980	28	—
Chicken Parmigiana	11¾ oz	410	20	1030	31	—
Chicken A La King	10¼ oz	330	13	830	29	—
Chicken Cordon Bleu	11 oz	460	20	850	47	—
Chicken In Wine Sauce	10 oz	280	7	680	27	—
Chopped Sirloin Beef	12¼ oz	430	24	1010	28	—
Entree LightStyle Chicken A La King	8¼ oz	240	5	670	29	—

FOOD	PORTION	CAL.	FAT	SOD.	CARB.	FIB.
Le Menu (CONT.)						
Entree LightStyle Chicken Dijon	8 oz	240	7	500	21	—
Entree LightStyle Empress Chicken	8¼ oz	210	5	690	26	—
Entree LightStyle Glazed Turkey	8¼ oz	260	6	720	34	—
Entree LightStyle Herb Roast Chicken	7¾ oz	260	6	500	29	—
Entree LightStyle Swedish Meatballs	8 oz	260	8	700	30	—
Entree LightStyle Traditional Turkey	8 oz	200	5	610	19	—
Ham Steak	10 oz	300	11	1500	31	—
LightStyle Glazed Chicken Breast	10 oz	230	3	480	25	—
LightStyle Herb Roasted Chicken	10 oz	240	7	400	18	—
LightStyle Salisbury Steak	10 oz	280	9	400	31	—
LightStyle Sliced Turkey	10 oz	210	5	540	21	—
LightStyle Sweet & Sour Chicken	10 oz	250	7	530	29	—
LightStyle Turkey Divan	10 oz	260	7	420	23	—
LightStyle Veal Marsala	10 oz	230	3	700	28	—
Pepper Steak	11½ oz	370	13	1020	36	—
Salisbury Steak	10½ oz	370	20	880	28	—
Sliced Breast Of Turkey w/ Mushroom Gravy	10½ oz	300	7	1020	38	—
Sweet & Sour Chicken	11¼ oz	400	18	1020	41	—
Veal Parmigiana	11½ oz	390	17	840	36	—
Yankee Pot Roast	10 oz	330	13	700	27	—
Lean Cuisine						
American Favorite Baked Chicken	1 pkg (8.6 oz)	230	4	520	31	5
American Favorite Baked Fish	1 pkg (9 oz)	270	6	540	36	3
American Favorite Beef Pot Roast	1 pkg (9 oz)	210	6	570	25	6
American Favorite Beef Tips Barbecue	1 pkg (8.75 oz)	290	6	560	47	7
American Favorite Chicken Medallions w/ Creamy Cheese	1 pkg (9.37 oz)	260	8	590	31	4

FOOD	PORTION	CAL.	FAT	SOD.	CARB.	FIB.
Lean Cuisine (CONT.)						
American Favorite Country Vegetables & Beef	1 pkg (9 oz)	210	4	590	33	3
American Favorite Honey Roasted Chicken	1 pkg (8.5 oz)	290	6	590	46	5
American Favorite Meatloaf & Whipped Potatoes	1 pkg (9.4 oz)	250	6	590	30	4
American Favorite Oven Roasted Beef	1 pkg (9.25 oz)	260	8	590	28	4
American Favorite Roasted Turkey Breast	1 pkg (9.75 oz)	270	3	590	49	5
American Favorite Salisbury Steak	1 pkg (9.5 oz)	280	8	590	29	4
American Favorite Scalloped Potatoes w/ Turkey Ham	1 pkg (10 oz)	250	6	590	38	6
Cafe Classics Chicken Carbonara	1 pkg (9 oz)	280	8	580	33	2
Cafe Classics Chicken Mediterranean	1 pkg (10.5 oz)	270	4	590	40	2
Cafe Classics Chicken Breast In Wine Sauce	1 pkg (8.1 oz)	210	6	560	23	2
Cafe Classics Chicken Parmesan	1 meal (10.9 oz)	220	5	560	27	4
Cafe Classics Chicken Piccata	1 pkg (9 oz)	270	6	530	41	2
Cafe Classics Chicken w/ Basil Cream Sauce	1 pkg (8.5 oz)	270	7	580	35	3
Cafe Classics Glazed Turkey	1 pkg (9 oz)	240	5	590	37	5
Cafe Classics Grilled Chicken Salsa	1 pkg (8.9 oz)	270	7	570	36	4
Cafe Classics Herb Roasted Chicken	1 pkg (8 oz)	210	5	540	27	3
Cafe Classics Honey Mustard Chicken	1 pkg (8 oz)	250	5	520	39	3
Cafe Classics Mesquite Beef w/ Rice	1 pkg (9 oz)	290	6	510	42	5
Cafe Classics Sirloin Beef Peppercorn	1 pkg (8.75 oz)	220	7	580	23	2
Chicken & Vegetables	1 pkg (10.5 oz)	250	6	590	31	4
Chicken A L'Orange	1 pkg (9 oz)	250	2	340	40	3

FOOD	PORTION	CAL.	FAT	SOD.	CARB.	FIB.
Lean Cuisine (CONT.)						
Chicken In Peanut Sauce	1 pkg (9 oz)	290	6	550	35	4
Fiesta Chicken w/ Rice & Vegetables	1 pkg (8.5 oz)	250	5	540	34	3
Glazed Chicken w/ Vegetable Rice	1 pkg (8.5 oz)	240	6	480	25	0
Homestyle Turkey	1 pkg (9.4 oz)	230	5	590	30	3
Mandarin Chicken	1 pkg (9 oz)	250	4	590	38	3
Oriental Beef	1 pkg (9.25 oz)	220	5	590	33	2
Stuffed Cabbage w/ Whipped Potatoes	1 pkg (9.5 oz)	170	5	380	24	5
Swedish Meatballs w/ Pasta	1 pkg (9.1 oz)	280	7	590	33	3
Life Choice						
Garden Potato Casserole	1 meal (13.4 oz)	160	1	590	37	9
Morton						
Breaded Chicken Pattie	1 meal (6.75 oz)	280	15	840	24	4
Chicken Nugget	1 meal (7 oz)	320	17	460	30	3
Fried Chicken	1 meal (9 oz)	420	25	1000	30	4
Meatloaf	1 meal (9 oz)	250	13	1110	24	5
Mexican	1 meal (10 oz)	260	7	1000	40	8
Salisbury Steak	1 meal (9 oz)	210	9	950	23	3
Turkey	1 meal (9 oz)	230	8	1090	27	5
Veal Parmagiana	1 meal (8.75 oz)	280	13	950	30	4
Western	1 meal (9 oz)	290	16	1210	26	6
Patio						
Chili	1 cup (8 oz)	260	13	1010	13	4
Ranchera	1 pkg (13 oz)	410	15	2400	14	14
Stouffer's						
Baked Chicken Breast w/ Mashed Potatoes	1 serv (12.2 oz)	330	14	1070	25	3
Beef Stroganoff	1 pkg (9.75 oz)	390	20	1100	30	2
Chicken A La King	1 pkg (9.5 oz)	350	13	800	41	2
Chicken Divan	1 pkg (8 oz)	210	10	570	10	1
Creamed Chicken	1 pkg (6.5 oz)	280	20	720	8	1
Creamed Chipped Beef	½ cup (4.5 oz)	150	11	690	6	1
Escalloped Chicken & Noodles	1 pkg (10 oz)	440	29	880	28	2
Green Pepper Steak	1 pkg (10.5 oz)	330	9	650	45	3
Homestyle Chicken Parmigiana	1 pkg (10.9 oz)	320	10	890	30	4
Homestyle Chicken Monterey	1 pkg (9.4 oz)	410	20	700	35	4

FOOD	PORTION	CAL.	FAT	SOD.	CARB.	FIB.
Stouffer's (CONT.)						
Homestyle Fish Filet With Macaroni & Cheese	1 pkg (9 oz)	430	21	930	37	2
Homestyle Fried Chicken	1 pkg (7.1 oz)	330	16	780	29	3
Homestyle Meatloaf	1 pkg (9.9 oz)	380	24	910	24	3
Homestyle Roast Turkey	1 pkg (7.9 oz)	280	11	950	25	1
Homestyle Salisbury Steak	1 pkg (9.6 oz)	370	19	1220	26	—
Homestyle Sliced Beef & Potatoes	1 pkg (8.1 oz)	270	10	900	25	2
Homestyle Veal Parmigiana	1 pkg (11.9 oz)	420	19	1200	43	6
Honestyle Baked Chicken	1 pkg (8.9 oz)	270	12	750	19	2
Lunch Express Mandarin Chicken	1 pkg (9.75 oz)	270	6	520	41	2
Lunch Express Mexican Style Rice With Chicken	1 pkg (9 oz)	270	8	390	39	3
Lunch Express Stir-Fry Rice & Chicken	1 pkg (9 oz)	280	9	590	39	3
Stuffed Pepper	1 pkg (10 oz)	200	8	900	24	1
Swedish Meatballs	1 pkg (9.25 oz)	440	23	840	36	3
Swanson						
Beans & Franks	10½ oz	440	19	900	53	—
Beef	11¼ oz	310	6	770	38	—
Beef In Barbecue Sauce	11 oz	460	17	860	51	—
Chicken Duet Gourmet Nuggets Pizza Style	3 oz	210	12	—	—	—
Chopped Sirloin Beef	10¾ oz	340	16	790	28	—
Fish 'n' Chips	10 oz	500	21	960	60	—
Fried Chicken Dark Meat	9¾ oz	560	28	1130	55	—
Fried Chicken White Meat	10¼ oz	550	25	1460	60	—
Homestyle Chicken Cacciatore	10.95 oz	260	8	1030	33	—
Homestyle Chicken Nibbles	4¼ oz	340	20	730	29	—
Homestyle Fish & Fries	6½ oz	340	16	670	37	—
Homestyle Fried Chicken	7 oz	390	21	1100	33	—
Homestyle Salisbury Steak	10 oz	320	16	980	22	—
Homestyle Scalloped Potatoes & Ham	9 oz	300	13	1080	26	—

FOOD	PORTION	CAL.	FAT	SOD.	CARB.	FIB.
Swanson (CONT.)						
Homestyle Seafood Creole With Rice	9 oz	240	6	810	40	—
Homestyle Sirloin Tips In Burgundy Sauce	7 oz	160	5	550	16	—
Homestyle Turkey With Dressing & Potatoes	9 oz	290	11	1010	30	—
Homestyle Veal Parmigiana	10 oz	330	13	960	33	—
Hungry-Man Boneless Chicken	17¾ oz	700	28	1530	65	—
Hungry-Man Chopped Beef Steak	16¾ oz	640	37	1600	41	—
Hungry-Man Fried Chicken Dark Meat	14¼ oz	860	45	1660	77	—
Hungry-Man Fried Chicken White Meat	14¼ oz	870	46	2150	80	—
Hungry-Man Salisbury Steak	16½ oz	680	41	1730	37	—
Hungry-Man Sliced Beef	15¼ oz	450	12	1060	49	—
Hungry-Man Turkey	17 oz	550	18	1810	61	—
Hungry-Man Veal Parmigiana	18¼ oz	590	26	1840	57	—
Loin Of Pork	10¾ oz	280	12	790	27	—
Macaroni & Beef	12 oz	370	15	930	48	—
Meatloaf	10¾ oz	360	15	960	41	—
Noodles & Chicken	10½ oz	280	8	740	45	—
Salisbury Steak	10¾ oz	400	17	880	43	—
Swedish Meatballs	8½ oz	360	20	790	26	—
Swiss Steak	10 oz	350	11	700	37	—
Turkey	8¾ oz	270	11	—	—	—
Turkey	11½ oz	350	11	1090	42	—
Veal Parmigiana	12¼ oz	430	20	1010	42	—
Western Style	11½ oz	430	19	1060	43	—
Tyson						
Beef Champignon	1 pkg (10.5 oz)	370	15	830	31	—
Chicken Picante	1 pkg (9 oz)	250	4	390	26	—
Chicken Supreme	1 pkg (9 oz)	230	6	480	23	—
Francais	1 pkg (9.5 oz)	280	14	1130	20	—
Glazed Chicken With Sauce	1 pkg (9.25 oz)	240	4	930	29	—
Grilled Chicken	1 pkg (7.75 oz)	220	3	520	22	—
Grilled Italian Chicken	1 pkg (9 oz)	210	3	420	19	—
Healthy Portions BBQ Chicken	1 pkg (12.5 oz)	400	8	600	56	—

FOOD	PORTION	CAL.	FAT	SOD.	CARB.	FIB.
Tyson (CONT.)						
Healthy Portions Chicken Marinara	1 pkg (13.75 oz)	340	7	590	37	—
Healthy Portions Herb Chicken	1 pkg (13.75 oz)	340	4	550	43	—
Healthy Portions Honey Mustard Chicken	1 pkg (13.75 oz)	390	6	520	52	—
Healthy Portions Italian Style Chicken	1 pkg (13.75 oz)	310	4	600	38	—
Healthy Portions Mesquite Chicken	1 pkg (13.25 oz)	330	5	600	38	—
Healthy Portions Salsa Chicken	1 pkg (13.75 oz)	370	6	470	52	—
Healthy Portions Sesame Chicken	1 pkg (13.5 oz)	400	6	400	59	—
Honey Roasted Chicken	1 pkg (9 oz)	220	4	500	23	—
Kiev	1 pkg (9.25 oz)	450	25	950	39	—
Marsala	1 pkg (9 oz)	200	4	670	19	—
Mexquite	1 pkg (9 oz)	320	8	660	39	—
Picatta	1 pkg (9 oz)	200	4	550	18	—
Roasted Chicken	1 pkg (9 oz)	200	2	430	21	—
Sweet & Sour	1 pkg (11 oz)	420	15	850	50	—
Turkey With Gravy	1 pkg (9.5 oz)	320	12	900	34	—
Ultra Slim-Fast						
Beef Pepper Steak	12 oz	270	4	590	36	0
Chicken Fettucini	12 oz	380	12	980	38	1
Chicken & Vegetable	12 oz	290	3	850	45	4
Country Style Vegetable & Beef Tips	12 oz	230	5	960	26	4
Mesquite Chicken	12 oz	360	1	300	61	5
Roasted Chicken In Mushroom Sauce	12 oz	280	6	830	30	0
Shrimp Creole	12 oz	240	4	730	45	5
Shrimp Marinara	12 oz	290	3	880	53	0
Sweet & Sour Chicken	12 oz	330	2	340	57	0
Turkey Medallions In Herb Sauce	12 oz	280	6	950	33	0
Weight Watchers						
Smart One Grilled Salisbury Steak	1 pkg (8.5 oz)	260	10	620	24	3
Smart Ones Fiesta Chicken	1 pkg (8.5 oz)	220	2	540	38	5
Smart Ones Honey Mustard Chicken	1 pkg (8.5 oz)	200	2	370	37	3

FOOD	PORTION	CAL.	FAT	SOD.	CARB.	FIB.
Weight Watchers (CONT.)						
Smart Ones Lemon Herb Chicken Piccata	1 pkg (8.5 oz)	200	2	460	34	3
Smart Ones Pepper Steak	1 pkg (10 oz)	240	5	690	33	4
Smart Ones Risotto w/ Cheese & Mushrooms	1 pkg (10 oz)	290	8	540	44	4
Smart Ones Roast Turkey Medallions & Mushrooms	1 pkg (8.5 oz)	190	2	530	32	2
Smart Ones Shrimp Marinara	1 pkg (9 oz)	190	2	470	35	4
Smart Ones Stuffed Turkey Breast	1 pkg (10 oz)	260	7	680	37	5
Smart Ones Swedish Meatballs	1 pkg (9 oz)	300	10	510	33	2
SHELF-STABLE						
My Own Meal						
Beef Stew	1 pkg (10 oz)	260	11	480	22	4
Chicken Mediterranean	1 pkg (10 oz)	270	9	320	28	4
Chicken Noodles	1 pkg (10 oz)	270	8	900	29	3
Chicken & Black Beans	1 pkg (10 oz)	240	5	460	30	6
Old World Stew	1 pkg (10 oz)	310	12	510	31	3
DIP						
Breakstone's						
Bacon & Onion	2 tbsp (1.1 oz)	60	5	180	2	0
Chesapeake Clam	2 tbsp (1.1 oz)	50	4	180	1	0
Free Creamy Salsa	2 tbsp (1.1 oz)	20	0	240	3	0
Free French Onion	2 tbsp (1.1 oz)	25	0	260	4	0
Free Ranch	2 tbsp (1.1 oz)	25	0	330	4	0
French Onion	2 tbsp (1.1 oz)	50	5	160	2	0
Cheez Whiz						
Medium Cheese & Salsa	2 tbsp (1.2 oz)	100	8	490	3	0
Mild Cheese & Salsa	2 tbsp (1.2 oz)	100	8	490	3	0
Chi-Chi's						
Fiesta Bean	2 tbsp (0.9 oz)	35	2	140	4	1
Fiesta Cheese	2 tbsp (0.9 oz)	40	3	270	3	0
Durkee						
Sour Cream as prep	2 tbsp	25	1	200	4	0
Frito Lay						
Picante Sauce	1 oz	10	0	160	3	—
Guiltless Gourmet						
Black Bean Mild	1 oz	25	0	80	5	1

FOOD	PORTION	CAL.	FAT	SOD.	CARB.	FIB.
Guiltless Gourmet (CONT.)						
Black Bean Spicy	1 oz	25	0	80	5	1
Pinto Bean	1 oz	25	0	80	5	1
Hain						
Hot Bean	4 tbsp	70	1	250	10	—
Mexican Bean	4 tbsp	60	1	260	9	—
Onion Bean	4 tbsp	70	1	270	10	—
Taco Dip & Sauce	4 tbsp	25	1	350	1	—
Heluva Good Cheese						
Bacon Horseradish	2 tbsp (1.1 oz)	60	5	200	2	0
Clam	2 tbsp (1.1 oz)	50	5	130	2	0
French Onion	2 tbsp (1.1 oz)	50	5	160	2	0
Homestyle Onion	2 tbsp (1.1 oz)	60	5	290	3	0
Light French Onion	2 tbsp (1.1 oz)	35	2	180	3	0
Light Jalapeno Cheddar	2 tbsp (1.1 oz)	40	2	160	3	0
Ranch	2 tbsp (1.1 oz)	60	5	180	2	0
Knudsen						
Free Creamy Salsa	2 tbsp (1.1 oz)	20	0	240	3	0
Free French Onion	2 tbsp (1.1 oz)	25	0	260	4	0
Free Ranch	2 tbsp (1.1 oz)	25	0	330	4	0
Kraft						
Avocado	2 tbsp (1.1 oz)	60	4	240	4	0
Bacon & Horseradish	2 tbsp (1.1 oz)	60	5	220	3	0
Clam	2 tbsp (1.1 oz)	60	4	250	3	0
Free French Onion	2 tbsp (1.1 oz)	25	0	260	4	0
Free Ranch	2 tbsp (1.1 oz)	25	0	330	4	0
Free Salsa	2 tbsp (1.1 oz)	20	0	240	3	0
French Onion	2 tbsp (1.1 oz)	60	4	230	4	0
Green Onion	2 tbsp (1.1 oz)	60	4	190	4	0
Jalapeno Cheese	2 tbsp (1.1 oz)	60	4	260	3	0
Premium Sour Cream	2 tbsp (1.1 oz)	50	4	180	1	0
Premium Sour Cream Bacon & Horseradish	2 tbsp (1.1 oz)	60	5	240	2	0
Premium Sour Cream Bacon & Onion	2 tbsp (1.1 oz)	60	5	180	2	0
Premium Sour Cream Creamy Onion	2 tbsp (1.1 oz)	45	4	160	2	0
Premium Sour Cream French Onion	2 tbsp (1.1 oz)	45	4	160	2	0
Premium Sour Cream Ranch	2 tbsp (1.1 oz)	50	4	230	2	0
Ranch	2 tbsp (1.1 oz)	60	5	210	3	0
Lay's						
Low Fat Sour Cream & Onion	2 tbsp (1 oz)	40	1	230	6	tr

FOOD	PORTION	CAL.	FAT	SOD.	CARB.	FIB.
Louise's						
Fat Free Honey Mustard	1 oz	40	0	170	9	0
Fat Free Sour Cream & Onion	1 oz	25	0	195	4	0
Fat Free White Cheese Peppercorn	1 oz	25	0	195	4	0
Marzetti						
Blue Cheese Veggie	2 tbsp	200	21	230	1	0
Lemon Dill Veggie	2 tbsp	140	14	190	2	0
Light Ranch Veggie	2 tbsp	60	7	290	5	1
Ranch Veggie	2 tbsp	140	14	200	1	0
Sour Cream & Onion	2 tbsp	130	14	200	2	0
Southwestern Veggie	2 tbsp	130	14	170	1	0
Spinach Veggie	2 tbsp	130	13	220	1	0
Old El Paso						
Black Bean	2 tbsp (1 oz)	20	0	150	4	1
Cheese 'n Salsa Medium	2 tbsp (1 oz)	40	3	300	3	0
Cheese 'n Salsa Mild	2 tbsp (1 oz)	40	3	300	3	0
Chunky Salsa Medium	2 tbsp (1 oz)	15	0	230	3	1
Chunky Salsa Mild	2 tbsp (1 oz)	15	0	230	3	1
Jalapeno	2 tbsp (1 oz)	30	1	125	4	2
Ruffles						
Low Fat French Onion	1 tbsp (1 oz)	40	1	230	6	tr
Snyder's						
Mustard Pretzel	2 tbsp (1.2 oz)	90	4	20	13	1
Taco Bell						
Fat Free Black Bean	2 tbsp (1.2 oz)	30	0	220	6	2
Salsa Con Queso Medium	2 tbsp (1.2 oz)	45	3	270	5	tr
Salsa Con Queso Mild	2 tbsp (1.2 oz)	45	3	270	5	tr
Tostitos						
Low Fat Con Queso	2 tbsp (1 oz)	40	2	180	5	tr
Wise						
Jalapeno Bean	2 tbsp	25	0	100	5	—
Taco	2 tbsp	12	0	115	3	—
DOCK						
fresh cooked	3½ oz	20	1	3	3	—
raw chopped	½ cup	15	tr	3	2	—
DOGFISH						
raw	3½ oz	193	15	14	0	—
DOLPHINFISH						
fresh baked	3 oz	93	1	96	0	—
fresh fillet baked	5.6 oz	174	1	179	0	—

FOOD	PORTION	CAL.	FAT	SOD.	CARB.	FIB.
DOUGHNUTS						
cake type unsugared	1 (1.6 oz)	198	11	257	23	1
chocolate glazed	1 (1.5 oz)	175	8	143	24	1
chocolate sugared	1 (1.5 oz)	175	8	143	24	1
chocolate coated	1 (1.5 oz)	204	13	185	21	1
creme filled	1 (3 oz)	307	21	262	26	—
french cruller glazed	1 (1.4 oz)	169	8	142	24	—
frosted	1 (1.5 oz)	204	13	185	21	1
honey bun	1 (2.1 oz)	242	14	205	27	1
jelly	1 (3 oz)	289	16	249	33	—
old fashioned	1 (1.6 oz)	198	11	257	23	1
sugared	1 (1.6 oz)	192	10	181	23	1
wheat glazed	1 (1.6 oz)	162	9	160	19	—
wheat sugared	1 (1.6 oz)	162	9	160	19	—
yeast glazed	1 (2.1 oz)	242	14	205	27	1
Drake's						
Old Fashion Donuts	1 (1.7 oz)	182	8	238	25	—
Powdered Sugar Donut Delites	7 (2.5 oz)	300	15	316	38	—
Dutch Mill						
Cider	1 (2.1 oz)	240	10	220	35	1
Cinnamon	1 (1.8 oz)	210	11	250	26	1
Donut Holes Double-Dipped Chocolate	3 (1.4 oz)	220	16	140	19	0
Donut Holes Shootin' Stars	3 (1.4 oz)	190	10	110	23	0
Double-Dipped Chocolate	1 (2.1 oz)	280	17	360	31	1
Glazed	1 (2.1 oz)	250	12	220	34	1
Glazed Chocolate	1 (2.4 oz)	270	11	380	40	1
Plain	1 (1.8 oz)	210	12	270	25	1
Sugared	1 (1.8 oz)	220	11	260	27	1
Entenmann's						
Crumb Topped	1 (2.1 oz)	260	12	220	34	—
Devil's Food Crumb	1 (2.1 oz)	250	12	200	34	—
Rich Frosted	1 (2 oz)	280	18	210	27	—
Freihofer's						
Assorted	1 (2 oz)	270	17	170	26	0
Hostess						
Assorted Regular	1 (1.6 oz)	200	11	230	23	tr
Cinnamon Family Pack	1 (1 oz)	110	5	140	15	tr
Cinnamon Swirl	1 (1.6 oz)	180	7	220	28	tr
Crumb Regular	1 (1 oz)	130	8	115	14	tr

FOOD	PORTION	CAL.	FAT	SOD.	CARB.	FIB.
Hostess (CONT.)						
Frosted Regular	1 (1.4 oz)	180	11	170	20	1
Gem Donettes Cinnamon	6 (3 oz)	320	11	390	53	1
Gem Donettes Frosted	6 (3 oz)	390	23	360	42	2
Gem Donettes Frosted Strawberry Filled	3 (3 oz)	240	13	210	29	1
Gem Donettes Powdered	6 (3 oz)	350	16	380	47	1
Gem Donettes Powdered Strawberry Filled	3 (3 oz)	210	9	210	31	tr
Glazed Party	1 (2.3 oz)	260	10	310	39	1
Jumbo Frosted	1 (2 oz)	260	16	240	28	1
Jumbo Plain	1 (1.1 oz)	140	7	190	16	tr
Jumbo Powdered	1 (1.3 oz)	160	9	170	19	tr
Mini Chocolate	5 (2 oz)	220	9	220	33	1
O's Raspberry Filled Powdered	1 (2.2 oz)	230	10	230	35	tr
Old Fashioned Glazed	1 (2.1 oz)	250	12	230	33	tr
Old Fashioned Glazed Honey Wheat	1 (2.1 oz)	250	12	270	33	1
Old Fashioned Plain	1 (1.5 oz)	170	9	230	21	tr
Plain Regular	1 (1 oz)	120	6	160	13	tr
Powdered Family Pack	1 (1 oz)	110	6	135	15	1
Little Debbie						
Donut Sticks	1 pkg (1.6 oz)	210	13	210	25	1
Donut Sticks	1 pkg (3 oz)	390	23	370	45	1
Donut Sticks	1 pkg (2.5 oz)	320	19	310	37	1
Donut Sticks	1 pkg (2 oz)	250	15	250	30	1
Tastykake						
Cinnamon	1 (47 g)	180	8	210	26	1
Frosted Rich	1 (57 g)	260	16	200	28	3
Frosted Rich Mini	1 (14 g)	44	3	60	8	1
Honey Wheat	1 (57 g)	210	8	200	32	1
Honey Wheat Mini	1 (12 g)	40	1	50	7	0
Orange Glazed	1 (57 g)	210	9	180	32	1
Plain	1 (47 g)	190	10	170	22	1
Powdered Sugar	1 (46 g)	180	9	220	24	1
Powdered Sugar Mini	1 (12 g)	40	1	70	7	0

DRESSING

(*see* STUFFING/DRESSING)

DRINK MIXERS

(*see also* SODA, MINERAL/BOTTLED WATER)

whiskey sour mix	2 oz	55	0	66	14	—
whiskey sour mix as prep	3.6 oz	169	0	48	16	—

FOOD	PORTION	CAL.	FAT	SOD.	CARB.	FIB.
Bacardi						
Margarita Mix w/ rum	8 fl oz	160	0	0	24	—
Margarita Mix w/o liquor	8 fl oz	100	0	0	25	—
Pina Colada	8 fl oz	140	0	10	34	—
Rum Runner	8 fl oz	140	0	10	35	—
Strawberry Daiquiri w/o liquor	8 fl oz	140	0	0	35	—
Canada Dry						
Collins Mixer	8 fl oz	120	0	20	25	0
Sour Mixer	8 fl oz	90	0	25	22	0
Libby						
Bloody Mary Mix	6 oz	40	0	1120	8	—
McIlhenny						
Tabasco Bloody Mary Mix	8 fl oz	56	tr	1548	11	1
Schweppes						
Collins Mixer	8 fl oz	100	0	55	24	0
Tabasco						
Bloody Mary Mix Extra Spicy	8 fl oz	58	tr	1645	11	2
DRUM						
freshwater fillet baked	5.4 oz	236	10	148	0	—
freshwater baked	3 oz	130	5	82	0	—
DUCK						
w/ skin roasted	1 cup (4.9 oz)	472	40	83	0	0
w/ skin w/ bone leg roasted	3 oz	184	10	94	0	—
w/ skin w/o bone breast roasted	3 oz	172	9	71	0	—
w/o skin roasted	1 cup (4.9 oz)	281	16	91	0	0
w/o skin w/ bone leg braised	1 cup (6.1 oz)	310	10	188	0	—
w/o skin w/o bone breast broiled	1 cup (6.1 oz)	244	4	183	0	—
wild w/ skin raw	½ duck (9.5 oz)	571	41	152	0	—
wild w/o skin breast raw	½ breast (2.9 oz)	102	4	47	0	—
DUMPLING						
FROZEN						
Pepperidge Farm						
Apple Dumpling	1 (3 oz)	260	13	230	33	—
DURIAN						
fresh	3½ oz	141	2	1	29	—

FOOD	PORTION	CAL.	FAT	SOD.	CARB.	FIB.
EEL						
fresh cooked	1 fillet (5.6 oz)	375	24	104	0	—
fresh cooked	3 oz	200	13	55	0	—
raw	3 oz	156	10	43	0	—
smoked	3.5 oz	330	28	—	0	0
EGG						
(*see also* EGG DISHES, EGG SUBSTITUTES)						
CHICKEN						
frozen	1 cup	363	24	307	3	—
frozen	1	75	5	63	1	—
hard cooked	1	77	5	62	1	—
hard cooked chopped	1 cup	210	14	169	2	—
poached	1	74	5	140	1	—
raw	1	75	5	63	1	—
scrambled plain	2	200	15	211	2	—
scrambled w/ whole milk & margarine	1 cup	365	27	616	5	—
white only	1 cup	121	0	399	2	—
white only	1	17	0	55	tr	—
EggsPlus						
Fresh	1 (1.8 oz)	70	5	65	0	0
OTHER POULTRY						
duck raw	1 (2.5 oz)	130	10	102	1	0
goose raw	1 (5 oz)	267	19	—	2	—
quail raw	1 (9 g)	14	1	—	tr	—
turkey raw	1 (2.7 oz)	135	9	—	1	—
EGG DISHES						
FROZEN						
Chefwich						
Cheese Omelet	5 oz	380	17	—	—	—
Ham & Cheese Omelet	5 oz	340	14	—	—	—
Sausage & Cheese Omelet	5 oz	400	19	—	—	—
Western Style Omelet	5 oz	350	13	—	—	—
Downyflake						
Scrambled Eggs With Ham & Hash Browns	1 pkg (6.25 oz)	360	26	730	17	—
Scrambled Eggs With Ham & Pecan Twirl	1 pkg (6.25 oz)	470	28	670	40	—
Scrambled Eggs With Hash Browns & Sausage	1 pkg (6.25 oz)	420	34	790	17	—
Scrambled Eggs With Sausage & Pecan Twirl	1 pkg (6.25 oz)	510	33	710	39	—

FOOD	PORTION	CAL.	FAT	SOD.	CARB.	FIB.
Great Starts						
Egg Sausage & Cheese	5½ oz	460	28	1310	35	—
Omelets With Cheese & Ham	7 oz	390	29	1220	15	—
Reduced Cholesterol Eggs With Mini Oatbran Muffins	4¾ oz	250	12	400	27	—
Scrambled Eggs & Bacon With Home Fries	5.6 oz	340	26	690	16	—
Scrambled Eggs & Home Fries	4.6 oz	260	19	380	14	—
Scrambled Eggs & Sausage With Hash Browns	6½ oz	430	34	760	19	—
Scrambled Eggs With Cheese & Cinnamon Pancakes	3.4 oz	290	23	380	14	—
Quaker						
Scrambled Eggs & Sausage With Hash Browns	1 pkg (5.7 oz)	290	20	810	14	—
Scrambled Eggs & Sausage With Pancakes	1 pkg (5.2 oz)	270	14	880	21	—
Scrambled Eggs Cheddar Cheese & Fried Potatoes	1 pkg (5.9 oz)	250	13	910	22	—
Weight Watchers						
Handy Ham & Cheese Omelet	1 (4 oz)	220	5	440	30	2
TAKE-OUT						
deviled	2 halves	145	13	180	1	—
salad	½ cup	307	28	565	2	—
sandwich w/ cheese	1	340	19	804	26	—
sandwich w/ cheese & ham	1	348	16	1005	31	—
scotch egg	1 (4.2 oz)	301	21	—	16	2
scrambled	2 eggs	202	14	342	2	—
sunny side up	1	91	7	162	1	—

EGG ROLLS

(*see also* ASIAN FOODS)

FOOD	PORTION	CAL.	FAT	SOD.	CARB.	FIB.
egg roll wrapper fresh	1	83	tr	162	16	—
Chun King						
Chicken	8 (4.4 oz)	270	9	350	40	4

FOOD	PORTION	CAL.	FAT	SOD.	CARB.	FIB.
Chun King (CONT.)						
Pork & Shrimp	8 (4.4 oz)	290	11	350	39	4
Shrimp	8 (4.4 oz)	260	8	480	39	4
Empire						
Large	1 (3 oz)	190	6	350	28	2
Miniature	6 (4.8 oz)	280	8	740	43	4
La Choy						
Almond Chicken Restaurant Style	1 (3 oz)	170	6	390	23	3
Chicken Mini	14 (7.25 oz)	430	11	900	67	6
Chicken Restaurant Style	1 (3 oz)	170	5	450	25	4
Lobster Mini	14 (7.25 oz)	410	11	690	65	9
Meat & Shrimp Mini	15 (3.75 oz)	240	9	350	31	3
Mu Sho Pork Restaurant Style	1 (3 oz)	190	7	330	25	2
Pork Restaurant Style	1 (3 oz)	150	5	480	20	—
Pork & Shrimp Mini	14 (7.25 oz)	430	12	890	65	7
Shrimp Mini	14 (7.25 oz)	410	9	990	68	7
Shrimp Restaurant Style	1 (3 oz)	150	4	420	24	3
Sweet & Sour Restaurant Style	1 (3 oz)	180	4	300	29	3
Lean Cuisine						
Vegetable	1 pkg (9 oz)	340	6	590	64	3
Lo-An						
White Meat Chicken	1 (2.7 oz)	140	4r	400	20	1
Luigino's						
Chicken	1 pkg (6 oz)	360	13	590	48	2
Pork & Shrimp	1 pkg (6 oz)	340	9	760	51	3
Shrimp	1 pkg (6 oz)	350	11	460	39	4
Sweet & Sour Chicken	1 pkg (6 oz)	400	12	460	59	4
Sweet & Sour Pork	1 pkg (6 oz)	360	10	270	56	4
Szechwan Vegetable	1 pkg (6 oz)	350	12	920	38	3
Worthington						
Vegetarian Egg Rolls	1 (85 g)	160	6	530	20	—
TAKE-OUT						
lobster	1 (4.8 oz)	270	7	460	43	6
meat & shrimp	1 (4.8 oz)	320	12	470	41	4
pork & shrimp	1 (5 oz)	300	10	890	41	7
shrimp	1 (3 oz)	170	5	420	24	5
spicy pork	1 (3 oz)	200	9	410	23	3
vegetable	1 (3 oz)	170	4	520	28	4

EGG SUBSTITUTES

frozen	¼ cup	96	7	120	2	—

FOOD	PORTION	CAL.	FAT	SOD.	CARB.	FIB.
frozen	1 cup	384	27	479	8	—
liquid	1½ oz	40	2	83	tr	—
liquid	1 cup (8.8 oz)	211	8	444	2	—
powder	0.7 oz	88	3	158	4	—
powder	0.35 oz	44	1	79	2	—
Egg Beaters						
Eggs Substitute	¼ cup	25	0	80	1	0
Omelette Cheese	½ cup	110	5	480	2	—
Omelette Vegetable	½ cup	50	0	170	5	—
Egg Watchers						
Egg Substitute	2 oz	50	2	100	2	—
Healthy Choice						
Cholesterol Free	¼ cup (2 oz)	25	0	95	tr	0
LaLoma						
Scramblers Links Muffins	1 pkg (4 oz)	220	10	400	22	—
Morningstar Farms						
Better'n Eggs	¼ cup (57 g)	30	0	100	1	—
Scramblers	¼ cup (57 g)	60	3	125	3	—
Scramblers Cheese Home Fries	1 pkg (5 oz)	210	9	310	20	—
Scramblers Links Hash Browns	1 pkg (5 oz)	240	13	580	20	—
Scramblers Sandwich w/ Cheese	1 (3.5 oz)	220	7	420	29	—
Scramblers Sandwich w/ Pattie	1 (4.5 oz)	300	12	590	29	—
Scramblers Sandwich w/ Pattie Cheese	1 (5 oz)	350	15	780	33	—
Second Nature						
No Cholesterol	2 fl oz	60	2	90	3	—
No Fat	2 fl oz	40	0	100	3	—
No Fat With Garden Vegetables	2.5 fl oz	40	0	100	4	—
Simply Eggs						
Egg Substitute	1.75 fl oz	35	1	130	1	1
EGGNOG						
eggnog	1 cup	342	19	138	34	—
eggnog	1 qt	1368	76	553	138	—
eggnog flavor mix as prep w/ milk	9 oz	260	8	163	39	—
Borden						
Eggnog	4 fl oz	160	9	80	16	—

FOOD	PORTION	CAL.	FAT	SOD.	CARB.	FIB.
Borden (CONT.)						
Light	½ cup	130	2	80	23	—
Hood						
Fat Free	4 fl oz	100	0	100	21	0
Golden	4 fl oz	180	8	100	22	0
Light	4 fl oz	120	2	105	23	0
Select	4 fl oz	210	12	100	22	0
EGGPLANT						
CANNED						
Progresso						
Appetizer	2 tbsp (1 oz)	30	2	130	2	2
FRESH						
cubed cooked	½ cup	13	tr	2	3	—
raw cut up	½ cup (1.4 oz)	11	tr	1	2	—
slices cooked	4 (7 oz)	38	0	—	0	—
whole peeled raw	1 (1 lb)	117	1	14	28	—
FROZEN						
Mrs. Paul's						
Parmigiana	5 oz	240	16	600	18	—
TAKE-OUT						
baba ghannouj	¼ cup	55	4	95	5	—
caponata	2 tbsp (1 oz)	30	2	115	3	—
ELDERBERRIES						
fresh	1 cup	105	1	—	27	—
ELDERBERRY JUICE						
elderberry	3½ oz	38	0	1	8	—
ELK						
roasted	3 oz	124	2	52	0	—
ENDIVE						
fresh	3½ oz	9	tr	53	tr	2
raw chopped	½ cup	4	tr	6	1	—

ENERGY BARS

(*see* BREAKFAST BARS, CEREAL BARS, GRANOLA BARS, NUTRITIONAL SUPPLEMENTS)

FOOD	PORTION	CAL.	FAT	SOD.	CARB.	FIB.
ENGLISH MUFFIN						
FROZEN						
Great Starts						
Egg Beefsteak & Cheese	5.9 oz	360	20	730	27	—
Egg Canadian Bacon & Cheese	4.1 oz	290	15	770	25	—

FOOD	PORTION	CAL.	FAT	SOD.	CARB.	FIB.
Weight Watchers						
Sandwich	1 (4 oz)	210	5	420	28	2
HOME RECIPE						
cinnamon raisin	1	186	3	123	38	—
english muffin	1	158	2	122	30	—
honey bran	1	153	3	154	30	—
whole wheat	1	167	tr	135	34	—
READY-TO-EAT						
apple cinnamon	1	138	2	255	28	—
granola	1	155	1	275	31	—
mixed grain	1	155	1	275	31	—
plain	1	134	1	265	26	—
plain toasted	1	133	1	262	26	—
raisin cinnamon	1	138	2	255	28	—
sourdough	1	134	1	265	26	—
wheat	1	127	1	218	26	—
whole wheat	1	134	1	420	27	4
Arnold						
Extra Crisp	l	130	1	230	26	1
Sourdough	1	130	1	250	25	1
Matthew's						
9 Grain & Nut	1	140	4	220	26	5
Cinnamon Raisin	1	160	2	290	33	4
Golden White	1	140	4	340	23	1
Whole Wheat	1	150	2	340	31	4
Pepperidge Farm						
Cinnamon Apple	1	140	1	210	27	—
Cinnamon Chip	1	160	3	180	28	—
Cinnamon Raisin	1	150	2	200	29	—
Plain	1	140	1	220	27	—
Sourdough	1	135	1	260	27	—
Roman Meal						
Engish Muffin	1 (2.2 oz)	135	1	332	25	3
Tastykake						
Cinnamon Raisin	1 (64 g)	150	1	150	31	—
English Muffin	1 (57 g)	130	1	240	26	—
Sourdough	1 (57 g)	130	1	210	25	—
Thomas'						
Honey Wheat	1	128	1	199	24	—
Oat Bran	1	116	1	192	26	3
Raisin Cinnamon	1	151	1	183	31	—
Regular	1	130	1	206	25	—
Sandwich Size	1 (92 g)	210	2	330	42	2
Sour Dough	1	131	1	210	25	—

FOOD	PORTION	CAL.	FAT	SOD.	CARB.	FIB.
Wonder						
English Muffin	1 (2 oz)	120	1	290	25	1
Raisin Rounds	1 (2.1 oz)	150	2	240	30	2
Sourdough	1 (2 oz)	120	1	290	25	1
REFRIGERATED						
Roman Meal						
English Muffin	½ muffin (1.1 oz)	66	tr	95	14	1
Honey Nut Oat Bran	½ muffin (1.1 oz)	81	1	114	16	1
TAKE-OUT						
w/ butter	1	189	6	386	30	—
w/ cheese & sausage	1	394	24	1036	29	—
w/ egg cheese & bacon	1	487	31	1135	31	—
w/ egg cheese & canadian bacon	1	383	20	785	31	—

EPPAW

raw	½ cup	75	1	6	16	—

FALAFEL

MIX						
Casbah						
as prep	5	130	3	530	20	2
TAKE-OUT						
falafel	3 (1.8 oz)	170	9	150	16	—
falafel	1 (1.2 oz)	57	3	50	5	—

FAT

(*see also* BUTTER, BUTTER BLENDS, BUTTER SUBSTITUTES, MARGARINE, OIL)

beef cooked	1 oz	193	20	12	0	—
beef suet	1 oz	242	27	—	0	—
beef tallow	1 tbsp (13 g)	115	13	0	0	—
chicken	1 cup	1846	205	—	0	—
chicken	1 tbsp	115	13	—	0	—
cocoa butter	1 tbsp	120	14	—	0	—
duck	1 tbsp (13 g)	115	13	0	0	0
goose	1 tbsp	115	13	—	0	—
goose	3.5 oz	900	100	—	0	—
lamb new zealand raw	1 oz	182	19	6	0	—
lard	1 cup (205 g)	1849	205	tr	0	—
lard	1 tbsp (13 g)	115	13	0	0	—
nutmeg butter	1 tbsp	120	14	—	0	—
pork backfat	1 oz	230	25	—	—	—
pork cooked	1 oz	200	21	9	0	—
pork cured	1 oz	164	17	—	—	—

FOOD	PORTION	CAL.	FAT	SOD.	CARB.	FIB.
pork cured roasted	1 oz	167	18	—	—	—
salt pork	1 oz	212	23	404	0	—
shortening	1 cup	1812	205	—	0	—
shortening	1 tbsp	113	13	—	0	—
turkey	1 tbsp	115	13	—	0	—
ucuhuba butter	1 tbsp	120	14	—	0	—
Crisco						
Butter Flavor	1 tbsp	110	12	0	0	—
Shortening	1 tbsp	110	12	0	0	—
Shortening	1 tbsp (0.4 oz)	110	12	0	0	—
Sticks	1 tbsp (0.4 oz)	110	12	0	0	0
Sticks Butter Flavor	1 tbsp (0.4 oz)	110	12	0	0	0
Empire						
Chicken Fat Rendered	1 tbsp (0.5 oz)	120	13	0	tr	0
Wesson						
Shortening	1 tbsp	100	12	0	0	0
FAT SUBSTITUTES						
Soy Is Us						
Fat Not! Organic	3 tbsp	66	1	3	7	4
FAVA BEANS						
Progresso						
Fava Beans	½ cup (4.6 oz)	110	1	250	20	5
FEIJOA						
fresh	1 (1.75 oz)	25	tr	2	5	—
puree	1 cup	119	2	7	26	—
FENNEL						
fresh bulb	1 (8.2 oz)	72	tr	122	17	—
fresh sliced	1 cup	27	tr	45	6	—
leaves	3.5 oz	24	tr	86	3	4
seed	1 tsp	7	tr	2	1	—
FENUGREEK						
seed	1 tsp	12	tr	2	2	—
FIBER						
Delta						
Natural Fiber	½ cup (1 oz)	20	tr	20	2	20
FIGS						
CANNED						
in heavy syrup	3	75	tr	1	19	—
in light syrup	3	58	tr	1	15	—
water pack	3	42	tr	1	11	—

FOOD	PORTION	CAL.	FAT	SOD.	CARB.	FIB.
S&W						
Kadota Figs Whole Fancy	½ cup	100	0	—	28	—
DRIED						
California	½ cup (3.5 oz)	200	1	11	58	17
cooked	½ cup	140	1	6	16	—
whole	10	477	2	20	122	17
Sonoma						
White Mission	3-4 (1.4 oz)	110	0	0	26	5
FRESH						
fig	1 med	50	tr	1	10	—

FISH

(*see also* FISH SUBSTITUTES, INDIVIDUAL NAMES, SUSHI)

FOOD	PORTION	CAL.	FAT	SOD.	CARB.	FIB.
CANNED						
Holmes						
Finest Kippered Snacks drained	1 can (3.2 oz)	135	8	470	0	0
Port Clyde						
Fish Steaks In Louisiana Hot Sauce	1 can (3.75 oz)	150	9	960	2	0
Fish Steaks In Mustard Sauce	1 can (3.75 oz)	140	7	540	1	0
Fish Steaks In Soybean Oil With Hot Chilies drained	1 can (3.3 oz)	155	8	420	0	0
Fish Steaks In Soybean Oil drained	1 can (3.3 oz)	220	17	360	0	0
FROZEN						
breaded fillet	1 (2 oz)	155	7	332	14	—
sticks	1 stick (1 oz)	76	3	163	7	—
Cajun Cookin'						
Seafood Gumbo	17 oz	330	7	1330	51	—
Gorton's						
Crispy Batter Dipped Fillets	2	290	19	550	18	—
Crispy Batter Sticks	4	260	18	480	16	—
Crunchy Fillets	2	230	13	420	16	—
Crunchy Sticks	4	210	13	240	15	—
Light Recipe Lightly Breaded Fish Fillets	1 fillet	180	8	380	16	—
Light Recipe Tempura Fillets	1 fillet	200	14	400	8	—
Microwave Crispy Batter Large Cut Fillets	1	320	21	680	20	—

FOOD	PORTION	CAL.	FAT	SOD.	CARB.	FIB.
Gorton's (CONT.)						
Microwave Entree Fillets In Herb Butter	1 pkg	190	8	450	3	—
Microwave Fillets	2	340	26	400	17	—
Microwave Larger Cut Fillets	1	320	22	500	20	—
Microwave Larger Cut Ranch Fillet	1	330	21	520	24	—
Microwave Sticks	6	340	22	420	24	—
Potato Crisp Fillets	2	300	20	360	18	—
Potato Crisp Sticks	4	260	16	390	21	—
Value Pack Portions	1 portion	180	11	490	13	—
Value Pack Sticks	4	190	9	420	17	—
Kineret						
Fish Sticks	5 pieces (4 oz)	280	14	430	27	1
Mrs. Paul's						
Buttered Fillet Microwave	1 fillet	80	4	130	10	—
Entree Light Seafood Dijon	8¾ oz	200	5	650	17	—
Entree Light Seafood Florentine	8 oz	220	8	820	10	—
Entree Light Seafood Mornay	9 oz	230	10	670	12	—
Fillet Sandwich Microwave	1	280	15	460	27	—
Fillets Microwave	1 fillet	280	19	390	16	—
Fish Cakes	2	190	7	690	24	—
Fish Fillets Batter Dipped	2 fillets	330	17	650	28	—
Fish Fillets Crispy Crunchy	2 fillets	220	9	380	23	—
Fish Fillets Crunchy Batter	2 fillets	280	14	730	26	—
Fish Sticks 40 Crunchy	4 (2.75 oz)	200	10	340	18	—
Fish Sticks Crispy Crunchy	4 sticks	190	8	560	18	—
Fish Sticks Microwave	5	290	20	330	18	—
In Butter Sauce Light Fillet	1 fillets	140	6	520	1	—
Portions Battered Fish	2 portions	300	19	540	21	—
Portions Crispy Crunchy Breaded Fish	2 portions	230	15	300	14	—
Seafood Platter Combination	9 oz	600	33	408	55	—

FOOD	PORTION	CAL.	FAT	SOD.	CARB.	FIB.
Mrs. Paul's (CONT.)						
Sticks Battered Fish	4 sticks	210	12	590	15	—
Sticks Crispy Crunchy Breaded Fish	4 sticks	140	6	340	14	—
Van De Kamp's						
Battered Fish Fillets	1 (2.6 oz)	180	11	340	12	0
Battered Fish Nuggets	8 (4 oz)	280	18	600	20	0
Battered Fish Portions	2 pieces (5 oz)	350	22	710	26	0
Battered Fish Sticks	6 (4 oz)	260	16	540	18	0
Breaded Fillets	2 (3.5 oz)	280	19	270	17	0
Breaded Fish Portions	3 pieces (4.5 oz)	330	21	410	23	0
Breaded Fish Sticks	6 (4 oz)	290	17	390	23	0
Breaded Mini Fish Sticks	13 (3.3 oz)	250	14	330	19	0
Crisp & Healthy Breaded Fillets	2 (3.5 oz)	150	3	380	20	0
Crisp & Healthy Fish Sticks	6 (4 oz)	180	3	440	26	0
Fish 'n Fries	1 pkg (6.6 oz)	380	18	370	41	2
MIX						
Golden Dipt						
Beer Batter Fry	1 oz	100	0	650	22	—
Cajun Style Fish Fry	⅔ oz	60	0	470	14	—
Fish & Chips Batter Mix	1¼ oz	120	0	910	27	—
Fish Fry	⅔ oz	60	0	430	14	—
Seafood Frying Mix	⅔ oz	60	0	600	14	—
Tempura Batter Mix	1 oz	100	0	130	22	—
TAKE-OUT						
fish cake	1 (4.7 oz)	166	7	—	6	—
jamaican brown fish stew	1 serv	426	22	419	9	2
kedgeree	5.6 oz	242	11	—	15	1
sandwich w/ tartar sauce	1	431	55	615	41	—
sandwich w/ tartar sauce & cheese	1	524	29	939	48	—
stew	1 cup (7.9 oz)	157	4	—	10	—
taramasalata	3.5 oz	446	46	—	4	—

FISH PASTE

fish paste	2 tsp	15	1	—	tr	0

FISH SUBSTITUTES

LaLoma						
Ocean Platter mix not prep	¼ cup (16 g)	50	0	260	5	—
Worthington						
Fillets	2 (85 g)	180	9	910	9	—

FOOD	PORTION	CAL.	FAT	SOD.	CARB.	FIB.
Worthington (CONT.)						
Tuno	2 oz (57 g)	100	7	310	3	—
FLAXSEED						
Arrowhead						
Flaxseed	3 tbsp (1 oz)	140	10	0	11	6
Stone-Buhr						
Flaxseed	1 tsp (1 oz)	150	10	20	11	5
FLOUNDER						
FRESH						
cooked	1 fillet (4.5 oz)	148	2	133	0	—
cooked	3 oz	99	1	89	0	—
FROZEN						
Gorton's						
Fishmarket Fresh	5 oz	110	1	170	1	—
Microwave Entree Stuffed	1 pkg	350	18	850	21	—
Mrs. Paul's						
Crunchy Batter Fillets	2 fillets	220	9	560	23	—
Light Fillets	1 fillet	240	10	450	20	—
Van De Kamp's						
Lightly Breaded Fillets	1 (4 oz)	230	11	400	19	0
Natural Fillets	1 (4 oz)	110	2	105	0	0
TAKE-OUT						
battered & fried	3.2 oz	211	11	484	15	—
breaded & fried	3.2 oz	211	11	484	15	—
FLOUR						
corn masa	1 cup	416	4	6	87	—
corn whole grain	1 cup	422	5	6	90	8
cottonseed lowfat	1 oz	94	tr	10	10	—
peanut defatted	1 cup	196	tr	108	21	—
peanut defatted	1 oz	92	tr	50	10	—
peanut lowfat	1 cup	257	13	0	19	—
potato	1 cup (6.3 oz)	628	1	61	143	—
rice brown	1 cup	574	4	12	121	4
rice white	1 cup	578	2	1	127	2
rye dark	1 cup	415	3	2	88	—
rye light	1 cup	374	1	2	82	7
rye medium	1 cup	361	2	3	79	7
sesame lowfat	1 oz	95	tr	11	10	—
triticale whole grain	1 cup	440	2	3	95	9
white all-purpose	1 cup	455	1	2	95	2
white bread	1 cup	495	2	2	99	—

FOOD	PORTION	CAL.	FAT	SOD.	CARB.	FIB.
white cake	1 cup	395	tr	2	85	—
white self-rising	1 cup	442	1	1587	93	—
whole wheat	1 cup	407	2	6	87	8
Arrowhead						
Kamut	¼ cup (1.2 oz)	110	1	0	25	4
Pastry	⅓ cup (1.1 oz)	100	1	0	22	3
Rye Whole Grain	¼ cup (1.6 oz)	160	1	0	34	6
Spelt	¼ cup (1.2 oz)	100	1	0	24	5
Teff	¼ cup (1.4 oz)	140	1	5	29	5
Unbleached White	⅓ cup (1.6 oz)	160	1	0	33	0
Whole Grain Wheat	¼ cup (1.6 oz)	160	1	0	34	7
Whole Wheat	¼ cup (1.2 oz)	130	1	0	25	4
Aunt Jemima						
Self-Rising	3 tbsp	90	0	310	20	1
Ballard						
All Purpose	1 cup	400	1	0	87	—
Self-Rising	1 cup	380	1	1290	84	—
Ceresota						
All Purpose	1 cup	390	1	0	83	—
Whole Wheat	1 cup	400	2	0	80	—
General Mills						
Drifted Snow	1 cup	400	1	—	—	—
Softasilk	¼ cup	100	0	—	—	—
Gold Medal						
All Purpose	1 cup	400	1	0	87	—
La Pina	1 cup	390	1	—	—	—
Oat Blend	1 cup	390	3	0	81	—
Self-Rising	1 cup	380	1	1520	83	—
Unbleached	1 cup	400	1	0	87	—
Whole Wheat	1 cup	350	2	0	78	10
Whole Wheat Blend	1 cup	380	2	0	84	8
Heckers						
All Purpose	1 cup	390	1	0	83	—
Whole Wheat	1 cup	400	2	0	80	—
Hodgson Mill						
50/50 Flour	¼ cup (1 oz)	100	1	0	21	2
Best For Bread	¼ cup (1 oz)	100	0	0	22	1
Buckwheat	⅓ cup (1.6 oz)	160	1	10	33	2
Oat Bran Blend	¼ cup (1 oz)	110	1	120	24	3
Oat Bran Flour	¼ cup (1 oz)	110	2	4	23	3
Rye	¼ cup (1 oz)	90	1	0	22	5
Seasoned Flour	¼ cup (1 oz)	90	0	1360	20	0
White	¼ cup (1 oz)	100	0	0	23	3
Whole Wheat	¼ cup (1 oz)	100	1	0	22	3

FOOD	PORTION	CAL.	FAT	SOD.	CARB.	FIB.
King Arthur						
All Purpose Unbleached	¼ cup (1 oz)	100	0	0	22	tr
Pillsbury						
All Purpose Best	1 cup	400	1	0	87	—
Bohemian Style Rye and Wheat Best	1 cup	400	1	0	86	—
Bread Best	1 cup	400	2	0	83	—
Rye Medium Best	1 cup	400	2	0	83	—
Self-Rising Best	1 cup	380	1	1290	84	—
Shake & Blend Best	2 tbsp	50	0	0	11	—
Unbleached Best	1 cup	400	1	0	86	—
Whole Wheat Best	1 cup	400	2	10	80	—
Red Band						
All-Purpose	1 cup	390	1	—	—	—
Self-Rising	1 cup	380	1	—	—	—
Robin Hood						
All Purpose	1 cup	400	1	0	85	—
Rye Stone Ground	1 cup	360	2	10	86	13
Self-Rising	1 cup	380	1	1520	83	—
Unbleached	1 cup	400	1	0	85	—
Stone Ground Mills						
White Unbleached Organic	¼ cup (1.4 oz)	130	0	0	25	1
Whole Wheat 100% Stone Ground	3 tbsp (1 oz)	90	1	0	20	3
White Deer						
All-Purpose	1 cup	400	1	—	—	—
Wondra						
Flour	1 cup	400	1	—	—	—

FRANKFURTER

(*see* HOT DOG)

FRENCH FRIES

(*see* POTATOES)

FRENCH BEANS

dried cooked	1 cup	228	1	11	43	—

FRENCH TOAST

FROZEN

french toast	1 slice (2 oz)	126	4	292	19	2
Aunt Jemima						
Cinnamon Swirl	2 pieces (4.1 oz)	240	6	330	37	2
Slices	2 pieces (4.1 oz)	240	6	360	38	1

FOOD	PORTION	CAL.	FAT	SOD.	CARB.	FIB.
Downyflake						
Extra Thick	1	150	9	340	11	—
French Toast	2 slices	270	12	380	34	—
Texas Style & Sausage	1 pkg (4.25 oz)	400	24	550	37	—
Great Starts						
Cinnamon Swirl With Sausage	5½ oz	390	21	530	37	—
French Toast With Sausage	5½ oz	380	21	550	35	—
Mini French Toast With Sausage	2½ oz	190	9	320	22	—
Oatmeal French Toast With Lite Links	4.65 oz	310	13	500	35	—
Healthy Starts						
French Toast With LeanLinks	6.5 oz	400	13	595	51	—
Quaker						
French Toast Sticks & Syrup	1 pkg (5.2 oz)	400	20	640	48	—
French Toast Wedges & Sausage	1 pkg (5.3 oz)	360	17	780	40	—
HOME RECIPE						
as prep w/ 2% milk	1 slice	149	7	311	16	—
as prep w/ whole milk	1 slice	151	7	311	16	—
TAKE-OUT						
w/ butter	2 slices	356	19	513	36	—

FROG'S LEGS

FOOD	PORTION	CAL.	FAT	SOD.	CARB.	FIB.
frog leg as prep w/ seasoned flour & fried	1 (0.8)	70	5	—	15	—

FROSTING

(*see* CAKE ICING)

FRUCTOSE

FOOD	PORTION	CAL.	FAT	SOD.	CARB.	FIB.
Estee						
Fructose	1 tsp (4 g)	15	0	0	4	—
Packet	1 pkg (3 g)	10	0	0	3	—

FRUIT DRINKS

(*see also individual names,* LEMONADE)

FOOD	PORTION	CAL.	FAT	SOD.	CARB.	FIB.
FROZEN						
citrus juice drink as prep	1 cup	114	0	7	28	—
citrus juice drink not prep	1 can (12 fl oz)	684	tr	12	171	—
fruit punch as prep w/water	1 cup	113	tr	11	29	—

FOOD	PORTION	CAL.	FAT	SOD.	CARB.	FIB.
fruit punch not prep	1 can (12 fl oz)	678	tr	34	173	—
limeade	1 can (6 oz)	408	tr	—	108	—
limeade as prep w/ water	1 cup	102	tr	6	27	—
Bright & Early						
Fruit Punch	8 fl oz	130	0	5	31	—
Dole						
100% Juice Blend Country Raspberry as prep	8 fl oz	140	0	30	34	0
100% Juice Blend Orchard Peach as prep	8 fl oz	140	0	30	34	0
Mountain Cherry 100% Juice Blend as prep	8 fl oz	120	0	30	30	0
Pineapple Grapefruit as prep	8 fl oz	130	0	20	29	0
Pineapple Orange as prep	8 fl oz	120	0	20	29	0
Pineapple Orange Banana as prep	8 fl oz	130	0	20	31	0
Pineapple Orange Guava as prep	8 fl oz	120	0	20	30	0
Pineapple Passion Banana as prep	8 fl oz	120	0	20	30	0
Tropical Fruit as prep	8 fl oz	140	0	30	34	0
Five Alive						
Berry Citrus	8 fl oz	120	0	0	30	—
Citrus	8 fl oz	120	0	0	30	—
Tropical Citrus	8 fl oz	120	0	25	29	—
Minute Maid						
Berry Punch	8 fl oz	130	0	5	31	—
Citrus Punch	8 fl oz	120	0	5	31	—
Fruit Punch	8 fl oz	120	0	5	31	—
Limeade	8 fl oz	100	0	0	26	—
Pineapple Orange	8 fl oz	120	0	0	31	—
Tropical Punch	8 fl oz	120	0	5	31	—
Seneca						
Cranberry-Apple Juice Cocktail frzn as prep	8 fl oz	140	0	0	33	0
Raspberry-Cranberry Juice Cocktail frzn as prep	8 fl oz	140	0	35	36	0
Tree Top						
Apple Citrus as prep	6 oz	90	0	10	22	—

FOOD	PORTION	CAL.	FAT	SOD.	CARB.	FIB.
Tree Top (CONT.)						
Apple Cranberry as prep	6 oz	100	0	10	25	—
Apple Grape as prep	6 oz	100	0	10	25	—
Apple Pear as prep	6 oz	90	0	10	22	—
Apple Raspberry as prep	6 oz	80	0	10	21	—
MIX						
fruit punch as prep w/water	9 oz	97	0	38	25	—
Crystal Light						
Fruit Punch as prep	1 serv (8 oz)	5	0	0	0	0
Lemon-Lime Drink as prep	1 serv (8 oz)	5	0	0	0	0
Passion Fruit Pineapple Drink as prep	1 serv (8 oz)	5	0	0	tr	0
Pineapple Orange Drink as prep	1 serv (8 oz)	5	0	0	0	0
Strawberry Orange Banana as prep	1 serv (8 oz)	5	0	0	0	0
Strawberry Kiwi as prep	1 serv (8 oz)	5	0	0	0	0
Watermelon Strawberry as prep	1 serv (8 oz)	5	0	0	0	0
Kool-Aid						
Cherry as prep	1 serv (8 oz)	60	0	0	16	0
Grape Berry Splash Drink as prep	1 serv (8 oz)	70	0	0	17	0
Grape Berry Splash Drink as prep w/ sugar	1 serv (8 oz)	100	0	0	25	0
Kickin' Kiwi Lime Drink as prep	1 serv (8 oz)	60	0	0	16	0
Kickin' Kiwi Lime Drink as prep w/ sugar	1 serv (8 oz)	100	0	10	25	0
Lemon-Lime Drink as prep w/ sugar	1 serv (8 oz)	100	0	5	25	0
Man-O-Mango Berry Drink as prep w/ sugar	1 serv (8 oz)	100	0	0	25	0
Mon-O-Mango Berry Drink as prep	1 serv (8 oz)	60	0	0	16	0
Oh Yeah Orange Pineapple Drink as prep w/ sugar	1 serv (8 oz)	100	0	0	25	0
Oh Yeah Orange Pineapple Drink as prep	1 serv (8 oz)	60	0	0	16	0

FOOD	PORTION	CAL.	FAT	SOD.	CARB.	FIB.
Kool-Aid (CONT.)						
Pina-Pineapple Drink as prep	1 serv (8 oz)	60	0	0	17	0
Pina-Pineapple Drink as prep w/ sugar	1 serv (8 oz)	100	0	0	25	0
Rainbow Punch	8 oz	98	0	—	25	—
Roarin' Raspberry Cranberry Drink as prep	1 serv (8 oz)	70	0	20	17	0
Roarin' Raspberry Cranberry Drink as prep w/ sugar	1 serv (8 oz)	100	0	10	25	0
Slammin' Strawberry Kiwi Drink as prep	1 serv (8 oz)	70	0	15	17	0
Slammin' Strawberry Kiwi Drink as prep w/ sugar	1 serv (8 oz)	100	0	15	25	0
Strawberry Raspberry Drink as prep	1 serv (8 oz)	60	0	0	16	0
Strawberry Raspberry Drink as prep w/ sugar	1 serv (8 oz)	100	0	0	25	0
Sugar Free Tropical Punch as prep	1 serv (8 oz)	5	0	10	0	0
Tropical Punch as prep	1 serv (8 oz)	60	0	0	16	0
Tropical Punch as prep w/ sugar	1 serv (8 oz)	100	0	15	25	0
Watermelon Cherry Drink as prep	1 serv (8 oz)	60	0	0	16	0
Watermelon Cherry Drink as prep w/ sugar	1 serv (8 oz)	100	0	10	25	0
Tang						
Orange Pineapple as prep	1 serv (8 oz)	100	0	45	24	0
READY-TO-DRINK						
cranberry apple drink	6 fl oz	123	0	4	32	—
cranberry apricot drink	6 fl oz	118	0	4	30	—
fruit punch	6 fl oz	87	tr	41	22	—
orange grapefruit juice	8 fl oz	107	tr	8	25	—
orange & apricot	8 fl oz	128	tr	—	32	—
pineapple & grapefruit	8 fl oz	117	tr	14	29	—
pineapple & orange drink	8 fl oz	125	0	9	29	—

FOOD	PORTION	CAL.	FAT	SOD.	CARB.	FIB.
After The Fall						
Amaretto Almond	1 can (12 oz)	170	0	25	42	0
American Pie Cherry	1 can (12 oz)	190	0	20	35	0
Apple Apricot	1 cup (8 oz)	100	0	20	26	0
Apple Raspberry	1 bottle (10 oz)	110	0	25	29	—
Apple Strawberry	1 bottle (10 oz)	120	0	23	30	—
Banana Casablanca	1 bottle (10 oz)	120	0	13	24	—
Berrymeister	1 can (12 oz)	160	0	25	40	0
Cranberry Meets Raspberry	1 bottle (10 oz)	120	0	25	29	—
Georgia Peach Blend	1 bottle (10 oz)	130	0	23	33	—
Mango Montage	1 bottle (10 oz)	140	0	15	33	—
Maui Grove	1 bottle (10 oz)	120	0	20	29	—
Nantucket Ginger Ale	1 can (12 oz)	140	0	25	35	0
Orange Icicle Cream	1 can (12 oz)	170	0	25	42	0
Oregon Berry	1 bottle (10 oz)	130	0	30	31	—
Passion Of The Islands	1 bottle (10 oz)	125	0	15	32	—
Peach Vanilla	1 can (12 oz)	170	0	35	42	0
Strawberry Vanilla	1 can (12 oz)	160	0	25	42	0
Twist O' Strawberry	1 can (12 oz)	190	0	25	37	0
Vanilla Bean Cream	1 can (12 oz)	170	0	25	42	0
Apple & Eve						
Apple Cranberry	6 fl oz	80	0	5	19	—
Apple Grape	6 fl oz	120	0	0	29	—
Cranberry Grape	6 fl oz	100	0	5	23	—
Fruit Punch	6 fl oz	78	0	0	18	—
Raspberry Cranberry	6 fl oz	90	0	10	21	—
BAMA						
Fruit Punch	8.45 fl oz	130	0	15	32	—
Boku						
White Grape Raspberry	16 fl oz	120	0	75	29	—
Capri Sun						
Fruit Punch	1 pkg (7 oz)	100	0	20	26	0
Maui Punch	1 pkg (7 oz)	100	0	20	27	0
Mountain Cooler	1 pkg (7 oz)	90	0	25	24	0
Pacific Cooler	1 pkg (7 oz)	100	0	20	26	0
Red Berry	1 pkg (7 oz)	100	0	20	26	0
Safari Punch	1 pkg (7 oz)	100	0	20	25	0
Strawberry Kiwi Drink	1 pkg (7 oz)	100	0	20	26	0
Surfer Cooler Drink	1 pkg (7 oz)	100	0	20	27	0
Chiquita						
Orange Banana	6 fl oz	90	0	—	—	—
Crystal Geyser						
Juice Squeeze Citrus Grape	1 bottle (12 fl oz)	145	0	20	35	—

FOOD	PORTION	CAL.	FAT	SOD.	CARB.	FIB.
Crystal Geyser (CONT.)						
Juice Squeeze Orange & Passion Fruit	1 bottle (12 fl oz)	130	0	20	31	—
Juice Squeeze Passion Fruit & Mango	1 bottle (12 fl oz)	125	0	20	31	—
Juice Squeeze Wild Berry	1 bottle (12 fl oz)	130	0	20	31	—
Crystal Light						
Fruit Punch	1 serv (8 oz)	5	0	20	0	0
Kiwi Strawberry	1 serv (8 oz)	5	0	20	0	0
Orange Strawberry Banana Drink	1 serv (8 oz)	5	0	20	0	0
Dole						
Pineapple Orange	6 fl oz	90	0	10	22	—
Pineapple Orange Banana	6 fl oz	100	0	10	23	—
Pineapple Orange Guava	6 fl oz	100	0	10	21	—
Pineapple Passion Banana	6 fl oz	100	0	10	21	—
Everfresh						
Cranberry-Apple Drink	1 can (8 oz)	120	0	0	31	0
Mandarin Orange Mango Drink	1 can (8 oz)	120	0	0	29	0
Orange Banana Strawberry Drink	1 can (8 oz)	120	0	19	30	0
Tropical Fruit Punch	1 can (8 oz)	120	0	0	30	0
Five Alive						
Citrus	1 bottle (16 fl oz)	120	0	25	31	—
Citrus	6 fl oz	90	0	20	22	—
Citrus	1 can (11.5 fl oz)	170	0	35	43	—
Citrus Chilled	8 fl oz	120	0	25	30	—
Fresh Samantha						
Banana Strawberry	1 cup (8 oz)	148	1	—	36	2
Beta Yet	1 cup (8 oz)	98	1	0	24	2
Carrot Orange	1 cup (8 oz)	107	1	—	24	1
Colossal C	1 cup (8 oz)	116	0	—	30	2
Desperately Seeking C	1 cup (8 oz)	129	1	0	30	3
Protein Blast	1 cup (8 oz)	156	1	—	30	2
Spirulina Fruit Blend	1 cup (8 oz)	129	1	—	30	2
Strawberry Orange	1 cup (8 oz)	120	1	0	27	1
The Big Bang	1 cup (8 oz)	97	1	0	24	2
Hawaiian Punch						
Fruit Juicy Red	6 fl oz	90	0	—	—	—
Island Fruit Cocktail	6 fl oz	90	0	—	—	—

FOOD	PORTION	CAL.	FAT	SOD.	CARB.	FIB.
Hawaiian Punch (CONT.)						
Lite Fruit Juicy Red	6 fl oz	60	0	—	—	—
Tropical Fruits	6 fl oz	90	0	—	—	—
Very Berry	6 fl oz	90	0	—	—	—
Wild Fruit	6 fl oz	90	0	—	—	—
Hi-C						
Boppin Berry Box	8.45 fl oz	140	0	30	33	—
Boppin' Berry	8 fl oz	130	0	30	32	—
Double Fruit Box	8.45 fl oz	130	0	35	32	—
Double Fruit Cooler	8 fl oz	130	0	30	31	—
Ecto Cooler	8 fl oz	130	0	25	32	—
Ecto Cooler	1 can (11.5 fl oz)	180	0	40	45	—
Ecto Cooler Box	8.45 fl oz	130	0	35	32	—
Fruit Punch	8 fl oz	130	0	30	32	—
Fruit Punch	1 can (11.5 fl oz)	190	0	40	46	—
Fruit Punch Box	8.45 fl oz	140	0	30	32	—
Fruity Bubble Gum	8 fl oz	120	0	25	30	—
Fruity Bubble Gum Box	8.45 fl oz	130	0	30	32	—
Hula Punch	8 fl oz	120	0	30	29	—
Hula Punch	1 can (11.5 fl oz)	170	0	40	42	—
Hula Punch Box	8.45 fl oz	120	0	30	30	—
Jammin' Apple Box	8.45 fl oz	130	0	30	33	—
Stompin' Banana Berry	8 fl oz	130	0	30	31	—
Stompin' Banana Berry Box	8.45 fl oz	130	0	30	32	—
Wild Berry	8 fl oz	120	0	30	30	—
Wild Berry Box	8.45 fl oz	130	0	30	32	—
Hood						
Natural Blenders Apple Cranberry Raspberry	1 cup (8 oz)	130	0	5	32	—
Natural Blenders Apple Grape Cherry	1 cup (8 oz)	130	0	5	32	—
Natural Blenders Apple Peach Pear	1 cup (8 oz)	120	0	5	30	—
Natural Blenders Apple Wild Blueberry Strawberry	1 cup (8 oz)	120	0	5	30	—
Natural Blenders Pineapple Orange Kiwi	1 cup (8 oz)	120	0	5	30	—
Juice Works						
Appleberry	6 fl oz	100	0	—	—	—
Juicy Juice						
Apple Grape	1 box (8.45 fl oz)	120	0	10	29	—
Berry	1 bottle (6 fl oz)	90	0	10	22	—

FOOD	PORTION	CAL.	FAT	SOD.	CARB.	FIB.
Juicy Juice (CONT.)						
Berry	1 box (8.45 fl oz)	130	0	15	30	—
Punch	1 bottle (6 fl oz)	100	0	10	23	—
Punch	1 box (8.45 fl oz)	140	0	10	33	—
Tropical	1 box (8.45 fl oz)	150	0	10	36	—
Tropical	1 bottle (6 fl oz)	110	0	10	26	—
Kern's						
Apple Strawberry Nectar	6 fl oz	110	0	0	26	—
Apricot Pineapple Nectar	6 fl oz	110	0	5	27	—
Banana Pineapple Nectar	6 fl oz	110	0	0	27	—
Coconut Pineapple Nectar	6 fl oz	140	0	25	26	—
Orange Banana Nectar	6 fl oz	110	0	0	25	—
Strawberry Banana Nectar	6 fl oz	110	0	0	28	—
Tropical Nectar	6 fl oz	110	0	5	27	—
Kool-Aid						
Bursts Great Bluedini	1 (7 oz)	100	0	30	24	0
Bursts Kickin' Kiwi Lime	1 (7 oz)	100	0	30	24	0
Bursts Oh Yeah Orange Pineapple	1 (7 oz)	100	0	30	24	0
Bursts Slammin' Strawberry Kiwi	1 (7 oz)	100	0	30	24	0
Bursts Tropical Punch	1 (7 oz)	100	0	30	24	0
Splash Grape Berry Punch	1 serv (8 oz)	120	0	35	31	0
Splash Kiwi Strawberry Drink	1 serv (8 oz)	110	0	35	29	0
Splash Tropical Punch	1 serv (8 oz)	120	0	35	31	0
Libby						
Strawberry Banana Nectar	1 can (11.5 fl oz)	220	0	10	51	—
Mauna La'i						
Island Guava Hawaiian Guava Fruit Juice Drink	8 fl oz	130	0	35	32	0
Mango & Hawaiian Guava Fruit Juice Drink	8 fl oz	130	0	35	33	0
Paradise Guava Hawaiian Guava & Passion Fruit Juice Drink	8 fl oz	130	0	35	32	0
Minute Maid						
Berry Punch Box	8.45 fl oz	130	0	25	31	—

FOOD	PORTION	CAL.	FAT	SOD.	CARB.	FIB.
Minute Maid (CONT.)						
Berry Punch Chilled	8 fl oz	130	0	25	31	—
Citrus Punch Chilled	8 fl oz	130	0	25	31	—
Fruit Punch Box	8.45 fl oz	120	0	25	31	—
Fruit Punch Chilled	8 fl oz	120	0	25	31	—
Juices To Go Citrus Punch	1 can (11.5 fl oz)	180	0	40	45	—
Juices To Go Citrus Punch	1 bottle (10 fl oz)	160	0	35	39	—
Juices To Go Concord Punch	1 can (11.5 fl oz)	180	0	40	46	—
Juices To Go Concord Punch	1 bottle (10 fl oz)	160	0	35	40	—
Juices To Go Concord Punch	1 bottle (16 fl oz)	130	0	25	32	—
Juices To Go Fruit Punch	1 bottle (10 fl oz)	160	0	35	39	—
Juices To Go Fruit Punch	1 can (11.5 fl oz)	180	0	40	44	—
Juices To Go Fruit Punch	1 bottle (16 fl oz)	120	0	25	31	—
Juices To Go Orange Blend	1 bottle (10 fl oz)	150	0	35	37	—
Juices To Go Orange Blend	1 can (11.5 fl oz)	170	0	40	43	—
Naturals Apple Cranberry	8 fl oz	170	0	25	42	—
Naturals Concord Medley	8 fl oz	130	0	25	32	—
Naturals Fruit Medley	8 fl oz	120	0	25	31	—
Naturals Orange Grape Medley	8 fl oz	120	0	25	30	—
Naturals Tropical Medley	8 fl oz	120	0	25	31	—
Tropical Punch Box	8.45 fl oz	130	0	25	32	—
Tropical Punch Chilled	8 fl oz	120	0	25	31	—
Mott's						
Apple Cranberry Blend	10 fl oz	180	0	15	44	0
Apple Cranberry From Concentrate as prep	8 fl oz	120	0	20	30	0
Apple Grape From Concentrate as prep	8 fl oz	120	0	20	30	0
Apple Raspberry Blend	10 fl oz	140	0	10	33	0
Apple Raspberry From Concentrate	8.45 fl oz	120	0	25	30	0
Fruit Basket Apple Raspberry Juice Cocktail as prep	8 fl oz	130	0	5	30	0

FOOD	PORTION	CAL.	FAT	SOD.	CARB.	FIB.
Mott's (CONT.)						
Fruit Basket Tropical Blend Juice Cocktail as prep	8 fl oz	120	0	5	30	0
Fruit Punch From Concentrate	10 fl oz	170	0	0	42	0
Fruit Punch From Concentrate	8.45 fl oz	120	0	20	29	0
Grape Apple	10 fl oz	170	0	10	41	0
Pineapple Orange	10 fl oz	170	0	15	42	0
Ocean Spray						
Cran.Blueberry	8 fl oz	160	0	35	41	0
Cran.Cherry	6 fl oz	160	0	35	39	0
Cran.Grape	8 fl oz	170	0	35	41	0
Cran.Raspberry	8 fl oz	140	0	35	36	0
Cran.Raspberry Reduced Calorie	8 fl oz	50	0	35	13	0
Cran.Strawberry	8 fl oz	140	0	35	36	tr
Cranapple	8 fl oz	160	0	35	41	tr
Cranapple Reduced Calorie	8 fl oz	50	0	35	13	0
Cranicot	8 fl oz	160	0	35	40	0
Crantastic	8 fl oz	150	0	35	37	0
Fruit Punch	8 fl oz	130	0	35	32	0
Lightstyle Low Calorie Cran.Grape	8 fl oz	40	0	35	9	0
Lightstyle Low Calorie Cran.Raspberry	8 fl oz	40	0	35	10	0
Refreshers Juice Drink Citrus Cranberry	8 fl oz	140	0	35	35	0
Refreshers Juice Drink Citrus Peach	8 fl oz	120	0	35	30	0
Refreshers Juice Drink Orange Cranberry	8 fl oz	130	0	35	33	0
Ruby Red & Tangerine Grapefruit Juice Cocktail	8 fl oz	130	0	35	32	0
Odwalla						
Boyzenberry Mango	8 fl oz	140	0	20	34	2
C Monster	16 fl oz	300	0	110	72	4
Fruitshake Blackberry	8 fl oz	160	0	50	39	3
Guanaba Dabba Doo!	8 fl oz	130	0	35	29	0
Lotta Colada	8 fl oz	160	3	45	33	2
Mango Tango	8 fl oz	150	3	55	37	6

FOOD	PORTION	CAL.	FAT	SOD.	CARB.	FIB.
Odwalla (CONT.)						
Mo Beta	16 fl oz	280	1	290	69	3
Raspberry Smoothie	8 fl oz	140	0	25	35	2
Strawberry Banana Smoothie	8 fl oz	100	0	10	26	2
Strawberry Go Man Go	8 fl oz	100	1	25	26	2
Super Protein	16 fl oz	400	6	250	40	5
Pek						
Mango Guava Ecstasy	1 bottle (20 fl oz)	110	0	20	27	0
Passionate Peach Grapefruit	8 fl oz	110	0	20	27	0
S&W						
Apricot Pineapple Nectar	6 fl oz	120	0	10	29	—
Apricot Pineapple Nectar Diet	6 fl oz	80	0	10	20	—
Shasta Plus						
Fruit Punch	1 can (11.5 oz)	160	0	45	39	0
Sipps						
Fruit Punch	8.45 oz	130	0	—	—	—
Lemon Lime Cooler	8.45 oz	130	0	—	—	—
Mixed Berry	8.45 oz	130	0	—	—	—
Sunshine Punch	8.45 oz	130	0	—	—	—
Smucker's						
Apple Cranberry	8 oz	120	0	10	32	—
Orange Banana	8 oz	120	0	10	30	—
Snapple						
Diet Kiwi Strawberry	8 fl oz	13	0	10	3	—
Fruit Punch	8 fl oz	120	0	5	29	—
Kiwi Strawberry Cocktail	8 fl oz	130	0	10	33	—
Melonberry Cocktail	8 fl oz	120	0	10	29	—
Vitamin Supreme	10 fl oz	150	0	20	38	—
Squeezit						
Berry B. Wild	1 (6.75 fl oz)	90	0	0	22	—
Chucklin' Cherry	1 (6.75 fl oz)	90	0	5	23	—
Grumpy Grape	1 (6.75 fl oz)	90	0	0	23	—
Mean Green Puncher	1 (6.75 fl oz)	90	0	0	23	—
Silly Billy Strawberry	1 (6.75 fl oz)	90	0	0	23	—
Smarty Arty Orange	1 (6.75 fl oz)	90	0	50	23	—
Sunny Delight						
Drink	6 fl oz	90	0	—	—	—
Tree Top						
Apple Citrus	6 fl oz	90	0	10	22	—
Apple Cranberry	6 fl oz	100	0	10	25	—
Apple Grape	6 fl oz	100	0	10	25	—

FOOD	PORTION	CAL.	FAT	SOD.	CARB.	FIB.
Tree Top (CONT.)						
Apple Pear	6 fl oz	90	0	10	22	—
Apple Raspberry	6 fl oz	80	0	10	21	—
Tropicana						
Berry Punch	8 fl oz	120	0	25	29	—
Citrus Punch	1 bottle (10 fl oz)	180	0	15	45	—
Citrus Punch	8 fl oz	140	0	20	36	—
Cranberry Punch	1 bottle (10 fl oz)	170	0	10	43	—
Cranberry Punch	1 can (11.5 fl oz)	200	0	15	49	—
Cranberry Punch	8 fl oz	140	0	10	34	—
Fruit Punch	8 fl oz	130	0	25	31	—
Fruit Punch	1 container (10 fl oz)	160	0	25	39	—
Fruit Punch	1 can (11.5 fl oz)	170	0	30	42	—
Fruit Punch	1 bottle (10 fl oz)	150	0	25	39	—
Orange Pineapple	8 fl oz	110	0	15	27	—
Orange Pineapple	1 bottle (10 fl oz)	130	0	15	32	—
Pineapple Punch	1 bottle (10 fl oz)	160	0	20	39	—
Pineapple Punch	8 fl oz	120	0	15	31	—
Season's Best Cranberry Medley	8 fl oz	120	0	20	29	—
Tropics Apple Cranberry Kiwi	8 fl oz	120	0	15	30	—
Tropics Orange Strawberry Banana	8 fl oz	110	0	5	27	—
Tropics Orange Kiwi Passion	8 fl oz	100	0	15	26	—
Tropics Orange Peach Mango	8 fl oz	110	0	15	28	—
Tropics Orange Pineapple	8 fl oz	110	0	15	27	—
Tropics Pineapple Passion	8 fl oz	120	0	25	30	—
Twister Apple Raspberry Blackberry	8 fl oz	120	0	20	31	—
Twister Apple Raspberry Blackberry	1 bottle (10 fl oz)	150	0	25	38	—
Twister Apple Raspberry Blackberry	1 can (11.5 fl oz)	180	0	25	44	—
Twister Cranberry Raspberry Strawberry	8 fl oz	120	0	5	31	—
Twister Cranberry Raspberry Strawberry	1 bottle (10 fl oz)	160	0	5	39	—
Twister Light Cranberry Raspberry Strawberry	8 fl oz	45	0	10	11	—

FOOD	PORTION	CAL.	FAT	SOD.	CARB.	FIB.
Tropicana (CONT.)						
Twister Light Cranberry Raspberry Strawberry	1 container (10 fl oz)	50	0	15	13	—
Twister Light Orange Cranberry	1 container (10 fl oz)	35	0	25	9	—
Twister Light Orange Cranberry	8 fl oz	30	0	20	7	—
Twister Light Orange Cranberry	1 container (10 fl oz)	35	0	25	9	—
Twister Light Orange Raspberry	8 fl oz	35	0	20	9	—
Twister Light Orange Raspberry	1 container (10 fl oz)	45	0	25	11	—
Twister Light Orange Strawberry Banana	1 container (10 fl oz)	45	0	25	11	—
Twister Orange Cranberry	1 bottle (10 fl oz)	140	0	20	36	—
Twister Orange Cranberry	8 fl oz	120	0	15	29	—
Twister Orange Peach	1 can (11.5 fl oz)	160	0	20	41	—
Twister Orange Peach	1 bottle (10 fl oz)	140	0	25	36	—
Twister Orange Peach	8 fl oz	120	0	20	29	—
Twister Orange Raspberry	1 bottle (10 fl oz)	140	0	20	36	—
Twister Orange Raspberry	8 fl oz	120	0	20	29	—
Twister Orange Strawberry Banana	1 container (10 fl oz)	140	0	20	35	—
Twister Strawberry Banana	1 bottle (10 fl oz)	140	0	20	35	—
Twister Strawberry Banana	8 fl oz	120	0	20	29	—
Twister Strawberry Banana	1 can (11.5 fl oz)	160	0	30	41	—
Twister Strawberry Guava	8 fl oz	110	0	20	28	—
Twister Strawberry Guava	1 bottle (10 fl oz)	140	0	25	35	—
Veryfine						
Apple Cherryberry	8 fl oz	130	0	<25	33	—
Apple Cranberry	8 fl oz	130	0	<10	33	—
Apple Raspberry	8 fl oz	110	0	<15	27	—
Fruit Punch	8 fl oz	130	0	<35	33	—
Guava Strawberry	8 fl oz	120	0	<25	30	—

FOOD	PORTION	CAL.	FAT	SOD.	CARB.	FIB.
Veryfine (CONT.)						
Lemon & Lime	8 fl oz	120	0	<10	30	—
Papaya Punch	8 fl oz	120	0	<10	30	—
Passionfruit Orange	8 fl oz	110	0	<25	26	—
Pineapple Orange	8 fl oz	130	0	<10	32	—
White House						
Apple Cherry	6 fl oz	90	0	10	22	0

FRUIT MIXED

(*see also individual names*)

FOOD	PORTION	CAL.	FAT	SOD.	CARB.	FIB.
CANNED						
fruit cocktail in heavy syrup	½ cup	93	tr	7	24	—
fruit cocktail juice pack	½ cup	56	tr	4	15	—
fruit cocktail water pack	½ cup	40	tr	5	10	—
fruit salad in heavy syrup	½ cup	94	tr	7	24	—
fruit salad in light syrup	½ cup	73	tr	7	19	—
fruit salad juice pack	½ cup	62	tr	7	16	—
fruit salad water pack	½ cup	37	tr	4	10	—
mixed fruit in heavy syrup	½ cup	92	tr	5	24	—
tropical fruit salad in heavy syrup	½ cup	110	tr	3	29	—
Del Monte						
Fruit Cocktail Fruit Naturals	½ cup (4.4 oz)	60	0	10	15	1
Fruit Cocktail In Heavy Syrup	½ cup (4.5 oz)	100	0	10	24	1
Fruit Cocktail Lite	½ cup (4.4 oz)	60	0	10	15	1
Lite Mixed Fruits Chunky	½ cup (4.4 oz)	60	0	10	15	1
Mixed Fruits Chunky Fruit Naturals	½ cup (4.4 oz)	60	0	10	15	1
Mixed Fruits Chunky In Heavy Syrup	½ cup (4.5 oz)	100	0	10	24	1
Snack Cups Mixed Fruit Fruit Naturals	1 serv (4.5 oz)	60	0	10	16	1
Snack Cups Mixed Fruit Fruit Naturals EZ-Open Lid	1 serv (4.5 oz)	60	0	10	15	1
Snack Cups Mixed Fruit In Heavy Syrup	1 serv (4.5 oz)	100	0	10	24	1
Snack Cups Mixed Fruit In Heavy Syrup EZ-Open Lid	1 serv (4.2 oz)	90	0	10	23	1
Snack Cups Mixed Fruit Lite	1 serv (4.5 oz)	60	0	10	16	1

FOOD	PORTION	CAL.	FAT	SOD.	CARB.	FIB.
Del Monte (CONT.)						
Snack Cups Mixed Fruit Lite EZ-Open Lid	1 serv (4.5 oz)	60	0	10	15	1
Dole						
Tropical Fruit Salad	½ cup	70	0	10	17	—
Hunt's						
Fruit Cocktail	½ cup (4.5 oz)	90	0	15	23	1
Libby						
Chunky Mixed Lite	½ cup (4.3 oz)	60	0	5	14	1
Fruit Cocktail Lite	½ cup (4.3 oz)	60	0	10	15	1
S&W						
Chunky Mixed Diet	½ cup	40	0	5	10	—
Chunky Mixed Natural Style	½ cup	90	0	5	21	—
Chunky Mixed Unsweetened	½ cup	40	0	5	10	—
Fruit Cocktail Diet	½ cup	40	0	5	10	—
Fruit Cocktail Heavy Syrup	½ cup	90	0	15	24	—
Fruit Cocktail Natural Lite	½ cup	60	0	5	15	—
Fruit Cocktail Natural Style	½ cup	90	0	5	21	—
Fruit Cocktail Unsweetened	½ cup	40	0	5	10	—
DRIED						
mixed	11 oz pkg	712	1	52	188	—
Del Monte						
Mixed	⅓ cup (1.4 oz)	110	0	50	30	5
Planters						
Fruit'n Nut Mix	1 oz	140	9	105	13	2
Sonoma						
Diced	⅓ cup (1.4 oz)	120	0	0	31	3
Mixed Fruit	5-8 pieces (1.4 oz)	120	0	0	30	3
FROZEN						
mixed fruit sweetened	1 cup	245	tr	8	61	—
Big Valley						
Burst O' Berries	⅔ cup (4.9 oz)	70	0	0	16	3
California Tropics	⅔ cup (4.9 oz)	60	0	0	15	2
Cup A Fruit	1 pkg (4 oz)	50	0	0	7	2
Mixed	4.9 oz	60	0	0	14	2
Birds Eye						
Mixed Fruit	½ cup	120	0	5	31	1

FOOD	PORTION	CAL.	FAT	SOD.	CARB.	FIB.
Dole						
Applesauce Strawberry	1 pkg (4 oz)	60	0	0	15	1
FRUIT SNACKS						
fruit leather	1 bar (0.8 oz)	81	1	18	18	—
fruit leather pieces	1 pkg (0.9 oz)	92	2	109	21	—
fruit leather pieces	1 oz	97	2	114	22	—
fruit leather rolls	1 lg (0.7 oz)	73	1	13	18	—
fruit leather rolls	1 sm (0.5 oz)	49	tr	8	12	—
Betty Crocker						
String Thing Berry 'N Blue	1 pkg (0.7 oz)	80	1	40	17	—
String Thing Cherry	1 pkg (0.7 oz)	80	1	40	17	—
String Thing Strawberry	1 pkg (0.7 oz)	80	1	40	17	—
Brock						
Beauty & The Beast	1 pkg (0.9 oz)	90	0	25	21	—
Cinderella	1 pkg (0.9 oz)	90	0	25	21	—
Dinosaurs	1 pkg (0.9 oz)	90	0	25	21	—
Ninja Trolls	1 pkg (0.9 oz)	90	0	25	21	—
Sharks	1 pkg (0.9 oz)	90	0	25	21	—
Del Monte						
Sierra Trail Mix	1 pkg (0.9 oz)	110	6	45	15	2
Sierra Trail Mix	¼ cup (1.2 oz)	150	8	65	20	3
Sierra Trail Mix	1 pkg (1 oz)	120	6	50	16	2
Fruit By The Foot						
Cherry	1	80	2	45	18	—
Grape	1	80	2	45	18	—
Strawberry	1	80	2	45	18	—
Fruit Roll-Ups						
Cherry	1 (½ oz)	50	tr	40	12	—
Crazy Colors	1 (½ oz)	50	tr	40	12	—
Fruit Punch	1 (½ oz)	50	tr	40	12	—
Grape	1 (½ oz)	50	tr	40	12	—
Raspberry	1 (½ oz)	50	tr	40	12	—
Strawberry	1 (½ oz)	50	tr	40	12	—
General Mills						
Garfield And Friends 1-2 Punch	1 pkg	100	1	60	22	—
Garfield And Friends Cat Cooler	1 pkg	100	1	60	22	—
Garfield And Friends Fat Cat Funnies	1 (½ oz)	50	tr	20	12	—
Garfield And Friends Fruit Party	1 (½ oz)	50	tr	40	12	—

FOOD	PORTION	CAL.	FAT	SOD.	CARB.	FIB.
General Mills (CONT.)						
Garfield And Friends Very Strawberry	1 pkg	100	1	60	22	—
Shark Bites & Berry Bears Assorted Fruit	1 pkg	100	tr	20	22	—
Shark Bites & Berry Bears Fruit Punch	1 pkg	100	tr	20	22	—
Surf's Up! Sun Splash	1 pkg	100	1	30	22	—
Surf's Up! Tutti Frutti	1 pkg	100	1	20	22	—
Thunder Jets Assorted Fruit Squadron	1 pkg	100	1	30	24	—
Thunder Jets Mach 1 Fruit Mix	1 pkg	100	1	30	24	—
Health Valley						
Bakes Apple	1 bar	100	3	25	16	3
Bakes Date	1 bar	100	3	25	16	3
Bakes Raisin	1 bar	100	3	20	16	3
Fat Free Fruit Bars 100% Organic Apple	1 bar	140	tr	10	33	4
Fat Free Fruit Bars 100% Organic Apricot	1 bar	140	tr	10	33	4
Fat Free Fruit Bars 100% Organic Date	1 bar	140	tr	10	33	4
Fat Free Fruit Bars 100% Organic Raisin	1 bar	140	tr	10	33	4
Fruit & Fitness Bars	2 bars	200	5	75	35	5
Oat Bran Bakes Apricot	1 bar	100	3	15	16	2
Oat Bran Bakes Fig & Nut	1 bar	110	3	10	16	2
Oat Bran Jumbo Fruit Bar Almond & Date	1 bar	170	5	10	28	7
Oat Bran Jumbo Fruit Bars Raisin & Cinnamon	1 bar	160	2	10	32	6
Rice Bran Jumbo Fruit Bars Almond & Date	1 bar	160	5	5	27	4
Seneca						
Apple Chips	12 chips (1 oz)	140	7	15	20	2
Sonoma						
Trail Mix	¼ cup (1.4 oz)	160	7	5	24	2
Sovex						
Fruit Bites Jungle Pals	1 pkg (0.9 oz)	90	1	15	21	—
Stretch Island						
Fruit Leather Berry Blackberry	2 pieces (1 oz)	90	0	0	24	3

FOOD	PORTION	CAL.	FAT	SOD.	CARB.	FIB.
Stretch Island (CONT.)						
Fruit Leather Chunky Cherry	2 pieces (1 oz)	90	0	0	24	2
Fruit Leather Great Grape	2 pieces (1 oz)	90	0	0	24	2
Fruit Leather Organic Apple	2 pieces (1 oz)	90	0	10	24	2
Fruit Leather Organic Grape	2 pieces (1 oz)	90	0	5	24	2
Fruit Leather Organic Raspberry	2 pieces (1 oz)	90	0	10	25	2
Fruit Leather Rare Raspberry	2 pieces (1 oz)	90	0	0	24	2
Fruit Leather Snappy Apple	2 pieces (1 oz)	90	0	0	25	3
Fruit Leather Tangy Apricot	2 pieces (1 oz)	90	0	0	23	2
Fruit Leather Truly Tropical	2 pieces (1 oz)	90	0	0	22	1
Sunbelt						
Fruit Boosters Apple	1 (1.3 oz)	130	2	60	27	0
Fruit Boosters Blueberry	1 (1.3 oz)	130	2	60	27	1
Fruit Boosters Strawberry	1 (1.3 oz)	130	2	65	27	0
Fruit Jammers	1 (1 oz)	100	1	20	23	0
Sunkist						
Fruit Roll Apple	1 (0.7 oz)	70	0	20	17	1
Fruit Roll Apricot	1	76	1	17	18	0
Fruit Roll Apricot	1 (0.5 oz)	70	0	15	17	2
Fruit Roll Cherry	1 (0.7 oz)	70	0	160	17	2
Fruit Roll Cherry	1 (0.5 oz)	50	0	10	11	1
Fruit Roll Fruit Punch	1 (0.7 oz)	70	0	25	17	2
Fruit Roll Grape	1	76	tr	13	19	0
Fruit Roll Grape	1 (0.5 oz)	50	0	25	11	1
Fruit Roll Grape	1 (0.7 oz)	80	0	0	17	2
Fruit Roll Raspberry	1 (0.7 oz)	70	0	20	17	1
Fruit Roll Raspberry	1 (0.5 oz)	45	0	15	11	1
Fruit Roll Strawberry	1 (0.7 oz)	70	0	20	17	2
Fruit Roll Strawberry	1 (0.5 oz)	45	0	15	11	1
Fruit Roll Strawberry	1	74	tr	11	18	0
Weight Watchers						
Apple & Cinnamon	1 pkg (0.5 oz)	50	0	125	13	2
Apple Chips	1 pkg (0.75 oz)	70	0	125	18	3
Cinnamon	1 pkg (0.5 oz)	50	0	125	13	2

FOOD	PORTION	CAL.	FAT	SOD.	CARB.	FIB.
Weight Watchers (CONT.)						
Peach & Strawberry	1 pkg (0.5 oz)	50	0	125	13	2
Strawberry	1 pkg (0.5 oz)	50	0	125	13	2

GARBANZO

(*see* CHICKPEAS)

GARLIC

(FAST FACT: Americans eat almost two pounds of garlic a year; garlic production is increasing at a rate of 10 percent a year. You love garlic, know that it's good for you but hate the thought of "garlic breath"? Try chewing on fresh parsley, roasted coffee beans, fresh mint, cardamon or caraway seeds.)

FOOD	PORTION	CAL.	FAT	SOD.	CARB.	FIB.
clove	1	4	tr	1	1	—
powder	1 tsp	9	tr	1	2	—
Watkins						
Garlic & Chive Seasoning	1 tbsp (7 g)	25	2	280	2	0
Garlic Lover's Herb Blend	¼ tsp (0.5 oz)	0	0	0	0	0
Liquid Spice	1 tbsp (0.5 oz)	120	14	0	0	0

GEFILTE FISH

READY-TO-EAT

FOOD	PORTION	CAL.	FAT	SOD.	CARB.	FIB.
sweet	1 piece (1.5 oz)	35	1	220	3	—
Manischewitz						
Gefilte Fish	1 piece	107	4	—	4	—
Gefiltefish & Pike	1 piece	99	4	—	5	—
Gefiltefish & Pike Sweet	1 piece	129	4	—	9	—
Homestyle	1 piece	111	4	—	6	—
Sweet	1 piece	132	4	—	9	—

GELATIN

(FAST FACT: Salt Lake City, Utah, ranks as the number one city in per capita consumption of Jell-O gelatin. Strawberry is the all-time favorite flavor.)

MIX

FOOD	PORTION	CAL.	FAT	SOD.	CARB.	FIB.
low calorie	½ cup	8	0	9	0	0
mix artifically sweetened as prep	½ cup (4.1 oz)	8	0	56	1	—
mix artifically sweetened as prep	1 pkg 4 serv (16.5 oz)	33	0	224	3	—
mix as prep	1 pkg 4 serv (19 oz)	319	0	227	76	—
mix as prep	½ cup (4.7 oz)	80	0	57	19	—
mix not prep	1 pkg (3 oz)	324	0	216	77	—
mix w/ fruit as prep	½ cup (3.7 oz)	73	tr	30	18	—

FOOD	PORTION	CAL.	FAT	SOD.	CARB.	FIB.
mix w/ fruit as prep	1 pkg 8 serv (19 oz)	588	2	242	144	—
powder unsweetened	1 oz	94	0	55	0	—
powder unsweetened	1 pkg (7 g)	23	0	14	0	—
Emes						
Kosher-Jel	½ cup (4 fl oz)	60	0	7	15	—
Kosher-Jel Plain	1 tbsp (7 g)	21	0	tr	5	1
Jell-O						
1-2-3-Brand Strawberry as prep	⅔ cup (5.2 oz)	130	2	50	26	0
Apricot as prep	½ cup (5 oz)	80	0	80	19	0
Berry Black as prep	½ cup (5 oz)	80	0	80	19	0
Berry Blue as prep	½ cup (5 oz)	80	0	80	19	0
Black Cherry as prep	½ cup (5 oz)	80	0	80	19	0
Cherry as prep	½ cup (5 oz)	80	0	100	19	0
Cranberry Raspberry as prep	½ cup (5 oz)	80	0	75	19	0
Cranberry Strawberry as prep	½ cup (5 oz)	80	0	75	19	0
Cranberry as prep	½ cup (5 oz)	80	0	75	19	0
Grape as prep	½ cup (5 oz)	80	0	80	19	0
Lemon as prep	½ cup (5 oz)	80	0	120	19	0
Lime as prep	½ cup (5 oz)	80	0	90	19	0
Mango as prep	½ cup (5 oz)	80	0	80	19	0
Mixed Fruit as prep	½ cup (5 oz)	80	0	80	19	tr
Orange as prep	½ cup (5 oz)	80	0	80	19	0
Peach as prep	½ cup (5 oz)	80	0	80	19	0
Peach Passion Fruit as prep	½ cup (5 oz)	80	0	80	19	0
Pineapple as prep	½ cup (5 oz)	80	0	80	19	0
Raspberry as prep	½ cup (5 oz)	80	0	80	19	0
Sparkling White Grape as prep	½ cup (5 oz)	80	0	80	19	0
Strawberry Banana as prep	½ cup (5 oz)	80	0	80	19	0
Strawberry Kiwi as prep	½ cup (5 oz)	80	0	80	19	0
Strawberry as prep	½ cup (5 oz)	80	0	90	19	0
Sugar Free Cherry as prep	½ cup (4.2 oz)	10	0	70	0	0
Sugar Free Cranberry as prep	½ cup (4.2 oz)	10	0	80	0	0
Sugar Free Lemon	½ cup (4.2 oz)	10	0	55	0	0
Sugar Free Lime as prep	½ cup (4.2 oz)	10	0	60	0	0
Sugar Free Mixed Fruit as prep	½ cup (4.2 oz)	10	0	50	0	0

FOOD	PORTION	CAL.	FAT	SOD.	CARB.	FIB.
Jell-O (CONT.)						
Sugar Free Orange as prep	½ cup (4.2 oz)	10	0	65	0	0
Sugar Free Raspberry as prep	½ cup (4.2 oz)	10	0	55	0	0
Sugar Free Strawberry Banana as prep	½ cup (4.2 oz)	10	0	50	0	0
Sugar Free Strawberry as prep	½ cup (4.2 oz)	10	0	55	0	0
Sugar Free Strawberry Kiwi as prep	½ cup (4.2 oz)	10	0	60	0	0
Sugar Free Watermelon as prep	½ cup (4.2 oz)	10	0	55	0	0
Watermelon as prep	½ cup (5 oz)	80	0	80	19	0
Wild Strawberry as prep	½ cup (5 oz)	80	0	120	19	0
Kojel						
Diet	1 serv	10	tr	16	4	—
Royal						
Apple	½ cup	80	0	95	19	—
Blackberry	½ cup	80	0	95	19	—
Cherry	½ cup	80	0	95	19	—
Cherry Sugar Free	½ cup	8	0	90	1	—
Concord Grape	½ cup	80	0	130	19	—
Fruit Punch	½ cup	80	0	90	19	—
Lemon	½ cup	80	0	250	19	—
Lemon-Lime	½ cup	80	0	95	19	—
Lime	½ cup	80	0	125	19	—
Lime Sugar Free	½ cup	8	0	100	1	—
Mixed Berry	½ cup	80	0	90	19	—
Orange	½ cup	80	0	95	19	—
Orange Sugar Free	½ cup	10	0	90	1	—
Peach	½ cup	80	0	95	19	—
Pineapple	½ cup	80	0	95	19	—
Raspberry	½ cup	80	0	125	19	—
Raspberry Sugar Free	½ cup	8	0	90	1	—
Strawberry	½ cup	80	0	105	19	—
Strawberry Banana Sugar Free	½ cup	8	0	85	1	—
Strawberry Orange	½ cup	80	0	110	19	—
Strawberry Sugar Free	½ cup	8	0	90	1	—
Tropical Fruit	½ cup	80	0	110	19	—
READY-TO-EAT						
Del Monte						
Gel Snack Cups Blue Berry	1 serv (3.5 oz)	70	0	40	19	tr

FOOD	PORTION	CAL.	FAT	SOD.	CARB.	FIB.
Del Monte (CONT.)						
Gel Snack Cups Cherry	1 serv (3.5 oz)	70	0	40	19	tr
Gel Snack Cups Orange	1 serv (3.5 oz)	70	0	40	19	tr
Gel Snack Cups Strawberry	1 serv (3.5 oz)	70	0	40	19	tr
Handi-Snacks						
Gels Blue Raspberry	1 serv (4 oz)	80	0	45	20	0
Gels Cherry	1 serv (4 oz)	80	0	45	20	0
Gels Orange	1 serv (3.5 oz)	80	0	45	20	0
Gels Strawberry	1 serv (3.5 oz)	80	0	40	20	0
Hunt's						
Snack Pack Juicy Gels Cherry	1 (4 oz)	100	0	42	25	0
Snack Pack Juicy Gels Lemon Lime	1 (4 oz)	100	0	42	25	0
Snack Pack Juicy Gels Mixed Fruit	1 (4 oz)	100	0	42	25	0
Snack Pack Juicy Gels Orange	1 (4 oz)	100	0	42	25	0
Snack Pack Juicy Gels Strawberry	1 (4 oz)	100	0	42	25	0
Jell-O						
Berry Black	1 serv (3.5 oz)	70	0	40	17	0
Berry Blue	1 serv (3.5 oz)	70	0	40	17	0
Cherry	1 serv (3.5 oz)	70	0	40	17	0
Orange	1 serv (3.5 oz)	70	0	40	17	0
Orange Strawberry Banana	1 serv (3.5 oz)	70	0	40	17	0
Raspberry	1 serv (3.5 oz)	70	0	40	17	0
Rhymin' Lymon	1 serv (3.5 oz)	70	0	40	17	0
Strawberry	1 serv (3.5 oz)	70	0	40	17	0
Strawberry Kiwi	1 serv (3.5 oz)	10	0	45	0	0
Sugar Free Orange	1 serv (3.2 oz)	10	0	45	0	0
Sugar Free Raspberry	1 serv (3.2 oz)	10	0	45	0	0
Sugar Free Strawberry	1 serv (3.2 oz)	10	0	45	0	0
Tropical Berry	1 serv (3.5 oz)	10	0	45	0	0
Tropical Fruit Punch	1 serv (3.5 oz)	70	0	40	17	0
Wild Watermelon	1 serv (3.5 oz)	70	0	40	17	0
Kozy Shack						
Gel Treat Cherry	1 pkg (4 oz)	100	0	25	25	1
Gel Treat Lemon Lime	1 pkg (4 oz)	100	0	25	25	1
Gel Treat Orange	1 pkg (4 oz)	100	0	25	25	1
Gel Treat Strawberry	1 pkg (4 oz)	100	0	25	25	1
Gel Treat Sugar Free Orange	1 pkg (4 oz)	10	0	25	2	

FOOD	PORTION	CAL.	FAT	SOD.	CARB.	FIB.
Kozy Shack (CONT.)						
Gel Treat Sugar Free Strawberry	1 pkg (4 oz)	10	0	25	2	1
GIBLETS						
capon simmered	1 cup (5 oz)	238	8	80	0	—
chicken floured & fried	1 cup (5 oz)	402	19	164	6	—
chicken simmered	1 cup (5 oz)	228	7	85	1	—
turkey simmered	1 cup (5 oz)	243	7	85	3	—
GINGER						
ground	1 tsp (1.8 g)	6	tr	1	1	—
root fresh	¼ cup	17	tr	3	4	—
root fresh	5 slices	8	tr	1	2	—
root fresh sliced	¼ cup	17	tr	3	4	—
Ka-Me						
Crystallized Slices	5 pieces (1 oz)	100	0	23	25	1
Sliced	20 pieces (0.5 oz)	0	0	70	0	0
GINKGO NUTS						
canned	1 oz	32	tr	87	6	—
dried	1 oz	99	tr	4	21	—
raw	1 oz	52	tr	1	11	—
GIZZARDS						
chicken simmered	1 cup (5 oz)	222	5	97	2	—
turkey simmered	1 cup (5 oz)	236	6	79	1	—
GOAT						
roasted	3 oz	122	3	73	0	—
GOOSE						
w/ skin roasted	6.6 oz	574	41	132	0	—
w/ skin roasted	½ goose (1.7 lbs)	2362	170	543	0	—
w/o skin roasted	½ goose (1.3 lbs)	1406	75	447	0	—
w/o skin roasted	5 oz	340	18	108	0	—
GOOSEBERRIES						
canned in light syrup	½ cup	93	tr	3	24	—
fresh	1 cup	67	1	1	15	—
GRANOLA						
BARS						
(*see also* CEREAL BARS, NUTRITIONAL SUPPLEMENTS)						
almond	1 (1 oz)	140	7	73	18	—
almond	1 (0.8 oz)	117	6	60	15	—
chewy chocolate coated chocolate chip	1 (1.25 oz)	165	9	71	23	1

FOOD	PORTION	CAL.	FAT	SOD.	CARB.	FIB.
chewy chocolate coated chocolate chip	1 (1 oz)	132	7	57	18	1
chewy chocolate coated peanut butter	1 (1 oz)	144	9	55	15	—
chewy chocolate coated peanut butter	1 (1.3 oz)	187	11	71	20	—
chewy raisin	1 (1 oz)	127	5	80	19	1
chewy raisin	1 (1.5 oz)	191	8	120	28	2
chocolate chip	1 (0.8 oz)	103	4	81	17	1
chocolate chip	1 (1 oz)	124	5	97	20	1
chocolate chip chewy	1 (1.5 oz)	178	7	116	29	2
chocolate chip chewy	1 (1 oz)	119	5	77	10	1
chocolate chip graham & marshmallow chewy	1 (1 oz)	121	4	90	20	1
nut & raisin chewy	1 (1 oz)	129	6	72	18	2
peanut	1 (1 oz)	136	6	79	18	—
peanut	1 (0.8 oz)	113	5	66	15	1
peanut butter	1 (1 oz)	137	7	80	18	—
peanut butter	1 (0.8 oz)	114	6	67	15	—
peanut butter chewy	1 (1 oz)	121	5	116	18	1
peanut butter & chocolate chip chewy	1 (1 oz)	122	6	93	18	1
plain	1 (0.9 oz)	115	4	72	19	1
plain	1 (1 oz)	134	7	83	18	2
plain chewy	1 (1 oz)	126	5	79	19	1
Carnation						
Chocolate Chunk	1 (1.26 oz)	140	5	65	23	1
Honey & Oats	1 (1.26 oz)	130	4	60	23	1
Fi-Bar						
Coconut	1	120	4	30	20	6
Peanut Butter	1	130	4	30	20	6
General Mills						
Nature Valley Cinnnamon	1	120	5	70	17	1
Nature Valley Oat Bran Honey Graham	1	110	4	90	16	1
Nature Valley Oats N'Honey	1	120	5	65	17	1
Nature Valley Peanut Butter	1	120	6	70	15	1
Nature Valley Rice Bran Cinnamon Graham	1	90	4	75	13	1
Grist Mill						
Chewy Apple Cinnamon	1 (1 oz)	120	4	35	21	1

FOOD	PORTION	CAL.	FAT	SOD.	CARB.	FIB.
Grist Mill (CONT.)						
Chewy Chocolate Chip	1 (1 oz)	130	4	30	21	1
Chewy Chunky Nut & Raisin	1 (1 oz)	130	6	35	18	1
Chewy Peanut Butter	1 (1 oz)	130	5	45	20	1
Chewy Peanut Butter Chocolate	1 (1 oz)	130	4	40	20	2
Chocolate Snack Chocolate Chip	1 (1.2 oz)	180	10	60	21	1
Chocolate Snack Nutty Fudge	1 (1.3 oz)	190	11	90	19	2
Crunchy Cinnamon	1 (0.8 oz)	110	5	60	16	1
Crunchy Oats 'N Honey	1 (0.8 oz)	110	5	60	15	1
Hershey						
Chocolate Covered Chocolate Chip	1 (1.2 oz)	170	8	50	22	—
Chocolate Covered Cocoa Creme	1 (1.2 oz)	180	9	50	22	—
Chocolate Covered Cookies & Creme	1 (1.2 oz)	170	8	50	22	—
Chocolate Covered Peanut Butter	1 (1.2 oz)	180	10	65	19	—
Kellogg's						
Low Fat Crunchy Almond & Brown Sugar	1 (0.7 oz)	80	2	60	16	1
Low Fat Crunchy Apple Spice	1 (0.7 oz)	80	2	60	16	1
Low Fat Crunchy Cinnamon Raisin	1 (0.7 oz)	80	2	60	16	1
Kudos						
Chocolate Chunk	1 (0.7 oz)	90	3	60	13	1
Chocolate Coated Chocolate Chip	1 (1 oz)	120	5	75	18	1
Chocolate Coated Milk & Cookies	1 (1 oz)	130	5	70	18	1
Chocolate Coated Nutty Fudge	1 (1 oz)	130	5	65	18	1
Chocolate Coated Peanut Butter	1 (1 oz)	130	5	85	18	1
Low Fat Blueberry	1 (0.7 oz)	90	2	90	15	1
Low Fat Strawberry	1 (0.7 oz)	80	2	90	15	1
New Country						
Chocolate Covered Cookies & Creme	1	200	11	85	23	—

FOOD	PORTION	CAL.	FAT	SOD.	CARB.	FIB.
Quaker						
Chewy Chocolate Chip	1	128	5	90	19	1
Chewy Chunky Nut & Raisin	1	131	6	86	17	2
Chewy Cinnamon Raisin	1	128	5	92	19	1
Chewy Honey & Oats	1	125	4	95	19	1
Chewy Peanut Butter	1	128	5	116	18	1
Chewy Peanut Butter Chocolate Chip	1	131	6	112	17	1
Dipps Caramel Nut	1	148	6	81	21	1
Dipps Chocolate Chip	1	139	6	78	19	1
Dipps Chocolate Fudge	1	160	8	74	20	—
Dipps Peanut Butter	1	170	9	74	9	1
Dipps Peanut Butter Chocolate Chip	1	174	10	102	10	—
Dipps Rocky Road	1	140	7	—	—	—
Sunbelt						
Chewy Chocolate Chip	1 (1.25 oz)	160	7	65	23	2
Chewy Chocolate Chip	1 (1.8 oz)	220	10	95	32	2
Chewy Oats & Honey	1 (1 oz)	130	5	65	19	1
Chewy Oats & Honey	1 (1.7 oz)	210	9	105	32	2
Chewy With Almonds	1 (1 oz)	130	7	60	17	2
Chewy With Almonds	1 (1.5 oz)	190	10	95	25	2
Chewy With Raisins	1 (1.2 oz)	150	6	65	25	2
Fudge Dipped Chewy Chocolate Chip	1 (1.5 oz)	190	8	80	28	2
Fudge Dipped Chewy Macaroo	1 bar (2 oz)	280	17	90	32	3
Fudge Dipped Chewy Macaroo	1 (1.4 oz)	200	13	60	22	2
Fudge Dipped Chewy With Peanuts	1 bar (1.5 oz)	210	12	65	24	2
Fudge Dipped Chewy With Peanuts	1 (2 oz)	270	15	95	32	2
CEREAL						
granola	¼ cup	138	8	3	16	—
Erewhon						
Date Nut	1 oz	130	6	45	17	—
Honey Almond	1 oz	130	6	65	17	—
Maple	1 oz	130	5	55	17	—
Spiced Apple	1 oz	130	6	55	17	—
Sunflower Crunch	1 oz	130	4	60	18	—
With Bran	1 oz	130	6	10	17	4

FOOD	PORTION	CAL.	FAT	SOD.	CARB.	FIB.
Good Shepherd						
Crunchy	1 oz	130	5	15	19	2
Honey Almond	1 oz	120	4	10	20	2
Organic 5 Grain Muesli	1 oz	160	3	55	27	3
Organic Brown Rice	1 oz	130	4	35	16	4
Organic Wheat Free	1 oz	90	3	3	39	2
Organic Wheat Free Apple Cinnamon	1 oz	125	4	35	20	3
Organic Wheat Free Blueberry Amaranth	1 oz	110	1	10	22	2
Organic Wheat Free Strawberry Amaranth	1 oz	110	1	12	22	2
Grist Mill						
Low-Fat With Raisins	⅔ cup (1.9 oz)	220	3	100	42	3
Kellogg's						
Low Fat	½ cup (1.9 oz)	210	3	120	43	3
Low Fat With Raisins	⅔ cup (1.9 oz)	210	3	135	43	3
Natural Valley						
Low Fat Fruit	⅔ cup (1.9 oz)	210	3	210	44	3
Nature Valley						
100% Natural Oat Cinnamon & Raisin	¾ cup (1.9 oz)	240	8	90	38	3
100% Natural Oat Fruit & Nut	⅔ cup (1.9 oz)	250	11	75	34	3
Stone-Buhr						
Hot Apple	⅓ cup (1.6 oz)	153	1	0	31	5
Sun Country						
100% Natural With Almonds	¼ cup	130	5	11	19	1
100% Natural With Raisins & Dates	¼ cup	123	5	9	20	2
With Raisins	¼ cup	125	5	10	19	2
Sunbelt						
Banana Nut	1.9 oz	250	9	60	37	4
Fruit & Nut	1.9 oz	230	7	100	38	4
Low Fat	1.9 oz	200	3	80	42	4
Uncle Roy's						
Cashew Raisin	½ cup (1.6 oz)	180	6	20	32	3
Fat Free Apple Cinnamon	½ cup (1.6 oz)	175	1	20	38	3
Fat Free Wild Cherry	½ cup (1.6 oz)	175	1	20	38	3
Fruit & Nut	½ cup (1.6 oz)	175	5	20	30	3
Low Fat Berries Jubilee	½ cup (1.6 oz)	175	3	20	34	3
Low Fat Crispy	½ cup (1.4 oz)	160	3	20	31	3

FOOD	PORTION	CAL.	FAT	SOD.	CARB.	FIB.
Uncle Roy's (CONT.)						
Low Fat Luscious Raspberry	½ cup (1.6 oz)	175	3	20	34	3
Low Fat True Blueberry	½ cup (1.6 oz)	175	3	20	34	3
Maple Date Nut	½ cup (1.6 oz)	180	6	20	29	3
Nut Butter & Almonds	½ cup (1.6 oz)	195	8	20	29	3
Organic Golden Honey	½ cup (1.6 oz)	190	6	20	30	3
Organic Maple Nut'N Rice	½ cup (1.4 oz)	170	6	20	27	3
Organic Maple Raisin	½ cup (1.6 oz)	190	6	20	30	3
GRAPE JUICE						
bottled	1 cup	155	tr	7	38	—
frzn sweetened as prep	1 cup	128	tr	5	32	—
frzn sweetened not prep	6 oz	386	1	15	96	—
grape drink	6 oz	84	0	12	22	—
BAMA						
Juice	8.45 fl oz	120	0	25	29	—
Bright & Early						
Frozen	8 fl oz	140	0	5	34	—
Capri Sun						
Drink	1 pkg (7 oz)	100	0	20	25	0
Everfresh						
Juice	1 can (8 oz)	150	0	10	38	0
Hawaiian Punch						
Drink	6 oz	90	0	—	—	—
Hi-C						
Box	8.45 fl oz	130	0	30	33	—
Drink	1 can (11.5 fl oz)	180	0	45	46	—
Drink	8 fl oz	130	0	30	32	—
Juice Works						
Drink	6 oz	100	0	—	—	—
Juicy Juice						
Drink	1 box	130	0	10	31	—
Drink	1 bottle (6 fl oz)	90	0	5	22	—
Kool-Aid						
Bursts Grape Drink	1 (7 oz)	100	0	30	25	0
Drink as prep w/ sugar	1 serv (8 oz)	100	0	10	25	0
Drink Mix as prep	1 serv (8 oz)	60	0	0	16	0
Sugar Free Drink Mix as prep	1 serv (8 oz)	5	0	0	0	0
Minute Maid						
Chilled	8 fl oz	130	0	5	33	—
Grape Punch frzn	8 fl oz	130	0	5	32	—

FOOD	PORTION	CAL.	FAT	SOD.	CARB.	FIB.
Minute Maid (CONT.)						
Punch Chilled	8 fl oz	130	0	25	32	—
Mott's						
Drink	10 fl oz	170	0	50	42	0
Fruit Basket Cocktail as prep	8 fl oz	130	0	5	32	0
S&W						
Concord Unsweetened	6 oz	100	0	9	25	—
Seneca						
Blush Grape Juice frzn as prep	8 fl oz	170	0	0	39	0
Fortified With Vitamin C frzn as prep	8 fl oz	170	0	24	39	0
Sweetened frzn as prep	8 fl oz	140	0	24	39	0
White Grape Juice frzn as prep	8 fl oz	140	0	0	33	0
Shasta Plus						
Grape Drink	1 can (11.5 oz)	160	0	45	39	0
Sippin' Pak						
100% Pure	8.45 fl	130	0	25	32	—
Sipps						
Juice	8.45 oz	130	0	—	—	—
Snapple						
Grapeade	8 fl oz	120	0	5	30	—
Tree Top						
Juice	6 oz	120	0	10	30	—
Sparkling Juice	6 oz	120	0	—	29	—
Tropicana						
Season's Best	8 fl oz	160	0	25	39	—
Veryfine						
100%	8 oz	153	0	<20	37	—
Grape Drink	8 oz	130	0	<10	34	—

GRAPE LEAVES

FOOD	PORTION	CAL.	FAT	SOD.	CARB.	FIB.
Cedar's						
Grape Leaves Stuffed With Rice	6 pieces (4.9 oz)	180	8	870	22	8

GRAPEFRUIT

CANNED

FOOD	PORTION	CAL.	FAT	SOD.	CARB.	FIB.
juice pack	½ cup	46	tr	9	11	—
unsweetened	1 cup	93	tr	3	22	—
water pack	½ cup	44	tr	2	11	—

FOOD	PORTION	CAL.	FAT	SOD.	CARB.	FIB.
S&W						
Sections In Light Syrup	½ cup	80	0	0	14	—
Sections Natural Style	½ cup	40	0	—	9	—
Sections Unsweetened	½ cup	40	0	0	9	—
FRESH						
pink	½	37	tr	0	9	1
pink sections	1 cup	69	tr	1	18	1
red	½	37	tr	0	9	—
red sections	1 cup	69	tr	1	18	—
white	½	39	tr	0	10	1
white sections	1 cup	76	tr	0	19	1
Chiquita						
Ruby Red	½ fruit	40	0	—	—	—
Dole						
Grapefruit	½	50	0	0	14	6
Ocean Spray						
Pink	½ med	50	0	0	13	—
White	½ med	45	0	0	12	—

GRAPEFRUIT JUICE

FOOD	PORTION	CAL.	FAT	SOD.	CARB.	FIB.
fresh	1 cup	96	tr	2	23	—
frzn as prep	1 cup	102	tr	2	24	—
frzn not prep	6 oz	302	1	6	72	—
sweetened	1 cup	116	tr	4	28	—
After The Fall						
Pink	1 bottle (10 oz)	100	0	10	23	—
Crystal Geyser						
Juice Squeeze	1 bottle (12 fl oz)	150	0	20	36	—
Del Monte						
Juice	8 fl oz	100	0	20	24	1
Everfresh						
Juice	1 can (8 oz)	90	0	0	22	0
Ruby Red Cocktail	1 can (8 oz)	130	0	0	32	0
Fresh Samantha						
Juice	1 cup (8 oz)	101	0	0	24	tr
Hood						
Select	1 cup (8 oz)	100	0	1	23	—
Minute Maid						
Frozen	8 fl oz	100	0	25	23	—
Juices To Go	1 can (11.5 fl oz)	140	0	40	33	—
Juices To Go	1 bottle (16 fl oz)	100	0	25	23	—
Juices To Go	1 bottle (10 fl oz)	120	0	35	29	—
Juices To Go Pink Cocktail	1 bottle (16 fl oz)	110	0	25	27	—
Juices To Go Pink Cocktail	1 bottle (10 fl oz)	140	0	35	34	—

FOOD	PORTION	CAL.	FAT	SOD.	CARB.	FIB.
Minute Maid (CONT.)						
Juices to Go Pink Cocktail	8 fl oz	160	0	40	39	—
Mott's						
From Concentrate as prep	8 fl oz	120	0	10	27	0
Ocean Spray						
100% Juice	8 oz	100	0	35	24	tr
Lightstyle Low Calorie Pink Cocktail	8 fl oz	40	0	35	9	0
Pink Juice Cocktail	8 oz	110	0	35	28	0
Ruby Red Drink	8 oz	130	0	35	33	0
Odwalla						
Juice	8 fl oz	90	0	5	20	—
S&W						
Unsweetened	6 oz	80	0	—	18	—
Snapple						
Juice	10 fl oz	110	0	45	25	—
Pink Grapefruit Cocktail	8 fl oz	120	0	5	31	—
Tree Of Life						
Juice	8 fl oz	100	0	10	26	0
Tree Top						
Juice	6 oz	80	0	0	19	—
Tropicana						
Juice	8 fl oz	90	0	0	23	—
Juice	1 container (6 fl oz)	80	0	0	19	—
Ruby Red	8 fl oz	100	0	0	25	—
Ruby Red	1 container (10 fl oz)	120	0	0	30	—
Season's Best	1 can (11.5 fl oz)	120	0	5	31	—
Season's Best	8 fl oz	90	0	5	22	—
Season's Best	1 bottle (10 fl oz)	110	0	5	27	—
Season's Best	1 bottle (7 fl oz)	80	0	5	19	—
Twister Light Pink	8 fl oz	40	0	20	10	—
Twister Light Pink	1 container (10 fl oz)	50	0	25	12	—
Twister Pink	1 can (11.5 fl oz)	160	0	30	40	—
Twister Pink	1 container (10 fl oz)	140	0	25	35	—
Twister Pink	8 fl oz	110	0	20	28	—
Veryfine						
100%	8 oz	101	0	<10	23	—

FOOD	PORTION	CAL.	FAT	SOD.	CARB.	FIB.
Veryfine (CONT.)						
Pink	8 oz	120	0	<20	29	—
GRAPES						
CANNED						
thompson seedless in heavy syrup	½ cup	94	tr	7	25	—
thompson seedless water pack	½ cup	48	tr	7	13	—
S&W						
Thompson Seedless Premium	½ cup	100	0	5	25	—
FRESH						
grapes	10	36	tr	1	9	tr
Dole						
Grapes	1½ cup	85	0	3	24	2
GRAVY (*see also* SAUCE)						
CANNED						
au jus	1 cup	38	tr	—	6	—
beef	1 cup	124	6	1305	11	—
beef	1 can (10 oz)	155	7	1630	14	—
chicken	1 cup	189	14	1375	13	—
mushroom	1 cup	120	6	1259	13	—
turkey	1 cup	122	5	—	12	—
Franco-American						
Au Jus	2 oz	10	0	330	2	—
Beef	2 oz	25	1	340	4	—
Chicken	2 oz	45	4	240	3	—
Chicken Giblet	2 oz	30	2	310	3	—
Cream	2 oz	35	2	220	4	—
Mushroom	2 oz	25	1	290	3	—
Pork	2 oz	40	3	330	3	—
Turkey	2 oz	30	2	290	3	—
Gravymaster						
Seasoning	¼ tsp	3	0	14	1	—
Rudy's Farm						
Sausage Gravy	¼ cup (2 oz)	50	1	330	7	0
MIX						
au jus as prep w/ water	1 cup	32	1	964	4	—
brown as prep w/ water	1 cup	75	2	1076	13	—
chicken as prep	1 cup	83	2	1133	14	—
mushroom as prep	1 cup	70	1	1402	14	—

FOOD	PORTION	CAL.	FAT	SOD.	CARB.	FIB.
onion as prep w/ water	1 cup	77	1	1013	16	—
pork as prep	1 cup	76	2	1235	13	—
turkey as prep	1 cup	87	2	1498	15	—
Bournvita						
Extract	2 heaping tsp	34	1	—	7	—
Bovril						
Extract	1 heaping tsp	9	0	—	tr	0
Cajun King						
Oil-Less Roux And Gravy Mix	3.5 oz	394	4	348	78	—
Durkee						
Au Jus as prep	¼ cup	5	0	320	1	0
Brown as prep	¼ cup	10	1	250	3	0
Brown Herb as prep	¼ cup	15	1	350	3	0
Brown Mushroom as prep	¼ cup	15	0	300	3	0
Brown Onion as prpe	¼ cup	15	0	290	4	0
Chicken as prep	¼ cup	20	1	350	4	0
Country as prep	¼ cup	35	2	370	5	0
Homestyle as prep	¼ cup	15	1	240	3	0
Mushroom as prep	¼ cup	15	0	230	3	0
Onion as prep	¼ cup	10	0	310	3	0
Pork as prep	¼ cup	10	0	240	3	0
Sausage as prep	¼ cup	35	2	570	5	0
Swiss Steak as prep	¼ cup	15	0	370	4	0
Turkey as prep	¼ cup	20	0	270	4	0
French's						
Au Jus as prep	¼ cup	5	0	220	1	0
Brown as prep	¼ cup	10	1	250	3	0
Chicken as prep	¼ cup	25	1	250	4	0
Country as prep	¼ cup	35	2	370	5	0
Herb Brown as prep	¼ cup	15	1	350	3	0
Homestyle as prep	¼ cup	10	1	230	3	0
Mushroom as prep	¼ cup	10	1	250	3	0
Onion	¼ cup	15	1	260	4	0
Pork as prep	¼ cup	10	1	250	3	0
Sausage as prep	¼ cup	35	2	570	5	0
Turkey as prep	¼ cup	20	0	270	4	0
Hain						
Brown	¼ pkg	16	0	600	3	—
LaLoma						
Brown Gravy Quik as prep	2 tsp	45	4	150	2	—
Chicken Gravy Quik as prep	2 tsp	45	4	180	2	—

FOOD	PORTION	CAL.	FAT	SOD.	CARB.	FIB.
LaLoma (CONT.)						
Country Quik Gravy as prep	2 tsp	10	tr	200	2	—
Mushroom Quik Gravy as prep	2 tsp	10	tr	160	2	—
Onion Quik Gravy as prep	2 tsp	10	tr	120	2	—
Marmite						
Extract	1 heaping tsp	9	0	—	tr	—
Pillsbury						
Brown	¼ cup	15	0	300	3	—
Chicken	¼ cup	25	1	230	4	—
Home Style	¼ cup	15	0	300	3	—
Weight Watchers						
Brown as prep	¼ cup	5	0	270	0	0
Brown With Mushrooms as prep	¼ cup	10	0	300	2	0
Brown With Onion as prep	¼ cup	10	0	300	2	0
Chicken as prep	¼ cup	10	0	400	1	0
GREAT NORTHERN BEANS						
CANNED						
great northern	1 cup	300	1	11	55	14
Allen						
Great Northern	½ cup (4.5 oz)	100	1	310	19	7
Green Giant						
Great Northern	½ cup	80	1	290	18	5
Hanover						
Great Northern	½ cup	110	0	—	—	—
Trappey						
With Sausage	½ cup (4.5 oz)	100	1	460	18	7
DRIED						
cooked	1 cup	210	1	4	37	—
Bean Cuisine						
Dried	½ cup	115	1	5	—	5
GREEN BEANS						
CANNED						
green beans	½ cup	13	tr	170	3	1
italian	½ cup	13	tr	170	3	1
italian low sodium	½ cup	13	tr	1	3	1
low sodium	½ cup	13	tr	1	3	1
Allen						
Cut	½ cup (4.2 oz)	30	1	320	6	3

FOOD	PORTION	CAL.	FAT	SOD.	CARB.	FIB.
Allen (CONT.)						
Cut No Added Salt	½ cup (4.2 oz)	15	0	10	3	2
French Style	½ cup (4.2 oz)	25	0	300	4	2
Italian	½ cup (4.2 oz)	35	1	320	7	3
Shell Outs	½ cup (4.5 oz)	30	0	460	6	2
Alma						
Cut	½ cup (4.2 oz)	30	1	320	6	3
Crest Top						
Cut	½ cup (4.2 oz)	30	1	320	6	3
Del Monte						
Cut	½ cup (4.3 oz)	20	0	360	4	2
Cut 50% Less Salt	½ cup (4.3 oz)	20	0	180	4	2
Cut Italian	½ cup (4.3 oz)	30	0	360	6	3
Cut No Salt Added	½ cup (4.3 oz)	20	0	10	4	2
French Style	½ cup (4.3 oz)	20	0	360	4	2
French Style 50% Less Salt	½ cup (4.3 oz)	20	0	180	4	2
French Style No Salt Added	½ cup (4.3 oz)	20	0	10	4	2
French Style Seasoned	½ cup (4.3 oz)	20	0	360	4	2
Whole	½ cup (4.3 oz)	20	0	360	4	2
GaBelle						
Cut	½ cup (4.2 oz)	30	1	320	6	3
Green Giant						
Almondine	½ cup	45	3	300	5	2
Cut	½ cup	16	0	300	4	1
French	½ cup	16	0	330	4	1
Kitchen Sliced	½ cup	16	0	280	4	1
Hanover						
Cut	½ cup	20	0	—	—	—
Owatonna						
Cut	½ cup	20	0	—	—	—
French	½ cup	20	0	—	—	—
S&W						
Cut Water Pack	½ cup	20	0	5	4	—
Cut Premium Blue Lake	½ cup	20	0	385	4	—
Dilled	½ cup	60	0	385	15	—
French Style Premium Blue Lake	½ cup	20	0	385	4	—
Green Beans & Wax Beans	½ cup	20	0	385	5	—
Whole Fancy Stringless	½ cup	20	0	385	4	—
Whole Vertical Pack	½ cup	20	0	385	4	—

FOOD	PORTION	CAL.	FAT	SOD.	CARB.	FIB.
Seneca						
Cut	½ cup	20	0	360	6	2
Cuts Natural Pack	½ cup	25	0	0	6	2
French	½ cup	20	0	360	6	2
French Natural Pack	½ cup	25	0	0	6	2
Whole	½ cup	20	0	360	6	2
Sunshine						
Cut	½ cup (4.2 oz)	30	1	320	6	3
Italian	½ cup (4.2 oz)	35	1	320	7	3
FRESH						
cooked	½ cup	22	tr	2	5	—
raw	½ cup	17	tr	3	4	1
FROZEN						
cooked	½ cup	18	tr	9	4	—
italian cooked	½ cup	18	tr	9	4	—
Birds Eye						
Cut	½ cup	25	0	0	6	2
Farm Fresh Whole	¾ cup	30	0	0	7	2
French Cut	½ cup	25	0	0	6	2
In Sauce French Green Beans With Toasted Almonds	½ cup	50	2	340	8	2
Italian	½ cup	30	0	0	7	3
Polybag Cut	½ cup	25	0	0	6	2
Polybag Deluxe Whole	½ cup	20	0	0	4	2
Polybag French Cut	½ cup	25	0	0	6	2
Whole Deluxe	½ cup	45	0	0	5	2
Fresh Like						
Cut	3.5 oz	29	tr	6	7	1
French	3.5 oz	29	tr	6	7	1
Italian	3.5 oz	35	tr	6	8	1
Whole	3.5 oz	29	tr	6	6	1
Green Giant						
Cut	½ cup	16	0	95	4	1
Cut In Butter Sauce	½ cup	30	1	230	4	2
Green Beans	½ cup	14	0	10	4	2
One Serve In Butter Sauce	1 pkg	60	2	370	8	3
Hanover						
Cut	½ cup	20	0	—	—	—
French Style Blue Lake	½ cup	25	0	—	—	—
Italian Cut	½ cup	35	0	—	—	—
Whole Blue Lake	½ cup	30	0	—	—	—

FOOD	PORTION	CAL.	FAT	SOD.	CARB.	FIB.
Southland						
Cut Beans	3 oz	25	0	—	—	—
French	3 oz	25	0	—	—	—
Stouffer's						
Green Bean Mushroom Casserole	½ cup (1.9 oz)	130	8	530	13	2
Tree Of Life						
Green Beans	⅔ cup (2.8 oz)	25	0	10	4	2
SHELF-STABLE						
Pantry Express						
Cut	½ cup	12	0	20	3	1

GREENS

FOOD	PORTION	CAL.	FAT	SOD.	CARB.	FIB.
CANNED						
Allen						
Mixed	½ cup (4.2 oz)	30	1	10	8	4
Sunshine						
Mixed	½ cup (4.2 oz)	30	1	10	8	4

GROUNDCHERRIES

FOOD	PORTION	CAL.	FAT	SOD.	CARB.	FIB.
fresh	½ cup	37	tr	—	8	—

GROUPER

FOOD	PORTION	CAL.	FAT	SOD.	CARB.	FIB.
cooked	1 fillet (7.1 oz)	238	3	107	0	—
cooked	3 oz	100	1	45	0	—
raw	3 oz	78	1	45	0	—

GUANABANA JUICE

FOOD	PORTION	CAL.	FAT	SOD.	CARB.	FIB.
Libby						
Nectar	1 can (11.5 fl oz)	210	0	25	50	—

GUAVA

FOOD	PORTION	CAL.	FAT	SOD.	CARB.	FIB.
fresh	1	45	1	2	11	—
guava sauce	½ cup	43	tr	4	11	—

GUAVA JUICE

FOOD	PORTION	CAL.	FAT	SOD.	CARB.	FIB.
Kern's						
Nectar	6 fl oz	110	0	0	28	—
Libby						
Nectar	6 oz	110	0	15	26	—
Nectar	1 can (11.5 fl oz)	220	0	10	54	—
Snapple						
Guava Mania	8 fl oz	110	0	0	29	—

GUINEA HEN

FOOD	PORTION	CAL.	FAT	SOD.	CARB.	FIB.
w/ skin raw	½ hen (12.1 oz)	545	22	—	0	—
w/o skin raw	½ hen (9.3 oz)	292	7	—	0	—

FOOD	PORTION	CAL.	FAT	SOD.	CARB.	FIB.
HADDOCK						
FRESH						
cooked	1 fillet (5.3 oz)	168	1	131	0	—
cooked	3 oz	95	1	74	0	—
raw	3 oz	74	1	58	0	—
roe raw	3½ oz	130	2	—	2	—
FROZEN						
Gorton's						
Fishmarket Fresh	5 oz	110	1	120	0	—
Microwave Entree Haddock In Lemon Butter	1 pkg	360	21	730	19	—
Mrs. Paul's						
Crunchy Batter Fillets	2 fillets	190	5	580	22	—
Light Fillets	1 fillet	220	9	350	15	—
Van De Kamp's						
Battered Fillets	2 (4 oz)	260	16	530	18	0
Breaded Fillets	2 (3.5 oz)	280	17	310	19	0
Lightly Breaded Fillets	1 (4 oz)	220	10	410	19	0
SMOKED						
smoked	3 oz	99	1	649	0	—
smoked	1 oz	33	tr	214	0	—
HAKE						
raw	3½ oz	84	1	101	0	—
HALIBUT						
FRESH						
atlantic & pacific cooked	½ fillet (5.6 oz)	223	5	110	0	—
atlantic & pacific cooked	3 oz	119	2	59	0	—
atlantic & pacific raw	3 oz	93	2	46	0	—
greenland baked	3 oz	203	15	87	0	—
greenland baked	5.6 oz	380	28	163	0	—
FROZEN						
Van De Kamp's						
Battered Fillets	3 (4 oz)	300	21	520	16	0
HALVA (*see* SESAME)						
HAM (*see also* HAM DISHES, PORK, TURKEY) (FAST FACT: Ham, unlike beef, does not have a lot of marbling. So once the visible fat is trimmed away, you've gotten rid of most of it.)						
boneless 11% fat	3 oz	151	8	—	—	—

FOOD	PORTION	CAL.	FAT	SOD.	CARB.	FIB.
boneless extra lean roasted	3 oz	140	7	—	—	—
canned 13% fat	1 oz	54	4	—	—	—
canned 13% fat	3 oz	192	13	800	tr	—
canned extra lean	1 oz	41	2	—	—	—
canned extra lean	3 oz	142	7	—	—	—
canned extra lean 4% fat	3 oz	116	4	965	tr	—
center slice lean & fat	4 oz	229	15	1566	tr	—
center slice lean only	4 oz	220	9	—	—	—
chopped	1 oz	65	5	389	0	—
chopped canned	1 oz	68	5	387	tr	—
ham & cheese loaf	1 oz	73	6	762	1	—
ham & cheese spread	1 tbsp	37	3	179	tr	—
ham & cheese spread	1 oz	69	5	339	1	—
ham salad spread	1 tbsp	32	2	137	2	—
ham salad spread	1 oz	61	4	259	3	—
minced	1 oz	75	6	353	1	—
patties uncooked	1 (2.3 oz)	206	18	—	—	—
patties grilled	1 patty (2 oz)	203	18	—	—	—
sliced extra lean 5% fat	1 oz	37	1	405	tr	—
sliced regular 11% fat	1 oz	52	3	373	1	—
steak boneless extra lean	1 oz	35	1	360	0	—
whole lean & fat roasted	3 oz	207	14	—	—	—
whole lean only roasted	3 oz	133	5	—	—	—
Alpine Lace						
Boneless Cooked	2 oz	60	2	440	1	0
Armour						
Chopped Ham canned	2 oz	120	9	880	2	—
Deviled Ham canned	1 pkg (3 oz)	200	16	800	0	—
Golden Star Boneless	1 oz	33	1	—	—	—
Golden Star Canned	1 oz	32	tr	—	—	—
Lower Salt 93% Fat Free	1 oz	35	1	221	—	—
Lower Salt Boneless	1 oz	34	1	—	—	—
Star Boneless	1 oz	41	2	—	—	—
Star Canned	1 oz	34	1	—	—	—
Star Speedy Cut	1 oz	44	3	—	—	—
1877 Boneless	1 oz	42	2	—	—	—
Black Label						
Chopped	2 oz	140	11	650	3	0
Carl Buddig						
Ham	1 oz	50	3	400	1	0
Honey Ham	1 oz	50	3	400	1	—
Hansel n'Gretel						
Baked Virginia	1 oz	34	1	245	2	—
Black Forest	1 oz	32	1	—	tr	—

FOOD	PORTION	CAL.	FAT	SOD.	CARB.	FIB.
Hansel n'Gretel (CONT.)						
Cappy	1 oz	31	1	—	1	—
Cooked Fresh	1 oz	33	1	120	tr	—
Deluxe	1 oz	31	1	245	1	—
Honey Valley	1 oz	31	1	260	1	—
Jalapeno	1 oz	25	1	260	1	—
Lessalt	1 oz	30	1	200	1	—
Lessalt Virginia	1 oz	32	1	190	1	—
Light AM	1 oz	27	1	200	1	—
Travane	1 oz	31	1	210	tr	—
Healthy Choice						
Baked Cooked	3 slices (2.2 oz)	70	2	560	1	0
Cooked	3 slices (2.2 oz)	70	2	580	1	0
Deli-Thin Baked Cooked With Natural Juices	6 slices (2 oz)	60	2	500	2	0
Deli-Thin Cooked	6 slices (2 oz)	60	2	510	1	0
Deli-Thin Honey With Natural Juices	6 slices (2 oz)	60	2	540	2	0
Deli-Thin Smoked With Natural Juices	6 slices (2 oz)	60	2	530	1	0
Fresh-Trak Cooked	1 slice (1 oz)	30	1	250	1	0
Fresh-Trak Honey	1 slice (1 oz)	30	1	250	1	0
Honey Boneless	3 oz	100	3	580	5	0
Smoked	3 slices (2.2 oz)	70	2	560	1	0
Variety Pack Regular	3 slice (2.2 oz)	70	2	570	1	0
Hillshire						
Brown Sugar	1 oz	40	2	440	2	—
Cooked Ham	1 oz	30	1	470	tr	—
Deli Select Baked Ham	1 slice	10	tr	95	tr	—
Deli Select Brown Sugar Baked	1 slice	10	tr	90	tr	—
Deli Select Cajun Ham	1 slice	10	tr	120	tr	—
Deli Select Honey Ham	1 slice	10	tr	100	tr	—
Deli Select Lower Salt	1 slice	10	tr	80	tr	—
Deli Select Smoked Ham	1 slice	10	tr	95	tr	—
Flavor Pack 90-99% Fat Free Brown Sugar Baked	1 slice (0.6 oz)	20	tr	170	1	—
Flavor Pack 90-99% Fat Free Honey Ham	1 slice (0.6 oz)	20	tr	180	1	—
Flavor Pack 90-99% Fat Free Smoked	1 slice (0.6 oz)	20	tr	170	tr	—
Genuine Baked	1 oz	35	1	290	1	—
Honey Ham	1 oz	40	2	440	2	—

FOOD	PORTION	CAL.	FAT	SOD.	CARB.	FIB.
Hillshire (CONT.)						
Lower Salt	1 oz	30	1	300	1	—
Lunch 'N Munch Cooked Ham/Swiss	1 pkg (4.5 oz)	360	22	1380	19	—
Lunch 'N Munch Cooked Ham/Swiss Oreo	1 pkg (4.125 oz)	370	21	1160	30	—
Lunch 'N Munch Cooked Ham/Swiss Snickers/ Hi-C	1 pkg (4.25 oz + 6 fl oz)	470	21	1180	54	—
Lunch 'N Munch Honey Ham/ Cheddar/ Snickers/Hi-C	1 pkg (4.25 oz + 6 fl oz)	500	23	1030	56	—
Hormel						
Black Label Canned (refrigerated)	3 oz	100	5	960	0	0
Black Label Canned (self stable)	3 oz	110	5	900	0	0
Canned Chunk	2 oz	90	6	600	0	0
Cure 81 Half Ham	3 oz	100	5	890	0	0
Curemaster	3 oz	80	3	940	0	0
Deli Cooked	1 oz	29	1	344	1	—
Deviled Ham	4 tbsp (2 oz)	150	12	430	1	0
Ham & Cheese Patties	1 patty (2 oz)	190	17	470	0	0
Light & Lean	3 oz	90	3	950	2	0
Light & Lean 97	3 oz	90	3	950	2	0
Light & Lean 97 Cuts	16 pieces (1 oz)	35	1	420	0	0
Light & Lean 97 Sliced	1 slice (1 oz)	25	1	340	0	0
Patties	1 patty (2 oz)	180	17	550	1	0
Primissimo Proscuitti	1 oz	70	5	540	0	0
Spread	4 tbsp (2 oz)	100	11	580	1	0
Supreme Cut Canned	1 oz	31	1	299	tr	—
Jones						
Family Ham	1 slice	40	2	290	tr	—
Ham Slices	1 slice	30	1	200	tr	—
Jordan's						
Healthy Trim 97% Fat Free Cooked	1 slice (1 oz)	30	1	180	2	0
Healthy Trim 97% Fat Free EZ Serve	1 slice (1 oz)	30	1	180	2	0
Healthy Trim 97% Fat Free Virginia	1 slice (1 oz)	30	1	180	2	0
Krakus						
Ham	1 oz	25	1	355	1	—

FOOD	PORTION	CAL.	FAT	SOD.	CARB.	FIB.
Louis Rich						
Carving Board Baked With Natural Juices	2 slices (1.6 oz)	45	1	510	1	0
Carving Board Carved Thin Honey With Natural Juices	6 slices (2.1 oz)	70	2	760	2	0
Carving Board Honey With Natural Juices	2 slices (1.6 oz)	50	2	530	1	0
Carving Board Smoked Cooked With Natural Juices	1 slice (1.6 oz)	50	2	560	0	0
Dinner Slices Baked	1 slice (3.3 oz)	80	2	1150	1	0
Mr. Turkey						
Deli Cuts Honey Cured	3 slices	35	1	300	1	—
Oscar Mayer						
Baked	3 slices (2.2 oz)	60	1	720	2	0
Boiled	3 slices (2.2 oz)	60	3	820	0	0
Chopped	1 slice (1 oz)	50	4	320	1	0
Deli-Thin Boiled	4 slices (1.8 oz)	50	2	680	0	0
Deli-Thin Honey Ham	4 slices (1.8 oz)	60	2	630	2	0
Deli-Thin Smoked	4 slices (1.8 oz)	50	2	620	0	0
Dinner Slice	3 oz	90	3	1030	0	0
Dinner Steaks	1 (2 oz)	60	2	750	0	0
Ham & Cheese Loaf	1 slice (1 oz)	70	5	350	1	0
Healthy Favorites Baked	4 slices (1.8 oz)	50	1	600	1	0
Healthy Favorites Honey Ham	4 slices (1.8 oz)	50	2	630	2	0
Healthy Favorites Smoked Cooked	4 slices (1.8 oz)	50	2	620	0	0
Honey Ham	3 slices (2.2 oz)	70	3	760	2	0
Lower Sodium	3 slices (2.2 oz)	70	3	520	2	0
Lunchables Cookies/ Ham/Swiss	1 pkg (4.2 oz)	360	19	1420	29	tr
Lunchables Dessert Chocolate Pudding/ Ham/American	1 pkg (6.2 oz)	390	20	1540	34	tr
Lunchables Ham/ Cheddar	1 pkg (4.5 oz)	340	20	1830	19	0
Lunchables Ham/Garden Vegetable Cheese	1 pkg (4.5 oz)	380	21	1240	36	1
Lunchables Honey Ham/ Herb & Chive Cheese	1 pkg (4.5 oz)	390	21	1270	37	1
Smoked Cooked	3 slices (2.2 oz)	60	3	750	0	0
Russer						
Baked	2 oz	70	3	750	4	—

FOOD	PORTION	CAL.	FAT	SOD.	CARB.	FIB.
Russer (CONT.)						
Canadian Brand Maple	2 oz	70	2	750	4	—
Chopped	2 oz	130	9	540	5	—
Cooked Ham	2 oz	60	2	650	2	—
Ham & Cheese Loaf	2 oz	120	8	600	5	—
Honey & Maple Cured	2 oz	70	2	550	3	—
Honey Cured	2 oz	60	3	600	2	—
Hot	2 oz	70	2	750	3	—
Light Cooked	2 oz	60	2	400	2	—
Light Smoked	2 oz	60	2	400	2	—
Smoked Virginia	2 oz	70	3	750	3	—
Spiced	2 oz	160	12	540	5	—
Sara Lee						
Bavarian Brand Baked	2 oz	80	4	610	1	—
Bavarian Brand Baked Honey	2 oz	80	4	490	2	—
Golden Cure Smoked	2 oz	80	4	650	1	—
Honey Ham	2 oz	60	2	520	2	—
Honey Roasted	2 oz	90	5	590	3	—
Spreadables						
Ham Salad	¼ can	100	6	—	—	—
Underwood						
Deviled	2.08 oz	220	19	430	tr	—
Deviled Light	2.08 oz	120	8	250	1	—
Deviled Smoked	2.08 oz	190	18	260	tr	—
Weight Watchers						
Deli Thin Oven Roasted	5 slices (⅓ oz)	12	tr	95	tr	—
Deli Thin Oven Roasted Honey Ham	5 slices (⅓ oz)	12	tr	95	tr	—
Deli Thin Premium Smoked	5 slices (⅓ oz)	12	tr	85	tr	—
Oven Roasted Honey Ham	2 slices (¾ oz)	25	1	220	tr	—
Oven Roasted Smoked	2 slices (¾ oz)	25	1	220	tr	—
Premium Cooked	2 slices (¾ oz)	25	1	220	tr	—

HAM DISHES

FROZEN

FOOD	PORTION	CAL.	FAT	SOD.	CARB.	FIB.
Croissant Pocket						
Stuffed Sandwich Ham & Cheddar	1 piece (4.5 oz)	360	17	710	39	5
Hot Pocket						
Stuffed Sandwich Ham & Cheese	1 (4.5 ox)	340	15	840	37	4

FOOD	PORTION	CAL.	FAT	SOD.	CARB.	FIB.
Ovenstuffs						
Ham/Turkey Deli Melt	1 (4.75 oz)	360	15	1050	35	—
TAKE-OUT						
croquettes	1 (3.1 oz)	217	14	475	11	tr
salad	½ cup	287	23	671	5	tr
sandwich w/ cheese	1	353	15	772	33	—

HAMBURGER
(*see also* BEEF)

FOOD	PORTION	CAL.	FAT	SOD.	CARB.	FIB.
FROZEN						
Jimmy Dean						
Burger	1 (2 oz)	220	21	380	0	0
Flamed Broiled Cheeseburger	1 (6.3 oz)	540	34	760	34	1
Mini Cheeseburger	2 (3 oz)	270	14	530	23	1
Kid Cuisine						
Beef Patty Sandwich w/ Cheese	1 (8.5 oz)	410	15	540	58	4
MicroMagic						
Cheeseburger	1 pkg (4.75 oz)	450	25	790	29	—
Hamburger	1 pkg (4 oz)	350	18	500	26	—
Rudy's Farm						
Mild Burger	1 (3 oz)	360	35	730	0	0
White Castle						
Cheeseburger	2 (3.6 oz)	310	17	480	23	6
Hamburger	2 (3.2 oz)	270	14	270	23	5
TAKE-OUT						
double patty w/ bun	1 reg	544	28	554	43	—
double patty w/ cheese & bun	1 reg	457	28	635	22	—
double patty w/ cheese & double bun	1 reg	461	22	892	44	—
double patty w/ cheese ketchup mayonnaise onion pickle tomato & bun	1 reg	416	21	1051	35	—
double patty w/ ketchup mayonnaise onion pickle tomato & bun	1 reg	649	35	920	53	—
double patty w/ ketchup cheese mayonnaise mustard pickle tomato & bun	1 lg	706	44	1149	40	—

FOOD	PORTION	CAL.	FAT	SOD.	CARB.	FIB.
double patty w/ ketchup mustard mayonnaise onion pickle tomato & bun	1 lg	540	27	791	40	—
double patty w/ ketchup mustard onion pickle & bun	1 reg	576	32	742	39	—
single patty w/ bacon ketchup cheese mustard onion pickle & bun	1 lg	609	37	1044	37	—
single patty w/ bun	1 reg	275	12	387	31	—
single patty w/ bun	1 lg	400	23	474	25	—
single patty w/ cheese & bun	1 reg	320	15	500	32	—
single patty w/ cheese & bun	1 lg	608	33	1589	47	—
single patty w/ ketchup cheese ham mayonnaise pickle tomato & bun	1 lg	745	48	1713	38	—
single patty w/ ketchup mustard mayonnaise onion pickle tomato & bun	1 reg	279	13	504	27	—
triple patty w/ cheese & bun	1 lg	769	51	1211	27	—
triple patty w/ ketchup mustard pickle & bun	1 lg	693	41	713	29	—
HAZELNUTS						
dried blanched	1 oz	191	19	1	5	—
dried unblanched	1 oz	179	18	1	4	—
dry roasted unblanched	1 oz	188	19	1	5	—
oil roasted unblanched	1 oz	187	18	1	5	2
Crumpy						
Chocolate Hazelnut Spread	1 tbsp (0.5 oz)	80	5	5	8	0
HEART						
beef simmered	3 oz	148	5	54	tr	—
chicken simmered	1 cup (5 oz)	268	11	69	tr	—
lamb braised	3 oz	158	7	54	2	—
pork braised	1 heart (4.3 oz)	191	7	—	—	—
turkey simmered	1 cup (5 oz)	257	9	79	3	—
veal braised	3 oz	158	6	50	tr	—

FOOD	PORTION	CAL.	FAT	SOD.	CARB.	FIB.
HEARTS OF PALM						
canned	1 cup (5.1 oz)	41	1	622	7	—
canned	1 (1.2 oz)	9	tr	141	2	—
HERBAL TEA						
(*see* TEA/HERBAL TEA)						
HERBS/SPICES						
(*see also individual names*)						
curry powder	1 tsp	6	tr	1	1	—
poultry seasoning	1 tsp	5	tr	tr	1	—
pumpkin pie spice	1 tsp	6	tr	1	1	—
Ac'cent						
Flavor Enhancer	½ tsp	5	0	300	0	0
Herbal All Purpose Seasoning	½ tsp	0	0	0	0	0
Golden Dipt						
All Purpose Seafood	¼ tsp	2	0	85	0	—
Blackened Redfish	¼ tsp	2	0	140	0	—
Broiled Fish	¼ tsp	2	0	125	0	—
Cajun Style Shrimp & Crab	¼ tsp	2	0	200	0	—
Lemon Pepper Seafood	¼ tsp	8	0	115	1	—
Ka-Me						
Five Spice Powder	¼ tsp (1 g)	0	0	0	1	0
Lawry's						
Seasoning Blend Sloppy Joe	1 pkg	126	tr	3442	28	1
McIlhenny						
Crab Boil	3 oz	378	17	95	40	32
Mrs. Dash						
Extra Spicy	⅛ tsp (0.02 oz)	2	0	1	tr	—
Garlic & Herb	⅛ tsp (0.02 oz)	2	tr	tr	tr	—
Lemon & Herb	⅛ tsp (0.02 oz)	2	0	1	tr	—
Low Pepper No Garlic	⅛ tsp (0.02 oz)	2	0	tr	tr	—
Original Blend	⅛ tsp (0.02 oz)	2	0	1	tr	—
Table Blend	⅛ tsp (0.02 oz)	2	0	1	tr	—
Watkins						
Apple Bake Seasoning	¼ tsp (0.5 g)	0	0	0	0	0
Barbecue Spice	¼ tsp (0.5 g)	0	0	30	0	0
Bean Soup Seasoning	¾ tsp (2 g)	5	0	150	1	0
Beef Jerky Seasoning	2 tsp (6 g)	15	0	600	3	0
Chicken Seasoning	½ tsp (1 g)	0	0	110	0	0
Cole Slaw Seasoning	½ tsp (1.5 g)	5	0	190	1	0
Egg Sensations	1 tsp (3 g)	10	0	180	1	0

FOOD	PORTION	CAL.	FAT	SOD.	CARB.	FIB.
Watkins (CONT.)						
Fajita Seasoning	½ tsp (3 g)	10	0	0	2	0
Grill Seasoning	¼ tsp (1 g)	0	0	210	0	0
Ground Beef Seasoning	⅛ tsp (0.5 g)	0	0	70	0	0
Italian Blend	1 tsp (3 g)	1	0	120	2	0
Meat Tenderizer	⅛ tsp (0.5 g)	0	0	140	0	0
Meatloaf Seasoning	½ tsp (5 g)	15	0	270	4	0
Mexican Blend	½ tbsp (4 g)	15	0	90	3	0
Omelet & Souffle Seasoning	¾ tsp (2 g)	5	0	110	1	0
Oriental Ginger Garlic Liquid Spice Blend	1 tbsp (0.5 oz)	120	14	0	0	0
Potato Salad Seasoning	¼ tsp (1 g)	0	0	135	0	0
Pumpkin Pie Spice	¼ tsp (0.5 g)	0	0	0	0	0
Smokehouse Liquid Blend	1 tbsp (0.5 oz)	120	14	0	0	0
Soup & Vegetable Seasoning	¼ tsp (0.5 g)	0	0	70	0	0
Spanish Seasoning Blend	¼ tsp (0.5 oz)	0	0	0	0	0

HERRING

FOOD	PORTION	CAL.	FAT	SOD.	CARB.	FIB.
CANNED						
roe	3.5 oz	118	3	—	tr	—
FRESH						
atlantic cooked	1 fillet (5 oz)	290	17	165	0	—
atlantic cooked	3 oz	172	10	98	0	—
atlantic raw	3 oz	134	8	76	0	—
pacific baked	3 oz	213	15	81	0	—
pacific fillet baked	5.1 oz	360	26	137	0	—
roe raw	3½ oz	130	2	—	2	—
TAKE-OUT						
atlantic kippered	1 fillet (1.4 oz)	87	5	367	0	—
atlantic pickled	½ oz	39	3	131	1	—

HICKORY NUTS

FOOD	PORTION	CAL.	FAT	SOD.	CARB.	FIB.
dried	1 oz	187	18	0	5	—

HOMINY

FOOD	PORTION	CAL.	FAT	SOD.	CARB.	FIB.
CANNED						
canned	½ cup	57	tr	168	11	—
Allen						
Golden	½ cup (4.5 oz)	120	1	340	27	4
Mexican	½ cup (4.5 oz)	120	1	340	25	3
White	½ cup (4.5 oz)	100	1	340	22	4

FOOD	PORTION	CAL.	FAT	SOD.	CARB.	FIB.
Uncle William						
Golden	½ cup (4.5 oz)	120	1	340	27	4
Mexican	½ cup (4.5 oz)	120	1	340	25	3
White	½ cup (4.5 oz)	100	1	340	22	4
Van Camp's						
Golden	½ cup (4.3 oz)	80	1	540	17	1
White	½ cup (4.3 oz)	80	1	530	15	1
HONEY						
honey	1 tbsp (0.7 oz)	64	0	1	17	—
honey	1 cup (11.9 oz)	1031	0	12	279	—
Burleson's						
Clover	1 tbsp	60	0	1	16	0
Creamed	1 tbsp	60	0	1	16	0
Natural	1 tbsp	60	0	1	16	0
Pure	1 tbsp	60	0	1	16	0
Raw	1 tbsp	60	0	1	16	0
Rocky Mountain Clover	1 tbsp	60	0	1	16	0
Golden Blossom						
Honey	1 tsp	20	0	tr	5	—
Smucker's						
Single Serving	½ oz	45	0	—	11	—
Tree Of Life						
Alfalfa	1 tbsp (0.7 oz)	60	0	0	17	—
Avocado	1 tbsp (0.7 oz)	60	0	0	17	—
Buckwheat	1 tbsp (0.7 oz)	60	0	0	17	—
Clover	1 tbsp (0.7 oz)	60	0	0	17	—
Honeybear Wildflower	1 tbsp (0.7 oz)	60	0	0	17	—
Orange	1 tbsp (0.7 oz)	60	0	0	17	—
Tupelo	1 tbsp (0.7 oz)	60	0	0	17	—
Wildflower	1 tbsp (0.7 oz)	60	0	0	17	—
HONEYDEW						
FRESH						
cubed	1 cup	60	tr	17	16	—
wedge	1/10	46	tr	13	12	—
Chiquita						
Fresh	1 cup	70	0	—	—	—
Dole						
Honeydew	1/10	50	0	50	12	1
FROZEN						
Big Valley						
Balls	¾ cup (4.9 oz)	45	0	16	11	1
HORSE						
roasted	3 oz	149	5	47	0	—

FOOD	PORTION	CAL.	FAT	SOD.	CARB.	FIB.
HORSERADISH						
Gold's						
Hot	1 tsp	4	tr	60	tr	—
Red	1 tsp	4	0	75	tr	—
White	1 tsp	4	tr	55	tr	—
Hebrew National						
White	1 tbsp	7	0	160	1	—
Heluva Good Cheese						
Horseradish	1 tsp (5 g)	0	0	6	0	—
Ka-Me						
Wasabi Powder	¼ tsp (1 g)	0	0	0	1	0
Kraft						
Cream Style	1 tsp (5 g)	0	0	50	0	0
Horseradish Sauce	1 tsp (5 g)	20	2	35	tr	0
Prepared	1 tsp (5 g)	0	0	50	0	0
Rosoff's						
Red	1 tbsp (0.5 oz)	8	0	160	2	—
White	1 tbsp (0.5 oz)	7	0	160	1	—
Schorr's						
Red	1 tbsp (0.5 oz)	8	0	160	2	—
White	1 tbsp (0.5 oz)	7	0	160	1	—

HOT CAKES

(*see* PANCAKES)

HOT COCOA

(*see* COCOA)

HOT DOG

(*see also* MEAT SUBSTITUTES, SAUSAGE, SAUSAGE SUBSTITUTES)

(FAST FACT: Although hot dogs are processed meat, they should not be eaten uncooked. Cooking the hot dogs until they are steaming hot throughout will kill the bacteria.)

FOOD	PORTION	CAL.	FAT	SOD.	CARB.	FIB.
beef	1 (2 oz)	180	16	585	1	—
beef	1 (1.5)	142	13	462	1	—
beef & pork	1 (2 oz)	183	17	639	1	—
beef & pork	1 (1.5 oz)	144	13	504	1	—
chicken	1 (1.5 oz)	116	9	617	3	—
pork cheesefurter smokie	1 (1.5 oz)	141	12	465	1	—
turkey	1 (1.5 oz)	102	8	642	1	—
Armour						
Lower Salt Jumbo	1	170	15	450	—	—
Lower Salt Jumbo Beef	1	170	15	460	—	—
Star Jumbo	1	190	18	590	—	—
Star Jumbo Beef	1	190	18	590	—	—

FOOD	PORTION	CAL.	FAT	SOD.	CARB.	FIB.
Chefwich						
Chili Dog	5 oz	380	15	—	—	—
Empire						
Chicken	1 (2 oz)	100	7	465	1	0
Turkey	1 (2 oz)	90	6	410	1	0
Health Valley						
Weiners	1	96	8	90	1	0
Weiners Turkey	1	96	8	112	1	0
Healthy Choice						
Beef	1 (1.8 oz)	60	2	480	5	0
Bunsize	1 (2 oz)	70	2	590	5	0
Franks	1 (1.6 oz)	50	2	450	4	0
Jumbo	1 (2 oz)	70	2	570	5	0
Hebrew National						
Beef	1 (1.7 oz)	150	14	370	—	—
Cocktail Beef	6 (1.8 oz)	160	15	410	—	—
Dinner Beef	1 (4 oz)	350	34	890	—	—
Reduced Fat Beef	1 (1.7 oz)	120	10	350	—	—
Hillshire						
Franks Bun Size Beef	2 oz	180	16	560	2	—
Light & Mild Franks Jumbo	1 link	110	8	570	2	—
Light & Mild Wieners	1 link	90	7	580	2	—
Lit'l Franks Beef	2 oz	180	16	580	1	—
Lit'l Wieners	2 oz	180	16	560	2	—
Weiners Natural Casing	2 oz	180	17	470	2	—
Wieners Bun Size	2 oz	180	16	550	2	—
Hormel						
Big 8	1 (2 oz)	170	15	480	1	0
Light & Lean 97	1 (1.6 oz)	45	1	490	4	0
Light & Lean 97 Beef	1 (1.6 oz)	45	1	490	4	—
Jordan's						
Healthy Trim Low Fat	1 (1.8 oz)	70	3	350	3	0
Healthy Trim Low Fat Skinless	1 (1.8 oz)	70	3	350	3	0
Louis Rich						
Bun Length	1 (2 oz)	110	8	630	2	0
Turkey	1 (1.6 oz)	90	7	500	1	0
Turkey	1 (1.5 oz)	80	6	480	1	0
Turkey Cheese	1 (1.6 oz)	90	7	490	2	0
Mr. Turkey						
Bun Size	1	130	11	670	2	—
Cheese	1	140	12	670	2	—
Hot Dog	1	110	9	540	2	—

FOOD	PORTION	CAL.	FAT	SOD.	CARB.	FIB.
Nathan's						
Natural Casing Franks	1	158	14	422	1	—
Skinless Franks	1	176	16	463	1	—
Oscar Mayer						
Beef	1 (1.6 oz)	150	13	450	1	0
Big & Juicy Deli Style Beef	1 (2.7 oz)	250	23	680	1	0
Big & Juicy Hot 'N Spicy	1 (2.7 oz)	220	20	770	1	0
Big & Juicy Original	1 (2.7 oz)	240	23	690	0	0
Big & Juicy Original Beef	1 (2.7 oz)	230	21	700	1	0
Big & Juicy Quarter Pound Beef	1 (4 oz)	350	32	1050	2	0
Big & Juicy Smokie Links	1 (2.7 oz)	200	18	770	1	0
Bun-Length Beef	1 (2 oz)	180	17	570	1	0
Cheese	1 (1.6 oz)	150	14	450	1	0
Free	1 (1.8 oz)	40	0	460	2	—
Healthy Favorites Turkey & Beef	1 (2 oz)	60	2	570	2	0
Light Beef	1 (2 oz)	110	8	620	2	0
Wieners Bun-Length Pork & Turkey	1 (2 oz)	180	17	570	1	0
Wieners Little	6 (2 oz)	170	16	540	1	0
Wieners Pork & Turkey	1 (1.6 oz)	150	13	450	1	0
Wieners Light Pork Turkey Beef	1 (2 oz)	110	8	580	2	0
Russer						
Lil'Salt Deli Franks	1 (2.67 oz)	160	11	640	3	—
Shofar						
Kosher Beef	1 (1.8 oz)	150	14	370	0	0
Kosher Beef Reduced Fat Reduced Sodium	1 (1.8 oz)	120	10	360	0	0
Tyson						
Chicken Cheese	1	145	11	680	1	—
Chicken Hot Dog	1	115	10	700	1	—
Wampler Longacre						
Chicken	1 (1.6 oz)	110	9	400	0	—
Chicken	1 (2 oz)	130	11	440	0	—
Turkey	1 (2 oz)	130	11	440	0	—
Turkey	1 (1.6 oz)	110	9	400	0	—
Wrangler						
Beef	1 (2 oz)	170	15	530	1	0
Cheese	1 (2 oz)	170	15	550	1	0
Smoked	1 (2 oz)	170	15	530	1	0

FOOD	PORTION	CAL.	FAT	SOD.	CARB.	FIB.
TAKE-OUT						
corndog	1	460	19	972	56	—
w/ bun chili	1	297	13	480	31	—
w/ bun plain	1	242	15	671	18	—
HUMMUS						
hummus	1 cup	420	21	599	50	—
Athenos						
Roasted Red Pepper	2 tbsp (1.1 oz)	60	4	210	6	1
Casbah						
Mix as prep	¼ cup	120	5	180	15	1
Cedar's						
No Salt Added Hommus Tahini	2 tbsp (1 oz)	50	2	70	5	3
TAKE-OUT						
hummus	⅓ cup	140	7	200	17	—
HYACINTH BEANS						
dried cooked	1 cup	228	1	13	40	—

ICE CREAM AND FROZEN DESSERTS

(*see also* ICES AND ICE POPS, PUDDING POPS, SHERBET, YOGURT FROZEN)

(FAST FACT: A national poll conducted by an ice cream company found that 88 percent of Americans reached for ice cream during times of stress. Chocolate was the favorite of those age 24 to 54 and butter pecan and other nut flavors preferred by those over 55. Three fourths of those polled chose ice cream, vanilla for men, women chocolate, after an amorous interlude.)

FOOD	PORTION	CAL.	FAT	SOD.	CARB.	FIB.
chocolate	½ cup (4 fl oz)	143	7	50	19	—
dixie cup chocolate	1 (3.5 fl oz)	125	6	44	16	—
dixie cup strawberry	1 (3.5 fl oz)	112	5	35	16	—
dixie cup vanilla	1 (3.5 fl oz)	116	6	46	14	—
freeze dried ice cream chocolate strawberry & vanilla	1 pkg (0.75 oz)	158	5	97	24	1
french vanilla soft serve	½ gal	3014	180	1228	306	—
french vanilla soft serve	½ cup (4 fl oz)	185	11	52	19	—
strawberry	½ cup (4 fl oz)	127	6	40	18	—
vanilla	½ cup (4 fl oz)	132	7	53	16	—
vanilla light	½ cup (2.3 oz)	92	3	56	15	—
vanilla rich	½ cup (2.6 oz)	178	12	41	17	—
vanilla soft serve	½ cup	111	2	62	19	—
vanilla 10% fat	½ gal	2153	115	929	254	—
vanilla 16% fat	½ gal	2805	190	868	256	—

FOOD	PORTION	CAL.	FAT	SOD.	CARB.	FIB.
vanilla light	1 cup	184	6	105	29	—
vanilla light	½ gal	1469	45	836	232	—
vanilla light soft serve	½ gal	1787	37	1303	307	—
vanilla light soft serve	1 cup	223	5	163	38	—
3 Musketeers						
Single Chocolate	1 (2 fl oz)	160	10	30	16	0
Single Vanilla	1 (2 fl oz)	160	10	30	16	0
Snack Chocolate	1 (0.72 fl oz)	60	4	10	6	0
Snack Vanilla	1 (0.72 fl oz)	60	4	10	6	0
Avari						
Creme Glace All Flavors	1 oz	10	0	35	3	—
Ben & Jerry's						
Banana Walnut	½ cup (3.9 oz)	290	21	50	26	1
Butter Pecan	½ cup (3.9 oz)	310	26	160	20	1
Cherry Garcia	½ cup (3.7 oz)	240	16	60	25	0
Cherry Vanilla	½ cup (3.9 oz)	240	15	60	26	0
Chocolate Chip Cookie Dough	½ cup (3.7 oz)	270	17	95	30	0
Chocolate Fudge Brownie	½ cup (3.7 oz)	250	14	100	31	2
Chunky Monkey	½ cup (3.7 oz)	280	19	50	29	1
Coconut Almond	½ cup (3.7 oz)	260	20	80	19	1
Coconut Almond Fudge Chip	½ cup (3.8 oz)	320	25	85	24	2
Coffee Almond Fudge	½ cup (3.7 oz)	290	20	85	24	2
Coffee Toffee Crunch	½ cup (3.7 oz)	280	19	120	28	0
English Toffee Crunch	½ cup (4 oz)	310	21	130	30	0
Mint Chocolate Cookie	½ cup (3.8 oz)	260	17	120	27	1
New York Super Fudge Chunk	½ cup (3.7 oz)	290	20	55	28	2
No Fat Strawberry	½ cup (3.3 oz)	140	0	60	31	0
No Fat Vanilla Fudge Swirl	½ cup (3.1 oz)	150	0	80	32	0
Peanut Butter Cup	½ cup (4.1 oz)	370	26	140	30	2
Pop Chocolate Chip Cookie Dough	1 (4.1 oz)	450	28	150	48	1
Pop English Toffee Crunch	1 (3.7 oz)	340	23	55	35	0
Pop Vanilla	1 (3.9 oz)	360	28	75	30	0
Rain Forest Crunch	½ cup (3.7 oz)	300	23	140	24	0
Smooth Aztec Harvest Coffee	½ cup (3.8 oz)	230	16	55	22	0
Smooth Deep Dark Chocolate	½ cup (3.9 oz)	260	15	55	32	2

FOOD	PORTION	CAL.	FAT	SOD.	CARB.	FIB.
Ben & Jerry's (CONT.)						
Smooth Double Chocolate Fudge	½ cup (4.1 oz)	280	16	60	35	3
Smooth Mocho Fudge	½ cup (4 oz)	270	18	65	30	1
Smooth Vanilla	½ cup (3.8 oz)	230	17	55	21	0
Smooth Vanilla Bean	½ cup (3.8 oz)	230	17	55	21	0
Smooth Vanilla Caramel Fudge	½ cup (4.1 oz)	280	17	75	33	1
Smooth White Russian	½ cup (3.8 oz)	240	16	55	23	0
Vanilla	½ cup (3.7 oz)	230	17	55	21	0
Wavy Gravy	½ cup (4.1 oz)	330	24	95	29	2
Bon Bons						
Vanilla With Milk Chocolate Coating	5 pieces	200	14	35	17	0
Vanilla With Milk Chocolate Coating	8 pieces	330	23	60	27	0
Borden						
Buttered Pecan	½ cup	180	12	65	16	—
Chocolate Swirl	½ cup	130	6	65	18	—
Dutch Chocolate Olde Fashioned Recipe	½ cup	130	6	65	16	—
Fat Free Black Cherry	½ cup	90	tr	40	21	—
Fat Free Chocolate	½ cup	100	tr	50	21	—
Fat Free Peach	½ cup	90	tr	40	21	—
Fat Free Strawberry	½ cup	90	tr	40	21	—
Fat Free Vanilla	½ cup	90	tr	50	20	—
Ice Milk Chocolate	½ cup	100	2	80	18	—
Ice Milk Strawberry	½ cup	90	2	65	17	—
Ice Milk Vanilla	½ cup	90	2	65	17	—
Strawberries 'N Cream Olde Fashioned Recipe	½ cup	130	5	55	19	—
Strawberry	½ cup	130	6	55	18	—
Sundae Cone	1	210	12	110	23	—
Vanilla Olde Fashioned Recipe	½ cup	130	7	55	15	—
Bounty						
Cherry/Dark	1 (0.84 fl oz)	70	5	20	8	0
Coconut/Dark	1 (0.84 fl oz)	70	5	20	7	0
Coconut/Milk	1 (0.84 fl oz)	70	5	20	7	0
Bresler's						
All Flavors Ice Cream	3.5 oz	230	12	—	23	—
All Flavors Royale Cremes	4 oz	260	16	—	24	—

FOOD	PORTION	CAL.	FAT	SOD.	CARB.	FIB.
Bresler's (CONT.)						
All Flavors Royale Lites	4 oz	217	0	—	49	—
Breyers						
Bar Vanilla	1 (2.7 oz)	250	17	45	21	tr
Bar Vanilla Carmel w/ Chocolate Brittle Coating	1 (2.7 oz)	260	15	65	26	0
Bar Vanilla With Chocolate Coating	1 (2.6 oz)	230	15	45	20	0
Butter Almond	½ cup	170	11	120	15	0
Butter Pecan	½ cup (2.6 oz)	180	12	125	15	0
Cherry Vanilla	½ cup	150	7	40	17	0
Chocolate	½ cup (2.6 oz)	160	8	30	19	1
Chocolate Chip	½ cup (2.5 oz)	170	10	40	18	0
Chocolate Chip Cookie Dough	½ cup (2.5 oz)	190	10	45	20	0
Chocolate Chocolate Chip	½ cup (2.5 oz)	180	10	30	21	1
Chocolate Peanut Butter Twirl	½ cup (2.6 oz)	220	13	75	20	1
Coffee	½ cup (2.6 oz)	150	8	45	15	0
Cookies n'Cream	½ cup (2.6 oz)	170	9	55	19	0
Deluxe Rocky Road	½ cup (2.5 oz)	190	9	30	24	1
French Vanilla	(2.5 oz)	170	10	45	15	0
Light Brownie Marble Fudge	½ cup (2.6 oz)	150	5	55	23	tr
Light Chocolate	½ cup (2.4 oz)	130	4	55	19	tr
Light Chocolate Fudge Twirl	½ cup (2.6 oz)	140	4	55	22	1
Light Heavenly Hash	½ cup (2.4 oz)	150	5	55	22	tr
Light Rocky Road Deluxe	½ cup (2.4 oz)	150	5	50	22	tr
Light Strawberry	½ cup (2.4 oz)	120	4	45	18	0
Light Toffee Fudge Parfait	½ cup (2.6 oz)	150	5	55	23	tr
Light Vanilla	½ cup (2.4 oz)	130	5	55	18	0
Light Vanilla Chocolate Strawberry	½ cup (2.4 oz)	120	4	50	18	0
Mint Chocolate Chip	½ cup (2.6 oz)	170	10	40	18	0
Mocha Almond Fudge	½ cup (2.7 oz)	190	10	45	20	1
Peach	½ cup (2.6 oz)	130	6	30	18	0
Reduced Fat Chocolate Chocolate Chip	½ cup (2.4 oz)	150	5	50	21	tr
Reduced Fat Heavenly Hash	½ cup (2.4 oz)	150	5	55	22	tr

FOOD	PORTION	CAL.	FAT	SOD.	CARB.	FIB.
Breyers (CONT.)						
Reduced Fat Mocha Almond Fudge	½ cup (2.5 oz)	160	6	55	20	tr
Reduced Fat Praline Almond Crunch	½ cup (2.4 oz)	140	5	70	20	tr
Reduced Fat Swiss Almond Fudge Twirl	½ cup (2.5 oz)	160	6	55	22	tr
Sandwich Vanilla	1 (2.8 oz)	250	11	160	32	1
Strawberry	½ cup (2.6 oz)	130	6	35	15	0
Toffee Bar Crunch	½ cup (2.5 oz)	180	11	65	18	0
Vanilla	½ cup (2.6 oz)	150	8	45	15	0
Vanilla Caramel Praline	½ cup (2.6 oz)	190	10	90	23	0
Vanilla Chocolate	½ cup (2.5 oz)	160	8	35	17	0
Vanilla Chocolate Strawberry	½ cup (2.5 oz)	150	8	35	16	0
Vanilla Fudge Twirl	½ cup (2.6 oz)	160	8	50	19	tr
Vanilla Peanut Butter Fudge Sundae	½ cup (2.5 oz)	170	9	65	18	0
Butterfinger						
Bar	1 (2.5 oz)	170	12	40	14	0
Nuggets	8	340	24	65	29	0
Carnation						
Berry Swirl Bar Raspberry	1 bar	70	3	—	—	—
Berry Swirl Bar Strawberry	1 bar	70	3	—	—	—
Cheesecake Bar Original	1 bar	120	6	—	—	—
Cheesecake Bar Strawberry	1 bar	125	6	—	—	—
Chocolate Malted Bar	1 bar	70	3	—	—	—
Creamy Lites Bar Chocolate	1 bar	50	2	—	—	—
Creamy Lites Bar Strawberry	1 bar	50	2	—	—	—
Sundae Cup Strawberry	1 (3.3 oz)	200	8	55	29	0
Chiquita						
Cherry & Ice Cream Swirl	1 bar	80	3	—	—	—
Mixed Berry & Ice Cream Swirl	1 bar	80	3	—	—	—
Orange & Ice Cream Swirl	1 bar	80	3	—	—	—
Raspberry & Ice Cream Swirl	1 bar	80	3	—	—	—

FOOD	PORTION	CAL.	FAT	SOD.	CARB.	FIB.
Chiquita (CONT.)						
Strawberry & Ice Cream Swirl	1 bar	80	3	—	—	—
Cool Creations						
Cookies & Cream Sandwich	1 (3.5 oz)	240	11	250	34	1
Mini Sandwich	1 (2.3 oz)	110	5	70	16	0
DoveBar						
Almond	1 (3.67 fl oz)	335	22	75	30	0
Bite Size Almond Praline	1 (0.75 fl oz)	80	5	15	8	0
Bite Size Cherry Royale	1 (0.75 fl oz)	70	5	10	8	0
Bite Size Classic Vanilla	1 (0.75 fl oz)	70	5	10	7	0
Bite Size French Vanilla	1 (0.75 fl oz)	70	5	10	7	0
Bite Size Mint Supreme	1 (0.75 fl oz)	80	5	5	8	0
Caramel Pecan	1 (3.67 fl oz)	350	35	85	35	0
Chocolate Milk Chocolate	1 (3.8 fl oz)	340	21	80	35	0
Coffee Cashew	1 (3.67 fl oz)	335	22	55	31	0
Crunchy Cookie	1 (3.8 fl oz)	340	21	65	35	0
Peanut	1 (3.8 fl oz)	380	25	100	35	0
Single Vanilla/Dark	1 (2 fl oz)	200	12	50	24	0
Vanilla Dark Chocolate	1 (3.8 fl oz)	340	22	65	34	0
Vanilla Milk Chocolate	1 (3.8 fl oz)	340	21	60	34	0
Drumstick						
Cone Chocolate	1 (4.6 oz)	340	19	95	37	2
Cone Chocolate Dipped	1 (4.6 oz)	340	17	95	41	1
Cone Vanilla	1 (4.6 oz)	350	20	95	36	2
Cone Vanilla Caramel	1 (4.6 oz)	360	20	100	39	6
Cone Vanilla Fudge	1 (4.6 oz)	370	21	105	40	2
Eagle Brand						
Vanilla	½ cup	150	9	55	16	—
Edy's						
American Dream Chocolate	3 oz	90	1	45	20	—
American Dream Chocolate Chip	3 oz	100	1	45	22	—
American Dream Cookies'N'Cream	3 oz	100	1	45	22	—
American Dream Mocha Almond Fudge	3 oz	110	1	45	24	—
American Dream Rocky Road	3 oz	110	1	45	24	—
American Dream Strawberry	3 oz	70	tr	40	16	—

FOOD	PORTION	CAL.	FAT	SOD.	CARB.	FIB.
Edy's (CONT.)						
American Dream Toasted Almond	3 oz	110	1	45	24	—
American Dream Vanilla	3 oz	80	tr	45	18	—
American Dream Vanilla Chocolate Strawberry	3 oz	80	1	45	18	—
Light Almond Praline	4 oz	140	5	50	18	—
Light Banana-Politan	4 oz	110	4	50	15	—
Light Butter Pecan	4 oz	140	5	50	18	—
Light Cafe Au Lait	4 oz	110	4	50	13	—
Light Candy Bar	4 oz	140	5	50	20	—
Light Chocolate Chip	4 oz	120	4	50	16	—
Light Chocolate Fudge Mousse	4 oz	130	5	50	18	—
Light Cookies'N'Cream	4 oz	120	5	50	18	—
Light Dreamy Caramel Cream	4 oz	140	4	50	16	—
Light Malt Ball 'N' Fudge	4 oz	140	5	50	20	—
Light Marble Fudge	4 oz	120	4	50	15	—
Light Mocha Almond Fudge	4 oz	140	5	50	19	—
Light Peanut Butter & Chocolate	4 oz	130	5	50	19	—
Light Raspberry Truffle	4 oz	110	5	50	19	—
Light Rocky Road	4 oz	130	5	50	17	—
Light Strawberry	4 oz	110	4	50	15	—
Light Vanilla	4 oz	100	4	50	13	—
Vanilla Chocolate Strawberry	4 oz	110	4	50	14	—
Fi-Bar						
Banana Cream	1 bar	93	tr	—	21	—
Cocoa-Fudge 'N Cream	1 bar	93	tr	—	21	—
Raspberries 'N Cream	1 bar	93	tr	—	21	—
Wildberry Cream	1 bar	93	tr	—	21	—
Flintstones						
Cool Cream	1 (2.75 oz)	90	2	30	18	0
Push-Up	1 (2.75 oz)	100	2	25	20	0
Friendly's						
Black Raspberry	½ cup	150	7	35	17	0
Chocolate Almond Chip	½ cup	170	10	45	18	0
Forbidden Chocolate	½ cup	150	9	40	14	0
Fudge Nut Brownie	½ cup	200	11	60	23	0
Heath English Toffee	½ cup (2.7 oz)	190	10	240	24	0
Purely Pistachio	½ cup	160	10	50	16	0

FOOD	PORTION	CAL.	FAT	SOD.	CARB.	FIB.
Friendly's (CONT.)						
Vanilla	½ cup	150	8	40	16	0
Vanilla Chocolate Strawberry	½ cup	150	8	35	16	tr
Vienna Mocha Chunk	½ cup	180	11	50	19	0
Frusen Gladje						
Butter Pecan	½ cup	280	21	160	16	—
Chocolate	½ cup	240	17	65	17	—
Good Humor						
Banana Bob	1 (3 fl oz)	155	7	55	22	0
Bar Classic Toasted Almond	1 (3.1 fl oz)	170	9	40	22	1
Bar Classic Vanilla	1 (3.1 fl oz)	190	10	35	22	0
Bar Classic Almond	1 (3.1 fl oz)	210	12	50	21	1
Bar Sidewalk Sundae	1	280	20	65	21	2
Bubble O'Bill	1 (3.6 fl oz)	170	10	45	20	1
Bubble Play	1	110	1	5	25	—
Chip Burrrger	1 (4.7 oz)	320	15	190	44	1
Chip Sandwich	1 (4.7 fl oz)	320	15	190	44	1
Choco Taco	1 (4.4 fl oz)	320	17	100	38	1
Chocolate Eclair Classic	1 (3.1 fl oz)	170	9	60	21	1
Classic Candy Center Crunch Vanilla	1	280	21	75	21	0
Colonel Crunch Chocolate	1 (3.1 oz)	160	7	60	21	1
Colonel Crunch Strawberry	1 (3.1 oz)	170	8	45	22	0
Combo Cup	1 (6.2 fl oz)	200	10	65	25	1
Cone Olde Nut Sundae	1 (3.9 oz)	230	9	100	32	2
Cone Sidewalk Sundae	1 (4.2 oz)	270	14	125	31	1
Creamee Burrrger	1 (4.7 oz)	310	17	150	40	1
Crunch Classic Candy Center	1 (3.1 fl oz)	260	19	60	21	1
Dinosaur Bar	1	110	2	5	25	—
Far Frog	1 (3.6 fl oz)	150	8	45	19	1
Fun Box Ice Cream Sandwich	1 (3.1 fl oz)	160	5	140	27	1
King Cone	1 (5.7 fl oz)	300	14	110	38	2
King Cone Classic Vanilla	1 (4.8 oz)	300	10	110	48	1
King Cone Strawberry	1 (5.7 oz)	250	10	105	38	1
Light Chocolate Chocolate Chip	½ cup (2.4 oz)	130	4	40	20	tr
Light Chocolate Chip	½ cup (2.4 oz)	130	4	45	20	0

FOOD	PORTION	CAL.	FAT	SOD.	CARB.	FIB.
Good Humor (CONT.)						
Light Coffee	½ cup (2.4 oz)	110	3	45	18	0
Light Cookies N'Cream	½ cup (2.4 oz)	130	3	70	21	0
Light Heavenly Hash	½ cup (2.4 oz)	140	4	45	23	tr
Light Praline Almond Crunch	½ cup (2.4 oz)	130	3	65	20	0
Light Toffee Bar Crunch	½ cup (2.4 oz)	130	4	55	20	0
Light Vanilla	½ cup (2.4 oz)	110	3	50	19	0
Light Vanilla Chocolate Strawberry	½ cup (2.4 oz)	110	3	45	19	0
Light Vanilla Fudge	½ cup (2.6 oz)	120	3	50	21	0
Magnum Almond	1 (4.2 fl oz)	270	12	50	35	5
Magnum Chocolate	1 (4.2 fl oz)	260	12	60	38	2
Number One Bar	1 (4.1 fl oz)	190	11	45	22	1
Popsicle Ice Cream Bar	1 (3.1 fl oz)	160	11	35	15	1
Popsicle Ice Cream Sandwich	1 (3.6 fl oz)	190	8	120	28	1
Sandwich Classic Chip Cookie	1 (4.1 fl oz)	300	13	215	43	1
Sandwich Giant Neapolitan	1 (5.2 fl oz)	260	10	150	39	1
Sandwich Giant Vanilla	1 (5.2 fl oz)	240	10	160	35	1
Sandwich Ice Cream	1	190	8	120	28	1
Sandwich Sidewalk Sundae	1 (3.1 oz)	160	5	140	27	1
Sandwich Sprinkle	1 (3.1 fl oz)	180	6	65	28	1
Strawberry Shortcake Bar Classic	1 (3.1 fl oz)	160	8	60	20	1
Sundae Twist Cup	1	160	3	100	33	0
Toffee Taco	1 (4.4 fl oz)	300	16	120	35	1
Viennetta Chocolate	1 (4.2 fl oz)	160	9	80	19	1
Viennetta Vanilla	1 (4.2 fl oz)	160	10	80	15	0
WWF Bar	1 (3.7 fl oz)	200	10	100	24	1
X-Men Bar	1 (3 fl oz)	150	6	90	23	0
Haagen-Dazs						
Baileys Original Irish Cream	½ cup (3.6 oz)	280	18	100	23	0
Brownies A La Mode	½ cup (3.7 oz)	280	18	130	25	0
Butter Pecan	½ cup (3.7 oz)	320	24	140	20	tr
Cappuccino Commotion	½ cup (3.6 oz)	310	21	105	25	1
Caramel Cone Explosion	½ cup (3.6 oz)	310	20	130	27	tr
Chocolate	½ cup (3.7 oz)	270	18	75	22	1
Chocolate Chocolate Chip	½ cup (3.7 oz)	300	20	70	26	2

FOOD	PORTION	CAL.	FAT	SOD.	CARB.	FIB.
Haagen-Dazs (CONT.)						
Coffee	½ cup (3.7 oz)	270	18	85	21	0
Cookie Dough Dynamo	½ cup (3.6 oz)	300	19	140	29	0
Cookies & Cream	½ cup (3.6 oz)	270	17	115	23	0
DiSaronno Amaretto	½ cup (3.6 oz)	260	15	80	26	0
Macadamia Brittle	½ cup (3.7 oz)	300	20	120	25	0
Multi Pack Bars Caramel Cone Explosion	1 (3.1 oz)	330	22	150	30	tr
Multi Pack Bars Chocolate & Dark Chocolate	1 (3.2 oz)	320	22	70	27	3
Multi Pack Bars Coffee & Almond Crunch	1 (3 oz)	290	21	70	22	tr
Multi Pack Bars Iced Cappuccino Explosion	1 (2.9 oz)	290	21	60	21	tr
Multi Pack Bars Triple Brownie Overload	1 (3 oz)	320	23	95	23	1
Multi Pack Bars Vanilla & Almonds	1 (3 oz)	300	22	65	21	1
Multi Pack Bars Vanilla & Dark Chocolate	1 (3.2 oz)	320	22	50	27	4
Multi Pack Bars Vanilla & Milk Chocolate	1 (3 oz)	280	20	65	20	0
Peanut Butter Burst	½ cup (3.6 oz)	330	22	150	26	1
Rum Raisin	½ cup (3.7 oz)	270	17	75	22	0
Single Pack Bars Caramel Cone Explosion	1 (3.3 oz)	350	23	160	32	tr
Single Pack Bars Chocolate & Dark Chocolate	1 (3.9 oz)	400	27	90	33	4
Single Pack Bars Coffee & Almond Crunch	1 (3.7 oz)	360	26	85	27	1
Single Pack Bars Cookie Dough Dynamo	1 (3.5 oz)	380	25	125	34	1
Single Pack Bars Iced Cappuccino	1 (3.4 oz)	330	24	70	24	tr
Single Pack Bars Triple Brownie Overload	1 (3.5 oz)	380	27	110	28	1
Single Pack Bars Vanilla & Almonds	1 (3.7 oz)	370	27	80	26	1

FOOD	PORTION	CAL.	FAT	SOD.	CARB.	FIB.
Haagen-Dazs (CONT.)						
Single Pack Bars Vanilla & Dark Chocolate	1 (3.9 oz)	400	27	65	33	4
Single Pack Bars Vanilla & Milk Chocolate	1 (3.5 oz)	330	25	75	24	tr
Strawberry	½ cup (3.7 oz)	250	16	80	23	tr
Strawberry Cheesecake Craze	½ cup (3.7 oz)	290	18	160	28	tr
Triple Brownie Overload	½ cup (3.5 oz)	300	20	100	26	0
Vanilla	½ cup (3.7 oz)	270	18	85	21	0
Vanilla Fudge	½ cup (3.7 oz)	280	18	105	25	0
Vanilla Swiss Almond	½ cup (3.7 oz)	310	21	80	23	1
Healthy Choice						
Black Forest	½ cup (2.5 oz)	120	2	50	23	1
Bordeaux Cherry Chocolate Chip	½ cup (2.5 oz)	110	2	55	19	tr
Butter Pecan Crunch	½ cup (2.5 oz)	120	2	60	22	1
Cappuccino Chocolate Chunk	½ cup (2.5 oz)	120	2	60	32	1
Cookies 'N Cream	½ cup (2.5 oz)	120	2	90	21	tr
Double Fudge Swirl	½ cup (2.5 oz)	120	2	50	21	1
Fudge Brownie	½ cup (2.5 oz)	120	2	55	22	2
Malt Caramel Cone	½ cup (2.5 oz)	120	2	60	22	1
Mint Chocolate Chip	½ cup (2.5 oz)	120	2	50	21	tr
Peanut Butter Cookie Dough 'N Fudge	½ cup (2.5 oz)	120	2	60	22	tr
Praline & Caramel	½ cup (2.5 oz)	130	2	70	25	tr
Rocky Road	½ cup (2.5 oz)	140	2	60	28	2
Vanilla	½ cup	100	2	50	18	1
Heath						
Bar	1 (2.5 oz)	160	12	35	13	0
Nuggets	8	180	11	45	18	0
Heaven						
Sundae Bars Chocolate Fudge	1 bar	150	9	—	—	—
Sundae Bars Vanilla Fudge	1 bar	150	9	—	—	—
Vanilla Caramel Nut	1 bar	225	15	—	—	—
Vanilla Nut Fudge	1 bar	222	15	—	—	—
Hood						
Bar Orange Cream	1 bar (1.8 oz)	90	2	30	18	0
Bar Vanilla	1 bar (1.6 oz)	160	12	45	11	0

FOOD	PORTION	CAL.	FAT	SOD.	CARB.	FIB.
Hood (CONT.)						
Caramel Butterscotch Blast	½ cup (2.3 oz)	160	8	70	20	0
Chocolate	½ cup (2.3 oz)	140	7	40	17	0
Chocolate Chip	½ cup (2.3 oz)	160	9	55	18	0
Chocolate Eclair	1 bar (1.6 oz)	150	10	45	14	0
Christmas Tree	½ cup (2.3 oz)	140	7	45	18	0
Coffee	½ cup (2.3 oz)	140	7	50	16	0
Cookie Dough Delight	½ cup (2.3 oz)	160	8	70	21	0
Cookies N Cream	½ cup (2.3 oz)	160	8	75	19	0
Cooler Cups	1 (2.1 oz)	80	1	25	18	0
Crispy Bar	1 (1.9 oz)	180	13	40	15	0
Egg Nog	½ cup (2.3 oz)	130	6	45	17	0
Fabulous Fudge & Peanut Butter Swirled Fudge Bars	1 bar (2.1 oz)	110	4	45	17	0
Fabulous Fudgies Assorted Bars	1 bar (2.1 oz)	100	3	50	19	0
Fat Free Chocolate Passion	½ cup (2.5 oz)	100	0	50	23	0
Fat Free Classic Harlequin	½ cup (2.5 oz)	100	0	50	23	0
Fat Free Double Brownie Sundae	½ cup (2.5 oz)	120	0	60	27	0
Fat Free Heavenly Hash	½ cup (2.5 oz)	120	0	75	27	0
Fat Free Mississippi Mud Pie	½ cup (2.5 oz)	130	0	75	29	0
Fat Free Praline Pecan Delight	½ cup (2.5 oz)	120	0	55	27	0
Fat Free Raspberry Blush	½ cup (2.5 oz)	120	0	55	26	0
Fat Free Super Strawberry Swirl	½ cup (2.5 oz)	100	0	40	23	0
Fat Free Vanilla Fudge Twist	½ cup (2.5 oz)	120	0	50	26	0
Fat Free Very Vanilla	½ cup (2.5 oz)	100	0	50	23	0
Fudge Bars	1 bar (2.7 oz)	100	1	80	21	0
Grasshopper Pie	½ cup (2.3 oz)	160	7	70	22	0
Heavenly Hash	½ cup (2.3 oz)	140	6	55	21	0
Hendrie's Cherry Chocolate Dips	1 bar (1.3 oz)	120	9	30	11	0
Hoodsie Cup Vanilla & Chocolate	1 (1.7 oz)	100	5	35	12	0
Light Almond Praline Delight	½ cup (2.4 oz)	110	5	75	23	0

FOOD	PORTION	CAL.	FAT	SOD.	CARB.	FIB.
Hood (CONT.)						
Light Brownie Nut Sundae	½ cup (2.4 oz)	140	5	55	22	0
Light Caribbean Coffee Royale	½ cup (2.4 oz)	110	4	50	18	0
Light Chocolate Almond Chip Sundae	½ cup (2.4 oz)	140	5	60	22	0
Light Chocolate Chocolate Chip Cookie Dough	½ cup (2.4 oz)	140	5	70	21	0
Light Cookies N Cream	½ cup (2.4 oz)	130	4	70	21	0
Light Heath Toffee Chunk Swirl	½ cup (2.4 oz)	140	5	95	23	0
Light Heavenly Hash	½ cup (2.4 oz)	130	4	55	22	0
Light Maple Sugar Shack	⅓ cup (2.4 oz)	130	4	65	23	0
Light Massachusetts Mud Pie	½ cup (2.4 oz)	140	5	60	20	0
Light Raspberry Swirl	½ cup (2.4 oz)	120	3	55	22	0
Light Strawberry Supreme	½ cup (2.4 oz)	110	3	45	19	0
Light Triple Nut Cluster Sundae	½ cup (2.4 oz)	140	5	50	22	0
Light Vanilla	½ cup (2.4 oz)	110	4	50	18	0
Light Vanilla Chocolate Strawberry	½ cup (2.4 oz)	110	4	45	18	0
Low Fat No Sugar Added Caramel Swirl	½ cup (2.4 oz)	120	3	80	18	0
Low Fat No Sugar Added Chocolate Supreme	½ cup (2.4 oz)	120	3	60	19	0
Low Fat No Sugar Added Mocha Fudge	½ cup (2.4 oz)	110	3	45	18	0
Low Fat No Sugar Added Raspberry Swirl	½ cup (2.4 oz)	110	3	45	17	0
Low Fat No Sugar Added Vanilla	½ cup (2.4 oz)	100	3	50	14	0
Maple Walnut	½ cup (2.3 oz)	160	9	45	16	0
Rockets	1 (2 oz)	120	5	50	18	1
Sandwich Light	1 (2.2 oz)	160	4	160	29	1
Sandwich Vanilla	1 (2.2 oz)	180	7	170	27	1
Sports Bar	1 (2.9 oz)	250	17	55	23	0
Spumoni	½ cup (2.3 oz)	140	9	45	17	0
Strawberry	½ cup (2.3 oz)	130	7	45	16	0
Super Sortment Chocolate & Banana Fudge Bar	1 bar (2.1 oz)	100	3	30	18	0

FOOD	PORTION	CAL.	FAT	SOD.	CARB.	FIB.
Hood (CONT.)						
Super Sortment Root Beer Float & Orange Cream Bar	1 bar (1.5 oz)	70	3	25	12	0
Vanilla	½ cup (2.3 oz)	140	7	50	16	0
Vanilla Chocolate Patchwork	½ cup (2.3 oz)	140	7	45	17	0
Vanilla Chocolate Strawberry	½ cup (2.3 oz)	140	7	45	16	0
Vanilla Fudge	½ cup (2.3 oz)	140	6	55	20	0
Klondike						
Almond Bar	1 (5.2 fl oz)	310	21	90	26	3
Caramel Crunch	1 (5.2 fl oz)	300	18	95	31	tr
Chocolate Chocolate Bar	1 (5.2 fl oz)	280	20	60	22	tr
Coffee Bar	1 (5.2 fl oz)	290	20	65	25	0
Dark Chocolate Bar	1 (5.2 fl oz)	290	20	75	24	tr
Gold Bar	1 (5.2 fl oz)	340	23	60	30	1
Krispy Bar	1 (5.2 fl oz)	300	20	85	28	0
Krunch	1 (3.1 fl oz)	200	13	160	17	1
Lite Bar	1 (2.3 fl oz)	110	6	55	14	1
Lite Bar Caramel	1 (2.4 fl oz)	120	6	65	18	1
Movie Bites Chocolate	8 pieces (4.6 fl oz)	340	26	50	22	1
Movie Bites Vanilla	8 pieces (4.6 fl oz)	320	22	60	27	1
Original Bar	1 (5.2 fl oz)	290	20	65	24	0
Sandwich Chocolate	1 (5.2 fl oz)	270	10	200	41	2
Sandwich Lite	1 (2.9 fl oz)	100	2	105	18	1
Sandwich Vanilla	1 (5.2 fl oz)	250	9	230	37	1
Mars						
Almond Bar	1 (1.85 fl oz)	210	14	45	20	0
Meadow Gold						
Sundae Cone	1	210	12	110	23	—
Milky Way						
Single Chocolate/Milk	1 (2 fl oz)	210	11	60	24	0
Snack Chocolate/Milk	1 (0.72 fl oz)	70	4	25	9	0
Snack Vanilla/Dark	1 (0.72 fl oz)	70	4	25	9	0
Mocha Mix						
Berry Berry Berry	½ cup	140	6	60	20	0
Dutch Chocolate	½ cup (2.3 oz)	140	8	80	16	0
Mocha Almond Fudge	½ cup (2.3 oz)	150	8	65	19	0
Neapolitan	½ cup (2.3 oz)	140	7	70	18	0
Strawberry Swirl	½ cup (2.3 oz)	140	6	55	20	0
Vanilla	½ cup (2.3 oz)	140	7	70	18	0
Nestle Crunch						
Chocolate	1 bar (3 oz)	200	14	40	18	0

FOOD	PORTION	CAL.	FAT	SOD.	CARB.	FIB.
Nestle Crunch (CONT.)						
Cones	1 (4.6 oz)	300	16	95	36	2
Crunch King	1 (4 oz)	270	19	45	21	0
Nuggets	8 pieces	140	9	30	12	0
Reduced Fat	1 (2.5 oz)	130	7	40	14	0
Vanilla	1 bar (3 oz)	200	14	40	17	0
Perry's						
No Fat No Sugar Added Caramel	½ cup (2.8 oz)	90	0	90	25	1
No Fat No Sugar Added Chocolate	½ cup (2.6 oz)	80	0	80	21	2
No Fat No Sugar Added Peach	½ cup (2.9 oz)	90	0	70	24	tr
No Fat No Sugar Added Strawberry	½ cup (2.8 oz)	90	0	75	23	tr
No Fat No Sugar Added Vanilla	½ cup (2.6 oz)	80	0	80	21	tr
Rice Dream						
Bar Chocolate	1	270	16	115	33	—
Bar Chocolate Nutty	1	330	23	110	29	—
Bar Strawberry	1	260	15	110	31	—
Bar Vanilla	1	275	16	120	33	—
Bar Vanilla Nutty	1	330	23	100	29	—
Cappuccino	½ cup	130	5	80	17	—
Carob	½ cup	130	5	80	20	—
Carob Almond	½ cup	140	6	80	20	—
Carob Chip	½ cup	140	6	80	20	—
Carob Chip Mint	½ cup	140	6	80	20	—
Cocoa Marble Fudge	½ cup	140	6	80	19	—
Dream Pie Chocolate	1	380	19	225	47	—
Dream Pie Mint	1	380	19	225	47	—
Dream Pie Mocha	1	380	19	225	47	—
Dream Pie Vanilla	1	380	19	225	47	—
Lemon	½ cup	130	5	80	17	—
Peanut Butter Fudge	½ cup	160	7	100	19	—
Strawberry	½ cup	130	5	80	17	—
Vanilla	½ cup	130	5	80	17	—
Vanilla Fudge	½ cup	140	6	80	21	—
Vanilla Swiss Almond	½ cup	140	6	80	20	—
Wildberry	½ cup	130	5	80	17	—
Sealtest						
American Glory	½ cup (2.4 oz)	130	6	45	17	0
Butter Pecan	½ cup (2.4 oz)	160	9	115	16	0
Candy Cane Crunch	½ cup (2.4 oz)	150	6	50	21	0

FOOD	PORTION	CAL.	FAT	SOD.	CARB.	FIB.
Sealtest (CONT.)						
Chocolate	½ cup (2.4 oz)	140	7	50	19	tr
Chocolate Butter Pecan	½ cup (2.4 oz)	150	8	85	17	0
Chocolate Chip	½ cup (2.4 oz)	150	8	50	18	0
Coconut Chocolate	½ cup (2.4 oz)	160	8	55	18	tr
Coffee	½ cup (2.4 oz)	140	7	55	16	0
Cupid's Scoops	½ cup (2.5 oz)	140	6	55	20	0
Dessert Bar Free Chocolate Fudge	1	90	0	30	19	—
Dessert Bar Free Vanilla Strawberry Swirl	1	80	0	40	17	—
Dessert Bar Free Vanilla Fudge	1	80	0	30	18	—
Free Black Cherry	½ cup	100	0	45	25	—
Free Chocolate	½ cup	100	0	50	23	—
Free Peach	½ cup	100	0	45	23	—
Free Strawberry	½ cup	100	0	40	23	—
Free Vanilla	½ cup	100	0	45	24	—
Free Vanilla Fudge Royale	½ cup	100	0	50	24	—
Free Vanilla Strawberry Royale	½ cup	100	0	35	25	—
French Vanilla	½ cup (2.4 oz)	140	8	50	16	0
Fudge Royale	½ cup (2.5 oz)	150	7	55	19	0
Heavenly Hash	½ cup (2.4 oz)	150	7	50	20	tr
Maple Walnut	½ cup (2.4 oz)	160	9	50	16	0
Strawberry	½ cup (2.4 oz)	130	6	45	19	0
Triple Chocolate Passion	½ cup (2.5 oz)	160	7	50	21	tr
Vanilla	½ cup (2.4 oz)	140	7	55	16	0
Vanilla Chocolate Strawberry	½ cup (2.4 oz)	140	6	50	18	0
Vanilla With Orange Sherbet	½ cup (2.7 oz)	130	4	45	22	0
Simple Pleasures						
Chocolate	4 oz	140	tr	—	25	—
Chocolate Caramel Sundae Light	4 oz	90	tr	—	20	—
Chocolate Chip	4 oz	150	3	—	25	—
Chocolate Light	4 oz	80	tr	—	16	—
Coffee	4 oz	120	tr	—	22	—
Cookies n' Cream	4 oz	150	2	—	25	—
Mint Chocolate Chip	4 oz	150	2	—	26	—
Peach	4 oz	120	tr	—	21	—
Pecan Praline	4 oz	140	2	—	25	—

FOOD	PORTION	CAL.	FAT	SOD.	CARB.	FIB.
Simple Pleasures (CONT.)						
Rum Raisin	4 oz	130	tr	—	35	—
Strawberry	4 oz	120	tr	—	22	—
Toffee Crunch	4 oz	130	tr	—	22	—
Vanilla	4 oz	120	tr	—	22	—
Vanilla Fudge Swirl Light	4 oz	90	tr	—	20	—
Vanilla Light	4 oz	80	tr	—	16	—
Snickers						
Single	1 (2 fl oz)	220	13	65	22	0
Snack	1 (1 fl oz)	110	7	35	11	0
Starbucks						
Biscotti Bliss	½ cup	240	12	70	30	—
Caffe Almond Fudge	½ cup	260	13	80	30	—
Caffe Almond Roast	1 bar	280	18	45	26	—
Dark Roast Expresso Swirl	½ cup	220	10	60	29	—
Frappuccino	1 bar (2.8 oz)	110	2	45	20	0
Italian Roast Coffee	½ cup	230	12	50	26	—
Javachip	½ cup	250	13	55	29	—
Low Fat Latte	½ cup	170	3	65	31	—
Low Fat Mocha Mambo	½ cup	170	3	75	32	—
Vanilla Mochachip	½ cup	270	16	60	27	—
Tofu Ice Creme						
Carob	4 fl oz	190	8	55	28	—
Vanilla	4 fl oz	190	8	55	28	—
Tofutti						
Frutti Vanilla Apple Orchard	4 fl oz	100	0	90	20	—
Turkey Hill						
Black Cherry	½ cup (2.3 oz)	140	7	30	18	0
Butter Pecan	½ cup (2.3 oz)	170	11	50	16	0
Choco Mint Chip	½ cup (2.3 oz)	160	10	45	17	0
Cookies 'N Cream	½ cup (2.3 oz)	160	9	60	19	0
Lite Butter Pecan	½ cup (2.3 oz)	130	6	80	17	0
Lite Choco Mint Chip	½ cup (2.3 oz)	140	5	75	19	0
Lite Cookies 'N Cream	½ cup (2.3 oz)	130	5	90	21	0
Lite Vanilla & Chocolate	½ cup (2.3 oz)	110	3	60	18	0
Lite Vanilla Bean	½ cup (2.3 oz)	110	3	65	18	0
Neapolitan	½ cup (2.3 oz)	150	8	30	18	0
Rocky Road	½ cup (2.3 oz)	170	8	40	23	0
Tin Roof Sundae	½ cup (2.3 oz)	160	9	70	19	0
Vanilla	½ cup (2.3 oz)	140	8	35	16	0
Vanilla & Chocolate	½ cup (2.3 oz)	150	8	35	17	0
Vanilla Bean	½ cup (2.3 oz)	140	8	35	16	0

FOOD	PORTION	CAL.	FAT	SOD.	CARB.	FIB.
Ultra Slim-Fast						
Bar Fudge	1	90	tr	50	17	2
Bar Vanilla Cookie Crunch	1	90	4	70	14	1
Chocolate	4 oz	100	tr	45	19	2
Chocolate Fudge	4 oz	120	tr	65	24	2
Peach	4 oz	100	tr	55	22	2
Pralines & Caramel	4 oz	120	tr	95	25	2
Sandwich Vanilla	1	140	2	220	28	1
Sandwich Vanilla Chocolate	1	140	2	220	28	1
Sandwich Vanilla Oatmeal	1	150	3	160	26	3
Vanilla	4 oz	90	tr	55	19	2
Vanilla Fudge Cookie	4 oz	110	tr	90	24	2
Weight Watchers						
Chocolate Dip	1 bar	100	6	15	11	0
Chocolate Mousse	1 bar	40	1	20	9	1
Chocolate Treat	1 bar	100	1	25	20	1
English Toffee Crunch	1 bar	110	6	30	12	1
Orange Vanilla Treat	1 bar	40	1	15	10	0
Vanilla Sandwich	1 bar	150	3	150	28	1
TAKE-OUT						
cone vanilla light soft serve	1 (4.6 oz)	164	6	92	24	—
gelato chocolate hazelnut	½ cup (5.3 oz)	370	29	49	26	2
gelato vanilla	½ cup (3 oz)	211	15	78	18	0
sundae caramel	1 (5.4 oz)	303	9	195	49	—
sundae hot fudge	1 (5.4 oz)	284	9	182	48	—
sundae strawberry	1 (5.4 oz)	269	8	92	45	—

ICE CREAM CONES AND CUPS

FOOD	PORTION	CAL.	FAT	SOD.	CARB.	FIB.
sugar cone	1	40	tr	32	8	tr
wafer cone	1	17	tr	6	3	tr
Comet						
Cups	1 (5 g)	20	0	20	1	tr
Sugar Cones	1 (12 g)	50	0	40	11	tr
Waffle Cone	1 (17 g)	70	1	30	14	1
Dutch Mill						
Chocolate Covered Wafer Cups	1 (0.5 oz)	80	5	—	8	0
Keebler						
Sugar Cones	1	45	tr	35	11	—
Vanilla Cups	1	15	tr	20	4	—
Oreo						
Chocolate Cones	1 (13 g)	50	1	110	10	tr

FOOD	PORTION	CAL.	FAT	SOD.	CARB.	FIB.
Teddy Grahams						
Cinnamon Cones	1 (0.5 oz)	60	1	55	13	tr
ICE CREAM TOPPINGS (*see also* SYRUP)						
butterscotch	2 tbsp (1.4 oz)	103	tr	143	27	—
caramel	2 tbsp (1.4 oz)	103	tr	143	27	—
marshmallow cream	1 oz	88	tr	13	23	—
marshmallow cream	1 jar (7 oz)	615	tr	90	157	—
pineapple	2 tbsp (1.5 oz)	106	0	26	28	—
pineapple	1 cup (11.5 oz)	861	—	214	226	—
strawberry	1 cup (11.5 oz)	863	1	73	225	—
strawberry	2 tbsp (1.5 oz)	107	tr	9	28	—
walnuts in syrup	2 tbsp (1.4 oz)	167	9	—	22	—
Ben & Jerry's						
Hot Fudge	(1.3 oz)	140	7	25	19	2
Crumpy						
Chocolate Hazelnut Spread	1 tbsp (0.5 oz)	80	5	5	8	0
Hershey						
Chocolate Fudge	2 tbsp	100	4	30	14	—
Chocolate Shoppe Candy Bar Sprinkles York	2 tbsp (1.1 oz)	170	8	0	22	2
Kraft						
Butterscotch	2 tbsp (1.4 oz)	130	2	150	28	0
Caramel	2 tbsp (1.4 oz)	120	0	90	28	0
Chocolate	2 tbsp (1.4 oz)	110	0	30	26	1
Hot Fudge	2 tbsp (1.4 oz)	140	5	100	24	tr
Pineapple	2 tbsp (1.4 oz)	110	0	15	28	0
Strawberry	2 tbsp (1.4 oz)	110	0	15	29	0
Marzetti						
Caramel Apple	2 tbsp	60	7	95	23	0
Caramel Apple Reduced Fat	2 tbsp	30	3	100	26	0
Peanut Butter Caramel	2 tbsp	60	6	135	21	1
Planters						
Nut	2 tbsp (0.5 oz)	100	9	0	3	1
Smucker's						
Butterscotch	2 tbsp	140	1	75	33	—
Butterscotch Special Recipe	2 tbsp	160	3	40	33	—
Caramel	2 tbsp	140	1	110	33	—
Chocolate	2 tbsp	130	0	35	27	—
Chocolate Fudge	2 tbsp	130	1	50	31	—

FOOD	PORTION	CAL.	FAT	SOD.	CARB.	FIB.
Smucker's (CONT.)						
Dark Chocolate Special Recipe	2 tbsp	130	1	45	31	—
Hot Caramel	2 tbsp	150	4	75	28	—
Hot Fudge	2 tbsp	110	4	55	18	—
Hot Fudge Light	2 tbsp	70	tr	35	19	—
Hot Fudge Special Recipe	2 tbsp	150	5	60	23	—
Hot Toffee Fudge	2 tbsp	110	4	55	18	—
Magic Shell Chocolate	2 tbsp	190	15	25	16	—
Magic Shell Chocolate Fudge	2 tbsp	190	15	50	16	—
Magic Shell Chocolate Nut	2 tbsp	200	16	40	25	—
Marshmallow	2 tbsp	120	0	0	29	—
Peanut Butter Caramel	2 tbsp	150	2	120	29	—
Pecans in Syrup	2 tbsp	130	1	0	28	—
Pineapple	2 tbsp	130	0	0	32	—
Strawberry	2 tbsp	120	0	0	30	—
Swiss Milk Chocolate Fudge	2 tbsp	140	1	70	31	—
Walnuts in Syrup	2 tbsp	130	1	0	27	—

ICED TEA

(*see also* TEA/HERBAL TEA)

FOOD	PORTION	CAL.	FAT	SOD.	CARB.	FIB.
MIX						
instant artifically sweetened lemon flavored as prep w/ water	8 oz	5	0	24	1	—
instant sweetened lemon flavor as prep w/ water	9 oz	87	tr	—	22	—
instant unsweetened lemon flavor as prep w/ water	8 oz	4	0	14	0	—
4C						
Instant	8 oz	90	0	0	22	—
Bigelow						
Nice Over Ice	5 fl oz	1	tr	1	tr	—
Celestial Seasonings						
Iced Delight	8 fl oz	4	tr	14	1	—
Crystal Light						
Decaffeinated as prep	1 serv (8 oz)	5	0	0	tr	0
Iced Tea as prep	1 serv (8 oz)	5	0	0	0	0
Peach Tea as prep	1 serv (8 oz)	5	0	0	0	0

FOOD	PORTION	CAL.	FAT	SOD.	CARB.	FIB.
Crystal Light (CONT.)						
Raspberry Tea as prep	1 serv (8 oz)	5	0	0	0	0
Lipton						
Calorie Free Decaf as prep	1 serv	0	0	0	0	0
Calorie Free as prep	1 serv	0	0	0	0	0
Citrus as prep	1 serv	90	0	0	22	0
Decaf Lemon as prep	1 serv	90	0	0	22	0
Family Size Bags Lemon as prep	1 qt	0	0	0	0	0
Family Size Bags Lemon Lime as prep	1 qt	0	0	0	0	0
Family Size Bags Peach as prep	1 qt	0	0	0	0	0
Lemon as prep	1 serv	90	0	0	22	0
Lemon Lime as prep	1 serv	90	0	0	22	0
No Lemon as prep	1 serv	80	0	0	19	0
Sugar Free Decaf as prep	1 serv	5	0	0	1	0
Sugar Free Lemon as prep	1 serv	5	0	0	1	0
Sugar Free No Lemon as prep	1 serv	0	0	0	1	0
Sugar Free Peach as prep	1 serv	5	0	0	2	0
Sugar Free Raspberry as prep	1 serv	5	0	0	1	0
Sugar Free Tropical as prep	1 serv	5	0	0	1	0
Tea & Lemonade as prep	1 serv	90	0	0	22	0
Tea Bag Herbal Iced Refresher as prep	1 serv	0	0	0	0	0
Tropical as prep	1 serv	90	0	0	22	0
Neștea						
100% Instant Tea as prep	8 oz	2	0	0	0	—
Ice Teasers Citrus	8 oz	6	0	0	1	—
Ice Teasers Lemon	8 oz	6	0	0	1	—
Ice Teasers Orange	8 oz	6	0	0	1	—
Ice Teasers Tropical	8 oz	6	0	0	1	—
Ice Teasers Wild Cherry	8 oz	6	0	0	1	—
Lemon as prep	8 oz	6	0	0	1	—
Peach as prep	8 oz	88	tr	25	22	—
Raspberry as prep	8 oz	88	tr	25	22	—
Sugarfree	8 oz	4	0	0	1	—

FOOD	PORTION	CAL.	FAT	SOD.	CARB.	FIB.
Nestea (CONT.)						
With Sugar & Lemon as prep	8 oz	70	0	0	19	—
READY-TO-DRINK						
Arizona						
Lemon	1 bottle (16 oz)	180	0	40	50	—
Raspberry	8 fl oz	95	0	20	25	—
Clearly Canadian						
Clearly Tea Original	8 fl oz	80	0	9	19	—
Clearly Tea Tangy Lemon	8 fl oz	80	0	9	19	—
Crystal Light						
Lemon	1 serv (8 oz)	5	0	40	0	0
Peach Tea	1 serv (8 oz)	5	0	40	0	0
Raspberry Tea	1 serv (8 oz)	5	0	40	0	0
Lipton						
Chilled Diet Lemon	8 fl oz	0	0	10	0	0
Chilled Lemon	8 fl oz	80	0	15	20	0
Chilled No Lemon	8 fl oz	90	0	15	24	0
Chilled Peach	8 fl oz	80	0	15	20	0
Chilled Raspberry	8 fl oz	80	0	15	20	0
Nestea						
With Sugar & Lemon	1 bottle (16 fl oz)	176	0	50	44	—
With Sugar & Lemon	1 can (11.5 fl oz)	127	0	36	32	—
Royal Mistic						
Diet	12 fl oz	8	0	34	2	—
Lemon	12 fl oz	144	0	26	36	—
Orange	12 fl oz	144	0	26	36	—
Wild Berry	12 fl oz	144	0	34	36	—
Schweppes						
Ice Tea	8 fl oz	90	0	60	22	0
Sipps						
Ice Tea	8.45 oz	100	0	—	—	—
Snapple						
Cranberry	8 fl oz	110	0	10	27	—
Diet	8 fl oz	0	0	10	1	—
Diet Peach	8 fl oz	0	0	10	1	—
Diet Raspberry	8 fl oz	0	0	10	1	—
Lemon	8 fl oz	110	0	10	27	—
Mango	8 fl oz	110	0	5	27	—
Mint	8 fl oz	120	0	10	29	—
Old Fashioned	8 fl oz	80	0	10	20	—
Orange	8 fl oz	110	0	10	27	—
Peach	8 fl oz	110	0	10	27	—
Raspberry	8 fl oz	120	0	10	29	—

FOOD	PORTION	CAL.	FAT	SOD.	CARB.	FIB.
Snapple (CONT.)						
Strawberry	8 fl oz	100	0	10	26	—
Tropicana						
Diet Lemon Fruit	8 fl oz	15	0	25	4	—
Lemon Fruit	8 fl oz	100	0	25	25	—
Peach Fruit	8 fl oz	120	0	15	28	—
Peach Fruit	1 bottle (10 fl oz)	140	0	20	35	—
Peach Fruit	1 can (11.5 fl oz)	160	0	20	41	—
Raspberry Fruit	1 bottle (10 fl oz)	140	0	20	34	—
Raspberry Fruit	8 fl oz	120	0	15	28	—
Raspberry Fruit	1 can (11.5 fl oz)	160	0	15	41	—
Tangerine Fruit	1 bottle (10 fl oz)	140	0	30	34	—
Tangerine Fruit	1 can (11.5 fl oz)	170	0	30	42	—
Tangerine Fruit	8 fl oz	110	0	20	27	—
Twister Apple Berry	8 fl oz	100	0	15	28	—
Twister Lemon Citrus	8 fl oz	110	0	5	28	—
Turkey Hill						
Diet Decaffeinated	1 cup (8 oz)	0	0	0	0	—
Raspberry Cooler	1 cup (8 oz)	110	0	0	28	—
Regular	1 cup (8 oz)	90	0	0	22	—
Veryfine						
With Lemon	8 oz	80	0	<10	16	—

ICES AND ICE POPS

(*see also* ICE CREAM AND FROZEN DESSERTS, PUDDING POPS, SHERBET, YOGURT FROZEN)

FOOD	PORTION	CAL.	FAT	SOD.	CARB.	FIB.
fruit & juice bar	1 (3 fl oz)	75	tr	3	19	—
gelatin pop	1 (1.5 oz)	31	0	20	7	—
ice coconut pineapple	½ cup (4 fl oz)	109	3	34	23	—
ice fruit w/ Equal	1 bar (1.7 oz)	12	0	3	3	—
ice lime	½ cup (4 fl oz)	75	0	—	31	—
ice pop	1 (2 fl oz)	42	0	7	11	—
Ben & Jerry's						
Cherry Pop	1	330	24	—	28	—
Bresler's						
All Flavors Ice	3.5 oz	120	0	—	30	—
Chiquita						
Fruit & Cream Banana	1 bar	80	2	—	—	—
Fruit & Cream Blueberry	1 bar	80	1	—	—	—
Fruit & Cream Peach	1 bar	80	1	—	—	—
Fruit & Cream Raspberry	1 bar	80	1	—	—	—
Fruit & Cream Strawberry	1 bar	80	1	—	—	—
Fruit & Cream Strawberry Banana	1 bar	80	2	—	—	—

FOOD	PORTION	CAL.	FAT	SOD.	CARB.	FIB.
Chiquita (CONT.)						
Fruit & Juice Bar Cherry	1 bar (2 oz)	50	0	—	—	—
Fruit & Juice Bar Raspberry	1 bar (2 oz)	50	0	—	—	—
Fruit & Juice Bar Raspberry Banana	1 bar (2 oz)	50	0	—	—	—
Fruit & Juice Bar Strawberry	1 bar (2 oz)	50	0	—	—	—
Fruit & Juice Bar Strawberry Banana	1 bar (2 oz)	50	0	—	—	—
Cool Creations						
10 Pack	1 pop (2 oz)	60	0	5	14	0
Lion King Cone	1 (4 oz)	280	14	90	36	1
Mickey Mouse Bar	1 (4 oz)	170	11	40	17	0
Mickey Mouse Bar	1 (2.5 oz)	110	7	25	12	0
Surprise Pops	1 (2 oz)	60	0	5	14	0
Dole						
Fruit 'N Juice Coconut	1 bar (4 oz)	210	7	50	33	0
Fruit 'N Juice Lemonade	1 bar (4 oz)	120	0	55	28	0
Fruit 'N Juice Lime	1 bar (4 oz)	110	0	55	28	0
Fruit 'N Juice Peach Passion	1 bar (2.5 oz)	70	0	5	17	0
Fruit 'N Juice Pineapple Coconut	1 bar (4 oz)	140	4	5	27	0
Fruit 'N Juice Pineapple Orange Banana	1 bar (2.5 oz)	70	0	5	16	0
Fruit 'N Juice Pineapple Orange Banana	1 bar (4 oz)	110	0	5	26	0
Fruit 'N Juice Raspberry	1 bar (2.5 oz)	70	0	5	16	0
Fruit 'N Juice Strawberry	1 bar (2.5 oz)	70	0	5	17	0
Fruit 'N Juice Strawberry	1 bar (4 oz)	110	0	5	26	0
Fruit Juice Grape	1 bar (1.75 oz)	45	0	5	11	0
Fruit Juice No Sugar Added Grape	1 bar (1.75 oz)	25	0	5	6	0
Fruit Juice No Sugar Added Strawberry	1 bar (1.75 oz)	25	0	5	6	0
Fruit Juice Raspberry	1 bar (1.75 oz)	25	0	5	6	0
Fruit Juice Raspberry	1 bar (1.75 oz)	45	0	5	11	0
Fruit Juice Strawberry	1 bar (1.75 oz)	45	0	5	11	0
Fi-Bar						
Juice Bar Lemoney-Lime	1 bar	63	tr	—	15	—
Juice Bar Strawberry Nectar	1 bar	63	tr	—	15	—
Juice Bar Tropical Delight	1 bar	63	tr	—	15	—

FOOD	PORTION	CAL.	FAT	SOD.	CARB.	FIB.
Flintstones						
Rock Pops	1 (3.5 oz)	80	0	5	20	0
Frozfruit						
Banana Cream	1 bar (4 oz)	150	7	20	20	1
Cantaloupe	1 bar (4 oz)	60	0	5	35	0
Cappuccino Cream	1 bar (3 oz)	140	6	20	18	0
Cherry	1 bar (4 oz)	70	0	0	18	1
Coconut Cream	1 bar (4 oz)	170	11	25	17	2
Kiwi Strawberry	1 bar (4 oz)	90	0	0	23	2
Lemon	1 bar (4 oz)	90	0	10	22	0
Lemon Iced Tea	1 bar (4 oz)	80	0	10	19	0
Lime	1 bar (4 oz)	90	0	10	21	0
Orange	1 bar (4 oz)	90	0	15	21	0
Pina Colada Cream	1 bar (4 oz)	170	8	20	23	1
Pineapple	1 bar (4 oz)	80	0	0	19	0
Raspberry	1 bar (4 oz)	80	0	5	20	1
Strawberry	1 (4 oz)	80	0	20	20	1
Strawberry Banana Cream	1 bar (4 oz)	140	6	20	22	1
Strawberry Cream	1 bar (4 oz)	130	5	20	21	1
Tropical	1 bar (4 oz)	90	0	0	23	1
Watermelon	1 bar (4 oz)	50	0	0	13	0
Good Humor						
Big Stick Cherry Pineapple	1 (3.6 fl oz)	50	0	—	12	0
Big Stick Popsicle	1 (3.6 fl oz)	50	0	5	12	—
Calippo Cherry	1 (3.8 fl oz)	100	0	5	23	—
Calippo Grape Lemon	1 (3.9 fl oz)	90	0	0	22	—
Calippo Orange	1 (3.9 fl oz)	90	0	0	23	—
Citrus Bites	1 (1.8 fl oz)	35	0	0	9	—
Creamsicle Orange	1 (1.8 fl oz)	70	2	15	13	0
Creamsicle Orange	1 (2.8 fl oz)	110	3	30	20	0
Creamsicle Orange Raspberry	1 (2.6 fl oz)	100	3	25	19	0
Creamsicle Sugar Free	1 (1.8 fl oz)	25	0	10	5	—
Flinstones Push-Up Yabba Dabba Doo Orange	1 (2.75 fl oz)	90	1	20	20	—
Fudgsicle Bar	1 (2.8 fl oz)	90	1	55	17	1
Fudgsicle Pop	1 (1.8 fl oz)	60	1	40	12	0
Fudgsicle Sugar Free	1 (1.8 fl oz)	40	1	35	8	1
Fun Box Fudge Bar	1 (2.3 fl oz)	80	1	65	16	0
Fun Box Pops	1 (2 fl oz)	35	0	5	10	—
Fun Box Twin Box Cherry	1 (2.6 fl oz)	50	0	10	14	—

FOOD	PORTION	CAL.	FAT	SOD.	CARB.	FIB.
Good Humor (CONT.)						
Fun Box Twin Pop Banana	1 (2.6 fl oz)	50	0	10	14	—
Fun Box Twin Pop Blue Raspberry	1 (2.6 fl oz)	50	0	10	14	—
Fun Box Twin Pop Cherry Lemon	1 (2.6 fl oz)	50	0	10	14	—
Fun Box Twin Pop Orange Cherry Grape	1 (2.6 oz)	50	0	10	14	—
Fun Box Twin Pop Root Beer	1 (2.6 fl oz)	50	0	10	14	—
Garfield Bar	1 (3.9 fl oz)	90	0	0	22	—
Great White	1 (3.1 fl oz)	70	1	0	18	—
Hyperstripe	1 (2.8 fl oz)	80	0	0	21	—
Ice Stripe Cherry Orange	1 (1.5 fl oz)	35	0	0	9	0
Jumbo Jet Star	1 (4.7 fl oz)	80	0	0	20	—
Laser Blazer	1 (2.6 oz)	70	0	5	16	—
Popsicle All Natural	1 (1.8 fl oz)	45	0	5	10	—
Popsicle Orange Cherry Grape	1 (1.8 fl oz)	45	0	0	11	—
Popsicle Rainbow Pops	1 (1.8 fl oz)	45	0	0	11	—
Popsicle Rootbeer Banana Lime	1 (1.8 fl oz)	45	0	0	11	—
Popsicle Strawberry Raspberry Wildberry	1 (1.8 fl oz)	45	0	0	11	—
Popsicle Supersicle Traffic Signal	1	80	0	0	20	—
Popsicle Twin Pop Cherry	1 (2.6 fl oz)	70	0	0	16	—
Popsicle Twin Pop Orange Cherry Grape Lime	1 (2.6 fl oz)	70	0	5	16	—
Snow Cone	1	60	0	5	14	—
Snowfruit Coconut Bar	1 (3.75 fl oz)	150	4	35	27	1
Snowfruit Orange Bar	1	140	0	10	34	tr
Snowfruit Strawberry Bar	1	120	0	15	31	tr
Snowfruit Tropical Fruit Bar	1	110	0	10	28	—
Sugar Free Pop Orange Cherry Grape	1 (1.8 fl oz)	15	0	0	3	—
Super Mario Bar	1	120	1	10	27	—
Supersicle Cherry Banana	1 (4.7 fl oz)	80	0	0	20	—

FOOD	PORTION	CAL.	FAT	SOD.	CARB.	FIB.
Good Humor (CONT.)						
Supersicle Cherry Cola	1 (4.7 fl oz)	80	0	0	20	—
Supersicle Double Fudge	1 (4.7 fl oz)	150	2	95	29	1
Supersicle Firecracker	1 (4.7 fl oz)	90	0	0	20	—
Supersicle Firecracker Jr.	1	72	0	0	10	—
Supersicle Sour Tower	1	80	0	0	20	—
Swirl Bubble Gum	1 (2.7 fl oz)	55	0	0	13	—
Swirl Cherry Banana	1 (2.7 fl oz)	55	0	0	13	—
Torpedo Cherry	1 (1.8 fl oz)	35	0	5	10	0
Twister Blue Raspberry Cherry Cherry Cola Cherry	1 (1.8 fl oz)	45	0	0	10	—
Twister Cherry Lemon Orange Lemon	1 (1.8 fl oz)	45	0	0	10	—
Vampire's Deadly Secret	1 (2.8 fl oz)	100	0	10	24	—
Watermelon Bar	1 (3.6 fl oz)	80	0	0	20	—
Haagen-Dazs						
Sorbet Banana Strawberry	½ cup (4 oz)	140	0	5	34	tr
Sorbet Chocolate	½ cup (4 oz)	130	0	80	30	2
Sorbet Manago	½ cup (4 oz)	120	0	0	30	tr
Sorbet Orchard Peach	½ cup (4 oz)	140	0	0	35	tr
Sorbet Raspberry	½ cup (4 oz)	120	0	5	29	1
Sorbet Strawberry	½ cup (4 oz)	130	0	0	33	1
Sorbet Zesty Lemon	½ cup (4 oz)	130	0	5	32	tr
Sorbet & Cream Blueberry	4 oz	190	8	35	25	—
Sorbet & Cream Keylime	4 oz	190	7	30	29	—
Sorbet & Cream Orange	½ cup (3.7 oz)	200	9	45	27	0
Sorbet & Cream Orange	4 oz	190	8	35	27	—
Sorbet & Cream Raspberry	½ cup (3.7 oz)	190	9	45	23	tr
Sorbet Bar Chocolate	1 (2.7 oz)	80	0	50	20	1
Sorbet Bar Wild Berry	1 (2.7 oz)	90	0	5	22	tr
Hood						
Hendrie's Sizzle'N Sour Stix	1 bar (2 oz)	80	tr	15	15	0
Hoodsie Pop	1 (3.3 oz)	60	0	0	16	—
Natural Blenders Pineappple	1 bar (1 oz)	60	0	0	16	—
Natural Blenders Raspberry	1 bar (1 oz)	60	0	0	16	—
Natural Blenders Strawberry	1 bar (1 oz)	60	0	0	16	—

FOOD	PORTION	CAL.	FAT	SOD.	CARB.	FIB.
Hood (CONT.)						
Pop Banana	1 (3.3 oz)	60	0	0	16	—
Pop Blue Raspberry	1 (3.3 oz)	60	0	0	16	—
Pop Cherry	1 (3.3 oz)	60	0	0	16	—
Pop Grape	1 (3.3 oz)	60	0	0	16	—
Pop Orange	1 (3.3 oz)	60	0	0	16	—
Pop Root Beer	1 (3.3 oz)	60	0	0	16	—
Super Sortment Juice Bars	1 bar (1.9 oz)	40	0	0	10	—
Lifesavers						
Ice Pops	1	35	0	0	9	0
Ice Pops	1 (1.75 oz)	35	0	0	9	0
Mr. Freeze						
Assorted	2 bars (3 oz)	45	0	20	11	0
Tropical	2 bars (3 oz)	45	0	20	11	0
Sunkist						
Orange Juice Bar	1 (3.4 fl oz)	80	1	5	19	—
Wildberry	1 (3.4 fl oz)	120	1	10	27	—
Tofutti						
Frutti Apricot Mango	4 fl oz	100	0	90	20	—
Frutti Three Berry	4 fl oz	100	0	90	20	—
Vitari						
Passion-Fruit	4 oz	80	0	—	—	—
Peach	4 oz	80	0	—	—	—

ICING

(*see* CAKE ICING)

INSTANT BREAKFAST

(*see* BREAKFAST DRINKS)

JACKFRUIT

fresh	3½ oz	70	tr	2	4	—

JALAPENO

(*see* PEPPERS)

JAM/JELLY/PRESERVES

all flavors jam	1 pkg (0.5 oz)	34	0	—	9	tr
all flavors jam	1 tbsp (0.7 oz)	48	0	—	13	tr
all flavors jelly	1 tbsp (0.7 oz)	52	0	—	14	tr
all flavors jelly	1 pkg (0.5 oz)	38	0	—	10	tr
all flavors preserve	1 pkg (0.5 oz)	34	0	—	9	tr
all flavors preserve	1 tbsp (0.7 oz)	48	0	—	13	tr
apple butter	1 tbsp (0.6 oz)	33	0	0	9	—
apple butter	1 cup (9.9 oz)	519	1	1	135	—

FOOD	PORTION	CAL.	FAT	SOD.	CARB.	FIB.
apple jelly	1 tbsp (0.7 oz)	52	0	7	14	tr
apple jelly	1 pkg (0.5 oz)	38	0	5	10	tr
apricot jam	3½ oz	250	0	—	62	—
blackberry jam	3½ oz	237	0	—	59	—
cherry jam	3½ oz	250	0	—	62	—
lingonberry jam	0.5 oz	23	tr	—	6	tr
orange jam	3½ oz	243	0	11	60	—
orange marmalade	1 pkg (0.5 oz)	34	0	8	9	—
orange marmalade	1 tbsp (0.7 oz)	49	0	11	13	—
plum jam	3½ oz	241	0	—	60	—
quince jam	3½ oz	236	0	—	59	—
raspberry jam	3½ oz	248	0	—	61	—
raspberry jelly	3½ oz	259	0	—	65	—
red currant jam	3½ oz	237	0	—	59	—
red currant jelly	3½ oz	265	0	4	66	—
rose hip jam	3½ oz	250	0	5	62	—
strawberry jam	1 tbsp (0.7 oz)	48	0	8	13	tr
strawberry jam	1 pkg (0.5 oz)	34	0	6	9	tr
strawberry preserve	1 tbsp (0.7 oz)	48	0	8	13	tr
strawberry preserve	1 pkg (0.5 oz)	34	0	6	9	tr
BAMA						
Apple Butter	2 tsp	25	0	5	6	—
Apple Jelly	2 tsp	30	0	5	8	—
Grape Jelly	2 tsp	30	0	5	8	—
Peach Preserves	2 tsp	30	0	5	8	—
Red Plum Jam	2 tsp	30	0	5	8	—
Strawberry Preserves	2 tsp	30	0	5	8	—
Eden						
Apple Butter	1 tbsp (0.5 fl oz)	25	0	0	3	0
Estee						
Apple Reduced Calorie	1 pkg (0.5 oz)	10	0	25	2	—
Apple Slice	1 tbsp (0.5 oz)	10	0	20	2	—
Apricot	1 tbsp (0.5 oz)	5	0	20	1	—
Blackberry	1 tbsp (0.5 oz)	5	0	25	1	—
Cherry	1 tbsp (0.5 oz)	5	0	20	1	—
Grape	1 tbsp (0.5 oz)	10	0	20	2	—
Orange	1 tbsp (0.5 oz)	10	0	20	2	—
Peach	1 tbsp (0.5 oz)	5	0	20	1	—
Red Raspberry	1 tbsp (0.5 oz)	5	0	25	1	—
Strawberry	1 tbsp (0.5 oz)	10	0	—	2	—
Harvest Moon						
Apricot Fruit Spread	1 tbsp (0.6 oz)	35	0	0	9	—
Blueberry Fruit Spread	1 tbsp (0.6 oz)	35	0	0	9	—
Cherry Fruit Spread	1 tbsp (0.6 oz)	35	0	0	9	—

FOOD	PORTION	CAL.	FAT	SOD.	CARB.	FIB.
Harvest Moon (CONT.)						
Grape Fruit Spread	1 tbsp (0.6 oz)	35	0	0	9	—
Peach Fruit Spread	1 tbsp (0.6 oz)	35	0	0	9	—
Raspberry Fruit Spread	1 tbsp (0.6 oz)	35	0	0	9	—
Strawberry Fruit Spread	1 tbsp (0.6 oz)	35	0	0	9	—
Home Brands						
All Flavors Jelly	2 tsp	35	0	—	—	—
All Flavors Preserves	2 tsp	35	0	—	—	—
Kraft						
Blackberry Preserves	1 tbsp (0.7 oz)	50	0	10	13	tr
Orange Marmalade	1 tbsp (0.7 oz)	50	0	10	14	0
Peach Preserves	1 tbsp (0.7 oz)	50	0	10	14	0
Pineapple Preserves	1 tbsp (0.7 oz)	50	0	10	14	0
Red Raspberry Preserves	1 tbsp (0.7 oz)	50	0	10	13	0
Strawberry Jelly	1 tbsp (0.7 oz)	60	0	10	14	0
Strawberry Preserves	1 tbsp (0.7 oz)	50	0	10	13	0
Red Wing						
Apple Jelly	1 tbsp (0.7 oz)	50	0	5	13	0
Apple Blackberry Jelly	1 tbsp (0.7 oz)	50	0	5	13	0
Apple Cherry Jelly	1 tbsp (0.7 oz)	50	0	10	13	0
Apple Currant Jelly	1 tbsp (0.7 oz)	50	0	15	13	0
Apple Grape Jelly	1 tbsp (0.7 oz)	50	0	10	13	0
Apple Raspberry Jelly	1 tbsp (0.7 oz)	50	0	5	13	0
Apple Strawberry Jelly	1 tbsp (0.7 oz)	50	0	5	13	0
Black Raspberry Jelly	1 tbsp (0.7 oz)	50	0	5	13	0
Blackberry Jelly	1 tbsp (0.7 oz)	50	0	5	13	0
Cherry Jelly	1 tbsp (0.7 oz)	50	0	5	13	0
Concord Grape Jelly	1 tbsp (0.7 oz)	50	0	5	13	0
Crabapple Jelly	1 tbsp (0.7 oz)	50	0	10	13	0
Cranberry Jelly	1 tbsp (0.7 oz)	50	0	10	13	0
Cranberry Grape Jelly	1 tbsp (0.7 oz)	50	0	10	13	0
Currant Jelly	1 tbsp (0.7 oz)	50	0	10	13	0
Damson Plum Jelly	1 tbsp (0.7 oz)	50	0	5	13	0
Elderberry Jelly	1 tbsp (0.7 oz)	50	0	5	13	0
Grape Jelly	1 tbsp (0.7 oz)	50	0	5	13	0
Mint Jelly	1 tbsp (0.7 oz)	50	0	5	13	0
Mint Apple Jelly	1 tbsp (0.7 oz)	50	0	5	13	0
Mixed Fruit Jelly	1 tbsp (0.7 oz)	50	0	5	13	0
Red Plum Jelly	1 tbsp (0.7 oz)	50	0	10	13	0
Red Raspberry Jelly	1 tbsp (0.7 oz)	50	0	5	13	0
Strawberry Jelly	1 tbsp (0.7 oz)	50	0	5	13	0
Strawberry Apple Jelly	1 tbsp (0.7 oz)	50	0	10	13	0

FOOD	PORTION	CAL.	FAT	SOD.	CARB.	FIB.
S&W						
Apricot Pineapple Reduced Calorie Preserves	1 tsp	4	0	0	1	—
Blueberry Reduced Calorie Jam	1 tsp	4	0	0	1	—
Concord Grape Reduced Calorie Jelly	1 tsp	4	0	0	1	—
Orange Marmalade Reduced Calorie	1 tsp	4	0	0	1	—
Red Raspberry Reduced Calorie Jam	1 tsp	4	0	0	1	—
Red Tart Cherry Reduced Calorie Preserves	1 tsp	4	0	0	1	—
Strawberry Reduced Calorie Jam	1 tsp	4	0	0	1	—
Smucker's						
All Flavors Jam	1 tsp	18	0	0	4	—
All Flavors Jelly	1 tsp	18	0	tr	4	—
All Flavors Low Sugar Spread	1 tsp	8	0	<10	2	—
All Flavors Preserves	1 tsp	18	0	0	4	—
All Flavors Simply Fruit	1 tsp	16	0	0	4	—
All Flavors Single Serving Jelly	½ oz	38	0	<10	9	—
All Flavors Single Serving Preserves	½ oz	38	0	<10	9	—
All Flavors Slenderella	1 tsp	7	0	0	2	—
Apple Butter Autumn Harvest	1 tsp	12	0	0	3	—
Apple Butter Simply Fruit	1 tsp	12	0	0	3	—
Apple Butter Natural	1 tsp	12	0	0	3	—
Apple Cider Butter	1 tsp	12	0	0	3	—
Blackberry Single Serving Imitation Jelly	1 pkg (0.4 oz)	4	0	<10	1	—
Cherry Singley Serving Imitation Jelly	1 pkg (0.4 oz)	4	0	<10	1	—
Grape Single Serving Imitation Jelly	1 pkg (0.4 oz)	4	0	<10	1	—
Orange Marmalade	1 tsp	18	0	0	4	—
Peach Butter	1 tsp	15	0	0	4	—
Pumpkin Butter Autumn Harvest	1 tsp	12	0	14	3	—

FOOD	PORTION	CAL.	FAT	SOD.	CARB.	FIB.
Tree Of Life						
Apricot Fruit Spread	1 tbsp (0.6 oz)	45	0	0	12	—
Blueberry Fruit Spread	1 tbsp (0.6 oz)	35	0	0	9	—
Cherry Fruit Spread	1 tbsp (0.6 oz)	40	0	0	10	—
Grape Fruit Spread	1 tbsp (0.6 oz)	35	0	0	8	—
Peach Fruit Spread	1 tbsp (0.6 oz)	45	0	0	12	—
Raspberry Fruit Spread	1 tbsp (0.6 oz)	30	0	0	7	—
Strawberry Fruit Spread	1 tbsp (0.6 oz)	35	0	0	9	—
Whistling Wings						
Blueberry Jam	1 oz	50	tr	2	12	tr
Raspberry Jam	1 oz	60	tr	1	14	1
White House						
Apple Butter	1 oz	50	0	5	12	1
JAPANESE FOOD						
(*see* ASIAN FOOD, SUSHI)						
JAVA PLUM						
fresh	1 cup	82	tr	18	21	—
fresh	3	5	tr	1	1	—
JELLY						
(*see* JAM/JELLY/PRESERVE)						
JERUSALEM ARTICHOKE						
(*see* ARTICHOKE, SUNCHOKE)						
JUJUBE						
fresh	3½ oz	105	tr	3	24	—
KALE						
FRESH						
chopped cooked	½ cup	21	tr	15	4	—
raw chopped	½ cup	21	tr	15	3	—
scotch chopped cooked	½ cup	18	tr	29	4	—
Dole						
Chopped	½ cup	17	1	15	3	—
FROZEN						
chopped cooked	½ cup	20	tr	10	4	—
KEFIR						
kefir	3½ oz	66	4	46	5	—
KETCHUP						
ketchup	1 tbsp	16	tr	178	4	tr
ketchup	1 pkg (0.2 oz)	6	tr	71	2	tr
low sodium	1 tbsp	16	tr	3	4	tr

FOOD	PORTION	CAL.	FAT	SOD.	CARB.	FIB.
Del Monte						
Ketchup	1 tbsp (0.5 oz)	15	0	190	4	0
Estee						
Imitation Sodium Free	1 pkg (0.5 oz)	15	0	0	3	—
Hain						
Natural	1 tbsp	16	0	155	4	—
Natural No Salt Added	1 tbsp	16	0	5	4	—
Healthy Choice						
Ketchup	1 tbsp (0.5 oz)	9	0	97	2	tr
Heinz						
Hot	1 tbsp	14	0	185	3	—
Lite	1 tbsp	8	0	115	2	—
Hunt's						
Ketchup	1 tbsp (0.6 oz)	16	tr	198	3	0
No Salt Added	1 tbsp (0.6 oz)	16	tr	6	3	0
McIlhenny						
Ketchup	1 tbsp (0.6 oz)	23	tr	128	5	tr
Spicy	1 tbsp (0.6 oz)	23	tr	128	5	tr
Muir Glen						
Organic	1 tbsp (0.6 oz)	15	0	190	3	0
Red Wing						
Extra Fancy	1 tbsp (0.6 oz)	20	0	190	5	0
Smucker's						
Ketchup	1 tsp	8	0	0	2	—
Tree Of Life						
Ketchup	1 tbsp (0.5 oz)	10	0	25	3	—
Salsa Ketchup	1 tbsp (0.5 oz)	10	0	50	3	—
KIDNEY						
beef simmered	3 oz	122	3	114	0	—
lamb braised	3 oz	117	3	128	1	—
pork braised	3 oz	128	4	—	—	—
veal braised	3 oz	139	5	93	0	—
KIDNEY BEANS						
CANNED						
kidney beans	1 cup	208	1	889	38	—
red	1 cup	216	1	873	40	—
B&M						
Red Baked Beans	½ cup (4.6 oz)	170	2	440	32	6
Eden						
Organic	½ cup (4.4 oz)	100	0	15	18	10
Friend's						
Red Baked Beans	½ cup (4.6 oz)	160	1	510	32	6

FOOD	PORTION	CAL.	FAT	SOD.	CARB.	FIB.
Goya						
Spanish Style	7.5 oz	140	1	760	29	10
Green Giant						
Dark Red	½ cup	90	0	250	20	5
Light Red	½ cup	90	0	250	20	5
Hanover						
Dark Red	½ cup	110	0	—	—	—
Light Red In Sauce	½ cup	120	0	—	—	—
Hunt's						
Red	½ cup (4.5 oz)	94	1	484	20	5
Luck's						
Seasoned w/ Pork	7.5 oz	220	6	—	—	—
Special Cook Red	7.5 oz	190	4	—	—	—
Progresso						
Red	½ cup (4.6 oz)	110	1	280	20	8
S&W						
Dark Red Lite 50% Less Salt	½ cup	120	0	355	22	—
Dark Red Premium	½ cup	120	1	—	22	—
Water Pack	½ cup	90	0	0	16	—
Trappey						
Dark Red	½ cup (4.5 oz)	130	1	310	22	8
Light Red	½ cup (4.5 oz)	120	1	340	22	8
Light Red New Orleans Style With Bacon	½ cup (4.5 oz)	110	1	410	20	6
Light Red With Jalapeno	½ cup (4.5 oz)	110	1	420	19	6
With Chili Gravy	½ cup (4.5 oz)	110	1	510	20	7
Van Camp's						
Dark Red	½ cup (4.6 oz)	90	0	760	20	6
Light Red	½ cup (4.6 oz)	90	0	390	20	6
DRIED						
california red cooked	1 cup	219	tr	7	40	—
cooked	1 cup	225	1	4	40	—
red cooked	1 cup	225	1	4	40	—
royal red cooked	1 cup	218	tr	8	39	—
Arrowhead						
Red	¼ cup (1.6 oz)	160	1	0	29	10
Hurst						
Kidney Beans	1.2 oz	120	1	10	21	10
SPROUTS						
cooked	1 lb	152	3	—	21	—
raw	½ cup	27	tr	—	4	—

KIWI JUICE

FOOD	PORTION	CAL.	FAT	SOD.	CARB.	FIB.
After The Fall						
Kiwi Bear	1 cup (8 oz)	100	0	15	24	0

FOOD	PORTION	CAL.	FAT	SOD.	CARB.	FIB.
KIWIS						
fresh	1 med	46	tr	4	11	3
Dole						
Fresh	2	90	1	0	18	4
Sonoma						
Dried	7-8 pieces (1 oz)	90	1	0	19	2
KNISH						
Joshua's						
Coney Island Potato	1 (4.6 oz)	280	8	610	52	1
TAKE-OUT						
cheese & blueberry	1 (7 oz)	378	13	—	40	—
cheese & cherry	1 (7 oz)	378	13	—	40	—
everything	1 (7 oz)	221	8	—	34	—
kashe	1 (7 oz)	270	8	—	45	—
potato	1 med (3.5 oz)	166	6	235	25	tr
potato	1 lg (7 oz)	332	12	470	49	1
potato w/ broccoli & cheese	1 (7 oz)	312	15	—	33	—
potato w/ spinach & mushroom	1 (7 oz)	214	8	—	32	—
KOHLRABI						
raw sliced	½ cup	19	tr	14	4	—
sliced cooked	½ cup	24	tr	17	5	—
KUMQUATS						
fresh	1	12	tr	1	3	—
LAMB						
(*see also* LAMB DISHES)						
FRESH						
cubed lean only braised	3 oz	190	7	60	0	—
cubed lean only broiled	3 oz	158	6	65	0	—
ground broiled	3 oz	240	17	69	0	—
leg lean & fat Choice roasted	3 oz	219	14	56	14	—
loin chop w/ bone lean & fat Choice broiled	1 chop (2.3 oz)	201	15	49	0	—
loin chop w/ bone lean only Choice broiled	1 chop (1.6 oz)	100	5	39	0	—
rib chop lean & fat Choice broiled	3 oz	307	25	64	0	—
rib chop lean only Choice broiled	3 oz	200	11	73	0	—
shank lean & fat Choice braised	3 oz	206	11	61	0	—

FOOD	PORTION	CAL.	FAT	SOD.	CARB.	FIB.
shank lean & fat Choice roasted	3 oz	191	11	55	0	—
shoulder chop w/ bone lean & fat Choice braised	1 chop (2.5 oz)	244	17	51	0	—
shoulder chop w/ bone lean only Choice braised	1 chop (1.9 oz)	152	8	41	0	—
sirloin lean & fat Choice roasted	3 oz	248	21	58	0	—
FROZEN						
New Zealand lean & fat cooked	3 oz	259	19	39	0	—
New Zealand lean only cooked	3 oz	175	8	43	0	—

LAMB DISHES

FOOD	PORTION	CAL.	FAT	SOD.	CARB.	FIB.
TAKE-OUT						
curry	¾ cup	345	17	258	22	—
moussaka	5.6 oz	312	21	—	16	1
stew	¾ cup	124	5	140	11	2

LAMBSQUARTERS

FOOD	PORTION	CAL.	FAT	SOD.	CARB.	FIB.
chopped cooked	½ cup	29	1	—	5	—

LECITHIN
(*see* SOY)

LEEKS

FOOD	PORTION	CAL.	FAT	SOD.	CARB.	FIB.
chopped cooked	¼ cup	8	tr	3	2	—
cooked	1 (4.4 oz)	38	tr	13	9	—
freeze dried	1 tbsp	1	0	0	tr	—
raw	1 (4.4 oz)	76	tr	25	18	—
raw chopped	¼ cup	16	tr	5	4	—

LEMON

FOOD	PORTION	CAL.	FAT	SOD.	CARB.	FIB.
fresh	1 med	22	tr	3	12	—
peel	1 tbsp	0	tr	0	1	—
wedge	1	5	tr	1	3	—
Dole						
Fresh	1	18	0	0	4	0

LEMON CURD

FOOD	PORTION	CAL.	FAT	SOD.	CARB.	FIB.
lemon curd made w/ egg	2 tsp	29	1	—	4	0
lemon curd made w/ starch	2 tsp	28	—	—	6	0

LEMON EXTRACT

FOOD	PORTION	CAL.	FAT	SOD.	CARB.	FIB.
Virginia Dare						
Extract	1 tsp	22	0	—	—	—

FOOD	PORTION	CAL.	FAT	SOD.	CARB.	FIB.
LEMON JUICE						
bottled	1 tbsp	3	tr	3	1	—
fresh	1 tbsp	4	0	0	1	—
frzn	1 tbsp	3	tr	0	1	—
After The Fall						
Spicy Lemon	1 can (12 oz)	150	0	35	37	0
Realemon						
Juice	1 fl oz	6	0	5	2	—
LEMONADE						
FROZEN						
as prep w/ water	1 cup	100	tr	8	26	—
not prep	1 can (6 oz)	397	tr	8	103	—
Bright & Early						
Lemonade	8 fl oz	120	0	5	30	—
Minute Maid						
Country Style	8 fl oz	120	0	0	30	—
Cranberry Lemonade	8 fl oz	80	0	0	30	—
Lemonade	8 fl oz	110	0	0	29	—
Pink	8 fl oz	120	0	0	30	—
Raspberry	8 fl oz	120	0	0	30	—
Seneca						
as prep	8 fl oz	110	0	0	27	1
MIX						
powder as prep w/ water	9 fl oz	113	tr	19	29	—
powder w/ equal	1 pitcher (67 oz)	40	0	58	10	—
4C						
Instant as prep	8 fl oz	80	0	0	20	—
Country Time						
Lem'n Berry Sippers Cranberry Raspberry Lemonade as prep	1 serv (8 oz)	90	0	0	21	0
Lem'n Berry Sippers Raspberry Lemonade as prep	1 serv (8 oz)	90	0	0	21	0
Lem'n Berry Sippers Strawberry Lemonade as prep	1 serv (8 oz)	90	0	0	21	0
Lem'n Berry Sippers Wildberry Lemonade as prep	1 serv (8 oz)	90	0	0	21	0
Lem'n Berry Sippers Sugar Free Strawberry Lemonade as prep	1 serv (8 oz)	5	0	0	0	0

FOOD	PORTION	CAL.	FAT	SOD.	CARB.	FIB.
Country Time (CONT.)						
Lemonade as prep	1 serv (8 oz)	70	0	15	17	0
Pink as prep	1 serv (8 oz)	70	0	15	17	0
Sugar Free Pink as prep	1 serv (8 oz)	5	0	0	0	0
Sugar Free as prep	1 serv (8 oz)	5	0	0	0	0
Crystal Light						
Lemonade as prep	1 serv (8 oz)	5	0	0	0	0
Pink as prep	1 serv (8 oz)	5	0	0	0	0
Kool-Aid						
Lemonade as prep	1 serv (8 oz)	70	0	0	17	0
Mix as prep w/ sugar	1 serv (8 oz)	100	0	10	25	0
Pink as prep w/ sugar	1 serv (8 oz)	100	0	10	25	0
Soarin' Strawberry Lemonade as prep	1 serv (8 oz)	70	0	15	17	0
Soarin' Strawberry Lemonade as prep w/ sugar	1 serv (8 oz)	100	0	0	25	0
Sugar Free Soarin' Strawberry Lemonade as prep	1 serv (8 oz)	5	0	0	0	0
Sugar Free Mix as prep	1 serv (8 oz)	5	0	0	0	0
READY-TO-DRINK						
After The Fall						
Apple Raspberry	1 bottle (10 oz)	120	0	15	29	—
Crystal Geyser						
Juice Squeeze Pink	1 bottle (12 fl oz)	140	0	20	34	—
Crystal Light						
Lemonade	1 serv (8 oz)	5	0	20	0	0
Pink	1 serv (8 oz)	5	0	20	0	0
Diet Rite						
Salt/Sodium Free	8 fl oz	2	0	0	1	—
Everfresh						
Lemonade	1 can (8 oz)	120	0	0	29	0
Ruby Red	1 can (8 oz)	110	0	0	27	0
Fruitopia						
Lemonade	8 fl oz	120	0	25	29	—
Minute Maid						
Chilled	8 fl oz	110	0	25	28	—
Cranberry Chilled	8 fl oz	120	0	25	31	—
Juices To Go	1 can (11.5 fl oz)	160	0	40	40	—
Juices To Go	1 bottle (16 fl oz)	110	0	25	28	—
Juices To Go Cranberry Lemonade	1 bottle (16 fl oz)	110	0	25	29	—
Juices To Go Raspberry Lemonade	1 bottle (16 fl oz)	120	0	25	29	—

FOOD	PORTION	CAL.	FAT	SOD.	CARB.	FIB.
Minute Maid (CONT.)						
Pink Chilled	8 fl oz	110	0	25	28	—
Raspberry Chilled	8 fl oz	120	0	0	30	—
Mott's						
Lemonade	10 fl oz	160	0	20	41	0
Nehi						
Lemonade	8 fl oz	130	0	35	35	—
Newman's Own						
Roadside Virginia	8 fl oz	100	tr	0	22	—
Ocean Spray						
Lemonade	8 fl oz	110	0	35	29	0
With Cranberry Juice	8 fl oz	110	0	35	26	0
With Raspberry Juice	8 fl oz	110	0	35	27	0
Odwalla						
Honey	8 fl oz	70	0	10	26	0
Strawberry	8 fl oz	150	0	35	40	2
Royal Mistic						
Lemonade Limeade	16 fl oz	230	0	19	57	—
Tropical Pink	16 fl oz	230	0	11	57	—
Santa Cruz						
Organic	8 oz	100	0	0	24	—
Shasta Plus						
Lemonade	1 can (11.5 oz)	160	0	45	40	0
Sipps						
Lemonade	8.45 fl oz	85	0	—	—	—
Snapple						
Diet Pink	8 fl oz	13	0	10	3	—
Lemonade	8 fl oz	110	0	10	29	—
Pink	8 fl oz	110	0	15	26	—
Strawberry	8 fl oz	110	0	5	26	—
Tropicana						
Lemonade	1 can (11.5 oz)	160	0	20	39	—
Lemonade	8 fl oz	110	0	20	28	—
Twister Wild Berry	8 fl oz	120	0	5	30	—
Turkey Hill						
Lemonade	8 fl oz	110	0	0	29	—
Veryfine						
Lemonade	8 fl oz	120	0	<25	30	—
LENTILS						
CANNED						
Health Valley						
Fast Menu Hearty Lentils Garden Vegetables	7½ oz	150	4	200	16	16

FOOD	PORTION	CAL.	FAT	SOD.	CARB.	FIB.
Health Valley (CONT.)						
Fast Menu Organic Lentils With Tofu Weiner	7½ oz	170	5	260	15	15
DRIED						
cooked	1 cup	231	1	4	40	—
Hurst						
Lentils	1.2 oz	120	1	5	20	11
FROZEN						
Natural Touch						
Lentil Rice Loaf	2.5 in slice (113 g)	200	11	420	18	—
MIX						
Casbah						
Pilaf as prep	1 cup	200	tr	400	38	2
SPROUTS						
raw	½ cup	40	tr	4	8	—
TAKE-OUT						
indian sambar	1 serv	236	5	189	37	9
LETTUCE						
(*see also* SALAD)						
bibb	1 head (6 oz)	21	tr	8	4	2
boston	1 head (6 oz)	21	tr	8	4	2
boston	2 leaves	2	tr	1	tr	tr
iceberg	1 leaf	3	tr	2	tr	tr
iceberg	1 head (19 oz)	70	1	48	11	5
looseleaf shredded	½ cup	5	tr	3	1	—
romaine shredded	½ cup	4	tr	2	1	tr
Dole						
Butter	1 head	21	tr	8	4	2
Iceberg	⅙ med head	20	0	10	4	1
Leaf shredded	1½ cup	12	0	40	1	1
Romaine shredded	1½ cups	18	1	40	2	1
Western Express						
Hearts Of Romaine	6 leaves (3 oz)	20	1	0	3	1
LIMA BEANS						
CANNED						
large	1 cup	191	tr	809	36	—
lima beans	½ cup	93	tr	309	17	—
Allen						
Green	½ cup (4.5 oz)	120	1	370	23	8
Green & White	½ cup (4.5 oz)	110	1	280	20	9
Del Monte						
Green	½ cup (4.4 oz)	80	0	360	15	4

FOOD	PORTION	CAL.	FAT	SOD.	CARB.	FIB.
Dennison's						
With Ham	7.5 oz	250	7	—	—	—
East Texas Fair						
Green	½ cup (4.5 oz)	120	1	370	23	8
Luck's						
Small Seasoned w/ Pork	7.5 oz	220	7	—	—	—
S&W						
Small Fancy	½ cup	80	0	390	16	—
Seneca						
Limas	½ cup	80	0	240	15	5
Trappey						
Baby Green With Bacon	½ cup (4.5 oz)	120	1	330	22	6
DRIED						
baby cooked	1 cup	229	1	5	42	17
cooked	½ cup	104	tr	14	20	—
large cooked	1 cup	217	1	4	39	14
FROZEN						
cooked	½ cup	94	tr	26	18	—
fordhook cooked	½ cup	85	tr	45	16	—
Birds Eye						
Baby	½ cup	130	0	115	24	—
Fordhook	½ cup	100	0	10	19	—
Fresh Like						
Baby	3.5 oz	138	1	106	25	2
Green Giant						
Harvest Fresh	½ cup	80	0	170	18	4
In Butter Sauce	½ cup	100	3	390	17	5
Hanover						
Baby	½ cup	110	0	—	—	—
Fordhook	½ cup	100	0	—	—	—
LIME						
fresh	1	20	tr	1	7	—
LIME JUICE						
bottled	1 tbsp	3	tr	2	1	—
fresh	1 tbsp	4	tr	0	1	—
After The Fall						
Caribbean Lime	1 can (12 oz)	170	0	25	42	0
Key West	1 cup (8 oz)	100	0	10	25	0
Odwalla						
Summertime Lime	8 fl oz	90	0	10	23	0
Realime						
Juice	1 oz	6	0	10	2	—

FOOD	PORTION	CAL.	FAT	SOD.	CARB.	FIB.
LING						
blue raw	3½ oz	83	1	—	0	—
fresh baked	3 oz	95	1	147	0	—
fresh fillet baked	5.3 oz	168	1	261	0	—
LINGCOD						
baked	3 oz	93	1	64	0	—
fillet baked	5.3 oz	164	2	114	0	—
LIQUOR/LIQUEUR						
(*see also* BEER AND ALE, CHAMPAGNE, DRINK MIXERS, MALT, WINE, WINE COOLERS						
anisette	⅔ oz	74	0	—	7	0
apricot brandy	⅔ oz	64	0	—	6	0
aquavit	3.5 oz	229	0	—	0	0
benedictine	⅔ oz	69	0	—	7	0
bloody mary	5 oz	116	tr	332	5	—
bourbon & soda	4 oz	105	0	16	0	—
coffee liqueur	1½ oz	174	tr	4	24	—
coffee w/ cream liqueur	1½ oz	154	7	43	10	—
cognac	3.5 oz	233	0	—	1	0
creme de menthe	1½ oz	186	tr	3	21	—
curacao liqueur	⅔ oz	54	0	—	6	0
daiquiri	2 oz	111	0	1	4	—
gin	1½ oz	110	0	1	0	—
gin & tonic	7.5 oz	171	0	10	16	—
gin ricky	4 oz	150	0	—	—	—
manhattan	2 oz	128	0	2	2	—
martini	2½ oz	156	0	2	tr	—
mint julep	10 oz	210	0	—	3	0
old-fashioned	2½ oz	127	0	—	3	0
pina colada	4½ oz	262	3	9	40	—
planter's punch	3½ oz	175	0	—	—	—
rum	1½ oz	97	0	0	0	—
screwdriver	7 oz	174	tr	2	18	—
sloe gin fizz	2½ oz	132	0	1	4	0
tequila sunrise	5½ oz	189	tr	7	15	—
tom collins	7½ oz	121	0	39	3	—
vodka	1½ oz	97	0	0	0	—
whiskey	1½ oz	105	0	0	tr	—
whiskey sour	3 oz	123	tr	10	5	—
whiskey sour mix not prep	1 pkg (0.6 oz)	64	0	46	16	—
LIVER						
(*see also* PATE)						
beef braised	3 oz	137	4	59	3	—

FOOD	PORTION	CAL.	FAT	SOD.	CARB.	FIB.
beef pan-fried	3 oz	184	7	90	7	—
chicken stewed	1 cup (5 oz)	219	8	71	1	—
duck raw	1 (1.5 oz)	60	2	—	2	—
goose raw	1 (3.3 oz)	125	4	132	6	—
lamb braised	3 oz	187	7	48	2	—
lamb fried	3 oz	202	11	105	3	—
pork braised	3 oz	141	4	42	3	—
sheep raw	3½ oz	131	4	95	0	—
turkey simmered	1 cup (5 oz)	237	8	89	5	—
veal braised	3 oz	140	6	45	2	—
veal fried	3 oz	208	10	112	3	—
Dakota Lean						
Beef raw	3 oz	100	1	—	8	—

LOBSTER

(*see also* CRAYFISH)

FOOD	PORTION	CAL.	FAT	SOD.	CARB.	FIB.
CANNED						
Progresso						
Rock Lobster Sauce	½ cup (4.3 oz)	100	7	430	6	2
FRESH						
northern cooked	1 cup	142	1	551	2	—
northern cooked	3 oz	83	1	323	1	—
northern raw	1 lobster (5.3 oz)	136	1	—	1	—
northern raw	3 oz	77	1	—	tr	—
spiny steamed	3 oz	122	2	193	3	—
spiny steamed	1 (5.7 oz)	233	3	370	5	—
FROZEN						
Cajun Cookin'						
Crawfish Etouffee	12 oz	390	10	1110	51	—
TAKE-OUT						
newburg	1 cup	485	27	127	13	—

LOGANBERRIES

FOOD	PORTION	CAL.	FAT	SOD.	CARB.	FIB.
frzn	1 cup	80	tr	1	19	—

LONGANS

FOOD	PORTION	CAL.	FAT	SOD.	CARB.	FIB.
fresh	1	2	0	0	tr	—

LOQUATS

FOOD	PORTION	CAL.	FAT	SOD.	CARB.	FIB.
fresh	1	5	tr	0	1	—

LOTUS

FOOD	PORTION	CAL.	FAT	SOD.	CARB.	FIB.
root raw sliced	10 slices	45	tr	33	14	—
root sliced cooked	10 slices	59	tr	40	14	—
seeds dried	1 oz	94	1	1	18	—

FOOD	PORTION	CAL.	FAT	SOD.	CARB.	FIB.
LOX						
(*see* SALMON)						
LUPINES						
dried cooked	1 cup	197	5	7	16	—
LYCHEES						
fresh	1	6	tr	0	2	—
Ka-Me						
Whole Pitted In Syrup	15 pieces (5 oz)	130	0	26	32	0
MACADAMIA NUTS						
dried	1 oz	199	21	1	4	—
oil roasted	1 oz	204	22	3	4	—
MacFarms of Hawaii						
Chocolate Covered	¼ cup (1.3 oz)	210	16	25	18	2
Dry Roasted Salted	¼ cup (1.3 oz)	220	23	65	4	3
Kona Coffee Dark Chocolate Covered	¼ cup (1.3 oz)	210	16	25	18	2
Mauna Loa						
Candy Glazed	1 oz	170	14	80	11	—
Chocolate Covered	1 oz	170	13	21	12	—
Honey Roasted	1 oz	200	17	80	8	—
Macadamia Nut Brittle	1 oz	150	8	140	19	—
Roasted & Salted	1 oz	210	21	75	4	—
MACARONI						
(*see* PASTA)						
MACE						
ground	1 tsp	8	1	1	1	—
MACKEREL						
CANNED						
jack	1 cup	296	12	720	0	—
jack	1 can (12.7 oz)	563	23	1368	0	—
Empress						
Jack	4 oz	140	8	480	0	—
FRESH						
atlantic cooked	3 oz	223	15	71	0	—
atlantic raw	3 oz	174	12	76	0	—
jack baked	3 oz	171	9	94	0	—
jack fillet baked	6.2 oz	354	18	194	0	—
king baked	3 oz	114	2	172	0	—
king fillet baked	5.4 oz	207	4	312	0	—
pacific baked	3 oz	171	9	94	0	—
pacific fillet baked	6.2 oz	354	18	194	0	—

FOOD	PORTION	CAL.	FAT	SOD.	CARB.	FIB.
spanish cooked	1 fillet (5.1 oz)	230	9	96	0	—
spanish cooked	3 oz	134	5	56	0	—
spanish raw	3 oz	118	5	50	0	—
MALANGA						
fresh	½ cup	137	tr	—	32	—
MALT						
nonalcoholic	12 fl oz	32	0	—	5	—
Bartles & Jaymes						
Malt Cooler Berry	12 fl oz	210	0	5	32	—
Malt Cooler Black Cherry	12 fl oz	190	0	5	30	—
Malt Cooler Light Berry	12 fl oz	140	0	0	29	—
Malt Cooler Mandarin Lemon	12 fl oz	210	0	5	34	—
Malt Cooler Margarita	12 fl oz	250	0	40	44	—
Malt Cooler Original	12 fl oz	180	0	0	27	—
Malt Cooler Peach	12 fl oz	200	0	5	31	—
Malt Cooler Pina Colada	12 fl oz	270	0	5	48	—
Malt Cooler Planter's Punch	12 fl oz	220	0	5	35	—
Malt Cooler Red Sangria	12 fl oz	190	0	5	29	—
Malt Cooler Strawberry	12 fl oz	200	0	5	31	—
Malt Cooler Strawberry Daiquiri	12 fl oz	220	0	5	35	—
Malt Cooler Tropical	12 fl oz	220	0	5	36	—
Olde English						
Malt	12 oz	163	0	—	10	—
Schaefer						
Malt	12 oz	165	0	20	12	—
Schlitz						
Malt	12 oz	177	0	21	15	—
MALTED MILK						
chocolate as prep w/ milk	1 cup	229	9	172	30	—
chocolate flavor powder	3 heaping tsp (¾ oz)	79	1	53	18	—
natural flavor as prep w/ milk	1 cup	237	10	223	27	—
natural flavor powder	3 heaping tsp (¾ oz)	87	2	103	19	—
Carnation						
Chocolate	3 heaping tsp (21 g)	79	tr	—	—	—
Original	3 heaping tsp (21 g)	90	2	—	—	—

FOOD	PORTION	CAL.	FAT	SOD.	CARB.	FIB.
MAMMY-APPLE						
fresh	1	431	4	127	106	—
MANGO						
fresh	1	135	1	4	35	—
CANNED						
Ka-Me						
Mango	4 pieces (5 oz)	102	0	10	25	0
DRIED						
Rainforest Farms						
Slices	6 slices (1.3 oz)	140	1	108	33	2
Sonoma						
Pieces	8 pieces (2 oz)	180	1	50	44	0
MANGO JUICE						
After The Fall						
Hawaiian Mango	1 can (12 oz)	180	0	20	45	0
Mango Ginger	1 can (12 oz)	150	0	25	35	0
Fresh Samantha						
Mango Mama	1 cup (8 oz)	125	1	0	33	2
Kern's						
Nectar	6 fl oz	100	0	0	28	—
Libby						
Nectar	1 can (11.5 fl oz)	210	0	10	52	—
Snapple						
Diet Mango Madness	8 fl oz	13	0	10	3	—
Mango Madness Cocktail	8 fl oz	110	0	10	29	—
Tang						
Drink Mix as prep	1 serv (8 oz)	100	0	0	25	0
MARGARINE (*see also* BUTTER BLENDS, BUTTER SUBSTITUTES)						
squeeze soybean & cottonseed	1 tsp	34	4	37	0	—
stick corn	1 tsp	34	4	44	0	—
stick corn	1 stick (4 oz)	815	91	1070	1	—
stick salted	1 stick (4 oz)	815	91	1069	1	—
stick salted	1 tsp	39	4	44	0	—
stick unsalted	1 tsp	34	4	tr	0	—
stick unsalted	1 stick (4 oz)	809	91	2	1	—
tub corn	1 tsp	34	4	51	0	—
tub corn	1 cup	1626	183	2449	1	—
tub diet	1 tsp	17	2	46	0	—
tub diet	1 cup	800	90	2226	1	—

FOOD	PORTION	CAL.	FAT	SOD.	CARB.	FIB.
tub safflower	1 tsp	34	4	51	0	—
tub safflower	1 cup	1626	183	2449	1	—
tub salted	1 cup	1626	183	2449	1	—
tub salted	1 tsp	34	4	51	0	—
tub soybean salted	1 tsp	34	4	51	0	—
tub soybean salted	1 cup	1626	183	2449	1	—
tub soybean unsalted	1 tsp	34	4	1	0	—
tub soybean unsalted	1 cup	1626	182	63	2	—
tub unsalted	1 tsp	34	4	1	0	—
tub unsalted	1 cup	1626	182	63	0	—
Blue Bonnet						
Stick	1 tbsp	100	11	95	0	—
Tub	1 tbsp	100	11	95	0	—
Whipped	1 tbsp	80	9	100	0	—
Chiffon						
Stick	1 tbsp	100	11	105	0	—
Tub	1 tbsp (0.5 oz)	100	11	105	0	0
Whipped	1 tbsp (0.3 oz)	70	7	70	0	0
Fleischmann's						
Stick	1 tbsp	100	11	95	0	—
Stick Light Corn Oil	1 tbsp	80	8	70	0	—
Stick Sweet Unsalted	1 tbsp	100	11	0	0	—
Hain						
Stick Safflower	1 tbsp	100	11	170	0	—
Stick Safflower Unsalted	1 tbsp	100	11	<5	0	—
Tub Safflower	1 tbsp	100	11	170	0	—
Hollywood						
Safflower	1 tbsp	100	11	130	0	—
Safflower Unsalted Sweet	1 tbsp	100	11	2	0	—
Soft Spread	1 tbsp	90	10	135	1	0
I Can't Believe It's Not Butter						
Tub	1 tbsp	90	10	—	—	—
Krona						
Stick	1 tbsp	100	11	—	—	—
Land O'Lakes						
Stick	1 tbsp (0.5 oz)	90	10	95	0	—
Stick With Sweet Cream	1 tbsp (0.5 oz)	90	10	95	0	—
Stick With Sweet Cream Unsalted	1 tbsp (0.5 oz)	90	10	0	0	—
Tub	1 tbsp (0.5 oz)	80	8	90	0	—
Tub With Sweet Cream	1 tbsp (0.5 oz)	80	8	70	0	—
Mazola						
Stick	1 cup (229 g)	1650	184	1650	3	—

FOOD	PORTION	CAL.	FAT	SOD.	CARB.	FIB.
Mazola (CONT.)						
Stick	1 tbsp (14 g)	100	11	100	0	·
Stick Unsalted	1 tbsp (14 g)	100	11	1	0	—
Stick Unsalted	1 cup (229 g)	1635	184	8	0	—
Tub Diet	1 tbsp (14 g)	50	6	130	0	—
Tub Diet	1 cup (235 g)	815	93	2160	1	—
Tub Light Corn Oil Spread	1 tbsp (14 g)	50	6	100	0	—
Mother's						
Stick Unsalted	1 tbsp	100	11	—	—	—
Sticks	1 tbsp	100	11	—	—	—
Tub Salted	1 tbsp	100	11	—	—	—
Tub Unsalted	1 tbsp	100	11	—	—	—
Nucanola						
Stick	1 tbsp	90	10	90	0	—
Parkay						
Squeeze	1 tbsp (0.5 oz)	80	9	120	0	0
Stick	1 tbsp (0.5 oz)	90	10	110	0	0
Stick ⅓ Less Fat	1 tbsp (0.5 oz)	70	7	120	0	0
Tub	1 tbsp (0.5 oz)	60	7	110	0	0
Tub Light	1 tbsp (0.5 oz)	50	6	120	0	0
Tub Soft	1 tbsp (0.5 oz)	100	11	105	0	0
Tub Soft Diet	1 tbsp (0.5 oz)	50	6	110	0	0
Whipped	1 tbsp (0.3 oz)	70	7	70	0	0
Promise						
Spread Soft	1 tbsp	80	8	—	—	—
Spread Stick	1 tbsp	90	10	—	—	—
Spread Light Soft	1 tbsp	50	6	—	—	—
Spread Light Stick	1 tbsp	50	6	—	—	—
Ultra Soft	1 tbsp	30	4	—	—	—
Ultra Spread Fat Free	1 tbsp	5	0	—	—	—
Smart Balance						
No Trans Fat	1 tbsp (0.5 oz)	120	14	0	0	—
No Trans Fat Light	1 tbsp (0.5 oz)	45	5	100	0	—
No Trans Fat Spread	1 tbsp (0.5 oz)	80	9	90	0	—
Smart Beat						
Light Unsalted	1 tbsp (0.5 oz)	25	3	0	0	—
Squeeze Fat Free	1 tbsp (0.5 oz)	5	0	100	1	—
Super Light Trans Fat Free	1 tbsp (0.5 oz)	20	2	105	0	—
Tub	1 tbsp	25	3	110	0	—
Tub Unsalted	1 tbsp	25	3	0	0	—
Touch Of Butter						
Squeeze	1 tbsp (0.5 oz)	80	9	115	0	0

FOOD	PORTION	CAL.	FAT	SOD.	CARB.	FIB.
Touch Of Butter (CONT.)						
Stick	1 tbsp (0.5 oz)	90	10	110	0	0
Tree Of Life						
Canola Soft	1 tbsp (0.5 oz)	100	11	110	0	—
Stick 100% Soy	1 tbsp (0.5 oz)	100	11	110	0	—
Stick 100% Soy Salt Free	1 tbsp (0.5 oz)	100	11	0	0	—
Stick Canola Soy	1 tbsp (0.5 oz)	100	11	110	0	—
Stick Canola Soy Salt Free	1 tbsp (0.5 oz)	100	11	0	0	—
Weight Watchers						
Light	1 tbsp	45	4	70	2	0
Light Sodium Free	1 tbsp	45	4	0	2	0
Reduced Fat Stick	1 tbsp	60	7	130	0	0
MARINADE						
(*see* SAUCE)						
MARJORAM						
dried	1 tsp	2	tr	tr	tr	—
MARSHMALLOW						
marshmallow	1 reg (0.3 oz)	23	0	3	6	—
marshmallow	1 cup (1.6 oz)	146	tr	22	37	—
Campfire						
Large	2	40	0	10	10	—
Miniature	24	40	0	10	10	—
Joyva						
Twists Chocolate Covered	2 (1.5 oz)	190	4	20	21	0
MATZO						
egg	1 (1 oz)	111	1	6	22	1
egg & onion	1 (1 oz)	111	1	81	22	1
plain	1 (1 oz)	112	tr	0	24	1
whole wheat	1 (1 oz)	99	tr	1	22	3
Goodman's						
Matzo Ball Mix 50% Less Salt	2 tbsp (0.5 oz)	50	0	150	11	0
Matzo Ball Mix as prep	2 tbsp (0.5 oz)	60	0	190	12	1
Horowitz Margareten						
Egg Milk Chocolate Coated	1 oz	97	4	7	16	1
Manischewitz						
American Matzo	1	115	2	—	22	—
Daily Thin Tea	1	103	tr	1	22	tr

FOOD	PORTION	CAL.	FAT	SOD.	CARB.	FIB.
Manischewitz (CONT.)						
Dietetic Thins	1	91	tr	tr	19	tr
Egg Dark Chocolate Coated	½ matzo (1 oz)	97	3	7	17	1
Egg n' Onion	1	112	tr	180	23	—
Matzo Cracker Miniatures	10	90	tr	—	20	—
Matzo Farfel	1 cup	180	1	2	60	—
Matzo Meal	1 cup	514	1	3	109	tr
Passover	1	129	tr	—	27	—
Passover Egg	1	132	2	—	27	—
Passover Egg Matzo Crackers	10	108	2	—	20	—
Salted Thin	1	100	tr	—	21	tr
Unsalted	1	110	tr	1	24	tr
Wheat Matzo Crackers	10	90	1	—	18	—
Whole Wheat w/ Bran	1	110	1	1	21	1
Streit's						
Dietetic	1 (1 oz)	100	0	0	23	1
Lightly Salted	1 (1 oz)	110	1	65	23	1
Matzoh Meal	¼ cup (1 oz)	110	1	0	24	1
Passover	1 (1 oz)	110	1	0	25	1
Unsalted	1 (0.9 oz)	100	1	0	22	1
Whole Wheat	1 (1 oz)	110	1	0	24	4
MAYONNAISE						
(*see also* MAYONNAISE TYPE SALAD DRESSING, RELISH)						
mayonnaise	1 cup	1577	175	1250	6	—
mayonnaise	1 tbsp	99	11	78	tr	—
reduced calorie	1 tbsp	34	3	75	2	—
reduced calorie	1 cup	556	46	1193	38	—
sandwich spread	1 tbsp	60	5	—	3	—
BAMA						
Mayonnaise	1 tbsp	100	11	65	0	—
Bennett's						
Mayonnaise	1 tbsp	110	12	65	1	—
Best Foods						
Cholesterol Free Reduced Calorie	1 cup (233 g)	760	75	1210	17	—
Cholesterol Free Reduced Calorie	1 tbsp (15 g)	50	5	80	1	—
Light	1 cup (233 g)	760	78	1815	16	—
Light	1 tbsp (15 g)	50	5	115	1	—
Real	1 tbsp	100	11	80	tr	—

FOOD	PORTION	CAL.	FAT	SOD.	CARB.	FIB.
Best Foods (CONT.)						
Real	1 cup	1570	175	1255	tr	—
Hain						
Canola	1 tbsp	60	5	160	2	—
Canola	1 tbsp	100	11	100	tr	—
Cold Processed	1 tbsp	110	12	70	0	—
Eggless No Salt Added	1 tbsp	110	12	<5	0	—
Light Low Sodium	1 tbsp	60	6	95	2	—
Real No Salt Added	1 tbsp	110	12	0	0	—
Safflower	1 tbsp	110	12	70	0	—
Hellman's						
Chlesterol Free Reduced Calorie	1 tbsp (15 g)	50	5	80	1	—
Cholesterol Free Reduced Calorie	1 cup (233 g)	760	75	1210	17	—
Light Reduced Calorie	1 tbsp (15 g)	50	5	115	1	—
Light Reduced Calorie	1 cup (233 g)	760	78	1815	16	—
Mayonnaise	1 cup (220 g)	1570	173	1255	1	—
Mayonnaise	1 tbsp	100	11	80	tr	—
Hollywood						
Canola	1 tbsp	100	11	100	tr	—
Mayonnaise	1 tbsp	110	12	80	0	—
Safflower	1 tbsp	100	12	75	0	—
Kraft						
Fat Free	1 tbsp (0.6 oz)	10	0	120	2	0
Light	1 tbsp (0.5 oz)	50	5	90	2	0
Real	1 tbsp (0.5 oz)	100	11	75	0	0
McIlhenny						
Spicy	1 tbsp (0.5 oz)	108	12	94	1	tr
Mother's						
Mayonnaise	1 tbsp	100	11	—	—	—
Red Wing						
"H" Style	1 tbsp (0.5 oz)	110	11	80	1	0
Smart Beat						
Canola Oil	1 tbsp	40	4	110	1	—
Corn Beat	1 tbsp	40	4	110	1	—
Fat Free	1 tbsp	10	0	135	3	—
Weight Watchers						
Fat Free	1 tbsp	10	0	105	3	0
Light	1 tbsp	25	2	130	1	0
Light Low Sodium	1 tbsp	25	2	40	1	0

MAYONNAISE TYPE SALAD DRESSING

(*see also* MAYONNAISE, RELISH)

home recipe	1 cup	400	24	1872	38	—

FOOD	PORTION	CAL.	FAT	SOD.	CARB.	FIB.
home recipe	1 tbsp	25	2	117	2	—
mayonnaise type salad dressing	1 cup	916	78	1670	56	—
mayonnaise type salad dressing	1 tbsp	57	5	—	4	—
reduced calorie w/o cholesterol	1 tbsp	68	7	49	2	—
reduced calorie w/o cholesterol	1 cup	1084	107	794	36	—
BAMA						
Dressing	1 tbsp	50	4	105	3	—
Bright Day						
Salad Dressing	1 tbsp	60	6	—	—	—
Miracle Whip						
Free	1 tbsp (0.5 oz)	15	0	125	2	0
Light	1 tbsp (0.5 oz)	35	3	130	2	0
Salad Dressing	1 tbsp (0.6 oz)	70	7	95	2	0
Nayonaise						
Cholesterol Free	1 tbsp (0.5 oz)	35	3	104	1	tr
Fat Free	1 tbsp (0.5 oz)	11	tr	107	2	tr
Spin Blend						
Cholesterol Free	1 tbsp	40	4	110	2	—
Dressing	1 tbsp	60	5	110	3	—
Weight Watchers						
Fat Free Whipped Dressing	1 tbsp	15	0	95	3	0

MEAT STICKS

FOOD	PORTION	CAL.	FAT	SOD.	CARB.	FIB.
jerky beef	1 lg piece (0.7 oz)	67	3	569	3	—
jerky beef	1 oz	96	4	815	4	—
smoked	1 oz	156	14	420	2	—
smoked	1 (0.7 oz)	109	10	293	1	—
Tombstone						
Beef Jerky	1 stick (0.5 oz)	35	0	310	tr	0
Beef Sticks	1 (0.8 oz)	110	10	270	0	0
Snappy Sticks	1 (0.8 oz)	110	10	260	tr	0

MEAT SUBSTITUTES

(*see also* BACON SUBSTITUTES, CHICKEN SUBSTITUTES, SAUSAGE SUBSTITUTES, TURKEY SUBSTITUTES)

FOOD	PORTION	CAL.	FAT	SOD.	CARB.	FIB.
simulated sausage	1 patty (38 g)	97	7	137	4	—
simulated sausage	1 link (25 g)	64	5	222	2	—
simulated meat product	1 oz	88	1	3	11	—
Boca Burgers						
Chef Max's Original	1 patty (2.5 oz)	110	2	296	9	4

FOOD	PORTION	CAL.	FAT	SOD.	CARB.	FIB.
Boca Burgers (CONT.)						
Hint Of Garlic	1 patty (2.5 oz)	110	2	296	9	4
Vegan Original	1 patty (2.5 oz)	84	0	269	9	5
Green Giant						
Harvest Burgers Original	1 (3 oz)	140	4	380	8	5
Harvest Direct						
TVP Beef Chunks	3.5 oz	280	1	15	32	18
TVP Beef Chunks Flavored	3.5 oz	250	1	2000	30	17
TVP Beef Strips	3.5 oz	280	1	15	32	18
TVP Ground Beef	3.5 oz	280	1	15	32	18
TVP Ground Beef Flavored	3.5 oz	250	1	2000	30	17
Jaclyn's						
Salisbury Steak Style Dinner	11 oz	260	8	320	37	—
Sirloin Strips Style Dinner	12 oz	290	6	320	37	—
Ken & Robert's						
Veggie Burger	1 (62 g)	110	2	390	19	—
Knox Mountain Farm						
Wheat Balls Mix	1 serv (1/10 pkg)	110	1	360	9	2
LaLoma						
Big Franks	1 (51 g)	110	6	190	2	—
Corn Dogs	1 (71 g)	190	8	400	15	—
Dinner Cuts	2 pieces (99 g)	110	1	340	2	—
Griddle Steaks	1 piece (54 g)	140	7	390	4	—
Nuteena	½ in slice (65 g)	160	12	110	6	—
Patty Mix	¼ cup (16 g)	50	0	200	4	—
Redi-Burger	½ in slice (68 g)	130	6	340	5	—
Sandwich Spread	3 tbsp (48 g)	70	4	300	4	—
Savory Dinner Loaf Mix not prep	¼ cup (16 g)	50	0	380	4	—
Savory Meatballs	7 (70 g)	190	8	420	7	—
Sizzle Burger	1 patty (71 g)	220	12	420	10	—
Sizzle Franks	2 (68 g)	170	13	340	3	—
Swiss Steak	1 piece (92 g)	170	10	360	7	—
Tender Bits	4 pieces (57 g)	80	3	260	5	—
Tender Rounds	6 pieces (73 g)	120	4	310	7	—
Vege-Burger	½ cup (108 g)	110	2	190	3	—
Vita-Burger Chunk	¼ cup (21 g)	70	0	150	6	—
Vita-Burger Granules	3 tbsp (21 g)	70	0	150	6	—
Lightlife						
American Grill	2.75 oz	110	3	325	8	—

FOOD	PORTION	CAL.	FAT	SOD.	CARB.	FIB.
Lightlife (CONT.)						
Barbecue Grill	2.75 oz	130	6	336	10	—
Smart Deli Slices	2 slices (1.5 oz)	44	0	290	1	—
Smart Dogs	1 (1.5 oz)	40	0	290	1	—
Smart Dogs To Go	1 (5 oz)	115	0	300	19	—
Tofu Pups	1 (1.5 oz)	92	5	—	—	—
Vegetarian Sloppy Joe	4.3 oz	130	6	310	11	—
Midland Harvest						
Burger n' Loaf Chili w/o Beans	0.8 oz	90	3	225	7	2
Burger n' Loaf Herbs & Spice	3.2 oz	140	5	250	7	4
Burger n' Loaf Italian	3.2 oz	140	5	375	7	4
Burger n' Loaf Original	3.2 oz	140	5	350	7	4
Burger n' Loaf Sloppy Joe w/o Sauce	0.8 oz	80	2	165	9	1
Burger n' Loaf Taco	2.7 oz	90	2	250	7	1
Morningstar Farms						
Breaded Cutlet	1 patty (71 g)	230	14	390	12	—
Deli Franks	1 (35 g)	90	6	420	2	—
Garden Grain Patties	1 pattie (2.5 oz)	120	3	280	18	4
Sandwich Burger Pattie w/ Cheese	1 (4.75 oz)	370	17	700	32	—
Sandwich Pattie Biscuit	1 (3.5 oz)	280	11	570	31	—
Natural Touch						
Dinner Entree	1 patty (85 g)	230	14	300	6	—
Garden Pattie	1 (67 g)	120	4	300	8	—
Loaf Mix as prep	4 oz	180	7	670	12	—
Okara Pattie	1 (64 g)	160	10	420	7	—
Stroganoff Mix as prep	4 oz	90	3	700	10	—
Taco Mix as prep	2 tbsp	90	2	210	6	—
NewMenu						
VegiBurger	1 patty (3 oz)	110	1	320	12	1
VegiDogs	1 (1.5 oz)	45	0	170	1	0
Quorn						
Burger	1 patty (3 oz)	100	4	420	9	4
Sovex						
Better Than Burger?	½ cup (1.9 oz)	165	2	52	25	9
Soy Is Us						
Beef Not!	½ cup (1.75 oz)	140	2	5	15	9
Spring Creek						
Soysage	1 patty (1.6 oz)	63	tr	237	11	—
Trader Joe's						
French Village Burger Champignon No Soy No Preservatives	1 patty (3.4 oz)	190	3	120	29	6

FOOD	PORTION	CAL.	FAT	SOD.	CARB.	FIB.
Veggie Patch						
Burgeriffics	1 (2.5 oz)	110	3	410	8	4
Perfectly Franks	1 (1.7 oz)	70	2	340	2	1
Veggie Rounds	1 (2.5 oz)	120	3	250	15	4
Veggitinos Meatballs	5 (2.8 oz)	120	4	470	10	3
White Wave						
Meatless Healthy Franks	1 (1.5 oz)	90	2	350	6	0
Meatless Jumbo Franks	1 (3 oz)	170	3	690	11	0
Meatless Sandwich Slices Beef	2 slices (1.6 oz)	90	0	270	8	1
Meatless Sandwich Slices Bologna	2 slices (1.6 oz)	120	8	370	5	1
Meatless Sandwich Slices Pastrami	2 slices (1.6 oz)	90	0	270	8	1
Meatless Healthy Franks	1 (1.5 oz)	90	2	350	6	—
Veggie Burger	1 patty (2.5 oz)	110	3	210	16	2
Worthington						
Beef Style Meatless	4 slices (70 g)	130	6	750	7	—
Bolono	2 slices (38 g)	60	2	390	2	—
Choplets	2 slices (92 g)	100	2	440	4	—
Corn Beef Sliced	4 slices (57 g)	120	6	740	8	—
Country Stew	9.5 oz (270 g)	220	10	760	23	—
Dinner Roast	2 oz	120	8	440	5	—
FriPats	1 (64 g)	180	12	360	5	—
Granburger not prep	6 tbsp (33 g)	110	1	730	7	—
Multigrain Cutlet	2 slices (92 g)	90	2	550	5	—
Non-Meat Balls	3 (54 g)	100	6	210	5	—
Numete	½ in slice (68 g)	150	11	410	7	—
Prime Stakes	1 piece (92 g)	160	10	410	7	—
Prosage Patties	2 (76 g)	210	14	780	4	—
Prosage Roll	2⅜ in slice (70 g)	180	12	570	4	—
Protose	½ in slice (76 g)	180	8	470	9	—
Salami Meatless	2 slices (38 g)	70	4	460	2	—
Savory Slices	2 slices (56 g)	100	6	340	4	—
Smoked Beef Slices	6 slices (56 g)	120	6	790	7	—
Stakelets	1 piece (71 g)	150	8	460	7	—
Veelets	1 patty (71 g)	230	14	390	12	—
Vegetable Skallops	½ cup (85 g)	90	2	430	4	—
Vegetable Skallops No Added Salt	½ cup (85 g)	80	1	80	4	—
Vegetable Steaks	2.5 pieces (90 g)	110	2	400	5	—
Vegetarian Burger	½ cup (113 g)	150	4	780	9	—
Vegetarian Burger No Added Salt	½ cup (113 g)	150	4	170	7	—

FOOD	PORTION	CAL.	FAT	SOD.	CARB.	FIB.
Worthington (CONT.)						
Vegetarian Beef Pie	1 (227 g)	360	16	1940	44	—
Wham	3 slices (68 g)	120	7	940	3	—
Zoglo's						
Crispy Vegetarian Cutlets	1 (3.5 oz)	200	10	300	10	2
Savory Vegetarian Kebabs	1 serv (2.8 oz)	135	5	240	5	2
Tender Vegetarian Burgers	1 (2.6 oz)	150	7	230	5	2
Vegetable Patties	1 (2.6 oz)	130	5	270	10	2
Vegetarian Franks	1 (2.6 oz)	125	5	240	5	2

MELON

(*see also individual names*)

FOOD	PORTION	CAL.	FAT	SOD.	CARB.	FIB.
FRESH						
Chiquita						
Cantalene	1 cup	60	0	—	—	—
Honey Mist	1 cup	80	0	—	—	—
FROZEN						
melon balls	1 cup	55	tr	53	14	—
Big Valley						
Mixed	¾ cup (4.9 oz)	40	0	16	10	1

MEXICAN FOOD

(*see* SALSA, SAUCE, SPANISH FOODS, TORTILLA)

MILK

(*see also* CHOCOLATE, COCOA, MILK DRINKS, MILKSHAKE)

(FAST FACT: Americans are drinking less milk: 28 gallons a year in 1974; 26 gallons in 1984 and 24 gallons in 1995.)

FOOD	PORTION	CAL.	FAT	SOD.	CARB.	FIB.
CANNED						
condensed sweetened	1 oz	123	3	49	21	—
condensed sweetened	1 cup	982	27	389	166	—
evaporated	½ cup	169	10	122	13	—
evaporated skim	½ cup	99	tr	147	14	—
Carnation						
Evaporated	2 tbsp	40	3	35	3	—
Evaporated Lowfat	2 tbsp	25	1	35	3	—
Lite Evaporated Skimmed	½ cup (4 fl oz)	100	tr	150	14	—
Sweetened Condensed	2 tbsp	130	3	45	22	—
Eagle						
Sweetened Condensed	⅓ cup	320	9	120	52	—
Pet						
Evaporated	½ cup	170	10	140	12	—

FOOD	PORTION	CAL.	FAT	SOD.	CARB.	FIB.
Pet (CONT.)						
Evaporated Filled	½ cup	150	8	140	12	—
Evaporated Light Skimmed	½ cup	100	tr	150	14	—
DRIED						
buttermilk	1 tbsp	25	tr	34	3	—
nonfat instantized	1 pkg (3.2 oz)	244	tr	499	47	—
Carnation						
Nonfat	⅓ cup dry	80	0	125	12	—
Nutra/Balance						
Lactose Reduced as prep	8 oz	80	tr	125	12	—
Sanalac						
As Prep	8 oz	80	tr	125	12	0
REFRIGERATED						
1%	1 cup	102	3	123	12	—
1%	1 qt	409	10	493	47	—
1% protein fortified	1 qt	477	12	574	54	—
1% protein fortified	1 cup	119	3	143	14	—
2%	1 cup	121	5	122	12	—
2%	1 qt	485	19	487	47	—
buffalo	3½ oz	112	8	40	5	—
buttermilk	1 cup	99	2	257	12	—
buttermilk	1 qt	396	9	1028	47	—
camel	3½ oz	80	4	30	5	—
donkey	3½ oz	43	1	—	6	—
goat	1 cup	168	10	122	11	—
goat	1 qt	672	40	486	43	—
human	1 cup	171	11	42	17	—
indian buffalo	1 cup	236	17	127	13	—
low sodium	1 cup	149	8	6	11	—
mare	3½ oz	49	2	—	6	—
nonfat	1 cup	86	tr	125	12	—
nonfat	1 qt	342	2	505	48	—
nonfat protein fortified	1 qt	400	2	578	55	—
nonfat protein fortified	1 cup	100	1	144	14	—
sheep	1 cup	264	17	108	13	—
whole	1 cup	150	8	120	11	—
BodyWise						
Nonfat	8 fl oz	100	0	150	14	0
Borden						
Acidophilus 1%	8 fl oz	100	2	130	11	—
Buttermilk Lowfat Golden Churn	8 fl oz	120	4	250	11	—

FOOD	PORTION	CAL.	FAT	SOD.	CARB.	FIB.
Borden (CONT.)						
Hi-Calcium	8 fl oz	150	8	130	11	—
Hi-Protein 2%	8 fl oz	140	5	150	13	—
Milk	8 fl oz	150	8	130	11	—
Skim	8 fl oz	90	1	130	12	—
Skim-line	8 fl oz	100	1	150	13	—
CalciMilk						
CalciMilk	8 fl oz	102	3	123	12	0
Farmland						
1%	8 fl oz	100	3	130	12	0
2%	8 fl oz	130	5	130	12	0
Cholesterol Reduced	8 oz	150	8	125	11	—
Easylac 1%	8 fl oz	100	2	125	11	—
Easylac Nonfat	8 fl oz	90	0	125	12	—
Skim	8 fl oz	80	0	130	12	0
Skim Plus	8 fl oz	110	0	170	17	0
Friendship						
Buttermilk	8 fl oz	120	4	125	12	0
Hood						
1%	1 cup (8 oz)	110	3	125	13	0
Better Taste 2%	1 cup (8 oz)	130	5	125	13	0
Buttermilk	1 cup (8 oz)	90	0	220	13	0
Whole	1 cup (8 oz)	150	8	125	12	0
Lactaid						
1%	8 fl oz	102	3	123	12	0
Nonfat	8 fl oz	86	tr	126	12	0
Nuform						
1%	1 cup (8 oz)	120	3	150	15	0
Skim	1 cup (8 oz)	100	0	150	15	0
Silovet						
Skim	1 cup (8 oz)	90	0	125	13	0
Viva						
2%	8 fl oz	120	5	125	11	—
Skim	8 fl oz	100	1	150	13	—
Weight Watchers						
Skim	1 cup	90	0	130	13	0
SHELF-STABLE						
Parmalat						
1%	1 cup (8 oz)	110	3	135	13	0
2%	1 cup (8 oz)	130	5	130	13	0
Skim	1 cup (8 oz)	90	1	130	13	0
Whole	1 cup (8 oz)	160	8	130	13	0

MILK DRINKS

(*see also* BREAKFAST DRINKS, CHOCOLATE, COCOA, MILKSHAKES)

chocolate milk	1 cup	208	8	149	26	—

FOOD	PORTION	CAL.	FAT	SOD.	CARB.	FIB.
chocolate milk	1 qt	833	34	596	103	—
chocolate milk 1%	1 cup	158	3	152	26	—
chocolate milk 1%	1 qt	630	10	607	104	—
chocolate milk 2%	1 cup	179	5	150	26	—
strawberry flavor mix as prep w/ whole milk	9 oz	234	8	128	33	—
Body Wise						
Chocolate Nonfat Milk	1 cup (8 fl oz)	180	0	170	35	1
Borden						
Chocolate Lowfat Dutch Brand	8 fl oz	180	5	180	25	—
Bosco						
Chocolate Milk	1 cup (8 fl oz)	230	8	110	33	—
Hershey						
Chocolate Milk 2%	1 cup	190	5	130	29	—
Whole Chocolate Milk	8 oz	210	9	120	28	—
Hood						
Chocolate Lowfat	1 cup (8 oz)	150	2	240	27	0
Lactaid						
Chocolate Milk 1%	8 fl oz	158	3	152	26	tr
Meadow Gold						
Chocolate Milk	8 fl oz	210	8	240	25	—
Parmalat						
Chocolate 2%	1 box (8 oz)	180	5	115	28	1
Quik						
Banana Lowfat Milk	8 oz	190	4	115	30	—
Chocolate Lowfat Milk	8 oz	200	5	150	29	—
Chocolate as prep w/ 2% milk	8 oz	210	5	150	31	—
Chocolate as prep w/ skim milk	8 oz	170	1	150	31	—
Chocolate as prep w/ whole milk	8 oz	230	9	140	31	—
Ready To Drink Chocolate	8 oz	230	9	120	30	—
Ready To Drink Lite Chocolate Lowfat	8 oz	130	5	150	13	—
Ready To Drink Strawberry	8 oz	230	8	140	32	—
Strawberry Lowfat Milk	8 oz	200	4	120	33	—
Strawberry as prep w/ 2% milk	8 oz	200	5	120	32	—
Strawberry as prep w/ skim milk	8 oz	160	0	125	32	—

FOOD	PORTION	CAL.	FAT	SOD.	CARB.	FIB.
Quik (CONT.)						
Strawberry as prep w/ whole milk	8 oz	220	8	120	32	—
Sugar Free Chocolate as prep w/ 2% milk	8 oz	140	5	150	15	—
Syrup Chocolate as prep w/ 2% milk	8 oz	220	5	160	34	—
Syrup Chocolate as prep w/ skim milk	8 oz	220	9	160	34	—
Syrup Chocolate as prep w/ whole milk	8 oz	240	9	160	33	—
Syrup Strawberry as prep w/ 2% milk	8 oz	220	5	120	36	—
Syrup Strawberry as prep w/ skim milk	8 oz	180	0	130	36	—
Syrup Strawberry as prep w/ whole milk	8 oz	240	8	120	36	—
Vanilla Lowfat Milk	8 oz	200	4	115	31	—
MILK SUBSTITUTES (*see also* COFFEE WHITENERS)						
imitation milk	1 cup	150	8	191	15	—
imitation milk	1 qt	600	33	764	60	—
Better Than Milk						
Carob	8 fl oz	130	5	175	20	—
Chocolate	8 fl oz	125	5	175	17	—
Light	8 fl oz	80	tr	120	15	—
Natural	8 fl oz	90	5	120	10	—
Eden						
Original	8 fl oz	130	4	105	13	0
Original	1 pkg (8.8 oz)	135	4	110	14	0
EdenBlend						
Original	8 fl oz	120	3	85	16	0
EdenRice						
Milk	8 fl oz	110	3	85	21	0
Edensoy						
Carob	8 fl oz	150	4	105	23	0
Extra Original	8 fl oz	130	5	100	12	0
Extra Original	1 pkg (8.8 oz)	140	5	105	13	0
Extra Vanilla	1 pkg (8.8 fl oz)	150	3	95	24	0
Extra Vanilla	8 fl oz	140	3	90	23	0
Vanilla	8 fl oz	150	3	90	23	0
Vanilla	1 pkg (8.8 fl oz)	150	3	95	24	0
Health Valley						
Soo Moo	1 cup	120	6	55	12	0

FOOD	PORTION	CAL.	FAT	SOD.	CARB.	FIB.
Rice Dream						
Carob Lite	8 fl oz	150	3	80	32	—
Chocolate	8 fl oz	190	3	80	44	—
Chocolate	8 fl oz	190	3	80	44	—
Lite Organic Original	8 fl oz	130	2	80	28	—
Lite Vanilla	8 fl oz	130	2	80	30	—
Spring Creek						
!Honey Vanilla	1 oz	23	5	7	3	—
Original	1 oz	21	5	6	3	—
Plain	1 oz	15	5	4	1	—
Vegelicious						
Milk	8 fl oz	100	2	125	18	—
Vitamite						
Non-Dairy 2% Fat	1 cup (8 oz)	110	5	120	14	0
Non-Diary Nonfat	1 cup (8 oz)	90	0	70	21	0
Vitasoy						
Carob Supreme	8 fl oz	210	6	160	32	1
Cocoa Light	8 fl oz	130	2	130	25	1
Original Creamy	8 fl oz	160	7	180	14	1
Original Light	8 fl oz	90	2	95	15	1
Rich Cocoa	8 fl oz	210	6	180	32	1
Vanilla Light	8 fl oz	110	2	95	20	1
Vanilla Delite	8 fl oz	190	6	130	27	1
Westsoy						
Cocoa Lite	8 fl oz	140	2	95	25	—
Plain Lite	8 fl oz	100	2	100	16	—
Vanilla Lite	8 fl oz	110	2	80	20	—
MILKFISH						
baked	3 oz	162	7	—	0	—
MILKSHAKE						
chocolate	10 oz	360	11	273	58	—
strawberry	10 oz	319	8	234	53	—
thick shake chocolate	10.6 oz	356	8	333	63	—
thick shake vanilla	11 oz	350	10	299	56	—
vanilla	10 oz	314	8	232	51	—
D'Frosta Shake						
Vanilla	1 serv (13.5 oz)	340	9	200	57	1
Freeze Flip						
Fruit Shake No Fat Lactose Free Black Raspberry	1 serv (6 oz)	150	0	25	37	1
Frostee						
Chocolate	8 fl oz	200	8	160	30	—

FOOD	PORTION	CAL.	FAT	SOD.	CARB.	FIB.
Frostee (CONT.)						
Strawberry	8 fl oz	180	7	150	27	—
Hood						
Shake Up Chocolate	1 cup (8 oz)	240	6	290	38	0
Shake Up Strawberry	1 cup (8 oz)	220	5	270	36	0
Shake Up Vanilla	1 cup (8 oz)	220	5	270	36	0
MicroMagic						
Chocolate	1 (10.5 oz)	290	8	90	46	—
Milky Way						
Shake	1 (10 fl oz)	390	16	235	54	0
Parmalat						
Shake A Shake Chocolate	1 box (6 oz)	180	4	140	29	1
Shake A Shake Orange Vanilla	1 box (6 oz)	110	3	55	14	0
Shake A Shake Vanilla	1 box (6 oz)	170	3	140	28	0
Weight Watchers						
Chocolate Fudge Shake Mix as prep	1 pkg	80	1	140	12	2
MILLET						
cooked	½ cup	143	1	2	28	—
MINERAL/BOTTLED WATER						
Canada Dry						
Sparkling Water	8 fl oz	0	0	10	0	0
Crystal Geyser						
Sparkling Natural Wild Cherry	1 bottle 12 fl oz	0	0	70	0	—
Sparkling Lemon	1 bottle (12 fl oz)	0	0	70	0	—
Sparkling Mineral	1 bottle (12 fl oz)	0	0	70	0	—
Sparkling Natural Cola Berry	1 bottle (12 fl oz)	0	0	70	0	—
Sparkling Orange	1 bottle (12 fl oz)	0	0	70	0	—
Diamond Spring						
Water	1 qt	0	0	—	—	—
Evian						
Water	1 liter	0	0	5	0	0
Glennpatrick						
Irish Spring Pure	8 oz	0	0	—	—	—
LaCroix						
Sparkling Berry	12 fl oz	0	0	—	—	—
Sparkling Lemon	12 fl oz	0	0	—	—	—
Sparkling Lime	12 fl oz	0	0	—	—	—
Sparkling Orange	12 fl oz	0	0	—	—	—

FOOD	PORTION	CAL.	FAT	SOD.	CARB.	FIB.
LaCroix (CONT.)						
Sparkling Regular	12 fl oz	0	0	—	—	—
Spring	1 bottle (12 oz)	0	0	<8	0	0
Mountain Valley						
Mineral Water	1 qt	0	0	—	—	—
Mt Shasta						
Natural Spring	1 bottle (20 oz)	0	0	<13	0	0
San Pellegrino						
Mineral Water	1 liter (33.8 oz)	0	0	41	0	—
Saratoga						
Sparkling	1 liter	0	0	19	0	—
Water Joe						
Caffeine Enhanced	8 fl oz	0	0	0	0	—
MISO						
miso	½ cup	284	8	5036	39	7
Eden						
Genmai Miso Organic	1 tbsp (0.5 oz)	25	1	810	3	tr
Hacho Miso Organic	1 tbsp (0.5 oz)	35	2	600	2	1
Kome Miso Organic	1 tbsp (0.6 oz)	25	1	850	3	tr
Mugi Miso Organic	1 tbsp (0.6 oz)	25	1	760	3	1
Shiro Miso Organic	1 tbsp (0.6 oz)	35	1	410	5	1
MOLASSES						
blackstrap	1 tbsp (0.7 oz)	47	0	11	12	—
blackstrap	1 cup (11.5 oz)	771	tr	180	199	—
molasses	1 tbsp (0.7 oz)	53	0	7	14	—
molasses	1 cup (11.5 oz)	873	1	120	226	—
Brer Rabbit						
Dark	2 tbsp	110	0	20	28	—
Light	2 tbsp	110	0	15	29	—
McIlhenny						
Molasses	1 tbsp (0.7 oz)	66	tr	9	16	tr
Tree Of Life						
Blackstrap	1 tbsp (0.5 oz)	45	0	15	11	—
MONKFISH						
baked	3 oz	82	2	20	0	—
MOOSE						
roasted	3 oz	114	1	58	0	—
MOTH BEANS						
dried cooked	1 cup	207	1	17	37	—
MOUSSE						
FROZEN						
Pepperidge Farm						
San Francisco Chocolate Mousse	1	490	34	75	41	—

FOOD	PORTION	CAL.	FAT	SOD.	CARB.	FIB.
Sara Lee						
Chocolate	1 slice (2.7 oz)	260	17	100	23	—
Chocolate Light	1 (3 oz)	170	8	60	20	—
Light Classics Strawberry	1 slice (53.8 g)	180	11	—	—	—
Weight Watchers						
Chocolate Mousse	1 (2.75 oz)	190	5	150	31	3
HOME RECIPE						
chocolate	½ cup (7.1 oz)	447	33	87	33	—
crab	¼ cup	364	20	—	—	—
orange	½ cup	87	5	24	19	—
MIX						
Knorr						
Dark Chocolate as prep	½ cup	90	5	50	10	—
Milk Chocolate as prep	½ cup	90	5	50	11	—
Unflavored as prep	½ cup	80	5	45	8	—
White Chocolate as prep	½ cup	80	4	50	10	—
Royal						
Chocolate Mousse No-Bake	⅛ pie	130	4	190	21	—
TAKE-OUT						
chocolate	½ cup (7.1 oz)	447	33	87	33	—

MUFFIN

FOOD	PORTION	CAL.	FAT	SOD.	CARB.	FIB.
FROZEN						
Health Valley						
Almond & Date Oat Bran Fancy Fruit	1	180	4	80	31	8
Fat Free Apple Spice	1	140	tr	110	30	5
Fat Free Banana	1	130	tr	110	29	5
Fat Free Raisin Spice	1	140	tr	100	32	5
Oat Bran Fancy Fruit Blueberry	1	140	4	100	32	8
Oat Bran Fancy Fruit Raisin	1	180	5	90	5	8
Rice Bran Fancy Fruit Raisin	1	210	7	125	7	6
Pepperidge Farm						
Banana Nut	1	170	6	220	28	—
Blueberry	1	170	7	250	27	1
Cholesterol Free Multi Grain Muesli	1	200	8	230	30	—
Cholesterol Free Oatbran With Apple	1	190	7	200	29	—

FOOD	PORTION	CAL.	FAT	SOD.	CARB.	FIB.
Pepperidge Farm (CONT.)						
Cholesterol Free Raisin Bran	1	170	6	280	30	—
Cinnamon Swirl	1	190	6	170	30	1
Corn	1	180	7	260	27	—
Sara Lee						
Apple Oat Bran	1	190	6	300	36	—
Apple Spice	1	220	8	280	36	—
Blueberry	1	200	8	290	34	—
Blueberry Free & Light	1	120	0	140	28	—
Cheese Streusel	1	220	11	170	27	—
Chocolate Chunk	1	220	8	210	33	—
Golden Corn	1	240	13	310	31	—
Oat Bran	1	210	8	320	35	—
Raisin Bran	1	220	7	400	37	—
Weight Watchers						
Chocolate Chocolate Chip	1 (2.5 oz)	190	2	350	39	4
Fat Free Banana	1 (2.5 oz)	170	0	310	41	3
Fat Free Blueberry	1 (2.5 oz)	160	0	290	38	2
Harvest Honey Bran	1 (2.5 oz)	220	4	150	43	10
HOME RECIPE						
blueberry as prep w/ 2% milk	1 (2 oz)	163	6	251	23	—
blueberry as prep w/ whole milk	1 (2 oz)	165	6	251	23	—
corn as prep w/ 2% milk	1 (2 oz)	180	7	334	25	—
corn as prep w/ whole milk	1 (2 oz)	183	7	333	25	—
plain as prep w/ 2% milk	1 (2 oz)	169	7	266	24	—
plain as prep w/ whole milk	1 (2 oz)	172	7	266	24	—
wheat bran as prep w/ 2% milk	1 (2 oz)	161	7	335	24	—
wheat bran as prep w/ whole milk	1 (2 oz)	164	7	335	24	—
MIX						
blueberry	1 (1¾ oz)	149	4	219	24	—
corn	1 (1.75 oz)	160	5	397	25	—
wheat bran as prep	1 (1¾ oz)	138	5	233	23	—
Arrowhead						
Bran	⅓ cup (1.4 oz)	150	2	160	26	7
Oat Bran Wheat Free	⅓ cup (1.5 oz)	160	4	310	23	7
Betty Crocker						
Apple Cinnamon	1	120	4	140	18	—
Apple Cinnamon No Cholesterol Recipe	1	110	2	140	18	—

FOOD	PORTION	CAL.	FAT	SOD.	CARB.	FIB.
Betty Crocker (CONT.)						
Banana Nut	1	120	5	140	17	—
Banana Nut No Cholesterol Recipe	1	110	4	140	17	—
Blueberry Streusel Bake Shop	1	210	8	230	31	—
Cinnamon Streusel	1	200	9	240	17	—
Oat Bran	1	190	8	240	25	—
Oat Bran No Cholesterol Recipe	1	180	7	240	25	—
Twice The Blueberries	1	120	4	140	18	—
Twice The Blueberries No Cholesterol Recipe	1	110	3	140	18	—
Wild Blueberry	1	120	4	150	18	—
Wild Blueberry Light	1	70	tr	140	16	—
Wild Blueberry Light No Cholesterol Recipe	1	70	tr	140	16	—
Wild Blueberry No Cholesterol Recipe	1	110	3	150	18	—
Dromedary						
Corn Muffin	1	120	4	270	20	—
Flako						
Corn	⅓ cup (1.4 oz)	160	4	380	29	1
Hain						
Oat Bran Apple Cinnamon	1	140	3	200	28	5
Oat Bran Banana Nut	1	140	4	190	26	4
Oat Bran Raspberry Spice	1	140	3	190	27	4
Jiffy						
Apple Cinnamon as prep	1	190	7	360	28	1
Banana Nut as prep	1	180	7	420	25	1
Blueberry as prep	1	190	7	288	28	1
Bran Date	1	110	—	—	—	—
Bran With Dates as prep	1	170	6	240	26	3
Corn as prep	1	180	4	320	28	1
Honey Date as prep	1	170	5	240	27	1
Oatmeal as prep	1	180	7	270	26	2
Wanda's						
Blue Corn	¼ cup mix per serv (1.2 oz)	130	1	350	25	1
READY-TO-EAT						
blueberry	1 (2 oz)	158	4	255	27	2
corn	1 (2 oz)	174	5	297	29	—

FOOD	PORTION	CAL.	FAT	SOD.	CARB.	FIB.
oat bran wheat free	1 (2 oz)	154	4	224	28	4
toaster type blueberry	1	103	3	158	18	—
toaster type corn	1	114	4	142	19	—
toaster type wheat bran w/ raisins	1 (1.3 oz)	106	3	178	19	—
Arnold						
Bran'nola	1 (2.3 oz)	160	1	220	30	2
Raisin	1 (2.3 oz)	160	1	220	33	2
Dutch Mill						
Apple Oat Bran	1 (2 oz)	180	5	210	31	1
Banana Walnut	1 (2 oz)	220	6	210	33	1
Carrot	1 (2 oz)	190	7	230	31	1
Corn	1 (2 oz)	190	6	280	31	1
Cranberry Orange	1 (2 oz)	170	6	290	26	1
Raisin Bran	1 (2 oz)	230	5	330	37	3
Entenmann's						
Blueberry	1 (2 oz)	200	8	250	29	—
Freihofer's						
Corn Toasters	1 (1.3 oz)	130	6	210	18	0
Hostess						
Mini Apple Cinnamon	5 (2 oz)	260	16	180	28	3
Mini Banana Nut	5 (2 oz)	260	16	160	28	tr
Mini Blueberry	5 (2 oz)	240	13	180	30	tr
Mini Chocolate Chip	5 (2 oz)	260	15	170	29	1
Muffin Loaf Blueberry	1 (3.8 oz)	440	19	460	62	2
Oat Bran	1 (1.5 oz)	160	8	150	22	tr
Oat Bran Banana Nut	1 (1.5 oz)	150	6	160	22	1
Weight Watchers						
Fat Free Apple Crisp	1 (2.5 oz)	160	0	290	37	1
Fat Free Cranberry Orange	1 (2.5 oz)	160	0	290	38	1
Fat Free Double Chocolate	1 (2.5 oz)	180	0	300	40	2
Fat Free Wild Blueberry	1 (2.5 oz)	160	0	280	36	1
Low Fat Apple Cinnamon	1 (2.5 oz)	170	3	200	35	2
Low Fat Blueberry	1 (2.5 oz)	180	3	200	37	2
Low Fat Carrot	1 (2.5 oz)	160	3	200	34	2
Low Fat Chocolate Chip	1 (2.5 oz)	180	3	200	38	2
Low Fat Lemon Poppy	1 (2.5 oz)	190	3	200	38	2
MULBERRIES						
fresh	1 cup	61	1	14	14	—
MULLET						
striped cooked	3 oz	127	4	61	0	—
striped raw	3 oz	99	3	55	0	—

FOOD	PORTION	CAL.	FAT	SOD.	CARB.	FIB.
MUNG BEANS						
DRIED						
cooked	1 cup	213	1	4	39	—
SPROUTS						
canned	½ cup	8	tr	—	1	—
cooked	½ cup	13	tr	6	3	—
raw	½ cup	16	tr	3	3	—
stir fried	½ cup	31	tr	—	7	—
MUNGO BEANS						
dried cooked	1 cup	190	1	13	33	—
MUSHROOMS						
CANNED						
chanterelle	3½ oz	12	1	165	tr	6
pieces	½ cup	19	tr	—	4	—
whole	1 (0.4 oz)	3	tr	—	1	—
B In B						
Mushrooms	¼ cup	12	0	240	2	1
With Garlic	¼ cup	12	0	200	2	1
Empress						
Button	2 oz	14	0	260	2	—
Button Sliced	2 oz	14	0	260	2	—
Pieces & Stems	2 oz	14	0	260	2	—
Straw Broken	2 oz	10	0	180	2	—
Green Giant						
Oriental Straw	¼ cup	12	0	290	2	1
Pieces And Stems	¼ cup	12	0	220	2	1
Sliced	¼ cup	12	0	220	2	1
Whole	¼ cup	12	0	220	2	1
Ka-Me						
Stir Fry	½ cup (4.5 oz)	20	0	380	3	2
Straw Whole Peeled	½ cup (4.5 oz)	20	0	380	3	2
Seneca						
Mushrooms	½ cup	25	0	552	3	2
DRIED						
chanterelle	3½ oz	89	2	32	2	60
shiitake	4 (½ oz)	44	tr	2	11	—
FRESH						
chanterelle	3½ oz	11	tr	3	tr	6
enoki raw	1 (4 in)	2	tr	0	tr	—
morel	3½ oz	9	tr	2	0	7
oyster	3.5 oz	11	tr	6	0	6
raw	1 (½ oz)	5	tr	1	1	tr
raw sliced	½ cup	9	tr	1	2	tr

FOOD	PORTION	CAL.	FAT	SOD.	CARB.	FIB.
shitake cooked	4 (2.5 oz)	40	tr	3	10	—
sliced cooked	½ cup	21	tr	2	4	1
whole cooked	1 (0.4 oz)	3	tr	0	1	—
Mother Earth						
Organic	4 oz	35	1	0	5	tr
FROZEN						
Empire						
Breaded	7 (2.8 oz)	90	1	390	16	1
Fresh Like						
Mushrooms	3.5 oz	28	tr	15	4	1
MUSKRAT						
roasted	3 oz	199	10	81	0	—
MUSSELS						
blue raw	3 oz	73	2	243	3	—
blue raw	1 cup	129	3	429	6	—
fresh blue cooked	3 oz	147	4	313	6	—
MUSTARD						
dry mustard seed yellow	1 tsp	15	1	tr	1	—
yellow ready-to-use	1 tsp	5	tr	63	tr	—
Blanchard & Blanchard						
Mustard	1 tsp (5 g)	0	0	45	0	0
Eden						
Hot Organic	1 tsp (5 g)	0	0	65	tr	0
Estee						
Sodium Free	1 pkg (0.5 oz)	5	1	0	tr	—
Grey Poupon						
Country Dijon	1 tsp	6	0	120	0	0
Dijon	1 tsp	6	0	120	0	0
Parisian	1 tsp	6	0	55	0	0
Gulden's						
Diablo	1 tsp	8	0	—	—	—
Mild	1 tsp	6	0	—	—	—
Spicy Brown	1 tsp	8	0	—	—	—
Hain						
Stone Ground	1 tbsp	14	1	185	1	—
Stone Ground No Salt Added	1 tbsp	14	1	10	1	—
Heinz						
Mild Yellow	1 tbsp	8	tr	175	1	—
Spicy Brown	1 tbsp	14	1	115	1	—
Ka-Me						
Hot Mustard Powder Chinese Style	¼ tsp (1 g)	5	0	0	1	1

FOOD	PORTION	CAL.	FAT	SOD.	CARB.	FIB.
Kosciuszko						
Spicy Brown	1 tsp	5	tr	60	tr	—
Kraft						
Horseradish Mustard	1 tsp (5 g)	0	0	55	0	0
Mustard	1 tsp (5 g)	0	0	60	0	0
McIlhenny						
Coarse Ground	1 tsp (0.2 oz)	4	tr	39	tr	tr
Spicy	1 tsp (0.2 oz)	6	tr	28	tr	1
Plochman						
Dijon	1 tsp (5 g)	7	tr	82	tr	—
Spoonable Salad	1 tsp (5 g)	4	tr	53	tr	—
Squeeze Salad	1 tsp (5 g)	4	tr	53	tr	—
Stone Ground	1 tsp (5 g)	6	tr	60	tr	—
Russer						
Deli	1 tsp (5 g)	4	0	65	0	—
Tree Of Life						
Dijon	1 tsp (5 g)	0	0	66	0	—
Dijon Imported	1 tsp (5 g)	5	0	120	tr	—
Low Sodium	1 tsp (5 g)	3	0	50	tr	—
Stone Ground	1 tsp (5 g)	0	0	55	0	—
Yellow	1 tsp (5 g)	0	0	55	0	—
Watkins						
Country Mill	1 tsp (7 g)	15	1	110	2	0
Dusseldorf	1 tsp (7 g)	10	0	110	1	0
Horseradish	1 tsp (7 g)	10	0	120	1	0
Jalapeno	1 tsp (7 g)	10	0	150	1	0
Onion	1 tsp (7 g)	10	0	110	1	0
Parisienne	1 tsp (7 g)	10	0	110	1	0
MUSTARD GREENS						
CANNED						
Allen						
Mustard Greens	½ cup (4.1 oz)	30	1	10	5	3
Sunshine						
Mustard Greens	½ cup (4.1 oz)	30	1	10	5	3
FRESH						
chopped cooked	½ cup	11	tr	11	1	—
raw chopped	½ cup	7	tr	7	1	—
FROZEN						
chopped cooked	½ cup	14	tr	19	2	—
NATTO						
natto	½ cup	187	10	6	13	—
NAVY BEANS						
CANNED						
navy	1 cup	296	1	1173	54	—

FOOD	PORTION	CAL.	FAT	SOD.	CARB.	FIB.
Allen						
Navy Beans	½ cup (4.5 oz)	110	1	380	19	6
Eden						
Organic	½ cup (4.3 oz)	100	1	15	18	7
Hanover						
Navy	½ cup	100	0	—	—	—
Luck's						
Seasoned w/ Pork	7.5 oz	230	7	—	—	—
Trappey						
With Bacon	½ cup (4.5 oz)	110	2	420	17	7
With Bacon & Jalapeno	½ cup (4.5 oz)	110	2	420	17	7
DRIED						
cooked	1 cup	259	1	2	48	—
SPROUTS						
cooked	3½ oz	78	1	—	—	—
raw	½ cup	35	tr	—	—	—

NECTARINE

fresh	1	67	1	0	16	2
Dole						
Nectarine	1	70	1	0	16	3

NEUFCHATEL

neufchatel	1 oz	74	7	113	1	—
neufchatel	1 pkg (3 oz)	221	20	339	3	—
Philadelphia						
Neufchatel	1 oz	70	6	120	tr	0
WisPride						
Garden Vegetable Cup	2 tbsp (1.1 oz)	60	5	180	2	0
Garlic & Herb Cup	2 tbsp (1.1 oz)	60	5	180	2	0

NON-DAIRY CREAMERS

(*see* COFFEE WHITENERS)

NON-DAIRY TOPPINGS

(*see* WHIPPED TOPPINGS)

NOODLE DISHES

(*see also* NOODLES AND PASTA DINNERS)

CANNED						
Van Camp's						
Noodlee Weenee	1 can (8 oz)	230	8	680	34	1
FROZEN						
Luigino's						
Stroganoff	1 pkg (8 oz)	310	17	920	25	2

FOOD	PORTION	CAL.	FAT	SOD.	CARB.	FIB.
MIX						
Kraft						
Noodle Classics Cheddar Cheese as prep	1 cup (7.4 oz)	400	19	760	47	1
Noodle Classics Savory Chicken as prep	1 cup (8.5 oz)	340	13	1370	46	2
La Choy						
Ramen Noodles Beef as prep	1 cup	200	8	865	33	4
Ramen Noodles Chicken as prep	1 cup	200	7	740	29	4
Lipton						
Noodles & Sauce Alfredo	⅔ cup (2.2 oz)	250	7	940	38	1
Noodles & Sauce Alfredo Broccoli as prep	⅔ cup (2.2 oz)	260	7	940	39	2
Noodles & Sauce Alfredo Carbonara	⅔ cup (2.2 oz)	260	7	890	38	2
Noodles & Sauce Beef	⅔ cup (2.1 oz)	220	4	930	42	2
Noodles & Sauce Butter	⅔ cup (2.2 oz)	260	8	910	40	2
Noodles & Sauce Butter & Herb	⅔ cup (2.2 oz)	250	7	860	41	2
Noodles & Sauce Cheddar & Bacon	⅔ cup (2.1 oz)	230	5	930	38	2
Noodles & Sauce Cheese	⅔ cup (2.3 oz)	250	5	850	44	1
Noodles & Sauce Chicken	⅔ cup (2.1 oz)	230	5	760	41	2
Noodles & Sauce Chicken Broccoli	⅔ cup (2.1 oz)	220	4	750	40	2
Noodles & Sauce Chicken Tetrazzini	⅔ cup (2 oz)	220	5	850	37	2
Noodles & Sauce Creamy Chicken	⅔ cup (2.1 oz)	230	6	710	39	2
Noodles & Sauce Parmesan	⅔ cup (2.1 oz)	250	8	750	37	2
Noodles & Sauce Romanoff	⅔ cup (2.3 oz)	260	7	920	41	2
Noodles & Sauce Sour Cream & Chive	⅔ cup (2.2 oz)	260	8	800	41	2
Noodles & Sauce Stroganoff	⅔ cup (2 oz)	210	4	850	37	2
Noodle Roni						
Chicken & Mushroom	½ cup	160	4	550	25	—
Fettuccini	½ cup	300	18	560	29	—
Herb & Butter	½ cup	160	7	290	19	—

FOOD	PORTION	CAL.	FAT	SOD.	CARB.	FIB.
Noodle Roni (CONT.)						
Parmesano	½ cup	240	13	140	23	—
Romanoff	½ cup	240	11	730	28	—
Stroganoff	½ cup	350	17	1190	37	—
Noodles By Leonardo						
Macaroni & Cheese as prep	1 cup (2.5 oz)	250	1	530	49	2
Ultra Slim-Fast						
Noodles & Alfredo Sauce	2.3 oz	240	4	1110	47	4
Noodles & Beef	2.3 oz	230	3	1070	45	4
Noodles & Cheese	2.3 oz	230	4	770	44	4
Noodles & Chicken Sauce	2.3 oz	220	3	980	45	4
Noodles & Tomato Herb Sauce	2.3 oz	220	3	1090	46	5
SHELF-STABLE						
Micro Cup Meals						
Noodles & Chicken	1 cup (7.5 oz)	180	8	1010	19	1
TAKE-OUT						
noodle pudding	½ cup	132	7	222	11	—
NOODLES						
cellophane	1 cup	492	tr	14	121	—
chow mein	1 cup	237	14	197	26	—
egg	1 cup (38 g)	145	2	8	27	—
egg cooked	1 cup	212	2	11	40	—
japanese soba cooked	½ cup	56	tr	34	12	—
japanese soba not prep	2 oz	192	tr	451	43	—
japanese somen cooked	½ cup	115	tr	142	24	—
japanese somen not prep	2 oz	203	tr	1049	42	—
spinach/egg cooked	1 cup	211	3	20	39	—
spinach/egg not prep	1 cup	145	2	27	27	—
Azumaya						
Chinese	4 oz	293	1	530	60	—
Japanese	4 oz	289	1	542	59	—
Creamette						
Egg	2 oz	221	3	—	—	—
Egg	2 oz	220	3	20	40	—
Golden Grain						
Egg	2 oz	210	2	10	39	2
Herb's						
Egg Fine	2 oz	220	2	5	42	2
Egg Medium	2 oz	220	2	5	42	2
Kluski Medium	2 oz	220	2	5	42	2

FOOD	PORTION	CAL.	FAT	SOD.	CARB.	FIB.
Herb's (CONT.)						
Kluski Wide	2 oz	220	2	5	42	2
Hodgson Mill						
Veggie Egg	2 oz	200	2	25	37	2
Whole Wheat Egg	2 oz	190	2	20	34	4
Whole Wheat Spinach Egg	2 oz	190	2	45	32	5
Ka-Me						
Chinese Egg	½ cup (2 oz)	210	2	3	40	2
Chinese Plain	½ cup (2 oz)	200	0	1	45	1
Chuka Soba Curly Noodles	2 oz	200	1	310	42	1
Lo Mein Wide Chinese	½ cup (2 oz)	200	0	1	45	1
Py Mai Fun Rice Sticks	2 oz	193	0	100	48	0
Sai Fun Bean Thread	1 cup (2 oz)	190	0	0	50	1
Soba Shin Shu Japanese Buckwheat	2 oz	200	1	80	40	2
Tomoshiraga Somen Noodles	2 oz	190	1	670	41	1
Udon Japanese Thick	2 oz	190	1	670	41	1
La Choy						
Chow Mein Narrow	½ cup	150	8	320	16	tr
Chow Mein Wide	½ cup	150	8	300	16	tr
Rice	½ cup	130	5	420	21	tr
Mueller's						
Egg	2 oz (57 g)	220	3	8	40	—
Noodle Trio	2 oz (57 g)	220	2	18	40	—
Noodles By Leonardo						
Egg Fine	2 oz	210	2	10	39	2
Egg Medium	2 oz	210	2	30	39	2
Egg Wide	2 oz	210	2	30	39	2
San Giorgio						
Egg	2 oz	210	3	15	38	—
Shofar						
No Yolks	2 oz	210	0	30	41	3
NOPALES						
cooked	1 cup (5.2 oz)	23	tr	30	5	—
raw sliced	1 cup (3 oz)	14	tr	19	3	—
raw sliced	½ cup (1.5 oz)	7	tr	9	1	—
NUTMEG						
ground	1 tsp	12	1	tr	1	—

FOOD	PORTION	CAL.	FAT	SOD.	CARB.	FIB.
Watkins						
Ground	¼ tsp (0.5 g)	0	0	0	0	0

NUTRITIONAL SUPPLEMENTS

(*see also* BREAKFAST BAR, BREAKFAST DRINKS, SPORTS DRINKS)

FOOD	PORTION	CAL.	FAT	SOD.	CARB.	FIB.
BeneFit						
Chocolate	1 serv	120	2	200	15	1
Nutrition Bar	1 (2 oz)	240	8	190	33	tr
Vanilla	1 serv	120	2	220	15	tr
Boost						
Chocolate	1 can (8 oz)	240	4	130	40	0
Vanilla	8 oz	240	4	130	40	0
Calorie Shed						
Shake Fat Free No Sugar Caramel Ripple	½ cup (4 fl oz)	70	0	45	21	2
Shake Fat Free No Sugar Chocolate	½ cup (4 fl oz)	70	0	45	21	2
Shake Fat Free No Sugar Marshmellow Nougat	½ cup (4 fl oz)	70	0	45	21	2
Dynatrim						
Dutch Chocolate as prep w/ 1% milk	8 oz	220	4	300	33	6
Strawberry Royale as prep w/ 1% milk	8 oz	220	4	300	33	6
Vanilla as prep w/ 1% milk	8 oz	220	4	300	33	6
Fi-Bar						
Apple	1 (1 oz)	90	3	12	15	5
Cocoa Almond	1	130	4	20	21	4
Cocoa Peanut	1	130	4	20	20	4
Cranberry & Wild Berries	1 (1 oz)	100	3	20	13	4
Lemon	1 (1 oz)	90	3	12	15	5
Mandarin Orange	1 (1 oz)	99	4	12	15	5
Nuggets Almond Cappuccino Crunch	1 pkg	136	6	—	18	—
Nuggets Almond Butter Crunch	1 pkg	163	11	—	12	—
Nuggets Coconut Almond Crunch	1 pkg	136	6	—	18	—
Nuggets Peanut Butter Crunch	1 pkg	160	10	—	12	—
Raspberry	1 (1 oz)	100	3	20	13	4
Strawberry	1 (1 oz)	100	3	20	13	4

FOOD	PORTION	CAL.	FAT	SOD.	CARB.	FIB.
Fi-Bar (CONT.)						
Treat Yourself Right Almond	1	152	6	38	22	5
Treat Yourself Right Peanutty Butter	1	152	5	56	18	5
Vanilla Almond	1	130	4	20	21	4
Vanilla Peanut	1	130	4	20	20	4
Figurines						
Chocolate	1 bar	100	5	45	11	—
Chocolate Caramel	1 bar	100	6	55	10	—
Chocolate Peanut Butter	1 bar	100	6	45	10	—
S'Mores	1 bar	100	5	54	11	—
Vanilla	1 bar	100	5	45	11	—
Gatorade						
GatorBar	1 (1.17 oz)	110	1	10	13	1
GatorLode	1 can (11.6 fl oz)	280	0	90	71	—
GatorPro	1 can (11 fl oz)	360	6	270	59	0
ReLode	1 pkt (0.75 oz)	80	0	25	17	—
GeniSoy						
Soy Protein Powder	1 scoop (0.6 oz)	60	0	180	0	—
Soy Protein Shake Chocolate	1 scoop (1.2 oz)	120	0	170	17	2
Soy Protein Shake Vanilla	1 scoop (1.2 oz)	130	0	180	18	—
Soy Protein Bar Chocolate	1 bar (2.2 oz)	210	0	190	36	1
Soy Protein Bar Chocolate Coated	1 bar (2.2 oz)	220	4	190	33	1
Gookinaid						
Lemonade	1 cup (8 fl oz)	45	0	70	12	—
Malsovit						
Mealwafers	2	152	8	—	—	—
Meal On The Go						
Apple	1 bar (3 oz)	294	5	114	50	5
Banana w/ Pecans	1 bar (3 oz)	289	10	109	50	8
Original	1 bar (3 oz)	286	9	119	52	7
Nancy Grey's						
Shake Hi-Protein Black Raspberry	1 cup (8 fl oz)	340	16	160	40	0
Shake Hi-Protein Chocolate	1 cup (8 fl oz)	340	15	140	42	—
Shake Hi-Protein Vanilla	1 cup (8 fl oz)	340	16	160	40	0
NiteBite						
Chocolate Fudge	1 bar (0.9 oz)	100	4	40	15	0

FOOD	PORTION	CAL.	FAT	SOD.	CARB.	FIB.
NiteBite (CONT.)						
Peanut Butter	1 bar (0.9 oz)	100	4	80	15	0
Nutra/Balance						
EggPro	4 oz	200	4	105	33	—
Frozen Pudding Butterscotch	4 oz	225	8	220	31	—
Frozen Pudding Chocolate	4 oz	225	8	220	31	—
Frozen Pudding Tapioca	4 oz	225	8	220	31	—
Frozen Pudding Vanilla	4 oz	225	8	220	31	—
NutraShake						
Chocolate	4 oz	200	6	55	31	—
Strawberry	4 oz	200	6	55	31	—
Vanilla	4 oz	200	6	55	31	—
With Fiber Strawberry	6 oz	300	2	110	60	—
With Fiber Vanilla	6 oz	300	2	110	60	—
Power Bar						
Malt-Nut	1 bar (2.3 oz)	230	3	90	45	3
Resource						
Fructose Sweetened	1 pkg (8 oz)	250	11	230	23	3
Fruit Beverage	1 pkg (8 oz)	180	0	55	36	—
Liquid Food	1 pkg (8 oz)	250	9	210	34	—
Plus Liquid Food	1 pkg (8 oz)	355	13	300	47	—
Sego						
Lite Chocolate	10 fl oz	150	3	480	20	—
Lite Dutch Chocolate	10 fl oz	150	3	480	20	—
Lite French Vanilla	10 fl oz	150	4	390	17	—
Lite Strawberry	10 fl oz	150	4	390	17	—
Lite Vanilla	10 fl oz	150	4	390	17	—
Very Chocolate	10 fl oz	225	1	450	43	—
Very Chocolate Malt	10 fl oz	225	1	450	43	—
Very Strawberry	10 fl oz	225	5	360	34	—
Very Vanilla	10 fl oz	225	5	360	34	—
Slim-Fast						
Powder Chocolate as prep w/ skim milk	8 oz	190	1	210	32	2
Powder Chocolate Malt as prep w/ skim milk	8 oz	190	tr	230	32	2
Powder Strawberry as prep w/ skim milk	8 oz	190	1	220	32	2
Powder Vanilla as prep w/ skim milk	8 oz	190	1	220	32	2
Sustacal						
Vanilla	8 oz	240	6	220	33	tr

FOOD	PORTION	CAL.	FAT	SOD.	CARB.	FIB.
Sweet Success						
Chewy Bar Chocolate Brownie	1 (1.6 oz)	120	4	35	28	3
Chewy Bar Chocolate Peanut Butter	1 (1.6 oz)	120	4	35	23	3
Chewy Bar Chocolate Raspberry	1 (1.6 oz)	120	4	35	23	3
Chewy Bar Chocolate Chip	1 (1.6 oz)	120	4	35	23	3
Chewy Bar Oatmeal Raisin	1 (1.6 oz)	120	4	30	23	3
Chocolate Raspberry Truffle	1 can (10 fl oz)	200	3	220	38	6
Chocolate Raspberry as prep w/ skim milk	9 fl oz	180	1	360	30	6
Chocolate Mocha Supreme	1 can (10 fl oz)	200	3	220	38	6
Chocolate Mocha Supreme as prep w/ skim milk	9 fl oz	180	tr	356	30	6
Classic Chocolate Chip as prep w/ skim milk	9 fl oz	180	1	288	30	6
Creamy Milk Chocolate	1 carton (12 fl oz)	220	2	300	45	6
Creamy Milk Chocolate	1 can (10 fl oz)	200	3	240	38	6
Creamy Milk Chocolate as prep w/ skim milk	9 fl oz	180	1	336	30	6
Creamy Vanilla Delight as prep w/ skim milk	9 fl oz	180	tr	312	33	6
Dark Chocolate Fudge	1 carton (12 fl oz)	220	2	310	45	6
Dark Chocolate Fudge	1 can (10 fl oz)	200	3	220	38	6
Dark Chocolate Fudge as prep w/ skim milk	9 fl oz	180	1	356	30	6
Rich Chocolate Almond	1 can (10 fl oz)	200	3	240	38	6
Rich Chocolate Almond	1 carton (12 fl oz)	220	2	300	45	6
Rich Chocolate Almond as prep w/ skim milk	9 fl oz	180	tr	356	30	6
Smooth Vanilla Creme	1 can (10 fl oz)	200	3	220	38	6
The Pumper						
Body Building MilkShake Chocolate	1 serv (13.5 oz)	390	2	260	80	5
Ultra Slim-Fast						
Cafe Mocha as prep w/ skim milk	8 oz	200	tr	280	38	6
Chocolate Royale as prep w/ skim milk	8 oz	200	1	230	36	5

FOOD	PORTION	CAL.	FAT	SOD.	CARB.	FIB.
Ultra Slim-Fast (CONT.)						
Crunch Bar Cocoa Almond	1	110	3	30	19	3
Crunch Bar Cocoa Raspberry	1	100	3	30	21	3
Crunch Bar Vanilla Almond	1	110	4	30	18	3
Dutch Chocolate as prep w/ water	8 oz	220	tr	260	40	5
French Vanilla as prep w/ skim milk	8 oz	190	tr	250	36	4
French Vanilla as prep w/ water	8 oz	220	tr	260	40	4
Fruit Juice Mix as prep w/ fruit juice	8 oz	200	tr	80	43	6
Nutrition Bar Dutch Chocolate	1	130	4	90	17	6
Nutrition Bar Peanut Butter	1	140	6	100	15	7
Pina Colada as prep w/ skim milk	8 oz	180	tr	250	36	6
Ready-To-Drink Chocolate Royale	12 oz	250	1	240	45	5
Ready-To-Drink Chocolate Royale	11 oz	230	3	220	42	5
Ready-To-Drink French Vanilla	11 oz	230	5	190	38	5
Ready-To-Drink French Vanilla	12 oz	220	tr	240	38	5
Ready-To-Drink Strawberry Supreme	12 oz	220	1	240	38	5
Strawberry Supreme as prep w/ water	8 oz	220	tr	260	40	4
Strawberry as prep w/ skim milk	8 oz	190	1	250	36	4
Vita-J						
Apple Juice	11.5 fl oz	8	0	25	2	—
Fruit Punch	11.5 fl oz	8	0	25	2	—
Grapefruit Cocktail w/ Raspberry	11.5 fl oz	8	0	25	2	—
Orange Juice	11.5 fl oz	8	0	25	2	—
NUTS MIXED (*see also individual names*)						
dry roasted w/ peanuts	1 oz	169	15	3	7	—

FOOD	PORTION	CAL.	FAT	SOD.	CARB.	FIB.
dry roasted w/ peanuts salted	1 oz	169	15	223	7	—
oil roasted w/ peanuts	1 oz	175	16	3	6	—
oil roasted w/ peanuts salted	1 oz	175	16	217	6	—
oil roasted w/o peanuts	1 oz	175	16	3	6	—
oil roasted w/o peanuts salted	1 oz	175	16	233	6	—
Fisher						
Mixed Deluxe Lightly Salted	1 oz	180	16	—	5	—
Mixed Deluxe Salted	1 oz	180	16	95	5	—
Mixed Oil Roasted 25% More Cashews Lightly Salted	1 oz	180	16	50	5	—
Mixed Oil Roasted 25% More Cashews Salted	1 oz	180	16	110	5	—
Nut & Fruit Pina Colada	1 oz	150	10	50	13	—
Nut & Fruit Raisin Cranberry	1 oz	150	10	70	12	—
Nut & Fruit Tropical Fruit	1 oz	140	8	90	15	—
Nut Toppings Oil Roasted With Peanuts	1 oz	190	17	150	6	—
Peanuts Cashews	1 oz	170	13	110	8	—
Guy's						
Mixed With Peanuts	1 oz	180	16	140	3	—
Tasty Mix	1 oz	130	7	510	14	—
Planters						
Cashews & Peanuts Honey Roasted	1 oz	150	12	125	10	2
Deluxe Oil Roasted	1 oz	170	16	110	6	2
Dry Roasted	1 oz	170	14	250	7	2
Honey Roasted	1 oz	140	13	85	9	2
Lightly Salted Oil Roasted	1 oz	170	15	55	6	2
No Brazils Lightly Salted Oil Roasted	1 oz	170	15	55	6	2
No Brazils Oil Roasted	1 oz	170	15	110	6	2
Oil Roasted	1 oz	170	15	115	5	2
Select Mix Cashews Almonds & Macadamias Oil Roasted	1 oz	170	16	90	6	2

FOOD	PORTION	CAL.	FAT	SOD.	CARB.	FIB.
Planters (CONT.)						
Select Mix Cashews Almonds & Pecans Oil Roasted	1 oz	170	15	95	7	2
Unsalted Oil Roasted	1 oz	170	15	0	6	3
OCTOBER BEANS						
Luck's						
Seasoned w/ Pork	7.25 oz	230	6	—	—	—
OCTOPUS						
fresh steamed	3 oz	140	2	—	4	—
OHELOBERRIES						
fresh	1 cup	39	tr	2	10	—
OIL						
(*see also* FAT)						
almond	1 cup	1927	218	—	0	—
almond	1 tbsp	120	14	—	0	—
apricot kernel	1 cup	1927	218	—	0	—
apricot kernel	1 tbsp	120	14	—	0	—
avocado	1 cup	1927	218	—	0	—
avocado	1 tbsp	124	14	—	0	—
babassu palm	1 tbsp	120	14	—	0	—
butter oil	1 tbsp	112	13	—	0	—
butter oil	1 cup	1795	204	—	0	—
canola	1 tbsp	124	14	—	0	—
canola	1 cup	1927	218	—	0	—
coconut	1 tbsp	117	14	—	0	—
corn	1 cup	1927	218	—	0	—
corn	1 tbsp	120	14	—	0	—
cottonseed	1 cup	1927	218	—	0	—
cottonseed	1 tbsp	120	14	—	0	—
cupu assu	1 tbsp	120	14	—	0	—
grapeseed	1 tbsp	120	14	—	0	—
hazelnut	1 tbsp	120	14	—	0	—
hazelnut	1 cup	1927	218	—	0	—
mustard	1 tbsp	124	14	—	0	—
mustard	1 cup	1927	218	—	0	—
oat	1 tbsp	120	14	—	0	—
olive	1 tbsp	119	14	0	0	—
olive	1 cup	1909	216	tr	0	—
palm	1 tbsp	120	14	—	0	—
palm	1 cup	1927	218	—	0	—
palm kernel	1 tbsp	117	14	—	0	—

FOOD	PORTION	CAL.	FAT	SOD.	CARB.	FIB.
palm kernel	1 cup	1879	218	—	0	—
peanut	1 cup	1909	216	tr	0	—
peanut	1 tbsp	119	14	tr	0	—
poppyseed	1 tbsp	120	14	—	0	—
poppyseed	3.5 fl oz	900	100	—	0	—
pumpkin seed	3½ oz	925	100	—	0	—
rice bran	1 tbsp	120	14	—	0	—
safflower	1 cup	1927	218	—	0	—
safflower	1 tbsp	120	14	—	0	—
sesame	1 tbsp	120	14	—	0	—
sheanut	1 tbsp	120	14	—	0	—
soybean	1 tbsp	120	14	0	0	—
soybean	1 cup	1927	218	tr	0	—
sunflower	1 tbsp	120	14	—	0	—
sunflower	1 cup	1927	218	—	0	—
teaseed	1 tbsp	120	14	—	0	—
tomatoseed	1 tbsp	120	14	—	0	—
vegetable soybean & cottonseed	1 tbsp	120	14	—	0	—
vegetable soybean & cottonseed	1 cup	1927	218	—	0	—
walnut	1 cup	1927	218	—	0	1
walnut	1 tbsp	120	14	—	0	—
wheat germ	1 tbsp	120	14	—	0	—
Arrowhead						
Flax Seed	1 tbsp (0.5 fl oz)	120	14	0	0	0
Hazelnut	1 tbsp (0.5 fl oz)	120	14	0	0	0
Bertolli						
Classico	1 tbsp	120	14	—	—	—
Extra Light	1 tbsp	120	14	—	—	—
Extra Virgin	1 tbsp	120	14	—	—	—
Crisco						
Corn Canola	1 tbsp (0.5 fl oz)	120	14	0	0	—
Oil	1 tbsp (0.5 fl oz)	120	14	0	0	—
Puritan Canola	1 tbsp (0.5 fl oz)	120	14	0	0	0
Eden						
Hot Pepper Sesame	1 tbsp (0.5 oz)	130	14	0	0	0
Toasted Sesame	1 tbsp (0.5 oz)	130	14	0	0	0
Hain						
All Blend	1 tbsp	120	14	0	0	—
Almond	1 tbsp	120	14	0	0	—
Apricot Kernel	1 tbsp	120	14	0	0	—
Avocado	1 tbsp	120	14	0	0	—
Canola	1 tbsp	120	14	0	0	—

FOOD	PORTION	CAL.	FAT	SOD.	CARB.	FIB.
Hain (CONT.)						
Canola Organic	1 tbsp	120	14	0	0	—
Coconut	1 tbsp	120	14	0	0	—
Corn	1 tbsp	120	14	0	0	—
Garlic & Oil	1 tbsp	120	14	0	0	—
Olive	1 tbsp	120	14	0	0	—
Peanut	1 tbsp	120	14	0	0	—
Rice Bran	1 tbsp	120	14	0	0	—
Safflower	1 tbsp	120	14	0	0	—
Safflower Hi-Oleic	1 tbsp	120	14	0	0	—
Safflower Organic	1 tbsp	120	14	0	0	—
Sesame	1 tbsp	120	14	0	0	—
Soy	1 tbsp	120	14	0	0	—
Sunflower	1 tbsp	120	14	0	0	—
Sunflower Organic	1 tbsp	120	14	0	0	—
Walnut	1 tbsp	120	14	0	0	—
Hollywood						
Canola	1 tbsp	120	14	0	0	—
Peanut	1 tbsp	120	14	0	0	—
Safflower	1 tbsp	120	14	0	0	—
Soy	1 tbsp	120	14	0	0	—
Sunflower	1 tbsp	120	14	0	0	—
House Of Tsang						
Hot Chili Sesame	1 tsp (5 g)	45	5	0	0	0
Mongolian Fire	1 tsp (5 g)	45	5	0	0	0
Pure Sesame	1 tsp (5 g)	45	5	0	0	0
Singapore Curry	1 tsp (5 g)	45	5	0	0	0
Wok Oil	1 tbsp (0.5 oz)	130	14	0	0	0
Italica						
Olive Oil	1 tbsp	120	9	—	0	—
Ka-Me						
Chili Hot	1 tbsp (0.5 fl oz)	130	14	0	0	0
Sesame	1 tbsp (0.5 fl oz)	130	14	0	0	0
Sesame Tempura	1 tbsp (0.5 fl oz)	130	14	0	0	0
Mazola						
No Stick	2.5 sec spray (0.2 g)	2	tr	0	0	—
Oil	1 tbsp (14 g)	120	14	0	0	—
Oil	1 cup (221 g)	1955	221	0	0	—
Orville Redenbacher's						
Oil	1 tbsp	120	14	0	0	0
Pam						
Butter	1 sec spray (0.266 g)	2	tr	0	0	—

FOOD	PORTION	CAL.	FAT	SOD.	CARB.	FIB.
Pam (CONT.)						
Cooking Spray	1 sec spray (0.266 g)	2	tr	0	0	—
Olive Oil	1 sec spray (0.266 g)	2	tr	0	0	—
Pump	1 spray (0.43 g)	4	tr	0	0	—
Planters						
Peanut	1 tbsp (0.5 oz)	120	14	0	0	—
Popcorn	1 tbsp (0.5 oz)	120	14	0	0	—
Pompeian						
Olive	1 tbsp	130	14	—	—	—
Progresso						
Olive Extra Light	1 tbsp	119	14	0	0	0
Olive Extra Mild	1 tbsp (0.5 oz)	120	14	0	0	0
Olive Extra Virgin	1 tbsp (0.5 oz)	120	14	0	0	0
Olive Riviera Blend	1 tbsp (0.5 oz)	120	14	0	0	0
Smart Beat						
Canola	1 tbsp	120	14	0	0	—
Oil	1 tbsp	120	14	0	0	—
Tree Of Life						
Almond	1 tbsp (0.5 g)	130	14	0	0	—
Apricot Kernel	1 tbsp (0.5 g)	130	14	0	0	—
Avocado	1 tbsp (0.5 g)	130	14	0	0	—
Macadamia Nut	1 tbsp (0.5 g)	130	14	0	0	—
Olive Extra Virgin Organic	1 tbsp (0.5 g)	130	14	0	0	—
Sesame	1 tbsp (0.5 g)	130	14	0	0	—
Toasted Sesame	1 tbsp (0.5 oz)	130	14	0	0	0
Weight Watchers						
Butter Spray	⅓ sec spray	0	0	0	0	0
Cooking Spray	⅓ sec spray	0	0	0	0	0
Wesson						
Canola	1 tbsp	120	14	0	0	0
Cooking Spray Lite	0.5 sec spray	0	0	0	0	0
Corn	1 tbsp	120	14	0	0	0
Olive	1 tbsp	120	14	0	0	0
Sunflower	1 tbsp	120	14	0	0	0
Vegetable	1 tbsp	120	14	0	0	0
FISH OIL						
cod liver	1 tbsp	123	14	—	0	—
herring	1 tbsp	123	14	—	0	—
menhaden	1 tbsp	123	14	—	0	—
salmon	1 tbsp	123	14	—	0	—
sardine	1 tbsp	123	14	—	0	—

FOOD	PORTION	CAL.	FAT	SOD.	CARB.	FIB.
shark	3½ oz	945	100	—	0	—
whale	3½ oz	945	100	—	0	—
Hain						
Cod Liver	1 tbsp	120	14	0	0	—
Cod Liver Cherry	1 tbsp	120	14	0	0	—
Cod Liver Mint	1 tbsp	120	14	0	0	—
OKRA						
CANNED						
Allen						
Cut	½ cup (4.4 oz)	25	0	400	6	3
McIlhenny						
Pickled	2 pieces (1 oz)	7	tr	18	1	1
Trappey						
Cocktail Hot	2 pieces (1 oz)	8	tr	139	2	1
Cocktail Mild	1 piece (1 oz)	9	tr	207	1	1
Creole Gumbo	½ cup (4.2 oz)	35	0	290	6	3
Cut	½ cup (4.4 oz)	25	0	400	6	3
FRESH						
raw	8 pods	36	tr	8	7	—
raw sliced	½ cup	19	tr	4	4	—
sliced cooked	½ cup	25	tr	4	6	—
sliced cooked	8 pods	27	tr	5	6	—
FROZEN						
sliced cooked	1 pkg (10 oz)	94	1	8	21	—
sliced cooked	½ cup	34	tr	3	8	—
Fresh Like						
Cut	3.5 oz	26	tr	3	6	1
Whole	3.5 oz	32	tr	2	7	1
Hanover						
Cut	½ cup	25	0	—	—	—
Whole	½ cup	35	0	—	—	—
OLIVES						
green	3 extra lg	15	2	312	tr	tr
green	4 med	15	2	312	tr	tr
ripe	1 lg	5	tr	38	tr	tr
ripe	1 sm	4	tr	28	tr	tr
ripe	1 colossal	12	1	136	1	—
ripe	1 jumbo	7	1	75	tr	—
Progresso						
Oil Cured	6 (0.5 oz)	80	6	330	3	1
Olive Salad (drained)	2 tbsp (0.8 oz)	25	3	360	1	1
S&W						
Ripe Extra Large	3.5 oz	163	18	760	1	—

FOOD	PORTION	CAL.	FAT	SOD.	CARB.	FIB.
S&W (CONT.)						
Ripe Pitted Large	3.5 oz	163	18	760	1	—
Tee Pee						
Spanish Green	2 oz	98	10	—	1	—
ONION						
CANNED						
chopped	½ cup	21	tr	416	5	—
whole	1 (2.2 oz)	12	tr	234	3	—
S&W						
Whole Small	½ cup	35	0	345	9	—
Vlasic						
Lightly Spiced Cocktail Onions	1 oz	4	0	365	1	—
Watkins						
Liquid Spice	1 tbsp (0.5 oz)	120	14	0	0	0
DRIED						
flakes	1 tbsp	16	tr	1	4	—
powder	1 tsp	7	tr	1	2	—
Watkins						
Flakes	¼ tsp (1 g)	0	0	0	0	0
FRESH						
chopped cooked	½ cup	47	tr	3	11	—
raw chopped	1 tbsp	4	tr	0	1	tr
raw chopped	½ cup	30	tr	2	7	—
scallions raw chopped	1 tbsp	2	tr	1	tr	tr
scallions raw sliced	½ cup	16	tr	8	4	1
welsh raw	3½ oz	34	tr	—	7	—
Antioch Farms						
Vidalia	1 med	60	0	10	14	3
Dole						
Green Chopped	1 tbsp	2	tr	0	tr	tr
Medium	1	60	0	10	14	3
FROZEN						
chopped cooked	½ cup	30	tr	12	7	—
chopped cooked	1 tbsp	4	tr	2	1	—
rings	7 (2.5 oz)	285	19	263	27	—
rings cooked	2 (0.7 oz)	81	5	75	8	—
whole cooked	3½ oz	28	tr	8	7	—
Birds Eye						
Polybag Whole Small	½ cup	30	0	10	8	2
Small With Cream Sauce	½ cup	100	3	340	12	1
Fresh Like						
Diced	3.5 oz	29	0	7	7	0

FOOD	PORTION	CAL.	FAT	SOD.	CARB.	FIB.
Fresh Like (CONT.)						
Whole	3.5 oz	37	tr	10	8	1
Kineret						
Rings	6 (3 oz)	200	10	310	25	0
Mrs. Paul's						
Crispy Onion Rings	2½ oz	190	12	230	19	—
Ore Ida						
Chopped	¾ cup (3 oz)	25	0	20	6	1
Onion Ringers	6 pieces (3 oz)	240	14	250	26	2
Southland						
Chopped	2 oz	15	0	—	—	—
TAKE-OUT						
fried	½ cup (7.5 oz)	176	11	—	17	—
rings breaded & fried	8 to 9	275	16	430	31	—
OPOSSUM						
roasted	3 oz	188	9	—	0	—
ORANGE						
CANNED						
Del Monte						
Mandarin In Heavy Syrup	½ cup (4.4 oz)	80	0	10	19	tr
Dole						
Mandarin Segments	½ cup	70	tr	10	19	—
Pineapple Mandarin Segments	½ cup	80	tr	5	19	—
Empress						
Mandarin	5.5 oz	100	0	10	25	—
Mandarin From Japan	5.5 oz	35	0	—	8	—
S&W						
Mandarin Natural Style	½ cup	60	0	10	15	—
Mandarin Selected Sections in Heavy Syrup	½ cup	76	0	10	20	—
Mandarin Unsweetened	½ cup	28	0	10	7	—
FRESH						
california navel	1	65	tr	1	16	3
california valencia	1	59	tr	0	14	3
florida	1	69	tr	1	17	4
peel	1 tbsp	6	tr	0	2	—
sections	1 cup	85	tr	0	21	4
Dole						
Orange	1	50	0	0	13	6

FOOD	PORTION	CAL.	FAT	SOD.	CARB.	FIB.
ORANGE EXTRACT						
Virginia Dare	1 tsp	22	0	—	—	—
ORANGE JUICE						
canned	1 cup	104	tr	6	25	—
chilled	1 cup	110	1	2	25	—
fresh	1 cup	111	tr	2	26	—
frzn as prep	1 cup	112	tr	2	27	1
frzn not prep	6 oz	339	tr	7	81	2
mandarin orange	3½ oz	47	tr	—	10	—
orange drink	6 oz	94	0	31	24	—
After The Fall						
Juice	1 bottle (10 oz)	110	0	10	26	—
Bright & Early						
Chilled	8 fl oz	120	0	30	30	—
Frozen	8 fl oz	120	0	10	30	—
Capri Sun						
Drink	1 pkg (7 oz)	100	0	20	25	0
Del Monte						
Juice	8 fl oz	110	0	25	27	tr
Everfresh						
Juice	1 can (8 oz)	100	0	0	24	0
Ruby Red Orange Drink	1 can (8 oz)	130	0	0	33	0
Fresh Samantha						
Juice	1 cup (8 oz)	109	1	0	24	1
Hawaiian Punch						
Drink	6 oz	100	0	—	—	—
Hi-C						
Box	8.45 fl oz	130	0	30	33	—
Drink	8 fl oz	130	0	25	32	—
Drink	1 can (11.5 fl oz)	180	0	40	45	—
Hood						
From Concentrate	1 cup (8 oz)	120	0	20	30	—
Select	1 cup (8 oz)	120	0	2	30	—
With Calcium	1 cup (8 oz)	120	0	20	30	—
Juice Works						
Drink	6 oz	90	0	—	—	—
Kool-Aid						
Drink Mix Orange as prep	1 serv (8 oz)	60	0	5	16	0
Orange Drink as prep w/ sugar	1 serv (8 oz)	100	0	10	25	0
Libby						
Juice	6 fl oz	80	0	0	20	—

FOOD	PORTION	CAL.	FAT	SOD.	CARB.	FIB.
Minute Maid						
Box	8.45 fl oz	120	0	25	28	—
Calcium Rich Chilled	8 fl oz	120	0	25	27	—
Calcium Rich frzn	8 fl oz	120	0	0	27	—
Chilled	8 fl oz	110	0	25	27	—
Country Style Chilled	8 fl oz	110	0	25	27	—
Country Style frzn	8 fl oz	110	0	0	27	—
Juices To Go	1 can (11.5 fl oz)	160	0	35	39	—
Juices To Go	1 bottle (10 fl oz)	140	0	30	34	—
Juices To Go	1 bottle (16 fl oz)	110	0	25	27	—
Orange Punch Box	8.45 fl oz	130	0	25	33	—
Premium Choice Chilled	8 fl oz	110	0	0	27	—
Pulp Free Chilled	8 fl oz	110	0	25	27	—
Pulp Free frzn	8 fl oz	110	0	0	27	—
Reduced Acid frzn	8 fl oz	110	0	0	27	—
Mott's						
From Concentrate	10 fl oz	130	1	20	29	0
Ocean Spray						
Juice	8 fl oz	120	0	35	31	0
Odwalla						
Juice	8 fl oz	110	1	25	25	1
S&W						
100% Unsweetened	6 oz	83	0	2	18	—
Shasta Plus						
Orange Drink	1 can (11.5 oz)	160	0	45	40	0
Sippin' Pak						
100% Pure	8.45 fl oz	110	0	25	26	—
Snapple						
Juice	10 fl oz	130	0	55	29	—
Orangeade	8 fl oz	120	0	10	31	—
Tang						
Orange Drink as prep	1 serv (8 oz)	90	0	0	23	0
Sugar Free Orange as prep	1 serv (8 oz)	5	0	0	0	0
Tree Of Life						
Juice	8 fl oz	110	0	10	27	0
Tree Top						
Juice	6 oz	90	0	5	22	—
Tropicana						
Double Vitamin C with Vitamin E	8 fl oz	110	0	0	26	—
Frozen as prep	6 fl oz	110	0	5	27	—
Juice	1 container (10 fl oz)	130	0	0	33	—

FOOD	PORTION	CAL.	FAT	SOD.	CARB.	FIB.
Tropicana (CONT.)						
Juice	1 container (8 fl oz)	110	0	0	27	—
Juice	1 container (6 fl oz)	80	0	0	20	—
Juice	8 fl oz	110	0	0	27	—
Prue Premium Calcium & Extra Vitamin C	8 fl oz	110	0	0	26	—
Prue Premium Vitamins C&E	8 fl oz	110	0	0	26	—
Season's Best	1 can (11.5 fl oz)	140	0	5	36	—
Season's Best	1 bottle (7 fl oz)	90	0	0	23	—
Season's Best	1 bottle (10 fl oz)	130	0	5	33	—
Season's Best Homestyle	8 fl oz	110	0	5	27	—
Veryfine						
100%	8 oz	121	0	<10	24	—
Orange Drink	8 oz	140	0	<70	33	—
OREGANO						
ground	1 tsp	5	tr	tr	1	—
Watkins						
Liquid Spice	1 tbsp (0.5 oz)	120	14	0	0	0
ORGAN MEATS						
(*see* BRAINS, GIBLETS, GIZZARD, HEART, KIDNEY, LIVER, SWEETBREADS)						
ORIENTAL FOOD						
(*see* ASIAN FOOD, EGG ROLLS, DINNER, NOODLES, RICE, SUSHI)						
OSTRICH						
ostrich	3 oz	127	3	—	—	—
OYSTERS						
CANNED						
eastern	3 oz	58	2	95	3	—
eastern	1 cup	170	6	277	10	—
Bumble Bee						
Whole	½ cup (3.5 oz)	100	4	490	6	0
Empress						
Whole	4 oz	100	4	390	8	—
S&W						
Fancy Whole	2 oz	95	3	—	4	—
FRESH						
eastern cooked	6 med	58	2	94	3	—
eastern cooked	3 oz	117	4	190	7	—
eastern raw	1 cup	170	6	277	10	—

FOOD	PORTION	CAL.	FAT	SOD.	CARB.	FIB.
eastern raw	6 med	58	2	94	3	—
pacific raw	3 oz	69	2	90	4	—
pacific raw	1 med	41	1	53	2	—
steamed	3 oz	138	4	180	8	—
steamed	1 med	41	1	53	2	—
TAKE-OUT						
battered & fried	6 (4.9 oz)	368	18	677	40	—
breaded & fried	6 (4.9 oz)	368	18	677	40	—
eastern breaded & fried	6 med (88 g)	173	11	367	10	—
eastern breaded & fried	3 oz	167	11	355	10	—
oysters rockefeller	3 oysters	66	2	80	5	—
stew	1 cup	278	18	928	15	tr

PANCAKE/WAFFLE SYRUP

(*see also* SYRUP)

FOOD	PORTION	CAL.	FAT	SOD.	CARB.	FIB.
low calorie	1 tbsp	12	0	—	3	0
maple	1 tbsp (0.8 oz)	52	0	2	13	—
maple	1 cup (11.1 oz)	824	1	27	212	—
pancake syrup	1 tbsp (0.7 oz)	57	0	17	15	—
pancake syrup	1 cup (11 oz)	903	0	290	238	—
pancake syrup light	1 oz	46	0	57	13	—
pancake syrup w/ butter	1 cup (11 oz)	933	5	307	234	—
pancake syrup w/ butter	1 tbsp (0.7 oz)	59	tr	20	15	—
Alaga						
Breakfast	2 tbsp	108	0	—	—	—
Butter Lite	2 tbsp	54	0	—	—	—
Honey Flavored	2 tbsp	124	0	—	—	—
Lite	2 tbsp	54	0	—	—	—
Aunt Jemima						
Butter Rich	¼ cup (2.8 oz)	210	0	170	52	—
Butterlite	¼ cup (2.5 oz)	100	0	150	26	—
Lite	¼ cup (2.5 oz)	100	0	160	27	—
Syrup	¼ cup (2.8 oz)	210	0	120	53	—
Brer Rabbit						
Dark	2 tbsp	120	0	0	31	—
Light	2 tbsp	120	0	0	31	—
Estee						
Lite Maple	¼ cup (2.4 oz)	80	0	125	20	—
Golden Griddle						
Syrup	1 tbsp (20 g)	50	0	55	14	—
Syrup	1 cup (321 g)	885	0	225	229	—
Karo						
Syrup	1 tbsp (21 g)	60	0	35	15	—
Log Cabin						
Country Kitchen	1 oz	103	0	22	27	—

FOOD	PORTION	CAL.	FAT	SOD.	CARB.	FIB.
Log Cabin (CONT.)						
Lite	1 oz	49	0	92	13	—
Mrs. Richardson's						
Lite	¼ cup (2.5 oz)	100	0	160	26	—
Original Recipe	¼ cup (2.8 oz)	210	0	115	52	—
Red Wing						
Lite	¼ cup (2 oz)	100	0	115	26	0
Syrup	¼ cup (2 oz)	210	0	30	53	0
Tastee						
Maple	2 tbsp	113	0	—	—	—
Syrup	2 tbsp	121	0	—	—	—
Tree Of Life						
Maple	¼ cup (2.1 oz)	200	0	7	53	—
Whitfield						
White Label	2 tbsp	121	0	—	—	—
Yellow Label	2 tbsp	125	0	—	—	—
Yellow Label Butter Flavor	2 tbsp	117	0	—	—	—
Yellow Label Maple Flavor	2 tbsp	117	0	—	—	—

PANCAKES

FROZEN

FOOD	PORTION	CAL.	FAT	SOD.	CARB.	FIB.
buttermilk	1 4 in diam (1.3 ox)	83	1	183	16	—
plain	1 4 in diam (1.3 oz)	83	1	183	16	—
Aunt Jemima						
Blueberry	3 (3.4 oz)	210	4	670	40	2
Buttermilk	3 (3 oz)	180	3	590	34	2
Lowfat	3 (3.4 oz)	130	2	580	33	8
Original	3 (3.4 oz)	200	3	700	40	2
Downyflake						
Blueberry	3	290	9	920	48	—
Buttermilk	3	280	9	920	45	—
Pancakes And Sausages	1 pkg (5.5 oz)	430	23	1170	47	—
Regular	3	280	9	920	45	—
Great Starts						
Pancakes And Sausages	6 oz	460	22	920	52	—
Pancakes With Bacon	4½ oz	400	20	1000	43	—
Silver Dollar Pancakes And Sausage	3¾ oz	310	14	680	37	—
Whole Wheat Pancakes With Lite Links	5½ oz	350	16	600	39	—
Healthy Starts						
Pancakes w/ LeanLinks	6 oz	360	8	490	48	—

FOOD	PORTION	CAL.	FAT	SOD.	CARB.	FIB.
Jimmy Dean						
Flapstick	1 (2.5 oz)	240	14	320	22	1
Flapstick Blueberry	1 (2.5 oz)	260	15	320	23	1
Morningstar Farms						
Pancakes/Links	1 pkg (4 oz)	240	8	700	31	—
Pillsbury						
Buttermilk Microwave	3	260	4	590	51	—
Harvest Wheat Microwave	3	240	4	420	48	—
Microwave	3	250	4	540	49	—
Original Microwave	3	240	4	550	47	—
Quaker						
Lite Pancakes & Lite Links	1 pkg (6 oz)	310	10	970	43	—
Lite Pancakes & Lite Syrup	1 pkg (6 oz)	260	3	860	53	—
Pancakes & Sausages	1 pkg (6 oz)	420	16	1140	57	—
HOME RECIPE						
plain	1 (4 in diam)	86	4	157	11	—
MIX						
buckwheat	1 (4 in diam)	62	2	160	9	—
buttermilk	1 4 in diam (1.3 oz)	74	1	239	14	tr
plain	1-4 in diam (1.3 oz)	74	1	239	14	tr
sugar free low sodium	1 (3 in diam)	44	tr	58	9	—
whole wheat	1 (4 in diam)	92	3	252	13	—
Arrowhead						
Multigrain Pancake & Waffle Mix	¼ cup (1.2 oz)	120	1	260	24	3
Aunt Jemima						
Buckwheat Pancake & Waffle Mix	¼ cup (1.4 oz)	120	1	560	28	4
Buttermilk Pancake & Waffle Mix	⅓ cup (1.9 oz)	190	2	480	38	2
Original Pancake & Waffle Mix	⅓ cup (1.6 oz)	150	1	620	34	1
Pancake & Waffle Mix Regular	⅓ cup (1.9 oz)	190	2	470	39	1
Pancake & Waffle Mix Whole Wheat	¼ cup (1.4 oz)	130	1	560	28	3
Betty Crocker						
Buttermilk	3 (4 in diam)	280	10	810	39	—
Bisquick						
Apple Cinnamon Shake 'N Pour	3 (4 in diam)	240	3	880	47	—

FOOD	PORTION	CAL.	FAT	SOD.	CARB.	FIB.
Bisquick (CONT.)						
Blueberry Shake 'N Pour	3 (4 in diam)	270	3	840	54	—
Buttermilk Shake 'N Pour	3 (4 in diam)	250	3	880	49	—
Original Shake 'N Pour	3 (4 in diam)	250	3	880	49	—
Estee						
Pancake Mix Fat Free as prep	4 (4 in diam)	180	0	255	40	1
Fast Shake						
Blueberry	1 serv (2.5 oz)	251	3	685	50	—
Buttermilk	1 serv (2.5 oz)	258	3	770	50	—
Original	1 serv (2.5 oz)	266	4	736	50	—
Health Valley						
Pancake Mix not prep	1 oz	100	1	170	20	3
Hodgson Mill						
Buckwheat	⅓ cup (1.8 oz)	160	1	550	35	1
Hungry Jack						
Blueberry	3 (4 in diam)	320	15	820	41	—
Buttermilk	3 (4 in diam)	240	11	820	29	—
Buttermilk Complete	3 (4 in diam)	180	1	710	39	—
Buttermilk Complete Packets	3 (4 in diam)	180	3	680	35	—
Extra Lights	3 (4 in diam)	210	7	490	30	—
Extra Lights Complete	3 (4 in diam)	190	2	700	37	—
Panshakes	3 (4 in diam)	250	6	880	43	—
Stone-Buhr						
Buckwheat	¼ cup (1.4 oz)	130	1	410	29	3
Oat Bran	¼ cup (1.4 oz)	130	0	330	30	2
Whole Wheat	¼ cup (1.4 oz)	120	1	330	25	3
Wanda's						
Blue Corn	⅓ cup mix per serv (1.7 oz)	170	2	480	32	2
TAKE-OUT						
blueberry	1 (4 in diam)	84	4	157	11	—
buckwheat	1 (4 in diam)	55	2	125	6	—
potato	1 (4 in diam)	78	6	238	4	tr
w/ butter & syrup	3	519	14	1103	91	—

PANCREAS

(*see* SWEETBREADS)

PAPAYA

FOOD	PORTION	CAL.	FAT	SOD.	CARB.	FIB.
CANNED						
Ka-Me						
Papaya	¾ cup	120	0	15	29	1
DRIED						
Sonoma						
Pieces	2 pieces (2 oz)	200	4	60	41	6

FOOD	PORTION	CAL.	FAT	SOD.	CARB.	FIB.
FRESH						
cubed	1 cup	54	tr	4	14	—
papaya	1	117	tr	8	30	—
PAPAYA JUICE						
nectar	1 cup	142	tr	14	36	—
Everfresh						
Premium Drink	1 can (8 oz)	140	0	0	35	0
Goya						
Nectar	6 oz	110	0	10	27	—
Kern's						
Nectar	6 fl oz	110	0	5	27	—
Libby						
Nectar	1 can (11.5 fl oz)	210	0	10	51	—
PAPRIKA						
paprika	1 tsp	6	tr	1	1	—
Watkins						
Ground	¼ tsp (0.5 oz)	0	0	0	0	0
PARSLEY						
dry	1 tsp	1	tr	1	tr	—
dry	1 tbsp	1	tr	2	tr	—
fresh chopped	½ cup	11	tr	17	2	—
Dole						
Chopped	1 tbsp	10	tr	4	1	tr
PARSNIPS						
fresh cooked	1 (5.6 oz)	130	tr	17	31	—
fresh sliced cooked	½ cup	63	tr	8	15	—
raw sliced	½ cup	50	tr	7	12	—
PASSION FRUIT						
purple fresh	1	18	tr	5	4	—
PASSION FRUIT JUICE						
purple	1 cup	126	tr	—	34	—
yellow	1 cup	149	tr	15	36	—
Snapple						
Passion Supreme	10 fl oz	160	0	20	39	—

PASTA

(*see also* NOODLES, PASTA DINNERS, PASTA SALAD)

(FAST FACT: The average American eats about 20 pounds of pasta a year. It is estimated that consumption will reach 30 pounds per person by the year 2000.)

FOOD	PORTION	CAL.	FAT	SOD.	CARB.	FIB.
DRY						
corn cooked	1 cup	176	1	1	39	—
elbows	1 cup	389	2	8	78	—
elbows cooked	1 cup	197	tr	1	40	—
protein fortified cooked	1 cup	188	tr	6	36	—

FOOD	PORTION	CAL.	FAT	SOD.	CARB.	FIB.
shells	1 cup	389	2	4	78	—
shells cooked	1 cup	197	tr	1	40	—
spaghetti	2 oz	211	tr	4	43	—
spaghetti cooked	1 cup	197	tr	1	40	—
spaghetti protein fortified cooked	1 cup	229	tr	7	44	—
spinach spaghetti	2 oz	212	tr	20	43	—
spinach spaghetti cooked	1 cup	183	tr	20	37	—
spirals	1 cup	389	2	8	78	—
spirals cooked	1 cup	197	tr	1	40	—
vegetable	1 cup	308	tr	36	63	—
vegetable cooked	1 cup	171	tr	9	36	—
whole wheat	1 cup	365	1	8	79	—
whole wheat cooked	1 cup (4.9 oz)	174	tr	4	37	—
whole wheat spaghetti	2 oz	198	tr	5	43	—
whole wheat spaghetti cooked	1 cup	174	tr	4	37	—
Anthony						
Pasta	2 oz	210	1	0	42	tr
Barilla						
Gemelli as prep	1 cup (2 oz)	200	1	0	42	2
Pennette Rigate	1 ⅓ cups (2 oz)	200	1	0	42	2
Bella Via						
Angel Hair	2 oz	200	0	0	40	—
Artichoke Angel Hair as prep	⅝ cup	200	0	0	40	—
Artichoke Spaghetti as prep	⅝ cup	200	0	0	40	—
Elbows	2 oz	200	0	0	40	—
Fettucini as prep	⅝ cup	200	0	0	40	—
Linguini	2 oz	200	0	0	40	—
Penne as prep	⅝ cup	200	0	0	40	—
Rotelli	2 oz	200	0	0	40	—
Shells	2 oz	200	0	0	40	—
Spaghetti	2 oz	200	0	0	40	—
Ziti	2 oz	200	0	0	40	—
Classico						
Gnocchi Di Toscana	1 cup (2 oz)	210	1	0	42	2
Creamette						
Elbow Macaroni not prep	2 oz	210	1	5	42	—
Linguini Egg	2 oz	221	3	—	—	—
Rotelle	2 oz	210	1	—	—	—
Rotini Rainbow	2 oz	210	1	—	—	—
Spaghetti Egg	2 oz	221	3	—	—	—
Spaghetti Thin	2 oz	210	1	—	—	—

FOOD	PORTION	CAL.	FAT	SOD.	CARB.	FIB.
Creamette (CONT.)						
Spaghetti not prep	2 oz	210	1	5	42	—
Spinach Ribbons not prep	2 oz	210	1	70	42	—
Ziti	2 oz	210	1	—	—	—
De Bole's						
Whole Wheat Organic Elbows	2 oz	210	2	0	40	5
DeFino						
Lasagna No Boil	1 oz	102	tr	2	20	—
Ribbons No Boil	2 oz	204	2	3	40	—
Delverde						
Spaghetti Whole Wheat	2 oz	206	1	1	42	5
Eden						
Elbows Whole Wheat Organic	2 oz	210	2	0	39	6
Elbows Whole Wheat Vegetable Organic	2 oz	210	2	0	39	6
Kudzu And Sweet Potato Pasta	2 oz	190	0	0	47	0
Kudzu Kiri Pasta	2 oz	190	0	0	47	0
Mung Bean Pasta Harusame	2 oz	190	0	5	47	0
Ribbons Durum Wheat Curry Organic	2 oz	220	1	0	44	3
Ribbons Durum Wheat Organic	2 oz	220	1	0	44	3
Ribbons Durum Wheat Paella Organic	2 oz	220	1	0	44	3
Ribbons Durum Wheat Parsley Garlic Organic	2 oz	220	1	0	44	3
Ribbons Durum Wheat Pesto Organic	2 oz	220	1	0	44	3
Ribbons Whole Wheat Spinach Organic	2 oz	200	2	10	40	7
Rice Pasta Bifun	2 oz	200	1	5	44	0
Shells Durum Wheat Vegetable Organic	2 oz	210	1	10	42	2
Soba 100% Buckwheat	2 oz	200	0	30	41	3
Soba 40% Buckwheat	2 oz	190	1	490	37	3
Soba Lotus Root	2 oz	190	1	470	37	4
Soba Mugwort	2 oz	190	1	550	37	2
Soba Wild Yam Jinenjo	2 oz	190	1	510	37	2
Spaghetti Durum Wheat Organic	2 oz	210	1	10	42	2

FOOD	PORTION	CAL.	FAT	SOD.	CARB.	FIB.
Eden (CONT.)						
Spaghetti Kamut Organic	2 oz	210	2	0	38	6
Spaghetti Pasley Garlic Organic	2 oz	210	1	10	42	2
Spaghetti Whole Wheat Organic	2 oz	210	2	0	39	6
Spirals Durum Wheat Vegetable Organic	2 oz	210	1	10	42	2
Spirals Kamut Organic	2 oz	210	2	0	38	6
Spirals Sesame Rice Organic	2 oz	200	2	0	37	6
Spirals Whole Wheat Vegetable Organic	2 oz	210	2	0	39	6
Udon	2 oz	190	1	660	37	3
Udon Brown Rice	2 oz	190	1	510	38	2
Gioia						
Pasta	2 oz	210	1	0	42	tr
Golden Grain						
Pasta	2 oz	203	1	26	41	0
Hanover						
Spaghetti Wheels	½ cup	90	0	—	—	—
Health Valley						
Lasagna Whole Wheat	2 oz	170	1	10	40	7
Lasagna Spinach Whole Wheat	2 oz	170	1	15	40	7
Spaghetti Amaranth	2 oz	170	1	10	40	9
Spaghetti Oat Bran	2 oz	120	1	2	23	4
Spaghetti Spinach Whole Wheat	2 oz	170	1	15	40	7
Spaghetti Whole Wheat	2 oz	170	1	10	40	7
Hodgson Mill						
Spaghetti Whole Wheat Spinach not prep	2 oz	190	2	25	35	5
Veggie Bows not prep	2 oz	200	1	15	41	1
Veggie Rotini not prep	2 oz	200	1	15	41	1
Veggie Wagon Wheels not prep	2 oz	200	1	15	41	1
Whole Wheat Spirals not prep	2 oz	190	1	10	34	6
La Molisana						
Radiatori	2 oz	230	1	30	48	—
Lupini						
Elbow uncooked	½ cup (2 oz)	190	2	0	37	5
Spaghetti Light uncooked	½ cup (2 oz)	190	2	0	37	5

FOOD	PORTION	CAL.	FAT	SOD.	CARB.	FIB.
Lupini (CONT.)						
Spaghetti With Triticale	1/7 pkg (2 oz)	190	3	5	38	6
Luxury						
Pasta	2 oz	210	1	0	42	tr
Merlino's						
Pasta	2 oz	210	1	0	42	tr
Mueller's						
Dinosaurs	2 oz (57 g)	210	1	3	42	—
Jungle Animals	2 oz (57 g)	210	1	3	42	—
Lasagne	2 oz (57 g)	210	1	4	42	—
Monsters	2 oz (57 g)	210	1	3	42	—
Outer Space	2 oz	210	1	3	42	—
Spaghetti	2 oz (57 g)	210	1	3	42	—
Teddy Bears	2 oz (57 g)	210	1	3	42	—
Twists Tri Color	2 oz (57 g)	210	1	10	41	—
Noodles By Leonardo						
Capellini	2 oz	200	1	10	40	2
Elbows not prep	½ cup (2 oz)	200	1	10	40	2
Fettucini	2 oz	200	1	10	40	2
Linguine not prep	½ cup (2 oz)	200	1	10	40	2
Rigatoni	2 oz	200	1	10	40	2
Rotini	2 oz	200	1	10	40	2
Shells not prep	½ cup (2 oz)	200	1	10	40	2
Spaghetti not prep	½ cup (2 oz)	200	1	10	40	2
Spaghettini	2 oz	200	1	10	40	2
Vermicelli not prep	½ cup (2 oz)	200	1	10	40	2
Penn Dutch						
Pasta	2 oz	210	1	0	42	tr
Pomi						
Capellini	2 oz	210	1	<5	41	—
Prince						
Egg	2 oz	221	3	3	40	1
Pasta	2 oz	210	1	0	42	tr
Rainbow	2 oz	210	1	5	42	1
Spinach Egg	2 oz	220	3	65	40	1
Pritikin						
Spaghetti Whole Wheat	⅛ box (2 oz)	190	1	0	40	—
Spiral	⅔ cup (2 oz)	190	1	10	40	—
Red Cross						
Pasta	2 oz	210	1	0	42	tr
Ronco						
Pasta	2 oz	210	1	0	42	tr
Ronzoni						
Elbows	¾ cup (2 oz)	210	1	0	40	—

FOOD	PORTION	CAL.	FAT	SOD.	CARB.	FIB.
Ronzoni (CONT.)						
Fettucini	¾ cup (2 oz)	210	1	0	40	—
Fusilli	¾ cup (2 oz)	210	1	0	40	—
Lasagne	¾ cup (2 oz)	210	1	0	40	—
Manicotti	¾ cup (2 oz)	210	1	0	40	—
Mostaccioli	¾ cup (2 oz)	210	1	0	40	—
Rigatoni	¾ cup (2 oz)	210	1	0	40	—
Rotelle uncooked	¾ cup (2 oz)	210	1	0	40	—
Rotini uncooked	¾ cup (2 oz)	210	1	0	40	—
Shells uncooked	¾ cup (2 oz)	210	1	0	40	—
Shells Jumbo	¾ cup (2 oz)	210	1	0	40	—
Spaghetti not prep	¾ cup (2 oz)	210	1	0	40	—
Tubettini	¾ cup (2 oz)	210	1	0	40	—
San Giorgio						
Bowties Egg	2 oz	210	3	15	38	—
Capellini	2 oz	210	1	0	40	2
Elbow Macaroni	2 oz	210	1	0	40	2
Fettuccine Egg	2 oz	210	3	15	38	—
Fettuccini Florentine	2 oz	210	3	15	38	—
Lasagne	2 oz	210	1	0	40	2
Linguini	2 oz	210	1	0	40	2
Manicotti	2 oz	210	1	0	40	2
Mostaccioli Rigati	2 oz	210	1	—	—	—
Rigatoni	2 oz	210	1	0	40	2
Rotini	2 oz	210	1	0	40	2
Shells	2 oz	210	1	0	40	2
Spaghetti	2 oz	210	1	0	40	2
Spaghetti Thin	2 oz	210	1	0	40	2
Vermicelli	2 oz	210	1	0	40	2
Ziti Cut	2 oz	210	1	0	40	2
Tree Of Life						
Cajun as prep	⅝ cup (4.9 oz)	200	1	50	40	1
Confetti as prep	⅝ cup (4.9 oz)	200	1	50	40	1
Garlic & Parsley as prep	⅝ cup (4.9 oz)	200	1	50	40	1
Jamaican Spice as prep	⅝ cup (4.9 oz)	200	1	50	40	1
Lemon Pepper as prep	⅝ cup (4.9 oz)	200	1	50	40	1
Spinach as prep	⅝ cup (4.9 oz)	200	1	50	40	1
Tex Mex as prep	⅝ cup (4.9 oz)	200	1	50	40	1
Thai as prep	⅝ cup (4.9 oz)	200	1	50	40	1
Tomato Basil as prep	⅝ cup (4.9 oz)	200	1	50	40	1
Vimco						
Pasta	2 oz	210	1	0	42	tr
FRESH						
plain made w/ egg cooked	2 oz	75	tr	3	14	—

FOOD	PORTION	CAL.	FAT	SOD.	CARB.	FIB.
spinach made w/ egg cooked	2 oz	74	tr	3	14	—
Contadina						
Angel's Hair	1¼ cup (2.8 oz)	240	3	30	43	2
Fettuccine	1¼ cup (2.9 oz)	250	4	30	45	2
Fettuccine Cholesterol Free	1 cup (2.9 oz)	240	3	16	46	2
Light Ravioli Cheese	1 cup (3.1 oz)	240	5	340	35	2
Light Ravioli Garden Vegetable	1¼ cup (3.8 oz)	290	6	370	43	3
Light Tortellini Garlic & Cheese	1 cup (3.6 oz)	280	5	390	50	3
Linguine	1¼ cup (3 oz)	260	4	30	47	2
Linguine Cholesterol Free	1¼ cup (3.1 oz)	250	3	20	49	2
Ravioli Beef And Garlic	1¼ cup (4 oz)	350	14	350	39	3
Ravioli Cheese	1 cup (3.1 oz)	280	12	350	31	2
Ravioli Chicken And Rosemary	1¼ cup (4 oz)	330	12	420	43	3
Tagliatelli Spinach	1¼ cup (3.1 oz)	270	4	110	46	4
Tortellini Spianch Three Cheese	¾ cup (3.1 oz)	280	5	380	38	3
Tortelloni Cheese	¾ cup (3 oz)	260	6	330	39	3
Tortelloni Cheese And Basil	1 cup (4 oz)	360	11	380	49	3
Tortelloni Chicken And Prosciutto	1 cup (3.8 oz)	360	13	440	46	3
Tortelloni Chicken And Vegetable	¾ cup (2.9 oz)	260	7	220	39	2
Tortelloni Spicy Italian Sausage And Bell Pepper	1 cup (3.6 oz)	330	10	280	47	3
Di Giorno						
Angel's Hair	1 cup	160	2	115	31	2
Beef & Roasted Garlic Tortellini	1 cup	340	11	390	46	1
Fettuccine	1 cup	200	2	140	38	2
Four Cheese Raviolo	1 cup	350	15	390	40	2
Herb Linguine	1 cup	200	2	140	38	2
Italian Sausage Ravioli In Green Bell Pepper Pasta	1¼ cup	350	12	570	45	3
Lemon Chicken Tortellini In Cracked Black Pepper Pasta	1 cup	270	5	290	42	1

FOOD	PORTION	CAL.	FAT	SOD.	CARB.	FIB.
Di Giorno (CONT.)						
Light Cheese Ravioli	1 cup	280	7	400	40	2
Linguine	1 cup	200	2	140	38	2
Mozzarella Garlic Tortelloni	1 cup	300	8	400	42	1
Pesto Tortelloni	1 cup	320	8	430	46	3
Portabello Mushroom Tortelloni	1 cup	310	7	490	48	3
Red Bell Pepper Fettuccine	1 cup	200	2	140	38	2
Spinach Fettuccine	1 cup	190	2	160	38	2
Sun-Dried Tomato Ravioli	1 ⅓ cup	380	14	600	48	3
Three Cheese Tortellini	¾ cup	250	7	300	37	2
Herb's						
Fettucine Bell Pepper Basil	2 oz	220	2	5	42	2
Fettucine Parsley Garlic	2 oz	220	2	5	42	2
Fettucine Spinach	2 oz	220	2	5	42	2
Ribbons Vegetable	2 oz	220	2	5	42	2
Ribbons Whole Wheat	2 oz	200	2	10	40	7
Rotini Mixed Vegetable	2 oz	210	1	10	42	2
Shells Mixed Vegetable	2 oz	210	1	10	42	2
Trios						
Ravioli Cracked Pepper Garlic Cheese	1 cup (4.3 oz)	340	9	380	48	0
HOME RECIPE						
made w/ egg cooked	2 oz	74	tr	47	13	—
made w/o egg cooked	2 oz	71	tr	42	14	—

PASTA DINNERS

(*see also* DINNER, PASTA SALAD)

FOOD	PORTION	CAL.	FAT	SOD.	CARB.	FIB.
CANNED						
Chef Boyardee						
ABC's & 1,2,3's In Cheese Flavor Sauce	7.5 oz	180	1	940	37	—
ABC's & 1,2,3's w/ Mini Meatballs	7.5 oz	260	11	1005	32	2
Beef Ravioli	7.5 oz	190	4	1160	31	2
Beefaroni	7.5 oz	220	7	1145	31	2
Cheese Ravioli In Meat Sauce	7.5 oz	200	3	1010	37	—
Dinosaurs In Cheese Flavor Sauce	7.5 oz	180	1	880	36	—

FOOD	PORTION	CAL.	FAT	SOD.	CARB.	FIB.
Chef Boyardee (CONT.)						
Dinosaurs w/ Meatballs	7.5 oz	240	9	900	32	4
Elbows In Beef Sauce	7.5 oz	210	7	1000	29	—
Lasagna	7.5 oz	230	9	1080	31	—
Lasagna In Garden Vegetable Sauce	7.5 oz	170	1	940	34	—
Macaroni & Cheese	7.5 oz	180	5	970	27	1
Pasta Rings & Meatballs	7.5 oz	220	8	990	33	4
Rigatoni	7.5 oz	210	6	1080	31	—
Rings & Franks	7.5 oz	190	5	980	31	3
Shells In Meat Sauce	7.5 oz	210	6	1090	32	—
Shells In Mushroom Sauce	7.5 oz	170	1	1080	35	—
Spaghetti & Meat Balls	7.5 oz	230	7	1060	29	—
Tic Tac Toes In Cheese Flavor Sauce	7.5 oz	170	1	930	36	3
Tic Tac Toes w/ Mini Meatballs	7.5 oz	250	10	1035	32	3
Turtles In Sauce	7.5 oz	160	1	870	33	2
Turtles w/ Meatballs	7.5 oz	210	8	990	30	2
Franco-American						
Beef RavioliO's In Meat Sauce	½ can (7½ oz)	250	8	920	35	—
CircusO's Pasta In Tomato & Cheese Sauce	½ can (7⅜ oz)	170	2	860	33	—
CircusO's Pasta With Meatballs In Tomato Sauce	½ can (7⅜ oz)	210	8	950	25	—
Macaroni & Cheese	½ can (7⅜ oz)	170	6	870	24	—
Spaghetti In Tomato Sauce w/ Cheese	½ can (7⅜ oz)	180	2	840	36	—
Spaghetti w/ Meatballs In Tomato Sauce	½ can (7⅜ oz)	220	8	870	28	—
SpaghettiO's With Meatballs	½ can (7⅜ oz)	220	9	950	25	—
SpaghettiO's With Sliced Franks	½ can (7⅜ oz)	220	9	1000	26	—
SpaghettiO's In Tomato & Cheese Sauce	½ can (7⅜ oz)	170	2	860	33	—
SportyO's In Tomato & Cheese Sauce	½ can (7½ oz)	170	2	860	33	—

FOOD	PORTION	CAL.	FAT	SOD.	CARB.	FIB.
Franco-American (CONT.)						
SportyO's Pasta With Meatballs In Tomato Sauce	½ can (7⅜ oz)	210	8	950	25	—
TeddyO's In Tomato & Cheese Sauce	½ can (7½ oz)	170	2	900	33	—
TeddyO's Pasta With Meatballs	½ can (7⅜ oz)	210	8	950	25	—
Hormel						
Lasagna	1 can (7.5 oz)	250	14	940	24	1
Spaghetti & Meatballs	1 can (7.5 oz)	210	7	940	28	2
Kid's Kitchen						
Cheezy Mac & Beef	1 cup (7.5 oz)	250	7	1180	34	0
Noodle Rings & Chicken	1 cup (7.5 oz)	150	5	860	16	1
Spaghetti Rings & Franks	1 cup (7.5 oz)	230	6	880	36	3
Progresso						
Beef Ravioli	1 cup (9.1 oz)	260	5	940	45	4
Cheese Ravioli	1 cup (9.1 oz)	220	2	930	43	4
Van Camp's						
Spaghetti Weenee	1 can (8 oz)	230	8	670	34	1
FROZEN						
Armour						
Classics Chicken Fettucini	1 meal (10 oz)	230	8	520	25	6
Banquet						
Family Entree Lasagna w/ Meat Sauce	1 serv (8 oz)	240	7	650	32	5
Family Entree Macaroni & Beef	1 serv (8 oz)	230	7	810	31	3
Family Entree Macaroni & Cheese	1 serv (8 oz)	300	10	1190	39	2
Family Entree Noodles & Chicken	1 serv (8 oz)	210	9	810	24	2
Family Entree Noodles & Beef	1 serv (7.47 oz)	140	4	1120	16	2
Birds Eye						
Easy Recipe Chicken Alfredo not prep	½ pkg	160	7	430	22	3
Easy Recipe Chicken Primavera not prep	½ pkg	80	3	540	14	7
Budget Gourmet						
Cheese Ravioli	1 meal (9.5 oz)	290	13	750	34	—
Lasagna Italian Sausage	1 meal (10 oz)	430	23	830	34	—

FOOD	PORTION	CAL.	FAT	SOD.	CARB.	FIB.
Budget Gourmet (CONT.)						
Lasagna Vegetable	1 meal (10.5 oz)	390	10	770	36	—
Lasagne Three Cheese	1 meal (10 oz)	390	17	640	26	—
Lasagne With Meat Sauce	1 meal (9.4 oz)	290	11	720	30	—
Linguini With Shrimp & Clams	1 meal (9.5 oz)	280	10	710	34	—
Linguini With Shrimp And Clams	1 meal (10 oz)	270	9	1160	35	—
Macaroni & Cheese	1 meal (5.75 oz)	230	12	570	22	—
Macaroni & Cheese With Cheddar & Parmesan	1 meal (10.5 oz)	330	8	760	49	—
Mainicotti Cheese	1 meal (10 oz)	440	24	740	36	—
Pasta Alfredo With Broccoli	1 meal (5.5 oz)	210	10	630	22	—
Penne Pasta With Chunky Tomato Sauce & Italian Sausage	1 meal (10 oz)	320	9	590	34	—
Rigatoni In Cream Sauce With Broccoli & Chicken	1 meal (10.8 oz)	290	7	710	44	—
Spaghetti With Chunky Tomato & Meat Sauce	1 meal (10 oz)	300	8	470	44	—
Tortellini Cheese	1 meal (5.5 oz)	200	8	530	25	—
Ziti In Marinara Sauce	1 meal (6.25 oz)	200	9	600	23	—
Dining Light						
Cheese Cannelloni	9 oz	310	9	650	38	—
Formagg						
Penne Pasta Alfredo	⅔ cup (5 oz)	190	2	470	35	0
Penne Pasta Primavera	⅔ cup (5 oz)	190	2	470	35	0
Vegetable Pasta & Caesar Italian Garden	⅔ cup (5 oz)	190	2	470	35	0
Green Giant						
Garden Gourmet Creamy Mushroom	1 pkg	220	11	860	29	3
Garden Gourmet Pasta Dijon	1 pkg	260	17	630	21	4
Garden Gourmet Pasta Florentine	1 pkg	230	9	840	27	4
Garden Gourmet Rotini Cheddar	1 pkg	230	10	570	32	5
One Serve Cheese Tortellini	1 pkg	260	9	660	37	—

FOOD	PORTION	CAL.	FAT	SOD.	CARB.	FIB.
Green Giant (CONT.)						
One Serve Macaroni & Cheese	1 pkg	230	9	590	28	—
One Serve Pasta Marinara	1 pkg	180	5	440	29	—
One Serve Pasta Parmesan With Green Peas	1 pkg	170	5	510	23	—
Pasta Accents Creamy Cheddar	½ cup	100	5	310	12	—
Pasta Accents Garden Herb	½ cup	80	3	220	11	—
Pasta Accents Garlic Seasoning	½ cup	110	5	280	13	—
Pasta Accents Pasta Primavera	½ cup	110	5	180	13	—
Healthy Choice						
Beef Macaroni Casserole	1 meal (8.5 oz)	200	1	450	34	5
Cheese Ravioli Parmigiana	1 meal (9 oz)	250	4	290	44	6
Chicken Broccoli Alfredo	1 meal (12.1 oz)	370	8	470	53	6
Chicken Fettucini Alfredo	1 meal (8.5 oz)	250	3	370	34	3
Classics Pasta Shells Marinara	1 meal (12 oz)	360	3	390	59	5
Classics Turkey Fettuccine Alla Crema	1 meal (12.5 oz)	350	4	370	50	5
Fettucini Alfredo	1 meal (8 oz)	240	5	430	39	3
Lasagna Roma	1 meal (13.5 oz)	390	5	580	60	9
Macaroni & Cheese	1 meal (9 oz)	290	5	580	45	4
Spaghetti Bolognese	1 meal (10 oz)	260	3	470	43	5
Three Cheese Manicotti	1 meal (11 oz)	310	9	450	41	7
Vegetable Pasta Italiano	1 meal (10 oz)	220	1	340	44	6
Zucchini Lasagna	1 meal (14 oz)	330	2	310	58	11
Kid Cuisine						
Macaroni & Cheese	1 pkg (10.6 oz)	420	12	920	68	3
Mini Cheese Ravioli	1 pkg (9.82 oz)	320	5	780	63	6
Le Menu						
Entree LightStyle Garden Vegetables Lasagna	10½ oz	260	8	500	35	—
Entree LightStyle Lasagna With Meat Sauce	10 oz	290	8	510	36	—
Entree LightStyle Meat Sauce & Cheese Tortellini	8 oz	250	8	480	34	—

FOOD	PORTION	CAL.	FAT	SOD.	CARB.	FIB.
Le Menu (CONT.)						
Entree LightStyle Spaghetti With Beef Sauce And Mushrooms	9 oz	280	6	450	45	—
LightStyle 3-Cheese Stuffed Shells	10 oz	280	8	690	34	—
LightStyle Cheese Tortellini	10 oz	230	6	460	35	—
Manicotto With Three Cheeses	11¾ oz	390	15	870	44	—
Lean Cuisine						
Alfredo Pasta Primavera	1 pkg (10 oz)	290	7	570	46	3
Angel Hair Pasta	1 pkg (10 oz)	220	3	420	41	6
Bow Tie Pasta & Creamy Tomato Sauce	1 pkg (9.5 oz)	260	6	550	43	6
Cafe Classics Bow Tie Pasta & Chicken	1 pkg (9.5 oz)	250	5	530	34	3
Cafe Classics Cheese Lasagna w/ Chicken Scaloppini	1 pkg (10 oz)	290	8	590	33	3
Cheddar Bake With Pasta	1 pkg (9 oz)	220	6	590	30	3
Cheese Cannelloni	1 pkg (9.1 oz)	230	4	570	28	3
Cheese Lasagna Casserole	1 pkg (10 oz)	270	6	590	40	5
Cheese Ravioli	1 pkg (8.5 oz)	270	7	580	40	5
Cheese Stuffed Shells	1 serv (8.9 oz)	230	5	590	34	3
Chicken Fettucini	1 pkg (9.25 oz)	280	6	590	36	4
Chicken Lasagna	1 pkg (10 oz)	270	8	590	30	5
Classic Cheese Lasagna	1 pkg (11.5 oz)	270	5	590	41	6
Fettucini Alfredo	1 pkg (9 oz)	300	7	550	47	2
Fettucini Primavera	1 pkg (10 oz)	270	7	580	38	4
Five Cheese Lasagna	1 serv (8 oz)	210	4	590	31	4
Lasagne With Meat Sauce	1 pkg (10.5 oz)	290	6	560	37	4
Macaroni & Beef	1 pkg (10 oz)	270	4	590	43	4
Macaroni & Cheese	1 pkg (10 oz)	290	7	590	43	4
Penne Pasta Bolognese	1 pkg (9.5 oz)	270	6	570	39	4
Penne Pasta w/ Tomato Basil Sauce	1 pkg (10 oz)	270	4	350	52	5
Spaghetti w/ Meat Sauce	1 pkg (11.5 oz)	290	5	570	50	7
Spaghetti w/ Meatballs	1 pkg (9.5 oz)	280	6	570	40	4
Vegetable Lasagna	1 pkg (10.5 oz)	260	7	590	35	5

FOOD	PORTION	CAL.	FAT	SOD.	CARB.	FIB.
Life Choice						
Linguini Roma	1 meal (13.2 oz)	230	1	580	48	6
Sun Dried Tomato Manicotti	1 meal (11.65 oz)	220	3	540	39	7
Vegetable Lasagna Primavera	1 meal (11.2 oz)	170	1	600	30	8
Lipton						
Golden Saute Angel Hair Parmesan	⅓ cup (2.2 oz)	240	5	890	42	2
Luigino's						
& Pomodoro Sauce With Meatballs	1 pkg (9 oz)	320	11	890	43	2
& Pomodoro Sauce With Meatballs	1 cup (6.3 oz)	270	9	740	36	2
Cheese Ravioli & Alfredo With Broccoli Sauce	1 pkg (8.5 oz)	420	25	890	30	2
Cheese Tortellini & Alfredo Sauce With Broccoli	1 pkg (8 oz)	390	24	840	28	2
Fettuccine Alfredo	1 pkg (9.4 oz)	390	14	630	45	4
Fettuccine Alfredo	1 cup (7.5 oz)	330	11	510	36	3
Fettuccine Alfredo With Broccoli	1 pkg (9.2 oz)	360	16	500	39	4
Fettuccine Carbonara	1 pkg (9 oz)	360	13	760	47	3
Lasagna Alfredo	1 cup (6.3 oz)	300	17	550	25	2
Lasagna Alfredo	1 pkg (9 oz)	360	20	660	30	2
Lasagna Pollo	1 pkg (9 oz)	320	14	610	33	3
Lasagna With Meat Sauce	1 pkg (9 oz)	290	10	820	36	2
Lasagna With Meat Sauce	1 cup (7.2 oz)	240	8	680	30	2
Lasagna With Vegetables	1 pkg (9 oz)	290	10	630	35	2
Linguini With Clams & Sauce	1 pkg (9 oz)	270	6	650	42	2
Linguini With Red Sauce &	1 pkg (9 oz)	260	6	540	41	3
Linguini With Seafood	1 pkg (9 oz)	290	8	740	45	4
Macaroni & Cheese	1 pkg (9 oz)	370	15	750	45	3
Macaroni & Cheese	1 cup (7.2 oz)	310	12	620	37	2
Marinara Sauce Penne Pasta Italian Sausage & Peppers	1 cup (7.4 oz)	290	14	730	27	2
Marinara Sauce Penne Pasta Italian Sausage & Peppers	1 pkg (9 oz)	350	17	880	32	2

FOOD	PORTION	CAL.	FAT	SOD.	CARB.	FIB.
Luigino's (CONT.)						
Meat Ravioli & Pomodoro Sauce	1 pkg (8.5 oz)	320	13	1060	37	3
Minestrone With Penne Pasta	1 cup (6.3 oz)	180	6	640	21	1
Penne Pollo	1 pkg (9 oz)	330	14	530	36	3
Penne Primavera	1 pkg (9 oz)	350	10	330	50	3
Rigatoni Pomodoro Italiano	1 pkg (9 oz)	290	8	710	40	4
Shells & Cheese With Jalapenos	1 pkg (8.5 oz)	360	15	700	41	2
Spaghetti Bolognese	1 pkg (9 oz)	270	8	820	38	4
Spaghetti Marinara	1 pkg (10 oz)	250	2	680	49	3
Spinach Ravioli & Primavera Sauce	1 pkg (8.5 oz)	360	17	800	36	2
Morton						
Macaroni & Cheese	1 serv (8 oz)	220	6	960	34	2
Mrs. Paul's						
Entrees Light Seafood Lasagne	9½ oz	290	8	750	39	—
Entrees Light Seafood Rotini	9 oz	240	6	570	34	—
Seafood Rotini	9 oz	240	6	570	34	—
Palmazone						
Macaroni 'n Cheese	½ pkg (6 oz)	260	7	320	36	—
Pasta Favorites						
Chicken Pasta Primavera	1 pkg (10.5 oz)	330	13	930	40	6
Fettuccini Alfredo	1 pkg (10.5 oz)	370	18	940	39	4
Italian Sausage & Peppers	1 pkg (10.5 oz)	340	13	840	43	7
Lasagna	1 pkg (10.5 oz)	290	9	900	39	6
Macaroni & Cheese	1 pkg (10.5 oz)	350	12	1070	47	5
Pasta Primavera	1 pkg (10.5 oz)	320	14	920	40	7
Spaghetti w/ Meatballs	1 pkg (10.5 oz)	370	16	1040	40	6
Vegetable Lasagna	1 pkg (10.5 oz)	260	6	850	41	7
White Cheddar & Rotini	1 pkg (10.5 oz)	350	12	900	48	6
Senor Felix's						
Lasagna Southwestern	1 serv (6 oz)	160	7	380	15	2
Stouffer's						
Cheddar Pasta w/ Beef & Tomatoes	1 pkg (11 oz)	450	19	1130	45	3
Cheese Manicotti	1 pkg (9 oz)	380	17	880	38	4
Cheese Ravioli	1 pkg (10.6 oz)	380	13	700	51	6
Chicken Lasagna	1 serv (7.8 oz)	320	17	750	29	4

FOOD	PORTION	CAL.	FAT	SOD.	CARB.	FIB.
Swanson						
Homestyle Lasagne With Meat Sauce	10½ oz	400	15	1070	39	—
Homestyle Macaroni & Cheese	10 oz	390	19	1150	37	—
Homestyle Spaghetti With Italian Style Meatballs	13 oz	490	18	940	60	—
Macaroni & Cheese	12¼ oz	370	15	1070	48	—
Macaroni & Cheese	7 oz	200	8	740	24	—
Spaghetti & Meatballs	12½ oz	390	17	1100	46	—
Tabatchnick						
Macaroni & Cheese	7.5 oz	280	12	840	30	2
Tyson						
Parmigiana	1 pkg (11.25 oz)	380	17	1100	37	—
Ultra Slim-Fast						
Pasta Primavera	12 oz	340	9	730	52	5
Spaghetti With Beef & Mushroom Sauce	12 oz	370	10	990	49	0
Weight Watchers						
Smart Ones Angel Hair Pasta	1 pkg (9 oz)	170	2	520	29	4
Smart Ones Bowtie Pasta & Mushrooms Marsala	1 pkg (9.65 oz)	280	9	560	36	5
Smart Ones Chicken Fettucini	1 pkg (10 oz)	290	7	590	39	4
Smart Ones Creamy Rigatoni w/ Broccoli & Chicken	1 pkg (9 oz)	230	2	670	40	4
Smart Ones Lasagna Florentine	1 pkg (10 oz)	200	2	500	34	5
Smart Ones Lasagna Alfredo	1 pkg (9 oz)	300	7	650	45	2
Smart Ones Lasagna w/ Meat Sauce	1 pkg (9 oz)	240	2	520	43	4
Smart Ones Lasagna w/ Meat Sauce	1 pkg (10.25 oz)	270	7	570	38	6
Smart Ones Macaroni & Cheese	1 pkg (9 oz)	220	2	640	42	4
Smart Ones Pasta & Spinach Romano	1 pkg (10.4 oz)	240	8	510	32	4
Smart Ones Pasta w/ Tomato Basil Sauce	1 pkg (9.6 oz)	260	9	360	33	5

FOOD	PORTION	CAL.	FAT	SOD.	CARB.	FIB.
Weight Watchers (CONT.)						
Smart Ones Penne Pasta w/ Sun-Dried Tomatoes	1 pkg (10 oz)	290	9	560	41	4
Smart Ones Penne Pollo	1 pkg (10 oz)	290	5	620	40	3
Smart Ones Ravioli Florentine	1 pkg (8.5 oz)	220	2	490	43	4
Smart Ones Spaghetti Marinara	1 pkg (9 oz)	280	7	690	46	5
Smart Ones Spaghetti w/ Meat Sauce	1 pkg (10 oz)	290	6	560	41	4
Smart Ones Spicy Penne & Ricotta	1 pkg (10.2 oz)	280	6	370	45	5
Smart Ones Tuna Noodle Casserole	1 pkg (9.5 oz)	270	7	670	39	4
Smart Ones Zita Mozzarella	1 pkg (9 oz)	280	6	430	45	4
HOME RECIPE						
macaroni & cheese	1 cup	430	22	1086	40	—
spaghetti w/ meatballs & tomato sauce	1 cup	330	12	1009	39	—
MIX						
Casbah						
Pasta Fasul	1 pkg (1.6 oz)	150	1	490	10	2
Golden Grain						
Macaroni & Cheese	½ cup	310	15	620	36	—
Hain						
Pasta & Sauce Creamy Parmesan	¼ pkg	150	3	400	22	—
Pasta & Sauce Creamy Swiss	¼ pkg	170	4	360	26	—
Pasta & Sauce Fettuccine Alfredo	¼ pkg	180	4	420	27	—
Pasta & Sauce Italian Herb	¼ pkg	110	2	160	17	—
Pasta & Sauce Primavera	¼ pkg	140	4	430	20	—
Pasta & Sauce Tangy Cheddar	¼ pkg	180	6	350	24	—
Kraft						
Deluxe Macaroni & Cheese Four Cheese Blend as prep	1 cup (6.2 oz)	320	10	910	44	1

FOOD	PORTION	CAL.	FAT	SOD.	CARB.	FIB.
Kraft (CONT.)						
Deluxe Macaroni & Cheese Original as prep	1 cup (6.1 oz)	320	10	730	44	1
Light Deluxe Macaroni & Cheese as prep	1 cup (6.5 oz)	290	5	810	48	1
Macaroni & Cheese All Shapes as prep	1 cup (6.9 oz)	410	18	750	49	1
Macaroni & Cheese Original as prep	1 cup (6.9 oz)	410	18	750	49	1
Macaroni & Cheese Original as prep light recipe	1 cup (6.4 oz)	290	6	580	48	2
Premium Macaroni & Cheese Cheesy Alfredo as prep	1 cup (6.9 oz)	410	19	810	49	2
Premium Macaroni & Cheese Mild White Cheddar as prep	1 cup (6.8 oz)	410	19	740	49	1
Premium Macaroni & Cheese Thick 'N Creamy as prep	1 cup (7.6 oz)	420	19	760	50	2
Premium Macaroni & Cheese Three Cheese as prep	1 cup (6.9 oz)	410	18	790	49	2
Spaghetti Classics Mild Italian as prep	1 cup (9.1 oz)	240	3	850	46	3
Spaghetti Classics Tangy Italian as prep	1 cup (8.9 oz)	240	2	830	46	3
Spaghetti Classics Zesty Cheese as prep	1 cup (8.6 oz)	240	2	800	46	3
Spaghetti Classics w/ Meat Sauce as prep	1 cup (8.2 oz)	330	10	810	47	3
Lipton						
Golden Saute Angel Hair Chicken	⅓ cup (2.1 oz)	210	2	850	44	2
Golden Saute Chicken Herb Parmesan	½ cup (2.2 oz)	230	3	830	45	3
Golden Saute Chicken Herb Parmesan	½ cup (2.2 oz)	230	2	830	46	2
Golden Saute Chicken Stir Fry	½ cup (2.2 oz)	220	2	850	45	2
Golden Saute Garlic Butter	½ cup (2.1 oz)	230	3	790	43	2

FOOD	PORTION	CAL.	FAT	SOD.	CARB.	FIB.
Lipton (CONT.)						
Golden Saute Penne Herb & Garlic	⅓ cup (2.1 oz)	230	3	810	44	2
Pasta & Sauce Cheddar Broccoli as prep	½ cup (2.4 oz)	260	4	870	46	1
Pasta & Sauce Cheese Bow Ties	½ cup (2 oz)	230	5	790	37	1
Pasta & Sauce Chicken Primavera as prep	½ cup (2 oz)	220	3	730	40	1
Pasta & Sauce Creamy Garlic as prep	½ cup (2.4 oz)	260	6	840	45	1
Pasta & Sauce Herb Tomato as prep	½ cup (2.3 oz)	240	2	690	48	3
Pasta & Sauce Primavera as prep	½ cup (2.2 oz)	240	5	880	42	2
Pasta & Sauce Three Cheese as prep	½ cup (2.2 oz)	240	5	870	41	1
Nile Spice						
Pasta'n Sauce Mediterranean	1 pkg	210	5	640	33	2
Pasta'n Sauce Parmesan	1 pkg	200	3	470	36	1
Pasta'n Sauce Primavera	1 pkg	200	4	610	34	2
Terrazza						
Pasta E Fagioli as prep	½ cup	150	3	135	23	—
Ultra Slim-Fast						
Macaroni & Cheese	2.3 oz	230	3	770	46	4
Uncle Ben						
Country Inn Pasta & Sauce Angel Hair Parmesan	1 serv (2.2 oz)	245	5	926	39	3
Country Inn Pasta & Sauce Broccoli & White Cheddar	1 serv (2.2 oz)	240	5	799	40	2
Country Inn Pasta & Sauce Butter & Herb	1 serv (2 oz)	230	6	885	36	1
Country Inn Pasta & Sauce Creamy Garlic	1 serv (2.4 oz)	261	5	599	45	2
Country Inn Pasta & Sauce Fettuccine Alfredo	1 serv (2.2 oz)	310	6	656	41	2
Country Inn Pasta & Sauce Herb Linguine	1 serv (2.2 oz)	240	3	654	43	2
Country Inn Pasta & Sauce Mushroom Fettuccine	1 serv (2.2 oz)	250	6	638	41	2

FOOD	PORTION	CAL.	FAT	SOD.	CARB.	FIB.
Uncle Ben (CONT.)						
Country Inn Pasta & Sauce Vegetable Alfredo	1 serv (2.2 oz)	240	5	548	42	2
Velveeta						
Rotini & Cheese w/ Broccoli as prep	1 cup (7.2 oz)	400	16	1230	47	2
Shells & Cheese Bacon as prep	1 cup (6.8 oz)	360	14	1140	43	1
Shells & Cheese Original as prep	1 cup (6.6 oz)	360	13	1030	44	1
Shells & Cheese Salsa as prep	1 cup (7.5 oz)	380	14	1180	47	2
SHELF-STABLE						
Chef Boyardee						
Microwave Main Meal Beans & Pasta	10.5 oz	200	1	1030	44	10
Microwave Main Meal Beef Ravioli Suprema	10.5 oz	290	4	1390	52	5
Microwave Main Meal Cheese Ravioli Suprema	10.5 oz	290	4	1360	52	5
Microwave Main Meal Fettuccine	10.5 oz	290	9	1010	46	6
Microwave Main Meal Lasagna	10.5 oz	290	8	1000	41	5
Microwave Main Meal Meat Tortellini	10.5 oz	220	4	980	53	6
Microwave Main Meal Noodles w/ Chicken	10.5 oz	170	1	1120	27	3
Microwave Main Meal Peas & Pasta	10.5 oz	190	2	1020	39	6
Microwave Main Meal Spaghetti Suprema	10.5 oz	200	7	1000	37	7
Microwave Main Meal Zesty Macaroni	10.5 oz	290	8	1300	40	5
Microwave Main Meal Ziti In Sauce	10.5 oz	210	tr	1030	52	7
Kid's Kitchen						
Microwave Meals Beefy Macaroni	1 cup (7.5 oz)	190	6	790	23	2
Microwave Meals Macaroni & Cheese	1 cup (7.5 oz)	260	11	690	30	1
Microwave Meals Mini Ravioli	1 cup (7.5 oz)	240	7	920	35	3

FOOD	PORTION	CAL.	FAT	SOD.	CARB.	FIB.
Kid's Kitchen (CONT.)						
Microwave Meals Spaghetti Ring & Meatballs	1 cup (7.5 oz)	250	7	1200	35	3
Lunch Bucket						
Elbows In Tomato Sauce	1 pkg (7.5 oz)	190	2	860	38	—
Lasagna With Meatsauce	1 pkg (7.5 oz)	220	4	870	38	—
Light'n Healthy Italian Style Pasta	1 pkg (7.5 oz)	130	1	630	23	—
Light'n Healthy Pasta In Wine Sauce	1 pkg (7.5 oz)	130	3	600	21	—
Light'n Healthy Pasta'n Garden Vegetables	1 pkg (7.5 oz)	150	1	630	30	—
Macaroni'n Cheese	1 pkg (7.5 oz)	210	9	990	24	—
Pasta'n Chicken	1 pkg (7.5 oz)	180	6	860	22	—
Spaghetti'n Meatsauce	1 pkg (7.5 oz)	240	5	870	39	—
Micro Cup Meals						
Lasagna	1 cup (7.5 oz)	230	7	650	34	2
Lasagna & Beef Tomato Sauce	1 cup	359	19	1384	34	3
Macaroni & Beef With Vegetables	1 cup	285	8	918	37	6
Macaroni & Cheese	1 cup (7.5 oz)	260	11	690	30	1
Ravioli Tomato Sauce	1 cup (7.5 oz)	260	10	990	34	3
Spaghetti & Meat Sauce	1 cup (7.5 oz)	220	5	670	33	4
My Own Meal						
Cheese Tortellini	1 pkg (10 oz)	340	10	1000	49	6
Top Shelf						
Italian Lasagna	1 bowl (10 oz)	350	15	860	29	3
Spaghetti With Meat Sauce	1 bowl (10 oz)	240	5	940	36	3
TAKE-OUT						
lasagna	1 piece (2.5 in x 2.5 in)	374	21	668	25	2
macaroni & cheese	1 cup	230	10	730	26	—
manicotti	¾ cup (6.4 oz)	273	12	414	28	2
rigatoni w/ sausage sauce	¾ cup	260	12	106	28	3
spaghetti w/ meatballs & cheese	1 cup	407	19	696	38	—

PASTA MACHINE MIX

FOOD	PORTION	CAL.	FAT	SOD.	CARB.	FIB.
Wanda's						
Dried Tomato	⅓ cup mix per serv (1.9 oz)	202	1	0	42	1

FOOD	PORTION	CAL.	FAT	SOD.	CARB.	FIB.
Wanda's (CONT.)						
Durum & Semolina	⅓ cup mix per serv (1.9 oz)	199	1	0	42	1
Semolina Blend	⅓ cup mix per serv (1.9 oz)	202	1	0	42	1
Spinach	⅓ cup mix per serv (1.9 oz)	202	1	0	42	1
Whole Wheat & Semolina	⅓ cup mix per serv (1.9 oz)	198	1	2	41	4
PASTA SALAD						
MIX						
Kraft						
Herb & Garlic as prep	¾ cup (4.9 oz)	280	14	670	34	2
Pasta Salad Classic Ranch w/ Bacon as prep	¾ cup (4.7 oz)	350	22	480	32	2
Pasta Salad Creamy Ceasar as prep	¾ cup (4.8 oz)	340	21	630	31	2
Pasta Salad Garden Primavera as prep	¾ cup (5 oz)	240	8	710	35	2
Pasta Salad Italian 97% Fat Free as prep	¾ cup (4.9 oz)	190	2	740	3534	2
Pasta Salad Parmesan Peppercorn as prep	¾ cup (4.9 oz)	360	23	570	29	2
Suddenly Salad						
Classic Pasta Low Fat Recipe as prep	¾ cup	180	3	830	34	1
Classic Pasta as prep	¾ cup	220	7	830	34	1
Garden Italian 98% Fat Free as prep	¾ cup	140	1	540	29	2
TAKE-OUT						
elbow macaroni salad	3.5 oz	160	5	590	26	—
italian style pasta salad	3.5 oz	140	7	480	15	—
mustard macaroni salad	3.5 oz	190	10	560	23	—
pasta salad w/ vegetables	3.5 oz	140	4	210	21	—
PASTRY						
(*see* BROWNIE, CAKE, DANISH PASTRY)						
PATE						
CANNED						
chicken liver	1 tbsp (13 g)	109	2	—	1	—
chicken liver	1 oz	238	4	—	2	—
goose liver smoked	1 tbsp (13 g)	60	6	—	1	—

FOOD	PORTION	CAL.	FAT	SOD.	CARB.	FIB.
goose liver smoked	1 oz	131	12	—	1	—
liver	1 oz	90	8	198	tr	—
liver	1 tbsp (13 g)	41	4	91	tr	—
Sells						
Liver	2.08 oz	190	16	470	4	—
PEACH						
CANNED						
halves in heavy syrup	1 half	60	tr	5	16	—
halves in light syrup	1 half	44	tr	4	12	—
halves juice pack	1 half	34	tr	3	9	—
halves water pack	1 half	18	tr	3	5	—
spiced in heavy syrup	1 cup	180	tr	9	49	—
spiced in heavy syrup	1 fruit	66	tr	3	18	—
Del Monte						
Halves Cling In Heavy Syrup	½ cup (4.5 oz)	100	0	10	24	1
Halves Cling Lite	½ cup (4.4 oz)	60	0	10	15	1
Halves Cling Melba In Heavy Syrup	½ cup (4.5 oz)	100	0	10	24	1
Halves Freestone In Heavy Syrup	½ cup (4.5 oz)	100	0	10	24	1
Sliced Cling Fruit Naturals	½ cup (4.4 oz)	60	0	10	15	1
Sliced Cling In Heavy Syrup	½ cup (4.5 oz)	100	0	10	24	1
Sliced Cling Lite	½ cup (4.4 oz)	60	0	10	15	1
Sliced Freestone In Heavy Syrup	½ cup (4.5 oz)	100	0	10	24	1
Sliced Freestone Lite	½ cup (4.4 oz)	60	0	10	14	1
Snack Cups Diced Fruit Naturals	1 serv (4.5 oz)	60	0	10	16	1
Snack Cups Diced Fruit Naturals EZ-Open Lid	1 serv (4.2 oz)	60	0	10	15	1
Snack Cups Diced In Heavy Syrup	1 serv (4.5 oz)	100	0	10	24	1
Snack Cups Diced In Heavy Syrup EZ-Open Lid	1 serv (4.2 oz)	90	0	10	23	1
Snack Cups Diced Lite	1 serv (4.5 oz)	60	0	10	16	1
Snack Cups Diced Lite EZ-Open Lid	1 serv (4.2 oz)	60	0	10	15	1
Whole Cling In Heavy Syrup	½ cup (4.2 oz)	100	0	10	24	tr

FOOD	PORTION	CAL.	FAT	SOD.	CARB.	FIB.
Hunt's						
Halves	½ cup (4.5 oz)	100	0	10	24	1
Slices	½ cup (4.5 oz)	100	0	10	24	1
Libby						
Halves Yellow Cling Lite	½ cup (4.4 oz)	60	0	10	13	1
Sliced Yellow Cling Lite	½ cup (4.4 oz)	60	0	10	13	1
S&W						
Halves Clingstone	½ cup	100	0	10	25	—
Halves Clingstone Diet	½ cup	30	0	5	8	—
Halves Clingstone Unsweetened	½ cup	30	0	5	8	—
Halves Freestone Diet	½ cup	30	0	10	7	—
Halves Freestone In Heavy Syrup	½ cup	100	0	10	26	—
Sliced Clingstone Diet	½ cup	30	0	5	8	—
Sliced Clingstone Unsweetened	½ cup	30	0	5	8	—
Sliced Freestone Diet	½ cup	30	0	10	7	—
Sliced Freestone In Heavy Syrup	½ cup	100	0	10	26	—
Sliced Yellow Cling Natural Style	½ cup	90	0	10	20	—
Sliced Yellow Cling Premium In Heavy Syrup	½ cup	100	0	10	25	—
Whole Yellow Cling Spiced In Heavy Syrup	½ cup	90	0	10	23	—
Yellow Cling Natural Lite	½ cup	50	0	10	13	—
DRIED						
halves	1 cup	383	1	12	98	13
halves	10	311	1	9	80	11
halves cooked w/ sugar	½ cup	139	tr	3	36	—
halves cooked w/o sugar	½ cup	99	tr	3	25	—
Del Monte						
Sun Dried	⅓ cup (1.4 oz)	90	0	0	28	5
Mariani						
Peaches	¼ cup	140	0	—	—	—
Sonoma						
Pieces	3-5 pieces (1.4 oz)	120	0	0	31	1
FRESH						
peach	1	37	tr	0	10	1
sliced	1 cup	73	tr	1	19	—

FOOD	PORTION	CAL.	FAT	SOD.	CARB.	FIB.
Dole						
Peach	2	70	0	0	19	1
FROZEN						
slices sweetened	1 cup	235	tr	16	60	—
Big Valley						
Freestone	⅔ cup (4.9 oz)	50	0	0	13	1
PEACH JUICE						
nectar	1 cup	134	tr	17	35	—
Goya						
Nectar	6 oz	110	0	30	27	—
Kern's						
Nectar	6 fl oz	110	0	0	26	—
Libby						
Nectar	1 can (11.5 fl oz)	210	0	5	52	—
Mott's						
Fruit Basket Orchard Peach Juice Cocktail as prep	8 fl oz	130	0	0	32	0
Smucker's						
Juice	8 oz	120	0	10	30	—
Snapple						
Dixie Peach	10 fl oz	140	0	20	39	—
PEANUT BUTTER						
chunky	2 tbsp	188	16	156	7	2
chunky	1 cup	1520	129	1255	56	17
chunky w/o salt	2 tbsp	188	16	5	7	2
chunky w/o salt	1 cup	1520	129	44	56	17
smooth	2 tbsp	188	16	153	7	2
smooth	1 cup	1517	128	1234	53	15
smooth w/o salt	1 cup	1517	129	44	53	15
smooth w/o salt	2 tbsp	188	16	5	7	2
Arrowhead						
Creamy	2 tbsp (1.1 oz)	200	15	0	6	1
Crunchy	2 tbsp (1.1 oz)	200	15	0	6	1
BAMA						
Creamy	2 tbsp	200	17	140	6	—
Crunchy	2 tbsp	200	17	115	6	—
Jelly & Peanut Butter	2 tbsp	150	7	75	20	—
Crazy Richard's						
Natural Creamy	2 tbsp (1.1 oz)	190	16	0	6	2
Erewhon						
Chunky	2 tbsp (32 g)	190	14	75	7	—
Chunky Unsalted	2 tbsp (32 g)	190	14	10	7	—

FOOD	PORTION	CAL.	FAT	SOD.	CARB.	FIB.
Erewhon (CONT.)						
Creamy	2 tbsp (32 g)	190	14	75	7	—
Creamy Unsalted	2 tbsp (32 g)	190	14	10	7	—
Estee						
Chunky Sodium Free	2 tbsp (1 oz)	190	15	0	7	2
Chunky Sodium Free Sorbitol Sweetened	2 tbsp (1 oz)	190	15	0	7	2
Creamy Sodium Free	2 tbsp (1 oz)	190	15	0	7	2
Creamy Sodium Free Sorbitol Sweetened	2 tbsp (1 oz)	190	15	0	7	2
Health Valley						
Chunky No Salt	2 tbsp	170	14	2	6	2
Creamy No Salt	2 tbsp	170	14	2	6	3
Hollywood						
Creamy	1 tbsp	35	3	25	1	1
Crunchy	1 tbsp	35	3	25	1	1
Unsalted	1 tbsp	35	3	0	1	1
Home Brand						
Natural Lightly Salted	2 tbsp	210	17	—	—	—
Natural Unsalted	2 tbsp	210	17	—	—	—
No-Sugar Added	2 tbsp	180	16	—	—	—
Peanut Butter	2 tbsp	210	17	—	—	—
Jif						
Creamy	2 tbsp (1.1 oz)	190	16	150	7	2
Extra Crunchy	2 tbsp (1.1 oz)	190	16	130	7	2
Reduced Fat	2 tbsp (1.3 oz)	190	12	250	15	2
Simply Creamy	2 tbsp (1.1 oz)	190	16	65	6	2
Simply Extra Crunchy	2 tbsp (1.1 oz)	190	16	50	6	2
Peter Pan						
Creamy	2 tbsp	190	16	150	6	2
Creamy Salt Free	2 tbsp	190	17	0	5	2
Crunchy	2 tbsp	190	16	150	6	2
Crunchy Salt Free	2 tbsp	190	17	0	5	2
Red Wing						
Creamy	2 tbsp (1.1 oz)	200	16	140	6	2
Crunchy	2 tbsp (1.1 oz)	200	16	120	6	2
Reese's						
Peanut Butter Chips	¼ cup (1.5 oz)	230	13	90	19	—
Skippy						
Creamy	1 cup (263 g)	1540	135	1240	38	—
Creamy w/ 2 slices white bread	1 sandwich	340	19	430	33	—
Reduced Fat Creamy	2 tbsp	190	12	200	13	1
Super Chunk	1 cup (260 g)	1540	138	1120	36	—

FOOD	PORTION	CAL.	FAT	SOD.	CARB.	FIB.
Skippy (CONT.)						
Super Chunk	2 tbsp (32 g)	190	17	130	4	—
Super Chunk w/ slices white bread	1 sandwich	340	19	410	32	—
Smucker's						
Goober Grape	2 tbsp	180	10	120	18	—
Honey Sweetened	2 tbsp	200	16	155	7	—
Natural	2 tbsp	200	16	125	6	—
Natural No-Salt Added	2 tbsp	200	16	<10	6	—
Tree Of Life						
Creamy	2 tbsp (1 oz)	190	15	150	7	1
Creamy No Salt	2 tbsp (1 oz)	190	15	0	7	1
Creamy Organic	2 tbsp (1 oz)	190	16	45	7	1
Creamy Organic No Salt	2 tbsp (1 oz)	190	16	0	7	1
Crunchy	2 tbsp (1 oz)	190	15	150	7	1
Crunchy No Salt	2 tbsp (1 oz)	190	15	0	7	1
Crunchy Organic	2 tbsp (1 oz)	190	16	45	7	1
Crunchy Organic No Salt	2 tbsp (1 oz)	190	16	0	7	1
Peanut Wonder 78% Less Fat	2 tbsp (1 oz)	100	4	250	11	1
PEANUTS						
chocolate coated	10 (1.4 oz)	208	13	16	20	—
chocolate coated	1 cup (5.2 oz)	773	50	61	74	—
cooked	½ cup	102	7	240	7	—
dry roasted	1 oz	164	14	228	6	2
dry roasted	1 cup	855	73	1187	31	12
oil roasted	1 oz	163	14	121	5	2
oil roasted	1 cup	837	71	624	27	13
oil roasted w/o salt	1 cup	837	71	9	27	13
oil roasted w/o salt	1 oz	163	14	2	5	2
spanish oil roasted	1 oz	162	14	121	5	2
spanish oil roasted w/o salt	1 oz	162	14	2	5	2
unroasted	1 oz	159	14	5	5	—
valencia oil roasted	1 oz	165	14	216	5	2
valencia oil roasted	1 cup	848	74	1111	23	9
valencia oil roasted w/o salt	1 oz	165	14	2	5	2
valencia oil roasted w/o salt	1 cup	848	74	9	23	9
virginia oil roasted	1 cup	826	70	619	28	—
virginia oil roasted	1 oz	161	14	121	5	—
Beer Nuts						
Peanuts	1 pkg (1 oz)	180	14	60	7	—
Fisher						
Party Peanuts	1 oz	160	14	—	—	—

FOOD	PORTION	CAL.	FAT	SOD.	CARB.	FIB.
Fisher (CONT.)						
Salted-In-Shell shelled	1 oz	170	14	170	6	—
Spanish Roasted	1 oz	180	16	130	6	—
Frito Lay						
Dry Roasted	1.2 oz	190	16	300	7	—
Salted	1 oz	170	15	170	6	—
Guy's						
Dry Roasted	1 oz	170	14	310	3	—
Spanish Salted	1 oz	170	14	170	3	—
Lance						
Honey Toasted	1 pkg (39 g)	230	17	240	11	—
Roasted w/ Shell	1 pkg (50 g)	190	15	0	8	—
Salted	1 pkg (32 g)	190	15	105	7	—
Salted Tube	1 pkg (42 g)	240	20	120	9	—
Little Debbie						
Salted	1 pkg (1.2 oz)	230	21	45	3	2
Pennant						
Oil Roasted	1 oz	170	14	115	6	3
Planters						
Cocktail Lightly Salted Oil Roasted	1 oz	170	15	55	5	2
Cocktail Oil Roasted	1 oz	170	14	115	6	3
Cocktail Unsalted Oil Roasted	1 oz	170	14	0	6	2
Dry Roasted	1 oz	160	13	250	6	3
Fun Size! Oil Roasted	2 pkg (1 oz)	170	15	140	6	2
Heat Hot Spicy Oil Roasted	1 pkg (1.7 oz)	290	25	370	9	4
Heat Hot Spicy Oil Roasted	1 oz	160	14	190	5	2
Heat Hot Spicy Oil Roasted	1 pkg (2 oz)	330	29	390	10	5
Heat Mild Spicy Oil Roasted	1 oz	160	14	130	5	2
Honey Roasted	1 oz	160	13	90	8	2
Honey Roasted Dry Roasted	1 pkg (1.7 oz)	260	19	260	17	3
Lightly Salted Dry Roasted	1 oz	160	14	110	5	3
Lightly Salted Dry Roasted	1 pkg (1.75 oz)	290	25	190	9	4
Lightly Salted Oil Roasted	1 pkg (1.8 oz)	300	27	95	8	4

FOOD	PORTION	CAL.	FAT	SOD.	CARB.	FIB.
Planters (CONT.)						
Munch'N Go Singles Heat Hot Spicy Oil Roasted	1 pkg (2.5 oz)	410	36	480	13	6
Reduced Fat Honey Roasted	⅓ cup (1 oz)	130	7	150	12	2
Salted Oil Roasted	1 pkg (1 oz)	170	15	110	5	2
Spanish Oil Roasted	1 oz	170	14	105	5	2
Spanish Raw	1 oz	150	13	5	6	3
Sweet N Crunchy	1 oz	140	7	20	16	2
Unsalted Dry Roasted	1 oz	160	14	0	6	3
Weight Watchers						
Honey Roasted	1 pkg (0.7 oz)	100	5	100	7	2

PEAR

CANNED

FOOD	PORTION	CAL.	FAT	SOD.	CARB.	FIB.
halves in heavy syrup	1 cup	188	tr	13	49	—
halves in heavy syrup	1 half	68	tr	4	15	—
halves in light syrup	1 half	45	tr	4	12	—
halves juice pack	1 cup	123	tr	10	32	—
halves water pack	1 half	22	tr	41	6	—
Del Monte						
Halves Fruit Naturals	½ cup (4.4 oz)	60	0	10	15	1
Halves In Heavy Syrup	½ cup (4.5 oz)	100	0	10	24	1
Halves Lite	½ cup (4.4 oz)	60	0	10	15	1
Sliced In Heavy Syrup	½ cup (4.5 oz)	100	0	10	24	1
Sliced Lite	½ cup (4.4 oz)	60	0	10	15	1
Snack Cups Diced In Heavy Syrup	1 serv (4.5 oz)	100	0	10	24	1
Snack Cups Diced In Heavy Syrup EZ-Open Lid	1 serv (4.2 oz)	90	0	10	23	1
Snack Cups Diced Lite	1 serv (4.5 oz)	60	0	10	15	1
Snack Cups Diced Lite EZ-Open Lid	1 serv (4.2 oz)	60	0	10	15	1
Libby						
Halves Lite	½ cup (4.3 oz)	60	0	10	13	1
Sliced Lite	½ cup (4.3 oz)	60	0	10	13	1
S&W						
Halves Bartlett In Heavy Syrup	½ cup	100	0	—	25	—
Halves Bartlett Peeled Unsweetened	½ cup	35	0	10	10	—
Halves Peeled Diet	½ cup	35	0	10	10	—

FOOD	PORTION	CAL.	FAT	SOD.	CARB.	FIB.
S&W (CONT.)						
Quartered Peeled Diet	½ cup	35	0	10	10	—
Sliced Natural Light Bartlett	½ cup	60	0	10	15	—
Sliced Natural Style	½ cup	80	0	10	20	—
DRIED						
halves	10	459	1	10	122	—
halves	1 cup	472	1	10	125	—
halves cooked w/ sugar	½ cup	196	tr	4	52	—
halves cooked w/o sugar	½ cup	163	tr	4	43	—
Mariani						
Pears	¼ cup	150	0	—	—	—
Sonoma						
Pieces	3-4 pieces (1.4 oz)	120	0	0	33	3
FRESH						
asian	1 (4.3 oz)	51	tr	0	13	—
pear	1	98	1	1	25	4
sliced w/ skin	1 cup	97	1	1	25	4
Dole						
Pear	1	100	1	1	25	4

PEAR JUICE

FOOD	PORTION	CAL.	FAT	SOD.	CARB.	FIB.
nectar	1 cup	149	tr	9	39	—
Goya						
Nectar	6 oz	120	0	15	29	—
Kern's						
Nectar	6 fl oz	120	0	0	28	—
Libby						
Nectar	1 can (11.5 fl oz)	220	0	5	54	3

PEAS

FOOD	PORTION	CAL.	FAT	SOD.	CARB.	FIB.
CANNED						
green	½ cup	59	tr	186	11	—
green low sodium	½ cup	59	tr	2	11	—
Allen						
Crowder	½ cup (4.5 oz)	110	1	460	19	8
Purple Hull	½ cup (4.4 oz)	120	1	350	21	6
Crest Top						
Early June	½ cup (4.5 oz)	100	1	300	20	6
Del Monte						
Sweet	½ cup (4.4 oz)	60	0	360	11	4
Sweet 50% Less Salt	½ cup (4.4 oz)	60	0	180	11	4
Sweet No Salt Added	½ cup (4.4 oz)	60	0	10	11	4
Sweet Very Young	½ cup (4.4 oz)	60	0	360	10	4

FOOD	PORTION	CAL.	FAT	SOD.	CARB.	FIB.
East Texas Fair						
Cream Peas	½ cup (4.4 oz)	120	1	420	20	5
Crowder	½ cup (4.5 oz)	110	1	460	19	8
Lady Peas With Snaps	½ cup (4.3 oz)	100	1	420	17	4
Peas 'n Pork	½ cup (4.5 oz)	110	2	540	19	5
Pepper Peas	½ cup (4.5 oz)	120	1	580	22	6
Purple Hull	½ cup (4.4 oz)	120	1	350	21	6
White Acre	½ cup (4.3 oz)	100	1	460	17	5
Green Giant						
Sweet	½ cup	50	0	320	11	4
Homefolks						
Crowder	½ cup (4.5 oz)	110	1	460	19	8
Purple Hull	½ cup (4.4 oz)	120	1	350	21	6
Luck's						
Crowder Peas Seasoned w/Pork	7.5 oz	200	7	—	—	—
Owatonna						
Early June or Sweet	½ cup	70	0	—	—	—
S&W						
Petit Pois	½ cup	70	0	330	12	—
Sweet	½ cup	70	0	330	12	—
Sweet Water Pack	½ cup	40	0	5	8	—
Veri-Green Sweet	½ cup	70	0	320	14	—
Seneca						
Natural Pack	½ cup	60	0	0	9	4
Peas	½ cup	50	0	360	9	5
Sunshine						
Field Peas	½ cup (4.4 oz)	120	1	350	21	6
Lady Peas	½ cup (4.3 oz)	100	1	460	17	5
Trappey						
Field Peas With Bacon	½ cup (4.5 oz)	90	1	380	15	5
Field Peas With Snaps And Bacon	½ cup (4.5 oz)	110	1	380	19	4
DRIED						
split cooked	1 cup	231	1	4	41	—
Bascom's						
Yellow Split as prep	½ cup	110	0	0	20	—
FRESH						
green cooked	½ cup	67	tr	2	13	—
green raw	½ cup	58	tr	3	11	—
snap peas cooked	½ cup	34	tr	3	6	2
snap peas raw	½ cup	30	tr	3	5	2
Dole						
Sugar Peas	½ cup	30	tr	3	5	2

FOOD	PORTION	CAL.	FAT	SOD.	CARB.	FIB.
FROZEN						
green cooked	½ cup	63	tr	70	11	—
snap peas cooked	½ cup	42	tr	4	7	—
snap peas cooked	1 pkg (10 oz)	132	1	12	23	—
Birds Eye						
Green	½ cup	80	0	130	13	4
In Butter Sauce	½ cup	80	2	170	12	3
Polybag Deluxe Tender Tiny	½ cup	60	0	120	11	4
Polybag Green	½ cup	70	0	125	12	2
Sugar Snap Deluxe	½ cup	45	0	5	9	4
Tender Tiny Deluxe	½ cup	60	0	120	11	4
Chun King						
Snow Pea Pods	½ pkg (3 oz)	35	2	0	4	2
Fresh Like						
Green	3.5 oz	85	1	79	14	2
Tiny Green	3.5 oz	63	tr	79	12	1
Green Giant						
Harvest Fresh Early June	½ cup	60	1	140	12	3
Harvest Fresh Sugar Snap	½ cup	30	0	100	8	2
Harvest Fresh Sweet	½ cup	50	0	95	12	3
In Butter Sauce	½ cup	80	2	410	14	4
One Serve In Butter Sauce	1 pkg	90	2	500	16	5
Sugar Snap Sweet Select	½ cup	30	0	0	8	2
Sweet	½ cup	50	0	95	11	4
Hanover						
Petite	½ cup	70	0	—	—	—
Snow Peas	½ cup	35	0	—	—	—
Sweet	½ cup	70	0	—	—	—
LeSueur						
Early In Butter Sauce	½ cup	80	2	440	14	3
Early Select	½ cup	60	0	115	13	4
Tree Of Life						
Peas	⅔ cup (3.1 oz)	70	0	100	12	1
SHELF-STABLE						
Green Giant						
Mini Sweet	½ cup	60	tr	240	12	4
SPROUTS						
raw	½ cup	77	tr	12	17	–
TAKE-OUT						
pea & potato curry	1 serv (7 oz)	284	22	—	19	6
pea curry	1 serv (4.4 oz)	438	42	—	11	4

FOOD	PORTION	CAL.	FAT	SOD.	CARB.	FIB.
PECANS						
dried	1 oz	190	19	0	5	2
dry roasted	1 oz	187	18	0	6	—
dry roasted salted	1 oz	187	18	260	6	—
halves dried	1 cup	721	73	1	20	7
oil roasted	1 oz	195	20	0	5	—
oil roasted salted	1 oz	195	20	252	5	—
Planters						
Chips	1 pkg (2 oz)	390	40	5	9	7
Gold Measure Halves	1 pkg (2 oz)	390	40	5	9	3
Halves	1 oz	190	20	0	4	2
Honey Roasted	1 oz	180	16	75	9	2
Pieces	1 oz	190	20	0	4	2
Pieces	1 pkg (2 oz)	390	40	5	9	3
PECTIN						
powder	1 pkg (1.75 oz)	163	tr	100	45	—
powder	¼ pkg (0.4 oz)	39	0	24	11	—
Slim Set						
Packet	1 pkg	208	0	42	44	14
Powder	1 tbsp	3	0	1	1	tr
Sure Jell						
For Lower Sugar Recipes	¼ tsp (0.7 g)	5	0	10	1	0
Pectin	¼ tsp (0.9 g)	5	0	0	1	0
PEPEAO						
pepeao dried	½ cup	36	tr	8	10	—
pepeao raw sliced	1 cup	25	tr	9	7	—
PEPPER						
black	1 tsp	5	tr	1	1	—
cayenne	1 tsp	6	tr	1	1	—
red	1 tsp	6	tr	1	1	—
white	1 tsp	7	tr	tr	2	—
Ac'cent						
Lemon	½ tsp	0	0	0	0	0
Seasoned	½ tsp	0	0	0	0	0
Lawry's						
Lemon	1 tsp	6	tr	340	1	tr
Watkins						
Black	¼ tbsp (0.5 g)	0	0	0	0	0
Cajun	¼ tbsp (0.5 g)	0	0	25	0	0
Cracked Black	¼ tbsp (0.5 g)	0	0	0	0	0
Dijon	¼ tbsp (0.5 g)	0	0	15	0	0

FOOD	PORTION	CAL.	FAT	SOD.	CARB.	FIB.
Watkins (CONT.)						
Garlic Peppercorn Blend	¼ tbsp (1 g)	0	0	0	0	0
Herb	¼ tbsp (0.5 g)	0	0	0	0	0
Italian	¼ tbsp (0.5 g)	0	0	0	0	0
Lemon	¼ tbsp (1 g)	0	0	55	0	0
Mexican	¼ tbsp (0.5 g)	0	0	0	0	0
Red Pepper Flakes	¼ tsp (0.5 oz)	0	0	0	0	0
Royal Pepper Blend	¼ tbsp (0.5 g)	0	0	0	0	0
PEPPERS						
CANNED						
chili green hot	1 (2.6 oz)	18	tr	—	4	—
chili green hot chopped	½ cup	17	tr	—	4	—
chili red hot	1 (2.6 oz)	18	tr	—	4	—
chili red hot chopped	½ cup	17	tr	—	4	—
green halves	½ cup	13	tr	958	3	—
jalapeno chopped	½ cup	17	tr	995	3	—
red halves	½ cup	13	tr	958	3	—
Chi-Chi's						
Chilies Diced Green	2 tbsp (1.2 oz)	10	0	5	1	0
Chilies Green Whole	¾ pepper (1 oz)	10	0	5	1	0
Jalapenos Green Wheels	1 oz	10	0	110	1	0
Jalapenos Green Whole	1 oz	10	0	110	2	0
Jalapenos Red Wheels	1 oz	10	0	110	1	0
Jalapenos Red Whole	1 oz	15	0	110	3	0
Del Monte						
Chilpotle In Spice Sauce	2 tbsp (1.1 oz)	20	1	430	4	1
Hot Chili	4 (1 oz)	10	0	610	3	tr
Jalapeno Nacho Pickled Sliced	2 tbsp (1 oz)	5	0	340	1	tr
Jalapeno Pickled Sliced	2 tbsp (1.1 oz)	5	0	530	1	tr
Jalapeno Pickled Whole	2 tbsp (1.1 oz)	5	0	560	1	tr
Jalapeno Whole	1 (0.7 oz)	3	0	230	tr	tr
Hebrew National						
Filet	¼ pepper (1 oz)	9	0	310	2	—
Hot Cherry	⅓ pepper (1 oz)	11	0	270	2	—
Red Filet	¼ pepper (1 oz)	9	0	310	2	—
McIlhenny						
Jalapeno Nacho Slices	12 slices (1.1 oz)	7	tr	70	1	1
Old El Paso						
Green Chilies Chopped	2 tbsp (1 oz)	5	0	110	1	1
Green Chilies Whole	1 (1.2 oz)	10	0	230	2	1
Jalapenos Peeled	3 (1 oz)	10	0	200	1	1
Jalapenos Pickled	2 (0.9 oz)	5	0	380	1	0

FOOD	PORTION	CAL.	FAT	SOD.	CARB.	FIB.
Old El Paso (CONT.)						
Jalapenos Slices	2 tbsp (1.1 oz)	15	0	400	3	1
Progresso						
Cherry (drained)	2 tbsp (0.9 oz)	30	2	30	2	1
Fried (drained)	2 tbsp (0.9 oz)	60	5	60	3	1
Hot Cherry	1 (1 oz)	15	0	250	0	0
Pepper Salad (drained)	2 tbsp (0.9 oz)	25	2	80	1	1
Roasted	½ piece (1 oz)	10	0	60	1	0
Tuscan (drained)	3 (1 oz)	10	0	330	1	1
Rosoff's						
Sweet	¼ pepper (1 oz)	9	0	310	2	—
Schorr's						
Filet Peppers	1 oz	9	0	310	2	—
Trappey						
Banana Mild	3 peppers (1 oz)	6	tr	100	1	1
Banana Sliced Rings	21 slices (1 oz)	6	tr	529	1	1
Cherry Hot	2 peppers (1 oz)	7	tr	373	1	1
Cherry Mild	2 peppers (1 oz)	10	tr	225	2	1
Dulcito Italian Pepperoncini	4 peppers (1 oz)	8	tr	178	2	1
In Vinegar Hot	15 peppers (1 oz)	9	tr	573	2	tr
Jalapeno Hot Sliced	21 slices (1 oz)	4	tr	296	1	1
Jalapeno Whole	2 peppers (1 oz)	11	0	658	2	1
Serano	7 peppers (1 oz)	7	tr	37	1	tr
Tempero Golden Greek Pepperoncini	4 peppers (1 oz)	7	tr	470	1	1
Torrido Santa Fe Grande	3 peppers (1 oz)	10	tr	492	2	tr
Vlasic						
Hot Banana Pepper Rings	1 oz	4	0	465	1	—
Hot Cherry	1 oz	10	0	425	2	—
Jalapeno Mexican Hot	1 oz	8	0	380	2	—
Mexican Tiny Hot	1 oz	6	0	430	2	—
Mild Cherry	1 oz	8	0	410	2	—
Mild Greek Pepperoncini Salad Peppers	1 oz	4	0	450	1	—
DRIED						
green	1 tbsp	1	tr	1	tr	—
red	1 tbsp	1	tr	1	tr	—
FRESH						
chili green hot raw	1	18	tr	3	4	—
chili green hot raw chopped	½ cup	30	tr	5	7	—
chili red hot raw	1 (1.6 oz)	18	tr	3	4	—

FOOD	PORTION	CAL.	FAT	SOD.	CARB.	FIB.
chili red raw chopped	½ cup	30	tr	5	7	—
green chopped cooked	½ cup	19	tr	1	5	—
green cooked	1 (2.6 oz)	20	tr	1	5	—
green raw	1 (2.6 oz)	20	tr	1	5	1
green raw chopped	½ cup	13	tr	1	3	1
red chopped cooked	½ cup	19	tr	1	5	—
red cooked	1 (2.6 oz)	20	tr	1	5	—
red raw	1 (2.6 oz)	20	tr	1	5	1
red raw chopped	½ cup	13	tr	1	3	1
yellow raw	10 strips	14	tr	1	3	—
yellow raw	1 (6.5 oz)	50	tr	3	12	—
Dole						
Medium	1	25	1	0	5	2
FROZEN						
green chopped not prep	1 oz	6	tr	1	1	—
red chopped	1 oz	6	tr	1	1	—
Southland						
Green Diced	2 oz	10	0	—	—	—
Sweet Red & Green Cut	2 oz	15	0	—	—	—
PERCH						
FRESH						
cooked	1 fillet (1.6 oz)	54	1	36	0	—
cooked	3 oz	99	1	67	0	—
ocean perch atlantic cooked	3 oz	103	2	82	0	—
ocean perch atlantic cooked	1 fillet (1.8 oz)	60	1	48	0	—
ocean perch atlantic raw	3 oz	80	1	64	0	—
raw	3 oz	77	1	52	0	—
red raw	3½ oz	114	4	80	0	—
FROZEN						
Gorton's						
Fishmarket Fresh Ocean Perch	5 oz	140	3	100	2	—
Van De Kamp's						
Battered Fillets	2 (4 oz)	300	20	480	19	0
PERSIMMONS						
dried japanese	1	93	tr	1	25	—
fresh	1	32	tr	0	8	—
fresh japanese	1	118	tr	3	31	—
Sonoma						
Dried	6-8 pieces (1.4 oz)	140	0	10	35	3

FOOD	PORTION	CAL.	FAT	SOD.	CARB.	FIB.
PHEASANT						
breast w/o skin raw	½ breast (6.4 oz)	243	6	60	0	—
leg w/o skin raw	1 (3.6 oz)	143	5	48	0	—
w/ skin raw	½ pheasant (14 oz)	723	37	161	0	—
w/o skin raw	½ pheasant (12.4 oz)	470	13	131	0	—
PHYLLO DOUGH						
phyllo dough	1 oz	85	2	137	15	—
sheet	1	57	1	92	10	—
Ekizian						
Sheets	½ lb	865	17	573	151	—
PICANTE						
(*see* SALSA)						
PICKLES						
(FAST FACT: Americans on the average eat 9 pounds of pickles a year.)						
dill	1 (2.3 oz)	12	tr	833	3	—
dill low sodium	1 (2.3 oz)	12	tr	12	3	1
dill low sodium sliced	1 slice	1	tr	1	tr	tr
dill sliced	1 slice	1	tr	77	tr	tr
gerkins	3½ oz	21	tr	960	4	—
kosher dill	1 (2.3 oz)	12	tr	833	3	1
polish dill	1 (2.3 oz)	12	tr	833	3	1
quick sour	1 (1.2 oz)	4	tr	423	1	—
quick sour low sodium	1 (1.2 oz)	4	tr	6	1	—
quick sour sliced	1 slice	1	tr	85	tr	—
sweet	1 (1.2 oz)	41	tr	328	11	tr
sweet gherkin	1 sm (½ oz)	20	tr	107	5	—
sweet low sodium	1 (1.2 oz)	41	tr	6	11	tr
sweet sliced	1 slice	7	tr	56	2	tr
Claussen						
Bread 'N Butter Slices	1 slice	7	tr	—	—	—
Dill Spears	1 spear	4	tr	—	—	—
Kosher Halves	1 half	9	tr	—	—	—
Kosher Slices	1 slice	1	tr	—	—	—
Kosher Whole	1	9	tr	—	—	—
No Garlic Dills	1	17	tr	—	—	—
Del Monte						
Dill Halves	¼ pickle (1 oz)	5	0	370	tr	tr
Dill Hamburger Chips	5 pieces (1 oz)	5	0	310	1	0
Dill Sweet Chips	5 pieces (1 oz)	40	0	210	10	tr
Dill Sweet Gherkin	2 pickles (1 oz)	40	0	210	10	tr

FOOD	PORTION	CAL.	FAT	SOD.	CARB.	FIB.
Del Monte (CONT.)						
Dill Sweet Midgets	3 pickles (1 oz)	40	0	210	10	tr
Dill Sweet Whole	2 pickles (1 oz)	40	0	210	10	tr
Dill Tiny Kosher	1½ pickle (1 oz)	5	0	240	1	tr
Dill Whole Pickles	1½ pickle (1 oz)	5	0	370	tr	tr
Hebrew National						
Half Sour	½ pickle (1 oz)	4	0	210	1	—
Kosher	⅓ pickle (1 oz)	4	0	260	1	—
Kosher Barrel Cured Dill	1 pkg	23	0	1570	4	—
Kosher Barrel Cured Hot Dill	1 pkg	23	0	1570	4	—
Kosher Chips	3 slices (1 oz)	4	0	300	1	—
Kosher Halves	⅓ pickle (1 oz)	4	0	290	1	—
Kosher Large	⅕ pickle (1 oz)	4	0	300	1	—
Kosher Spears	½ spear (1 oz)	4	0	260	1	—
Sour Garlic	⅓ pickle (1 oz)	3	0	250	1	—
McIlhenny						
Hot N' Sweet	4 (1 oz)	42	tr	28	10	tr
Rosoff's						
Half Sour	⅓ pickle (1 oz)	4	0	210	1	—
Half Sour Spears	½ spear (1 oz)	4	0	200	1	—
Kosher	⅓ pickle (1 oz)	4	0	260	1	—
Kosher Halves	⅓ pickle (1 oz)	4	0	290	1	—
Schorr's						
Garlic	⅓ pickle (1 oz)	3	0	250	1	—
Half Sour	⅓ pickle (1 oz)	4	0	210	1	—
Half Sour	½ spear (1 oz)	4	0	200	1	—
Kosher Deli	½ pickle (1 oz)	4	0	160	1	—
Kosher Halves	⅓ pickle (1 oz)	4	0	290	1	—
Kosher Spears	½ spear (1 oz)	4	0	260	1	—
Kosher Whole	⅓ pickle (1 oz)	4	0	260	1	—
Vlasic						
Bread & Butter Chips	1 oz	30	0	160	7	—
Bread & Butter Chunks	1 oz	25	0	120	6	—
Bread & Butter Stixs	1 oz	18	0	110	5	—
Deli Bread & Butter	1 oz	25	0	120	6	—
Deli Dill Halves	1 oz	4	0	290	1	—
Half-The-Salt Hamburger Dill Chips	1 oz	2	0	175	1	—
Half-The-Salt Kosher Crunchy Dills	1 oz	4	0	125	1	—
Half-The-Salt Kosher Dill Spears	1 oz	4	0	120	1	—
Half-The-Salt Sweet Butter Chips	1 oz	30	0	80	7	—

FOOD	PORTION	CAL.	FAT	SOD.	CARB.	FIB.
Vlasic (CONT.)						
Hot & Spicy Garden Mix	1 oz	4	0	380	1	—
Kosher Baby Dills	1 oz	4	0	210	1	—
Kosher Crunchy Dills	1 oz	4	0	210	1	—
Kosher Dill Gherkins	1 oz	4	0	210	1	—
Kosher Dill Spears	1 oz	4	0	175	1	—
Kosher Snack Chunks	1 oz	4	0	220	1	—
No Garlic Dill Spears	1 oz	4	0	210	1	—
Original Dills	1 oz	2	0	375	1	—
Polish Snack Chunk Dills	1 oz	4	0	300	1	—
Zesty Crunchy Dills	1 oz	4	0	250	1	—
Zesty Dill Snack Chunks	1 oz	4	0	290	1	—
Zesty Dill Spears	1 oz	4	0	230	1	—

PIE

(*see also* PIE CRUST)

FOOD	PORTION	CAL.	FAT	SOD.	CARB.	FIB.
CANNED FILLING						
apple	⅛ can (2.6 oz)	74	tr	32	19	1
apple	1 can (21 oz)	599	1	259	156	6
cherry	1 can (21 oz)	683	1	54	175	—
cherry	⅛ can (2.6 oz)	85	tr	7	22	—
pumpkin pie mix	1 cup	282	tr	561	71	—
Libby						
Pumpkin Pie Mix	½ cup	100	0	150	25	2
None Such						
Mincemeat Condensed	¼ pkg	220	2	310	50	—
Mincemeat Ready-to-Use	⅓ cup	200	1	360	48	—
Mincemeat Ready-to-Use With Brandy & Rum	⅓ cup	220	2	260	48	—
S&W						
Mincemeat Old Fashioned	½ cup	206	2	206	49	—
FROZEN						
apple	⅛ of 9 in pie (4.4 oz)	297	14	333	43	2
blueberry	⅛ of 9 in pie (4.4 oz)	289	13	406	44	—
cherry	⅛ of 9 in pie (4.4 oz)	325	14	308	50	1
chocolate creme	⅙ of 8 in pie (4 oz)	344	22	153	38	—
coconut creme	⅙ of 7 in pie (2.2 oz)	191	11	163	24	1

FOOD	PORTION	CAL.	FAT	SOD.	CARB.	FIB.
lemon meringue	1/6 of 8 in pie (4.5 oz)	303	10	165	53	1
peach	1/6 of 8 in pie (4.1 oz)	261	12	316	39	—
Banquet						
Apple	1/5 pie (4 oz)	300	13	370	41	2
Banana Cream	1/3 pie (4.7 oz)	350	21	290	39	1
Cherry	1/5 pie (4 oz)	290	14	310	39	2
Chocolate Cream	1/3 pie (4.7 oz)	360	20	240	43	3
Coconut Cream	1/3 pie (4.7 oz)	350	20	250	39	2
Lemon Cream	1/3 pie (4.7 oz)	360	20	240	43	2
Mincemeat	1/5 pie (4 oz)	310	13	430	46	2
Peach	1/5 pie (4 oz)	260	12	340	36	2
Pumpkin	1/6 pie (4 oz)	250	8	340	40	3
Kineret						
Apple Homestyle	1/6 pie (4 oz)	313	16	175	41	1
McMillin's						
Apple	4 oz	430	23	340	51	—
Berry	4 oz	430	23	410	52	—
Cherry	4 oz	430	24	350	51	—
Chocolate Pudding	4 oz	420	21	350	54	—
Coconut Pudding	4 oz	450	26	420	50	—
Lemon	4 oz	450	25	330	52	—
Peach	4 oz	430	24	370	52	—
Strawberry	4 oz	400	20	370	50	—
Mrs. Smith's						
Apple	1/8 of 9 in pie (4.6 oz)	370	18	430	50	2
Apple	1/6 of 8 in pie (4.3 oz)	270	11	300	41	1
Apple	1/10 of 10 in pie (4.6 oz)	280	12	310	43	1
Apple Cranberry	1/6 of 8 in pie (4.3 oz)	280	11	290	43	1
Apple Lattice Ready To Serve	1/5 of 8 in pie (4.6 oz)	310	13	350	45	2
Banana Cream	1/4 of 8 in pie (3.4 oz)	250	9	170	40	1
Berry	1/6 of 8 in pie (4.3 oz)	280	11	340	44	0
Blackberry	1/6 of 8 in pie (4.3 oz)	280	11	320	43	1
Blueberry	1/6 of 8 in pie	260	11	320	39	1
Boston Cream	1/8 of 8 in pie (2.4 oz)	170	5	140	29	0

FOOD	PORTION	CAL.	FAT	SOD.	CARB.	FIB.
Mrs. Smith's (CONT.)						
Cherry	1/10 of 10 in pie (4.6 oz)	410	18	—	—	—
Cherry	1/6 of 8 in pie	270	11	320	41	1
Cherry	1/8 of 9 in pie (4.6 oz)	320	13	350	48	1
Cherry Lattice Ready To Serve	1/5 of 8 in pie (4.6 oz)	320	13	340	47	1
Chocolate Cream	1/4 of 8 in pie (3.4 oz)	290	14	180	37	1
Coconut Cream	1/4 of 8 in pie (3.4 oz)	280	14	160	36	0
Coconut Custard	1/5 of 8 in pie (5 oz)	280	12	350	35	0
Dutch Apple	1/10 of 10 in pie (4.6 oz)	320	12	270	50	1
Dutch Apple	1/6 of 8 in pie	310	13	270	48	1
Dutch Apple	1/9 of 9 in pie (4.5 oz)	300	12	240	48	2
French Silk Cream	1/5 of 8 in pie (4.8 oz)	410	21	250	55	1
Hearty Pumpkin	1/5 of 8 in pie (5.2 oz)	280	10	350	46	2
Lemon Cream	1/4 of 8 in pie (3.4 oz)	270	13	150	36	0
Lemon Meringue	1/5 of 8 in pie (4.8 oz)	300	8	220	54	0
Mince	1/6 of 8 in pie (4.3 oz)	300	11	400	48	2
Peach	1/6 of 8 in pie	260	11	310	38	1
Peach	1/8 of 9 in pie (4.6 oz)	310	13	350	46	1
Pecan	1/8 of 10 in pie (4.5 oz)	500	23	460	68	1
Pumpkin	1/9 of 10 in pie (5.1 oz)	250	8	330	42	1
Pumpkin	1/5 of 8 in pie (5.2 oz)	270	8	350	44	1
Red Raspberry	1/6 of 8 in pie (4.3 oz)	280	11	310	43	0
Strawberry Rhubarb	1/6 of 8 in pie (4.3 oz)	280	11	380	44	0
Strawberry Rhubarb	1/5 of 8 in pie (4.8 oz)	520	23	450	73	1

FOOD	PORTION	CAL.	FAT	SOD.	CARB.	FIB.
Pepperidge Farm						
Hyannis Boston Cream Pie	1	230	10	125	34	2
Mississippi Mud	1	310	23	45	23	—
Pet-Ritz						
Apple	⅙ pie (4.33 oz)	330	12	385	53	—
Banana Cream	⅙ pie (2.33 oz)	170	9	155	22	—
Blueberry	⅙ pie (4.33 oz)	370	12	330	50	—
Cherry	⅙ pie (4.33 oz)	300	12	330	48	—
Chocolate Cream	⅙ pie (2.33 oz)	190	8	145	27	—
Coconut Cream	⅙ pie (2.33 oz)	190	8	145	27	—
Egg Custard	⅙ pie (4.0 oz)	200	8	—	28	—
Lemon Cream	⅙ pie (2.33 oz)	190	9	150	26	—
Mince	⅙ pie (4.33 oz)	280	9	—	48	—
Neapolitan Cream	⅙ pie (2.33 oz)	180	10	185	17	—
Peach	⅙ pie (4.33 oz)	320	12	320	51	—
Pumpkin Custard	⅙ pie (4.33 oz)	250	9	—	39	—
Strawberry Cream	⅙ pie (2.33 oz)	170	9	145	20	—
Sweet Potato	⅙ pie (3.33 oz)	150	7	110	21	—
Sara Lee						
Apple Homestyle	1 slice (4 oz)	280	12	220	42	—
Apple Homestyle High	1 slice (4.9 oz)	400	23	450	46	—
Apple Streusel Free & Light	1 slice (2.9 oz)	170	2	140	36	—
Blueberry Homestyle	1 slice (4 oz)	300	12	210	45	—
Cherry Homestyle	1 slice (4 oz)	270	13	270	37	—
Cherry Streusel Free & Light	1 slice (3.6 oz)	160	2	140	34	—
Dutch Apple Homestyle	1 slice (4 oz)	300	12	310	45	—
Mince Homestyle	1 slice (4 oz)	300	13	340	43	—
Peach Homestyle	1 slice (3.4 oz)	280	12	170	41	—
Pecan Homestyle	1 slice (3.4 oz)	400	18	290	56	—
Pumpkin Homestyle	1 slice (4 oz)	240	10	250	34	—
Raspberry Homestyle	1 slice (4 oz)	280	13	150	39	—
Weight Watchers						
Mississippi Mud	1 piece (2.45 oz)	160	5	120	24	5
HOME RECIPE						
apple	⅛ of 9 in pie (5.4 oz)	411	19	327	58	3
banana cream	⅛ of 9 in pie (5.2 oz)	398	20	355	49	—
blueberry	⅛ of 9 in pie (5.2 oz)	360	18	272	49	—

FOOD	PORTION	CAL.	FAT	SOD.	CARB.	FIB.
butterscotch	⅛ of 9 in pie (4.5 oz)	355	18	335	42	—
cherry	⅛ of 9 in pie (6.3 oz)	486	22	343	69	—
coconut creme	⅛ of 9 in pie (4.7 oz)	396	21	356	46	—
custard	⅛ of 9 in pie (4.5 oz)	262	11	256	34	2
lemon meringue	⅛ of 9 in pie (4.5 oz)	362	16	307	50	2
mince	⅛ of 9 in pie (5.8 oz)	477	18	419	79	—
pecan	⅛ of 9 in pie (4.3 oz)	502	27	320	64	4
pumpkin	⅛ of 9 in pie (5.4 oz)	316	14	349	41	4
vanilla cream	⅛ of 9 in pie (4.4 oz)	350	18	327	41	—
MIX						
banana cream no-bake	⅛ of 9 in pie (3.2 oz)	231	12	267	29	—
chocolate mousse no-bake	⅛ of 9 in pie (3.3 oz)	247	15	437	28	—
coconut creme no-bake	⅛ of 9 in pie (3.3 oz)	259	17	309	27	—
Betty Crocker						
Boston Cream Classic Dessert	⅛ pie	270	6	390	50	—
Jell-O						
No Bake Chocolate Silk as prep	⅙ pie (4.4 oz)	320	16	490	37	tr
Royal						
Key Lime Pie Filling	mix for 1 serv	50	0	120	13	—
Lemon Pie Filling	mix for 1 serv	50	0	120	13	0
Lemon Meringue No-Bake	⅛ pie	210	5	170	38	—
READY-TO-EAT						
Entenmann's						
Apple Homestyle	1 serv (2.1 oz)	140	7	150	21	—
Coconut Custard	1 serv (1.8 oz)	140	8	160	16	—
SNACK						
apple	1 (3 oz)	266	14	325	33	—
apple fried	1 (6.4 oz)	404	21	479	55	3
blueberry fried	1 (6.4 oz)	404	21	479	55	3

FOOD	PORTION	CAL.	FAT	SOD.	CARB.	FIB.
cherry	1 (3 oz)	266	14	325	33	—
cherry fried	1 (6.4 oz)	404	21	479	55	3
lemon	1 (3 oz)	266	14	325	33	—
lemon fried	1 (6.4 oz)	404	21	479	55	3
peach fried	1 (6.4 oz)	404	21	479	55	3
strawberry fried	1 (6.4 oz)	404	21	479	55	3
Drake's						
Apple	1 (2 oz)	210	10	135	29	—
Blueberry	1 (2 oz)	210	10	135	30	—
Cherry	1 (2 oz)	220	10	135	30	—
Lemon	1 (2 oz)	210	11	115	27	—
Lance						
Pecan	1 (38 g)	350	15	70	51	—
Little Debbie						
Marshmallow Banana	1 pkg (1.4 oz)	160	5	95	27	0
Marshmallow Banana	1 pkg (2 oz)	240	8	140	40	0
Marshmallow Banana	1 pkg (2.7 oz)	320	11	190	54	0
Marshmallow Chocolate	1 pkg (1.4 oz)	160	5	95	27	1
Marshmallow Chocolate	1 pkg (2.7 oz)	320	11	190	53	1
Marshmallow Chocolate	1 pkg (2 oz)	240	9	135	40	1
Oatmeal Creme	1 pkg (1.3 oz)	170	8	200	25	1
Oatmeal Creme	1 pkg (3 oz)	360	14	400	58	2
Oatmeal Creme	1 pkg (2.5 oz)	300	11	330	48	1
Raisin Creme	1 pkg (1.2 oz)	140	5	120	23	1
Raisin Creme	1 pkg (2.5 oz)	290	12	240	47	0
Tastykake						
Apple	1 pkg (113 g)	300	12	340	46	2
Banana Creme	1 pkg (120 g)	380	16	430	54	2
Blueberry	1 pkg (113 g)	310	9	410	55	2
Cherry	1 pkg (113 g)	300	10	310	49	2
Coconut Creme	1 pkg (113 g)	380	20	420	46	2
French Apple	1 pkg (120 g)	350	11	220	63	2
Lemon	1 pkg (113 g)	320	13	380	48	2
Lemon Lime	1 pkg (113 g)	320	13	310	49	1
Peach	1 pkg (113 g)	300	12	360	47	—
Pineapple Cheese	1 pkg (120 g)	340	13	410	54	2
Pumpkin	1 pkg (4 oz)	320	14	520	46	2
Strawberry	1 pkg (113 g)	340	11	300	57	1
Tasty Klair	1 pkg (113 g)	400	20	320	51	2
TAKE-OUT						
coconut custard	⅙ of 8 in pie (3.6 oz)	271	14	348	32	—
custard	⅙ pie 9 in	330	17	436	36	—
pecan	⅙ of 8 in pie (4 oz)	452	21	480	65	4

FOOD	PORTION	CAL.	FAT	SOD.	CARB.	FIB.
pumpkin	1/6 of 8 in pie (3.8 oz)	229	10	308	30	3
PIE CRUST (*see also* PIE)						
FROZEN						
baked	1/8 of 9 in pie (0.6 oz)	82	5	104	8	—
baked	9 in shell (4.4 oz)	647	41	815	63	—
puff pastry baked	1 shell (1.4 oz)	223	15	101	18	—
Oronoque						
Deep Dish	1/6 pie (1.41 oz)	200	13	200	16	—
Pie Crust	1/6 pie (1.23 oz)	170	12	170	14	—
Pepperidge Farm						
Patty Shells	1	210	15	180	16	—
Puff Pastry Sheets	1/4 sheet	260	17	290	22	—
Pet-Ritz						
Deep Dish	1/6 pie (1 oz)	130	8	120	12	—
Graham Cracker	1/6 pie (0.83 oz)	110	6	80	8	—
Regular	1/6 pie (0.83 oz)	110	7	110	11	—
Tart Shells	1	150	10	150	12	—
HOME RECIPE						
9-inch crust	1	900	60	1100	79	—
baked	1/8 of 9 in crust (0.8 oz)	119	8	122	11	—
baked	9 in shell (6.3 oz)	949	62	975	86	—
MIX						
as prep	9 in crust (5.6 oz)	801	49	1167	81	—
as prep	1/8 of 9 in pie (0.7 oz)	100	6	146	10	—
Betty Crocker						
Pie Crust	1/16 pkg	120	8	140	10	—
Sticks	1/16 pkg	120	8	140	10	—
Flako						
Mix	1/4 cup (0.9 oz)	130	8	170	13	1
Jiffy						
As prep	1/7 crust	180	10	250	19	tr
Pillsbury						
Mix	1/6 of 2 crust pie	270	17	420	25	—
Stick	1/6 of a 2 crust pie	270	17	420	25	—
READY-TO-EAT						
chocolate cookie crumb baked	9 in crust (7.7 oz)	1130	69	1502	122	—
chocolate cookie crumb baked	1/8 of 9 in pie (1 oz)	139	9	185	15	—

FOOD	PORTION	CAL.	FAT	SOD.	CARB.	FIB.
chocolate cookie crumb chilled	9 in crust (7.8 oz)	1127	69	1499	121	—
chocolate cookie crumb chilled	⅛ of 9 in pie (1 oz)	142	9	188	15	—
graham cracker baked	9 in crust (8.4 oz)	1181	60	1365	156	—
graham cracker baked	⅛ of 9 in pie (1 oz)	148	8	171	20	—
graham cracker chilled	9 in crust (8.6 oz)	1182	60	1365	155	—
graham cracker chilled	⅛ of 9 in pie (1 oz)	150	8	173	20	—
vanilla wafer cracker crumbs baked	⅛ of 9 in pie (0.8 oz)	119	8	116	11	—
vanilla wafer cracker crumbs baked	9 in crust (6.1 oz)	937	64	909	89	—
vanilla wafer cracker crumbs chilled	9 in crust (6.2 oz)	934	64	906	88	—
vanilla wafer cracker crumbs chilled	⅛ of 9 in pie (0.8 oz)	117	8	113	11	—
Generic Label						
Graham	⅛ pie (0.7 oz)	110	5	110	14	1
Honey Maid						
Graham	⅙ crust (1 oz)	140	7	125	18	tr
Nabisco						
Nilla	⅙ crust (1 oz)	140	8	65	18	0
Oreo						
Crumb Crust	⅙ crust (1 oz)	140	11	180	18	tr
Ready Crust						
Chocolate	⅛ pie 9 in	100	5	120	14	—
Chocolate	1 (3 in diam)	110	5	135	15	—
Graham	1 (3 in diam)	110	5	145	15	—
Graham	⅛ pie 9 in	100	5	130	13	—
REFRIGERATED						
Pillsbury						
All Ready	⅛ of 2 crust pie	240	15	200	24	—

PIEROGI

FOOD	PORTION	CAL.	FAT	SOD.	CARB.	FIB.
FROZEN						
Empire						
Potato Cheese	3 (4.6 oz)	260	6	200	40	5
Potato Onion	3 (4.6 oz)	250	5	210	43	4
Golden						
Potato Cheese	3 (4 oz)	250	8	260	38	—
Potato Onion	3 (4 oz)	210	6	220	36	—
Mrs. T's						
Potato And Cheddar Cheese	1 (1.3 oz)	60	tr	170	11	—

FOOD	PORTION	CAL.	FAT	SOD.	CARB.	FIB.
Mrs. T's (CONT.)						
Potato And Onion	1 (1.3 oz)	50	tr	140	10	—
Sauerkraut	1	60	0	—	—	—
TAKE-OUT						
pierogi	¾ cup (4.4 oz)	307	19	369	24	—
PIG'S EARS AND FEET						
ears frzn simmered	1 ear (3.7 oz)	183	12	183	0	—
feet pickled	1 oz	58	5	—	tr	—
feet pickled	1 lb	923	73	—	tr	—
feet simmered	2.5 oz	138	9	—	0	—
Hormel						
Pickled Feet	2 oz	80	6	530	0	0
Pickled Hocks	2 oz	110	8	530	0	0
PIGEON						
w/ skin & bone	3.5 oz	169	10	90	0	—
PIGEON PEAS						
dried cooked	½ cup	102	tr	5	20	—
dried cooked	1 cup	204	1	9	39	—
PIGNOLIA						
(*see* PINE NUTS)						
PIKE						
northern cooked	½ fillet (5.4 oz)	176	1	76	0	—
northern cooked	3 oz	96	1	42	0	—
northern raw	3 oz	75	1	33	0	—
roe raw	3½ oz	130	2	—	2	—
walleye baked	3 oz	101	1	56	0	—
walleye fillet baked	4.4 oz	147	2	81	0	—
PILLNUTS						
canarytree dried	1 oz	204	23	1	1	—
PIMIENTOS						
canned	1 slice	0	0	0	tr	—
canned	1 tbsp	3	tr	2	1	—
Dromedary						
Pimientos	1 oz	10	0	5	2	—
PINE NUTS						
pignolia dried	1 tbsp	51	5	0	1	—
pignolia dried	1 oz	146	14	1	4	—
pinyon dried	1 oz	161	17	20	5	—

FOOD	PORTION	CAL.	FAT	SOD.	CARB.	FIB.
Progresso						
Pignoli	1 jar (1 oz)	170	13	0	2	0
PINEAPPLE						
CANNED						
chunks in heavy syrup	1 cup	199	tr	3	52	—
chunks juice pack	1 cup	150	tr	4	39	—
crushed in heavy syrup	1 cup	199	tr	3	52	—
slices in heavy syrup	1 slice	45	tr	1	12	—
slices in light syrup	1 slice	30	tr	1	8	—
slices juice pack	1 slice	35	tr	1	9	—
slices water pack	1 slice	19	tr	1	5	—
tidbits in heavy syrup	1 cup	199	tr	3	52	—
tidbits in juice	1 cup	150	tr	4	19	—
tidbits in water	1 cup	79	tr	3	20	—
Del Monte						
Chunks In Heavy Syrup	½ cup (4.3 oz)	90	0	10	24	1
Chunks In Its Own Juice	½ cup (4.4 oz)	70	0	5	17	1
Crushed In Heavy Syrup	½ cup (4.4 oz)	90	0	10	24	1
Crushed In Its Own Juice	½ cup (4.3 oz)	70	0	10	17	1
Sliced In Heavy Syrup	½ cup (4.1 oz)	90	0	10	23	1
Sliced In Its Own Juice	½ cup (4 oz)	60	0	10	16	1
Snack Cups Tidbits In Juice	1 serv (4.5 oz)	70	0	10	18	1
Snack Cups Tidbits In Juice EZ-Open Lid	1 serv (4.2 oz)	60	0	10	17	1
Spears In Its Own Juice	½ cup (4.3 oz)	70	0	5	17	1
Tidbits In Its Own Juice	½ cup (4.3 oz)	70	0	5	17	1
Wedges In Its Own Juice	½ cup (4.3 oz)	70	0	5	17	1
Dole						
All Cuts Juice Pack	½ cup	70	tr	10	18	—
All Cuts Syrup Pack	½ cup	90	0	10	23	—
Empress						
Chunk	4 oz	70	0	—	18	—
Crushed	4 oz	70	0	—	18	—
Sliced	4 oz	70	0	—	18	—
Libby						
Crushed	1 cup with juice	140	0	10	35	—
Sliced In Unsweetened Juice	1 cup with juice	140	0	<10	35	—
S&W						
Hawaiian Slice In Heavy Syrup	½ cup	90	0	0	23	—
Hawaiian Slice Juice Pack	½ cup	70	0	10	17	—

FOOD	PORTION	CAL.	FAT	SOD.	CARB.	FIB.
S&W (CONT.)						
Sliced Unsweetened	½ cup	60	0	10	15	—
DRIED						
Sonoma						
Pieces	2 pieces (1.4 oz)	140	2	30	30	2
FRESH						
diced	1 cup	77	tr	1	19	2
slice	1 slice	42	tr	1	10	1
Chiquita						
Fresh	1 cup	90	1	—	—	—
Dole						
Pineapple	2 slices	90	1	10	21	2
FROZEN						
chunks sweetened	½ cup	104	tr	2	27	—
PINEAPPLE JUICE						
canned	1 cup	139	tr	2	34	—
frzn as prep	1 cup	129	tr	3	32	—
frzn not prep	6 oz	387	tr	6	96	—
After The Fall						
Mandarin Pineapple	1 can (12 oz)	150	0	25	37	0
Bright & Early						
Frozen	8 fl oz	120	0	10	30	—
Del Monte						
Juice	6 fl oz	80	0	5	20	0
Juice	1 serv (11.5 oz)	190	0	15	45	1
Juice	8 fl oz	110	0	10	26	0
Dole						
100% frzn as prep	8 fl oz	130	0	20	30	0
Chilled	6 fl oz	90	0	5	22	—
Minute Maid						
Box	8.45 fl oz	130	0	25	33	—
Frozen	8 fl oz	110	0	5	28	—
S&W						
Unsweetened	6 oz	100	0	0	25	—
Tree Top						
Juice	6 oz	100	0	0	24	—
Veryfine						
100%	8 oz	125	0	<10	31	—
PINK BEANS						
CANNED						
Goya						
Spanish Style	7.5 oz	140	tr	800	32	10

FOOD	PORTION	CAL.	FAT	SOD.	CARB.	FIB.
DRIED						
cooked	1 cup	252	1	3	47	—

PINTO BEANS

FOOD	PORTION	CAL.	FAT	SOD.	CARB.	FIB.
CANNED						
pinto	1 cup	186	1	998	35	—
Allen						
Pinto Beans	½ cup (4.5 oz)	110	1	290	20	7
Brown Beauty						
Pinto Beans	½ cup (4.5 oz)	110	1	290	20	7
East Texas Fair						
Pinto Beans	½ cup (4.5 oz)	110	1	290	20	7
Eden						
Organic	½ cup (4.4 oz)	90	1	15	17	6
Gebhardt						
Pinto Beans	4 oz	100	tr	600	19	5
Goya						
Spanish Style	7.5 oz	140	1	860	31	10
Green Giant						
Picante	½ cup	100	1	580	21	6
Pinto Beans	½ cup	90	1	280	20	5
Luck's						
Seasoned w/ Pork w/ Onions	7.5 oz	220	6	—	—	—
Old El Paso						
Pinto Beans	½ cup (4.6 oz)	110	1	420	19	7
Progresso						
Pinto Beans	½ cup (4.6 oz)	110	1	250	18	7
Trappey						
Jalapinto With Bacon	½ cup (4.5 oz)	120	1	540	22	8
With Bacon	½ cup (4.5 oz)	120	1	270	20	7
DRIED						
cooked	1 cup	235	1	3	44	—
Arrowhead						
Dried	¼ cup (1.5 oz)	150	1	0	27	8
Bean Cuisine						
Dried	½ cup	115	1	5	—	5
Hurst						
Pinto Beans	1.2 oz	120	1	5	22	10
With Spanish Seasoning	1.3 oz	120	1	350	22	6
FROZEN						
cooked	3 oz	152	tr	—	29	—
SPROUTS						
cooked	3½ oz	22	tr	—	4	—
raw	3½ oz	62	1	—	12	—

FOOD	PORTION	CAL.	FAT	SOD.	CARB.	FIB.
PINYON						
(*see* PINE NUTS)						
PISTACHIOS						
dried	1 cup	739	62	7	32	14
dried	1 oz	164	14	2	7	3
dry roasted	1 oz	172	15	2	8	—
dry roasted salted	1 cup	776	68	1040	35	—
dry roasted salted	1 oz	172	15	260	8	—
Dole						
Shelled	1 oz	163	14	—	7	—
Shells On	1 oz	90	7	250	3	—
Fisher						
Red Tint	1 oz	170	15	220	6	—
Lance						
Pistachios	1 pkg (32 g)	100	8	100	4	—
Planters						
Munch'N Go Singles Shelled Dry Roasted	1 pkg (2 oz)	330	29	450	14	6
Red Salted Dry Roasted	1 pkg	160	14	250	7	3
Uncolored Dry Roasted	½ cup	160	14	180	7	3
Sonoma						
Salted Shelled	¼ cup (1 oz)	190	14	220	9	3
PITANGA						
fresh	1 cup	57	1	5	13	—
fresh	1	2	tr	0	1	—
PIZZA						
DOUGH						
Boboli						
Shell + Sauce	⅛ lg shell (2.6 oz)	170	3	460	28	1
Shell + Sauce	⅙ sm shell (2.6 oz)	170	3	540	29	1
House of Pasta						
Frozen	⅛ of 14 in pie (1.9 oz)	140	1	140	27	1
Jiffy						
As prep	¼ crust	180	3	264	33	2
Sassafras						
Cornmeal Pizza Crust	1 slice (1.4 oz)	140	0	240	30	1
Italian Pizza Crust Mix	1 slice (1.4 oz)	140	0	135	30	1
Wanda's						
Crust Mix Oregano & Basil	1/10 pie (1.4 oz)	149	0	227	32	1
Crust Mix Oregano & Basil Whole Wheat	1/10 pie (1.4 oz)	141	1	227	30	5

FOOD	PORTION	CAL.	FAT	SOD.	CARB.	FIB.
Watkins						
Crust Mix	1/8 pkg (1.8 oz)	180	1	60	36	2
FROZEN						
Celeste						
Italian Bread Deluxe	1 (5.1 oz)	290	11	1000	36	3
Italian Bread Garlic & Herb Zesty Chicken	1 (5 oz)	260	8	960	34	3
Italian Bread Pepperoni	1 (5 oz)	320	13	1140	37	3
Italian Bread Zesty Four Cheese	1 (4.6 oz)	300	12	820	32	3
Large Cheese	1/4 pie (4.4 oz)	320	16	590	32	3
Large Deluxe	1/4 pie (5.5 oz)	350	18	880	35	4
Large Pepperoni	1/4 pie (4.7 oz)	350	20	990	33	3
Large Suprema With Meat	1/5 pie (4.6 oz)	290	16	770	27	3
Large Zesty Four Cheese	1/4 pie (4.4 oz)	330	16	610	34	3
Small Cheese	1 (7.5 oz)	540	25	1090	60	4
Small Deluxe	1 (8.2 oz)	540	29	1320	53	6
Small Hot & Zesty Four Cheese	1 (7 oz)	530	27	1090	50	4
Small Original Four Cheese	1 (7 oz)	540	30	1040	47	4
Small Pepperoni	1 (6.7 oz)	520	27	1280	53	4
Small Sausage	1 (7.5 oz)	530	27	1400	52	5
Small Suprema Vegetable	1 (7.5 oz)	480	23	1270	52	5
Small Suprema With Meat	1 (9 oz)	580	31	1480	56	7
Small Zesty Four Cheese	1 (7 oz)	530	27	1090	50	4
Croissant Pocket						
Stuffed Sandwich Pepperoni Pizza	1 piece (4.5 oz)	350	15	870	39	3
Di Giorno						
Rising Crust 12 inch Four Cheese	1/6 pie (4.9 oz)	320	11	870	39	3
Rising Crust 12 inch Italian Sausage	1/6 pie (5.3 oz)	360	14	1000	40	3
Rising Crust 12 inch Pepperoni	1/6 pie (5.2 oz)	370	16	1080	40	3
Rising Crust 12 inch Supreme	1/6 pie (5.8 oz)	380	17	1100	40	3
Rising Crust 12 inch Three Meat	1/6 pie (5.4 oz)	380	16	1100	40	3
Rising Crust 12 inch Vegetable	1/6 pie (5.6 oz)	310	10	830	41	3

FOOD	PORTION	CAL.	FAT	SOD.	CARB.	FIB.
Pappalo's (CONT.)						
French Bread Pepperoni	1 pizza	410	20	1130	41	—
French Bread Sausage	1 pizza	410	18	1000	41	—
Pan Combination	1/6 pizza	340	15	700	34	—
Pan Hamburger	1/6 pizza	310	12	580	34	—
Pan Pepperoni	1/6 pizza	330	14	710	34	—
Pan Sausage	1/6 pizza	360	18	550	34	—
Thin Crust Combination	1/6 pizza	260	10	590	29	—
Thin Crust Hamburger	1/6 pizza	240	8	470	28	—
Thin Crust Pepperoni	1/6 pizza	270	11	600	28	—
Thin Crust Sausage	1/6 pizza	250	9	490	28	—
Pepperidge Farm						
Croissant Pastry Cheese	1	430	23	640	41	—
Croissant Pastry Deluxe	1	440	23	790	43	—
Croissant Pastry Pepperoni	1	420	22	690	43	—
Pillsbury						
Microwave Cheese	1/2 pizza	240	10	540	28	—
Microwave Combination	1/2 pizza	310	15	780	29	—
Microwave French Bread	1 pizza	370	15	680	41	—
Microwave French Bread Pepperoni	1 pizza	430	19	940	46	—
Microwave French Bread Sausage	1 pizza	410	16	860	48	—
Microwave French Bread Sausage & Pepperoni	1 pizza	450	21	950	47	—
Microwave Pepperoni	1/2 pizza	300	15	790	29	—
Microwave Sausage	1/2 pizza	280	13	680	29	—
Small World						
Four Cheese	1 (4 oz)	240	6	350	38	1
Special Delivery						
Organic	1/3 pizza (5.3 oz)	320	9	500	46	1
Organic Soy Kaas	1/3 pizza (5.3 oz)	320	7	600	47	1
Stouffer's						
French Bread Bacon Cheddar	1 piece (5.8 oz)	440	22	940	44	4
French Bread Cheese	1 piece (5.2 oz)	350	14	660	42	3
French Bread Cheeseburger	1 piece (6 oz)	440	26	1110	31	5
French Bread Deluxe	1 piece (6.2 oz)	440	22	980	42	5
French Bread Double Cheese	1 piece (5.9 oz)	420	19	790	44	5
French Bread Garden Vegetable	1 piece (5.8 oz)	340	12	540	45	4

FOOD	PORTION	CAL.	FAT	SOD.	CARB.	FIB.
Stouffer's (CONT.)						
French Bread Pepperoni	1 piece (5.6 oz)	420	20	930	42	3
French Bread Pepperoni & Mushroom	1 piece (6.1 oz)	430	21	1000	43	3
French Bread Sausage	1 piece (6 oz)	420	20	900	41	4
French Bread Sausage & Pepperoni	1 piece (6.25 oz)	460	25	1130	45	4
French Bread Vegetable Deluxe	1 piece (6.4 oz)	380	17	830	43	5
French Bread White Pizza	1 piece (5.1 oz)	460	28	760	43	5
Tombstone						
Double Top Pepperoni	⅙ pie (4.5 oz)	340	19	810	24	2
Double Top Sausage	⅙ pie (4.6 oz)	320	17	760	25	2
Double Top Sausage & Pepperoni	⅙ pie (4.6 oz)	340	19	820	25	2
Double Top Supreme	⅙ pie (4.7 oz)	330	18	780	25	2
Double Top Two Cheese	⅙ pie (5.2 oz)	380	19	760	29	2
For One ½ Less Fat Cheese	1 pie (6.5 oz)	460	10	940	43	3
For One ½ Less Fat Vegetable	1 pie (7.2 oz)	360	9	860	48	5
For One Extra Cheese	1 pie (6.9 oz)	520	28	940	47	3
For One Pepperoni	1 pie (6.9 oz)	550	32	1160	41	3
For One Supreme	1 pie (7.5 oz)	550	32	1090	42	3
Light Supreme	⅕ pie (4.8 oz)	270	9	720	30	3
Light Vegetable	⅕ pie (4.6 oz)	240	7	500	31	3
Original 12 inch Canadian Bacon	¼ pie (5.5 oz)	350	14	890	36	3
Original 12 inch Deluxe	⅕ pie (4.8 oz)	310	14	690	29	3
Original 12 inch Extra Cheese	¼ pie (5.1 oz)	350	15	680	35	3
Original 12 inch Hamburger	⅕ pie (4.4 oz)	310	15	670	29	2
Original 12 inch Pepperoni	¼ pie (5.3 oz)	400	21	930	35	3
Original 12 inch Sausage	⅕ pie (4.4 oz)	300	14	680	29	2
Original 12 inch Sausage & Mushroom	⅕ pie (4.6 oz)	300	14	680	29	3
Original 12 inch Sausage & Pepperoni	⅕ pie (4.4 oz)	320	16	740	29	2
Original 12 inch Supreme	⅕ pie (5.1 oz)	320	16	730	29	2

FOOD	PORTION	CAL.	FAT	SOD.	CARB.	FIB.
Tombstone (CONT.)						
Original 9 inch Deluxe	⅓ pie (4.4 oz)	280	13	630	27	2
Original 9 inch Extra Cheese	½ pie (5.6 oz)	380	19	740	40	3
Original 9 inch Hamburger	⅓ pie (4 oz)	280	13	600	27	2
Original 9 inch Pepperoni	⅓ pie (4 oz)	300	15	680	27	2
Original 9 inch Pepperoni & Sausage	⅓ pie (4.1 oz)	300	15	710	27	2
Original 9 inch Sausage	⅓ pie (4 oz)	280	13	610	27	2
Original 9 inch Supreme	⅓ pie (4.4 oz)	310	16	720	27	2
Oven Rising Italian Sausage	⅙ pie (5.1 oz)	320	13	700	35	2
Oven Rising Pepperoni	⅙ pie (4.9 oz)	340	15	750	34	2
Oven Rising Supreme	⅙ pie (5.1 oz)	320	14	720	34	2
Oven Rising Three Cheese	⅙ pie (4.8 oz)	320	13	580	34	2
Oven Rising Three Meat	⅙ pie (5.1 oz)	340	15	750	34	2
Thin Crust Four Meat Combo	¼ pie (5 oz)	380	23	890	26	2
Thin Crust Italian Sausage	¼ pie (5 oz)	370	22	840	26	2
Thin Crust Pepperoni	¼ pie (4.8 oz)	400	25	920	25	2
Thin Crust Supreme	¼ pie (5 oz)	380	22	840	26	2
Thin Crust Supreme Taco	¼ pie (5.1 oz)	370	23	740	27	2
Thin Crust Three Cheese	¼ pie (4.7 oz)	360	21	690	25	2
Totino's						
Microwave Cheese	1 pizza	250	8	760	34	—
Microwave Pepperoni	1 pizza	280	12	880	34	—
Microwave Sausage	1 pizza	320	16	870	33	—
Microwave Sausage Pepperoni Combination	1 pizza	310	15	970	31	—
My Classic Deluxe Cheese	⅙ pizza	210	9	420	23	—
My Classic Deluxe Combination	⅙ pizza	270	14	630	23	—
My Classic Deluxe Pepperoni	⅙ pizza	260	13	630	23	—
Pan Pepperoni	⅙ pizza	330	14	730	34	—

FOOD	PORTION	CAL.	FAT	SOD.	CARB.	FIB.
Totino's (CONT.)						
Pan Sausage	⅙ pizza	320	13	630	34	—
Pan Sausage & Pepperoni Combination	⅙ pizza	340	15	720	34	—
Pan Three Cheese	⅙ pizza	290	10	510	33	—
Party Bacon	½ pizza	370	20	1030	35	—
Party Canadian Bacon	½ pizza	310	14	1150	35	—
Party Cheese	½ pizza	340	17	1000	34	—
Party Combination	½ pizza	380	21	1230	35	—
Party Hamburger	½ pizza	370	19	1060	35	—
Party Mexican Style	½ pizza	380	21	970	35	—
Party Pepperoni	½ pizza	370	20	1310	35	—
Party Sausage	½ pizza	390	21	1180	35	—
Party Vegetable	½ pizza	300	13	910	36	—
Slices Cheese	1	170	7	350	20	—
Slices Combination	1	200	10	630	20	—
Slices Pepperoni	1	190	9	530	20	—
Slices Sausage	1	200	10	540	20	—
Weight Watchers						
Smart Ones Deluxe Combo	1 (6.57 oz)	380	11	550	47	6
Smart Ones Pepperoni	1 (5.56 oz)	390	12	650	46	4
SAUCE						
Boboli						
Sauce	¼ cup (2.5 oz)	40	0	410	9	1
Sauce	1 pkg (1.2 oz)	20	0	200	4	1
Contadina						
Flavored With Pepperoni	¼ cup	40	2	420	6	1
Pizza Sauce	¼ cup	35	2	350	6	1
Squeeze	¼ cup	35	2	350	6	1
With Italian Cheeses	¼ cup	40	2	420	6	1
Eden						
Pizza Pasta Sauce	½ cup (4.4 oz)	80	3	320	12	3
Muir Glen						
Organic	¼ cup (2.2 oz)	40	1	230	6	2
Progresso						
Pizza Sauce	¼ cup (2.2 oz)	35	1	140	5	1
Ragu						
Quick Traditional	3 tbsp (1.7 oz)	35	2	330	3	—
Tree Of Life						
Sauce	¼ cup (1.9 oz)	30	1	120	5	—
TAKE-OUT						
cheese	⅛ of 12 in pie	140	3	336	21	—

FOOD	PORTION	CAL.	FAT	SOD.	CARB.	FIB.
cheese	12 in pie	1121	26	2680	164	—
cheese deep dish individual	1 (5.5 oz)	460	24	750	47	2
cheese meat & vegetables	12 in pie	1472	43	3054	170	—
cheese meat & vegetables	1/8 of 12 in pie	184	5	382	21	—
pepperoni	1/8 of 12 in pie	181	7	267	20	—
pepperoni	12 in pie	1445	56	2133	157	—
PLANTAINS						
fresh uncooked	1 (6.3 oz)	218	1	7	57	—
sliced cooked	1/2 cup	89	tr	4	24	—
Chifles						
Plantain Chips	1 pkg (2 oz)	170	11	14	17	2
TAKE-OUT						
ripe fried	2.8 oz	214	7	—	38	4
PLUMS						
CANNED						
purple in heavy syrup	3	119	tr	26	31	—
purple in heavy syrup	1 cup	320	tr	50	60	—
purple in light syrup	1 cup	158	tr	50	41	—
purple in light syrup	3	83	tr	26	22	—
purple juice pack	3	55	tr	1	14	—
purple juice pack	1 cup	146	tr	3	38	—
purple water pack	3	39	tr	1	10	—
purple water pack	1 cup	102	tr	2	27	—
S&W						
Halves Purple Fancy Unpeeled In Extra Heavy Syrup	1/2 cup	135	0	25	35	—
Whole Purple Fancy Unpeeled In Extra Heavy Syrup	1/2 cup	135	0	25	35	—
Whole Unpeeled Diet	1/2 cup	52	0	0	13	—
FRESH						
plum	1	36	tr	0	9	—
sliced	1 cup	91	1	1	21	—
Dole						
Plums	2	70	1	0	17	1
POI						
poi	1/2 cup	134	tr	14	33	—
POKEBERRY SHOOTS						
cooked	1/2 cup	16	tr	—	3	—
raw	1/2 cup	18	tr	—	3	—

FOOD	PORTION	CAL.	FAT	SOD.	CARB.	FIB.
Allen						
Pokeberry Shoots	½ cup (4.1 oz)	35	1	5	5	3
POLENTA						
(*see* CORNMEAL)						
POLLACK						
altantic fillet baked	5.3 oz	178	2	166	0	—
atlantic baked	3 oz	100	1	94	0	—
Mrs. Paul's						
Fillets Light frzn	1 fillet (4.5 oz)	240	11	530	18	—
POMEGRANATES						
pomegranate	1	104	tr	5	26	—
POMPANO						
florida cooked	3 oz	179	10	65	0	—
florida raw	3 oz	140	8	55	0	—
POPCORN						
(*see also* CHIPS, POPCORN CAKES, PRETZELS, SNACKS)						
air-popped	1 cup (0.3 oz)	31	tr	0	6	2
air-popped	1 oz	108	1	1	22	4
caramel coated	1 oz	122	4	58	22	1
caramel coated	1 cup (1.2 oz)	152	5	72	28	2
caramel coated w/ peanuts	⅔ cup (1 oz)	114	2	84	23	1
cheese	1 oz	149	9	252	15	3
cheese	1 cup (0.4 oz)	58	4	98	6	1
oil popped	1 oz	142	8	251	16	3
oil popped	1 cup (0.4 oz)	55	3	97	6	1
Barrel O' Fun						
Baked Curl	1 oz	150	9	260	17	0
Caramel Corn	1 oz	115	1	170	25	1
Corn Pop	1 oz	190	16	230	10	0
Popcorn	1 oz	160	12	240	13	1
White Cheddar Pops	1 oz	170	13	370	11	0
Cheetos						
Cheddar Cheese	0.5 oz	80	6	160	6	—
Chesters						
Microwave	3 cups	110	7	170	13	—
Microwave Butter	3 cups	120	7	180	13	—
Microwave Cheese	3 cups	110	8	230	11	—
Popcorn	0.5 oz	70	3	200	9	—
Cracker Jack						
Original	1 oz	120	3	85	22	—
Estee						
No Sugar Added Caramel	1 cup (1 oz)	120	2	90	26	1

FOOD	PORTION	CAL.	FAT	SOD.	CARB.	FIB.
Greenfield						
Caramel	1 cup (1 oz)	120	2	100	22	—
Herr's						
Regular	3 cups (1 oz)	140	11	250	11	3
Jiffy Pop						
Bag Butter	3 cups	90	5	140	11	2
Bag Lite	3 cups	70	3	110	11	2
Bag Regular	3 cups	100	6	140	11	2
Glazed Popcorn Clusters	1 oz	120	2	120	25	1
Microwave Butter	4 cup	140	7	270	17	3
Microwave Regular	4 cup	140	7	270	17	3
Pan Butter	4 cup	130	6	270	16	2
Pan Regular	4 cup	130	6	270	16	2
Lance						
Cheese	1 pkg (25 g)	130	8	280	13	—
Plain	1 pkg (25 g)	140	9	210	13	—
White Cheddar Cheese	1 pkg (25 g)	140	9	170	12	—
Louise's						
Fat-Free Apple Cinnamon	1 oz	100	0	80	24	1
Fat-Free Buttery Toffee	1 oz	100	0	80	24	1
Fat-Free Caramel	1 oz	100	0	80	24	1
Newman's Own						
Oldstyle Picture Show	3 ⅓ cups	80	1	0	16	—
Oldstyle Picture Show Microwave Natural Butter	3 cups	150	8	200	18	4
Oldstyle Picture Show Microwave No Salt	3 cups	150	8	0	18	4
Oldstyle Picture Show Microwave Light Butter	3 cups	90	3	100	18	4
Oldstyle Picture Show Microwave Light Natural	3 cups	90	3	100	18	4
Orville Redenbacher's						
Gourmet Hot Air	3 cups	40	tr	0	10	3
Gourmet Original	3 cups	80	4	0	10	3
Gourmet White	3 cups	80	4	0	10	3
Microwave Gourmet	3 cups	100	6	200	11	3
Microwave Gourmet Butter	3 cups	100	6	240	11	3
Microwave Gourmet Butter Toffee	2½ cups	210	12	85	26	2

FOOD	PORTION	CAL.	FAT	SOD.	CARB.	FIB.
Orville Redenbacher's (CONT.)						
Microwave Gourmet Caramel	2½ cups	240	14	90	29	2
Microwave Gourmet Cheddar Cheese	3 cups	130	8	280	14	3
Microwave Gourmet Frozen	3 cups	100	6	200	11	3
Microwave Gourmet Frozen Butter	3 cups	100	6	240	11	3
Microwave Gourmet Light	3 cups	70	3	115	8	3
Microwave Gourmet Light Butter	3 cups	70	3	110	8	3
Microwave Gourmet Salt Free	3 cups	100	6	0	11	3
Microwave Gourmet Salt Free Butter	3 cups	100	6	0	11	3
Microwave Gourmet Sour Cream 'n Onion	3 cups	160	12	270	12	3
Pillsbury						
Microwave Butter	3 cups	210	13	410	20	—
Microwave Original	3 cups	210	13	410	20	—
Microwave Salt Free	3 cups	170	7	0	23	—
Pop Secret						
Butter Flavor	3 cups	100	6	170	11	2
Butter Flavor Singles	6 cups	250	16	310	23	4
Light Butter Flavor	3 cups	70	3	115	12	2
Light Butter Flavor Singles	6 cups	140	6	190	23	4
Light Natural Flavor	3 cups	70	3	160	12	2
Light Natural Flavor Singles	6 cups	150	6	320	23	4
Natural Flavor	3 cups	100	6	170	11	2
Natural Flavor Salt Free	3 cups	100	6	<5	11	2
Pop Chips	1½ cups (1 oz)	130	4	400	23	1
Pop Qwiz Butter Flavor	3 cups	100	6	170	11	2
Pop Qwiz Natural Flavor	3 cups	100	6	170	11	2
Smartfood						
Cheddar Cheese	0.5 oz	80	5	130	7	—
Lowfat Toffee Crunch	¾ cup	110	2	200	24	1
Reduced Fat White Cheddar	¾ cup	130	6	260	17	3
Snyder's						
Butter	1 oz	140	9	140	13	3

FOOD	PORTION	CAL.	FAT	SOD.	CARB.	FIB.
Ultra Slim-Fast						
Lite N' Tasty	½ oz	60	2	150	10	2
Weight Watchers						
Butter	1 pkg (0.66 oz)	90	3	100	14	3
Butter Toffee	1 pkg (0.9 oz)	110	3	90	21	1
Butter Toffee	1 pkg (0.9 oz)	110	3	90	21	1
Caramel	1 pkg (0.9 oz)	100	1	45	22	1
Microwave	1 pkg (1 oz)	100	1	0	22	7
White Cheddar Cheese	1 pkg (0.66 oz)	90	4	125	12	2
Wise						
Tender Eating	0.5 oz	70	6	120	4	—
With Real Premium White Cheddar Cheese	0.5 oz	70	5	170	4	—
POPCORN CAKES						
popcorn cake	1 (0.3 oz)	38	tr	29	8	—
General Mills						
Popcorn Bars Caramel	1 (0.6 oz)	70	1	55	16	0
Lundberg						
Organic Lightly Salted	1	60	1	140	12	—
Organic Unsalted	1	60	1	3	12	—
Rye With Caraway Lightly Salted	1	59	0	5	14	—
Mother's						
Butter Flavor	1 (0.3 oz)	35	0	0	7	0
Unsalted	1 (0.3 oz)	35	0	0	7	0
Orville Redenbacher's						
Chocolate Peanut Crunch Mini	6 pieces (0.5 oz)	60	1	20	12	1
Peanut Caramel Crunch	6 (0.5 oz)	60	1	30	13	1
Quaker						
Blueberry Crunch	1 (0.5 oz)	50	0	0	11	—
Butter Mini	6 (0.5 oz)	50	1	140	11	2
Butter Popped	1 (0.3 oz)	35	0	45	7	—
Caramel	1 (0.5 oz)	50	0	30	12	—
Caramel Mini	5 (0.5 oz)	50	1	70	12	1
Cheddar Cheese Mini	6 (0.5 oz)	50	1	200	11	1
Lightly Salted Mini	7 (0.5 oz)	50	1	120	12	2
Monterey Jack	1 (0.4 oz)	40	0	80	8	—
Strawberry Crunch	1 (0.5 oz)	50	0	0	11	—
White Cheddar	1 (0.4 oz)	40	0	90	8	—
POPOVER						
home recipe as prep w/ 2% milk	1 (1.4 oz)	87	3	82	11	—

FOOD	PORTION	CAL.	FAT	SOD.	CARB.	FIB.
home recipe as prep w/ whole milk	1 (1.4 oz)	90	3	82	11	—
mix as prep	1 (1.2 oz)	67	2	143	10	—
POPPY SEEDS						
poppy seeds	1 tsp	15	1	1	1	—
PORK						
(*see also* BACON, BACON SUBSTITUTES, CANADIAN BACON, DELI MEATS/COLD CUTS, HAM, PORK DISHES, SAUSAGE)						
CANNED						
Hormel						
Pickled Tidbits	2 oz	100	8	530	0	0
FRESH						
blade chop roasted	1 (3.1 oz)	321	27	54	0	—
center loin chop broiled	1 (3.1 oz)	275	24	61	0	—
center loin roasted	3 oz	259	18	54	0	—
center loin chop lean & fat braised	1 chop (2.6 oz)	266	19	—	—	—
center loin chop lean & fat broiled	1 chop (3.1 oz)	275	19	—	—	—
center loin chop lean & fat panfried	1 chop (3.1 oz)	333	27	—	—	—
center loin chop lean & fat roasted	1 chop (3.1 oz)	268	19	—	—	—
center loin chop lean only braised	1 chop (2.1 oz)	166	8	—	—	—
center loin chop lean only broiled	1 chop (2.5 oz)	166	8	—	—	—
center loin chop lean only panfried	1 chop (2.4 oz)	178	11	—	—	—
center loin chop lean only roasted	1 chop (2.4 oz)	180	10	—	—	—
center loin lean & fat braised	3 oz	301	22	—	—	—
center loin lean & fat panfried	3 oz	318	26	—	—	—
center loin lean only broiled	3 oz	196	9	—	—	—
center loin lean only panfried	3 oz	226	14	—	—	—
center loin lean only roasted	3 oz	204	11	—	—	—
chop loin bone-in lean & fat roasted	3 oz	199	11	54	0	—
chop rib bone-in lean & fat roasted	3 oz	217	13	36	0	—

FOOD	PORTION	CAL.	FAT	SOD.	CARB.	FIB.
ham fresh rump half lean & fat roasted	3 oz	233	23	—	—	—
ham fresh rump half lean only roasted	3 oz	187	9	—	—	—
ham fresh shank half lean & fat roasted	3 oz	258	19	—	—	—
ham fresh shank half lean only roasted	3 oz	183	9	—	—	—
ham fresh whole lean & fat roasted	3 oz	250	18	—	—	—
ham fresh whole lean only roasted	3 oz	187	9	—	—	—
leg loin & shoulder lean only roasted	3 oz	198	11	—	—	—
loin blade chop lean & fat braised	1 chop (2.4 oz)	275	23	—	—	—
loin blade chop lean & fat braised	1 chop (3.1 oz)	321	27	—	—	—
loin blade chop lean & fat panfried	1 chop (3.1 oz)	368	33	—	—	—
loin blade chop lean only braised	1 chop (1.8 oz)	156	10	—	—	—
loin blade chop lean only broiled	1 chop (2.1 oz)	177	13	—	—	—
loin blade chop lean only panfried	1 chop (2.2 oz)	175	12	—	—	—
loin blade chop lean only roasted	1 chop (2.5 oz)	198	14	—	—	—
loin blade lean & fat braised	3 oz	348	29	—	—	—
loin blade lean & fat broiled	3 oz	334	29	—	—	—
loin blade lean & fat panfried	3 oz	352	31	—	—	—
loin blade lean & fat roasted	3 oz	310	26	—	—	—
loin blade lean only brolied	3 oz	255	18	—	—	—
loin blade lean only panfried	3 oz	240	17	—	—	—
loin blade lean only roasted	3 oz	238	16	—	—	—
loin chop lean & fat braised	1 chop (2.5 oz)	261	20	—	—	—
loin chop lean & fat roasted	1 chop (2.9 oz)	262	20	—	—	—
loin chop lean & fat braised	1 chop (2.3 oz)	267	20	—	—	—
loin chop lean & fat broiled	1 chop (2.7 oz)	295	23	—	—	—
loin chop lean & fat panfried	1 chop (2.9 oz)	337	29	—	—	—

FOOD	PORTION	CAL.	FAT	SOD.	CARB.	FIB.
loin chop lean & fat roasted	1 chop (2.8 oz)	274	21	—	—	—
loin chop lean only braised	1 chop (1.8 oz)	147	8	—	—	—
loin chop lean only broiled	1 chop (2.1 oz)	165	10	—	—	—
loin chop lean only panfried	1 chop (2 oz)	157	9	—	—	—
loin chop lean only roasted	1 chop (2.3 oz)	167	9	—	—	—
loin lean & fat braised	3 oz	312	24	—	—	—
loin lean & fat broiled	3 oz	294	23	—	—	—
loin lean only braised	3 oz	232	12	—	—	—
loin lean only broiled	3 oz	218	13	—	—	—
loin lean only roasted	3 oz	204	12	—	—	—
loin w/ fat roasted	3 oz	271	21	53	0	—
lungs braised	3 oz	84	3	—	—	—
pancreas braised	3 oz	186	9	—	—	—
rib chop lean only braised	1 chop (1.8 oz)	147	8	—	—	—
rib chop lean only panfried	1 chop (2 oz)	160	9	—	—	—
rib chop lean only roasted	1 chop (2.2 oz)	162	9	—	—	—
rib chop lean & fat braised	1 chop (2.2 oz)	246	18	—	—	—
rib chop lean & fat broiled	1 chop (2.6 oz)	264	20	—	—	—
rib chop lean & fat roasted	1 chop (2.6 oz)	252	19	—	—	—
shoulder arm picnic cured lean & fat roasted	3 oz	238	18	—	—	—
shoulder arm picnic cured lean only roasted	3 oz	145	6	1046	0	—
shoulder arm picnic lean only braised	3 oz	211	10	—	—	—
shoulder arm picnic lean only roasted	3 oz	194	11	—	—	—
shoulder arm picnic lean & fat braised	3 oz	293	22	—	—	—
shoulder arm picnic lean & fat roasted	3 oz	281	22	—	—	—
shoulder blade boston steak lean & fat braised	1 steak (5.6 oz)	594	46	—	—	—
shoulder blade boston steak lean & fat broiled	1 steak (6.5 oz)	647	53	—	—	—
shoulder blade boston steak lean & fat roasted	1 steak (6.5 oz)	594	47	—	—	—
shoulder blade boston steak lean only braised	1 steak (4.6 oz)	382	23	—	—	—
shoulder blade boston steak lean only broiled	1 steak (5.3 oz)	413	28	—	—	—
shoulder blade boston steak lean only roasted	1 steak (5.5 oz)	404	27	—	—	—

FOOD	PORTION	CAL.	FAT	SOD.	CARB.	FIB.
shoulder blade roll cured lean & fat	3 oz	304	25	1412	0	—
shoulder boston blade lean & fat braised	3 oz	316	24	—	—	—
shoulder boston blade lean & fat broiled	3 oz	297	24	—	—	—
shoulder boston blade lean & fat roasted	3 oz	273	21	—	—	—
shoulder boston blade lean only braised	3 oz	250	15	—	—	—
shoulder boston blade lean only broiled	3 oz	233	16	—	—	—
shoulder boston blade lean only roasted	3 oz	218	14	—	—	—
shoulder whole lean only roated	3 oz	207	13	—	—	—
shoulder whole roasted	3 oz	277	22	58	0	—
sirloin chop lean & fat braised	1 chop (2.4 oz)	250	18	—	—	—
sirloin chop lean & fat broiled	1 chop (2.8 oz)	278	21	—	—	—
sirloin chop lean & fat roasted	1 chop (2.8 oz)	244	17	—	—	—
sirloin chop lean only braised	1 chop (1.9 oz)	149	7	—	—	—
sirloin chop lean only broiled	1 chop (2.3 oz)	165	9	—	—	—
sirloin chop lean only roasted	1 chop (2.5 oz)	175	10	—	—	—
spareribs braised	3 oz	338	26	79	0	—
spleen braised	3 oz	127	3	—	0	—
tail simmered	3 oz	336	30	—	—	—
tenderloin lean only roasted	3 oz	141	4	57	0	—
Oscar Mayer						
Sweet Morsel Smoked Boneless Pork Shoulder	3 oz	180	15	990	0	0
PORK DISHES						
Jimmy Dean						
BBQ Pork Rib Sandwich	1 (5.4 oz)	440	23	970	36	1
TAKE-OUT						
pork roast	2 oz	70	3	390	0	—
tourtiere	1 piece (4.9 oz)	451	34	—	21	—

FOOD	PORTION	CAL.	FAT	SOD.	CARB.	FIB.
POSOLE						
(*see* HOMINY)						
POT PIE						
Award Brand						
Beef	1 (7 oz)	350	18	1130	37	3
Chicken	1 (7 oz)	350	19	1140	39	3
Banquet						
Family Entree Chicken Pie	1 serv (8 oz)	450	30	1010	39	6
Macaroni & Cheese	1 pkg (6.5 oz)	200	3	600	35	2
Vegetable & Cheese	1 (7 oz)	390	18	1000	49	3
Vegetable Pie w/ Beef	1 (7 oz)	330	15	1000	38	3
Vegetable Pie w/ Chicken	1 (7 oz)	350	18	950	36	3
Vegetable Pie w/ Turkey	1 (7 oz)	370	20	850	38	3
Empire						
Chicken	1 (8.1 oz)	440	21	960	41	11
Turkey	1 (8.1 oz)	470	23	820	46	11
Great Value						
Beef	1 (7 oz)	390	19	940	38	3
Chicken	1 (7 oz)	380	20	900	39	2
Turkey	1 (7 oz)	400	22	910	42	3
Morton						
Beef	1 (7 oz)	310	17	1380	34	2
Chicken	1 (7 oz)	320	18	1020	32	3
Macaroni & Cheese	1 (6 oz)	160	3	640	30	3
Turkey	1 (7 oz)	300	18	1060	29	2
Ozark Valley						
Chicken	1 (7 oz)	330	19	1010	32	2
Macaroni & Cheese	1 (6.5 oz)	160	3	780	29	0
Turkey	1 (7 oz)	280	16	1030	29	2
Stouffer's						
Beef Pie	1 pkg (10 oz)	450	26	1140	36	3
Chicken Pie	1 pkg (10 oz)	520	33	1000	37	3
Turkey	1 pkg (10 oz)	530	33	1040	36	3
Turkey	1 cup (8 oz)	500	31	910	36	3
Swanson						
Beef	7 oz	370	19	730	36	—
Beef Hungry Man	16 oz	610	31	1360	58	—
Chicken	7 oz	380	22	760	35	—
Chicken Homestyle	8 oz	410	21	1030	41	—
Hungry Man Chicken	16 oz	630	35	1600	57	—
Hungry Man Turkey	16 oz	650	36	1470	57	—
Turkey	7 oz	380	21	720	36	—

FOOD	PORTION	CAL.	FAT	SOD.	CARB.	FIB.
TAKE-OUT						
beef	⅓ of 9 in pie (7.4 oz)	515	30	596	39	—
chicken	⅓ of 9 in pie (8.1 oz)	545	31	594	42	—

POTATO

(*see also* CHIPS, KNISH, PANCAKES)

(FAST FACT: One quarter of all the fruits and vegetables eaten are potatoes, fresh and frozen. Along with ketchup, they make up one third of all vegetables eaten.)

FOOD	PORTION	CAL.	FAT	SOD.	CARB.	FIB.
CANNED						
potatoes	½ cup	54	tr	—	12	—
Allen						
Refried Potatoes	½ cup (4.5 oz)	150	3	360	24	11
Butterfield						
Diced	⅔ cup (5.7 oz)	100	0	350	22	3
Sliced	½ cup (5.7 oz)	100	0	390	22	4
Whole	2½ pieces (5.6 oz)	90	0	330	20	2
Del Monte						
New Sliced	⅔ cup (5.4 oz)	60	0	360	13	2
New Whole	⅔ cup (5.5 oz)	60	0	360	13	2
Hormel						
Au Gratin & Bacon	1 can (7.5 oz)	250	14	840	23	2
Scalloped & Ham	1 can (7.5 oz)	260	16	920	20	1
S&W						
New Potatoes Extra Small	½ cup	45	0	310	9	—
Seneca						
Potatoes	½ cup	80	0	264	15	2
Sunshine						
Whole	2½ pieces (5.6 oz)	90	0	330	20	2
FRESH						
baked skin only	1 skin (2 oz)	115	tr	12	27	2
baked w/ skin	1 (6.5 oz)	220	tr	16	51	—
baked w/o skin	1 (5 oz)	145	tr	8	34	2
baked w/o skin	½ cup	57	tr	3	13	1
boiled	½ cup	68	tr	3	16	1
microwaved	1 (7 oz)	212	tr	16	49	—
microwaved w/o skin	½ cup	78	tr	5	18	—
raw w/o skin	1 (3.9 oz)	88	tr	7	20	—
Yukon Gold						
Fresh	1 (5.3 oz)	110	0	—	—	—
FROZEN						
french fries	10 strips	111	4	15	17	2

FOOD	PORTION	CAL.	FAT	SOD.	CARB.	FIB.
french fries thick cut	10 strips	109	4	23	17	—
hashed brown	½ cup	170	9	27	22	—
potato puffs	½ cup	138	7	462	19	—
potato puffs as prep	1	16	1	52	2	—
Budget Gourmet						
Baked With Broccoli And Cheese	1 pkg (10.5 oz)	300	10	740	40	—
Cheddared Potatoes	1 pkg (5.5 oz)	260	16	600	22	—
Cheddared Potatoes With Broccoli	1 pkg (5 oz)	150	7	410	14	—
Three Cheese Potatoes	1 pkg (5.75 oz)	220	11	470	23	—
Empire						
Crinkle Cut French Fries	½ cup (3 oz)	90	2	20	18	7
Latkes Potato Pancakes	1 (2 oz)	80	2	200	15	8
Latkes Mini Potato Pancakes	2 (2 oz)	90	3	160	16	6
Golden						
Potato Pancakes	1 (1.33 oz)	71	3	187	10	—
Green Giant						
One Serve Au Gratin	1 pkg	200	10	560	20	—
One Serve Potatoes & Broccoli In Cheese Sauce	1 pkg	130	5	720	19	—
Healthy Choice						
Cheddar Broccoli Potatoes	1 meal (10.5 oz)	310	5	550	53	8
Garden Potato Casserole	1 meal (9.25 oz)	200	4	520	30	6
Kineret						
Crinkle Cut	18 pieces (3 oz)	120	4	260	20	2
Kugel	1 piece (2.5 oz)	150	10	160	13	1
Latkes	1 (1.5 oz)	90	5	150	9	2
Latkes Mini	10 (3 oz)	160	9	240	18	2
Lean Cuisine						
Deluxe Cheddar	1 pkg (10.4 oz)	270	7	590	40	6
Roasted Potatoes w/ Broccoli & Cheddar Cheese Sauce	1 pkg (10.25 oz)	260	6	590	39	7
MicroMagic						
French Fries Low Fat	1 pkg (3 oz)	130	3	35	23	3
Skinny Fries	1 pkg (3 oz)	350	15	40	49	—
Oh Boy!						
Stuffed With Cheddar Cheese	1 (6 oz)	130	4	310	20	4
Stuffed With Real Bacon	1 (6 oz)	120	3	300	20	4

FOOD	PORTION	CAL.	FAT	SOD.	CARB.	FIB.
Ore Ida						
Cheddar Browns	1 patty (3 oz)	90	3	350	14	1
Cottage Fries	14 pieces (3 oz)	130	4	20	21	1
Crispers!	17 pieces (3 oz)	220	13	510	24	2
Crispers! Nacho	10 pieces (3 oz)	170	9	360	21	2
Crispers! Texas	3 oz	170	10	270	19	2
Crispy Crowns!	12 pieces (3 oz)	100	11	450	21	2
Crispy Crunchies	12 pieces (3 oz)	160	9	370	18	2
Deep Fries Crinkle Cuts	18 pieces (3 oz)	160	7	15	23	2
Deep Fries French Fries	22 pieces (3 oz)	160	7	20	22	2
Dinner Fries Country Style	8 pieces (3 oz)	110	3	20	19	1
Fast Fries	23 pieces (3 oz)	140	6	230	20	2
Fast Fries Ranch	22 pieces (3 oz)	150	7	430	21	1
Golden Crinkles	16 pieces (3 oz)	120	4	25	20	2
Golden Fries	16 pieces (3 oz)	120	4	25	20	1
Golden Patties	1 (2.5 oz)	140	7	280	16	1
Golden Twirls	28 pieces (3 oz)	160	7	25	22	2
Hash Browns Country Style	1 cup (2.6 oz)	60	0	10	13	1
Hash Browns Shredded	1 patty (3 oz)	70	0	25	15	1
Hash Browns Southern Style	¾ cup (3 oz)	70	0	25	17	2
Hot Tots	9 pieces (3 oz)	150	6	380	21	2
Mashed Natural Butter	½ cup (2.1 oz)	80	2	140	14	tr
Microwave Crinkle Cuts	1 pkg (3.5 oz)	180	8	10	26	2
Microwave Hash Browns	1 patty (2 oz)	110	6	150	13	tr
Microwave Tater Tots	1 pkg (3.75 oz)	190	10	420	26	2
O'Brien Potatoes	¾ cup (3 oz)	60	0	15	13	2
Pixie Crinkles	33 pieces (3 oz)	140	5	25	21	3
Shoestrings	38 pieces (3 oz)	150	5	20	22	2
Snackin' Fries	1 pkg (5 oz)	180	20	590	36	3
Snackin' Fries Extra Zesty	1 pkg (5 oz)	180	20	510	35	4
Tater ABC's	10 pieces (3 oz)	190	11	310	20	2
Tater Tots	9 pieces (3 oz)	160	8	340	21	2
Tater Tots Bacon	9 pieces (3 oz)	150	7	490	20	1
Tater Tots Onion	9 pieces (3 oz)	150	7	370	20	2
Toaster Hash Browns	2 patties (3.5 oz)	190	12	550	21	1
Topped Broccoli & Cheese	½ (6 oz)	150	4	410	24	4
Topped Salsa & Cheese	½ (5.5 oz)	160	5	430	25	3
Topped Vegetable Primavera	1 (6.13 oz)	160	5	390	23	—

FOOD	PORTION	CAL.	FAT	SOD.	CARB.	FIB.
Ore Ida (CONT.)						
Twice Baked Butter	1 (5 oz)	200	9	350	27	4
Twice Baked Cheddar Cheese	1 (5 oz)	190	8	460	27	3
Twice Baked Ranch	1 (5 oz)	180	6	400	27	3
Twice Bakes Sour Cream & Chives	1 (5 oz)	180	6	370	28	3
Waffle Fries	15 pieces (3 oz)	140	5	35	22	2
Wedges With Skin	9 pieces (3 oz)	110	3	15	19	2
Zesties!	12 pieces (3 oz)	160	9	370	21	1
Stouffer's						
Au Gratin	½ cup (2.25 oz)	130	6	590	15	1
Baked Cheddar Cheese & Bacon	1 pkg (9.4 oz)	380	22	900	31	5
Scalloped	½ cup (2.25 oz)	130	6	450	17	2
Weight Watchers						
Smart Ones Baked Broccoli & Cheese	1 pkg (10 oz)	250	7	590	35	6
HOME RECIPE						
au gratin	½ cup	160	9	528	14	—
mashed w/ whole milk & margarine	⅓ cup	66	tr	182	13	—
scalloped	½ cup	105	5	409	13	—
MIX						
au gratin as prep	4½ oz	127	6	601	18	—
instant mashed flakes as prep w/ whole milk & butter	½ cup	118	6	349	16	—
instant mashed flakes not prep	½ cup	78	tr	24	18	—
instant mashed granules as prep w/ whole milk & butter	½ cup	114	5	270	15	—
instant mashed granules not prep	½ cup	372	1	67	86	—
scalloped as prep	4½ oz	127	6	467	18	—
Betty Crocker						
Au Gratin as prep	½ cup	110	3	610	22	1
Cheddar & Bacon as prep	½ cup	120	3	630	21	1
Cheddar & Sour Cream as prep	½ cup	130	3	580	25	1
Chicken & Vegetable as prep	⅔ cup	130	3	520	24	1

FOOD	PORTION	CAL.	FAT	SOD.	CARB.	FIB.
Betty Crocker (CONT.)						
Chicken & Vegetable as prep	⅔ cup	140	4	540	24	1
Creamy Garlic as prep	⅔ cup	150	5	490	24	1
Hash Browns as prep	½ cup	200	8	590	31	2
Homestyle Broccoli Au Gratin as prep	½ cup	110	3	510	21	2
Homestyle Broccoli Au Gratin Stove Top Recipe as prep	½ cup	130	4	560	21	2
Homestyle Cheddar Cheese Stove Top Recipe as prep	½ cup	140	5	680	21	1
Homestyle Cheddar Cheese as prep	½ cup	120	3	600	21	1
Homestyle Cheesy Scalloped Stove Top Recipe as prep	½ cup	130	5	590	20	1
Homestyle Cheesy Scalloped as prep	½ cup	120	3	520	20	1
Julienne as prep	½ cup	110	3	600	20	1
Mashed Butter & Herb Reduced Fat Recipe as prep	½ cup	130	5	480	20	1
Mashed Butter & Herb as prep	½ cup	160	8	510	20	1
Mashed Potato Buds Reduced Fat Recipe as prep	⅔ cup	120	4	420	19	1
Mashed Potato Buds Sour Cream 'N Chive as prep	⅔ cup	190	11	560	23	1
Mashed Potato Buds Sour Cream 'N Chive Reduced Fat as prep	⅔ cup	160	7	520	23	1
Mashed Potato Buds as prep	⅔ cup	160	8	460	19	1
Mashed Roasted Garlic Reduced Fat Recipe as prep	½ cup	130	5	380	19	1
Mashed Roasted Garlic as prep	½ cup	160	8	410	19	1
Mashed Sour Cream & Chives Reduced Fat Recipe as prep	½ cup	130	4	440	21	1

FOOD	PORTION	CAL.	FAT	SOD.	CARB.	FIB.
Betty Crocker (CONT.)						
Mashed Sour Cream & Chives as prep	½ cup	160	7	470	21	1
Potato Shakers Original Low Fat Recipe as prep	⅔ cup	120	2	560	23	2
Potato Shakers Original as prep	⅔ cup	140	4	560	23	2
Potato Shakers Parmesan & Herb Low Fat Recipe as prep	⅔ cup	120	2	490	23	2
Potato Shakers Parmesan & Herb as prep	⅔ cup	140	4	490	23	2
Potato Shakers Zesty Cheddar Low Fat Recipe as prep	⅔ cup	120	2	490	22	2
Potato Shakers Zesty Cheddar as prep	⅔ cup	140	5	490	22	2
Ranch as prep	½ cup	130	2	600	25	1
Scalloped Potatoes & Ham as prep	½ cup	120	3	540	21	1
Scalloped as prep	½ cup	130	3	600	23	1
Smokey Cheddar as prep	½ cup	120	3	570	22	1
Sour Cream 'n Chive as prep	½ cup	120	3	530	22	1
Three Cheese as prep	½ cup	120	3	580	23	1
Twice Baked Cheddar & Bacon Low Fat Recipe as prep	⅔ cup	130	3	540	22	1
Twice Baked Cheddar & Bacon as prep	⅔ cup	210	11	610	22	1
White Cheddar as prep	½ cup	120	3	540	22	1
Country Store						
Mashed not prep	⅓ cup	70	0	10	15	—
French's						
Cheddar & Bacon Casserole	½ cup	130	5	390	18	—
Creamy Italian Scalloped	½ cup	120	3	430	19	—
Creamy Stroganoff	½ cup	130	4	520	20	—
Crispy Top Scalloped With Savory Onion	½ cup	140	5	390	20	—
Real Cheese Scalloped	½ cup	140	5	380	19	—

FOOD	PORTION	CAL.	FAT	SOD.	CARB.	FIB.
French's (CONT.)						
Real Sour Cream & Chives	½ cup	150	7	550	19	—
Spuds Mashed	½ cup	140	7	380	17	—
Tangy Au Gratin	½ cup	130	5	460	20	—
Hungry Jack						
Mashed Flakes	½ cup	40	7	380	17	—
Shake 'N Bake						
Perfect Potatoes Crispy Cheddar	⅙ pkg (7 g)	30	2	380	2	0
Perfect Potatoes Herb & Garlic	⅙ pkg (7 g)	20	0	380	5	0
Perfect Potatoes Home Fries	⅙ pkg (7 g)	20	0	410	5	0
Perfect Potatoes Parmesan Peppercorn	⅙ pkg (7 g)	25	1	300	3	0
Perfect Potatoes Savory Onion	⅙ pkg (7 g)	20	0	280	5	0
REFRIGERATED						
Simply Potatoes						
Au Gratin	¼ pkg (3 oz)	130	8	370	13	—
Hash Browns	⅕ pkg (4 oz)	100	tr	410	23	—
Hash Browns Onion	⅕ pkg (4 oz)	120	tr	380	26	—
Hash Browns Southwest Style	⅕ pkg (4 oz)	100	tr	410	23	—
Mashed	⅕ pkg (4 oz)	90	2	150	15	—
Scalloped	¼ pkg (3 oz)	100	5	390	11	—
SHELF-STABLE						
Lunch Bucket						
Scalloped	1 pkg (7.5 oz)	160	7	770	20	—
Micro Cup Meals						
Scalloped Potatoes & Ham	1 cup (10.4 oz)	360	23	1280	28	3
Scalloped Potatoes With Ham	1 cup (7.5 oz)	260	16	920	20	2
Pantry Express						
Augratin	½ cup	120	5	430	17	2
TAKE-OUT						
au gratin w/ cheese	½ cup	178	10	548	17	—
baked topped w/ cheese sauce	1	475	29	381	47	—
baked topped w/ cheese sauce & bacon	1	451	26	973	44	—
baked topped w/ cheese sauce & broccoli	1	402	14	484	47	—

FOOD	PORTION	CAL.	FAT	SOD.	CARB.	FIB.
baked topped w/ cheese sauce & chili	1	481	22	701	56	—
baked topped w/ sour cream & chives	1	394	22	182	50	—
curry	1 serv (6 oz)	292	16	—	36	4
french fried in beef tallow	1 reg	237	12	124	29	—
french fried in beef tallow	1 lg	358	19	187	44	—
french fried in vegetable oil	1 reg	235	12	124	29	—
french fried in vegetable oil	1 lg	355	19	187	44	—
hash brown	½ cup	163	11	19	17	2
indian yogurt potatoes	1 serv	315	9	216	52	0
mashed	½ cup	111	4	309	18	—
mustard potato salad	3.5 oz	120	6	393	16	—
o'brien	1 cup	157	3	421	30	—
potato dumpling	3½ oz	334	1	1	74	3
potato pancakes	1 (1.3 oz)	101	7	188	11	—
potato salad	½ cup	179	10	661	14	—
potato salad	⅓ cup	108	6	312	13	—
potato salad w/ vegetables	3.5 oz	120	3	390	20	—
scalloped	½ cup	127	5	435	18	—
POTATO STARCH						
potato starch	3½ oz	335	tr	8	83	—
Manischewitz						
Potato Starch	1 cup	570	0	1	137	—
POUT						
ocean baked	3 oz	86	1	66	0	—
ocean fillet baked	4.8 oz	139	2	107	0	—
PRESERVE						
(*see* JAM/JELLY/PRESERVE)						
PRETZELS						
(*see also* CHIPS, POPCORN, SNACKS)						
chocolate covered	1 oz	130	5	—	20	—
chocolate covered	1 (0.4 oz)	50	2	—	8	—
dutch twist	4 (2.1 oz)	229	2	1029	48	2
pretzels	1 oz	108	1	486	23	1
rods	4 (2 oz)	229	2	1029	48	2
sticks	10	10	tr	48	2	—
sticks	120 (2 oz)	229	2	1029	48	2
twist	1 (½ oz)	65	1	258	13	—
twists	10 (2.1 oz)	229	2	1029	48	2
whole wheat	2 med (2 oz)	205	2	115	46	—
whole wheat	2 sm (1 oz)	103	1	58	23	—

FOOD	PORTION	CAL.	FAT	SOD.	CARB.	FIB.
Barrel O' Fun						
Mini	1 oz	110	1	100	23	1
Sticks	1 oz	110	1	100	23	1
Twists	1 oz	110	1	100	23	1
Estee						
Dutch Unsalted	2 (1.1 oz)	130	1	40	26	1
Nuggets Ranch Reduced Sodium	23 (1 oz)	130	2	240	24	tr
Nuggets Reduced Sodium	30 (1 oz)	120	2	180	24	1
Unsalted	23 (1 oz)	120	1	30	25	1
Formagg						
Pretzel Nuts	1 oz	120	4	390	21	tr
Herr's						
Hard Sourdough	1 (1 oz)	100	0	450	23	2
J&J						
Soft	1 (2.25 oz)	170	0	140	37	—
Soft Bites	5 bites	110	0	95	23	—
Lance						
Twist	1 pkg (42 g)	150	1	700	30	—
Manischewitz						
Bagel Pretzels Original	4 (1 oz)	110	0	260	22	1
Mister Salty						
Chips	16 (1 oz)	110	3	620	21	tr
Dutch	2 (1.1 oz)	120	1	580	25	1
Fat Free Chips	16 (1 oz)	100	0	620	22	1
Mini	22 (1 oz)	110	1	440	22	1
Sticks Fat Free	47 (1 oz)	110	0	370	23	1
Twist Fat Free	9 (1 oz)	110	0	380	23	1
Mr. Phipps						
Chips Lower Sodium	16 (1 oz)	120	3	410	21	tr
Chips Original	16 (1 oz)	120	3	630	21	tr
Chips Original Fat Free	16 (1 oz)	100	0	630	22	tr
Newman's Own						
Salted Rounds Organic	1 pkg (1.4 oz)	150	2	530	31	1
Planters						
Twists	1 pkg (1.5 oz)	160	1	640	35	1
Twists	1 oz	100	1	420	23	1
Quinlan						
Beers	1 oz	110	2	550	22	1
Hard Sourdough	1 oz	110	2	550	22	1
Logs	1 oz	110	2	550	22	1
Nuggets	1 oz	110	2	550	22	1
Rods	1 oz	110	2	550	22	1

FOOD	PORTION	CAL.	FAT	SOD.	CARB.	FIB.
Quinlan (CONT.)						
Sticks	1 oz	110	2	550	22	1
Thins	1 oz	110	2	550	22	1
Rold Gold						
Bavarian	3 pieces (1 oz)	120	2	430	22	—
Fat Free Hard Sour Dough	1	80	0	270	19	1
Fat Free Thins	12 pieces (1 oz)	110	0	460	23	1
Fat Free Tiny Twists	18 pieces (1 oz)	110	0	430	23	1
Pretzel Chips	1 oz	110	1	310	22	—
Pretzel Chips Cheese	1 oz	120	3	240	22	—
Rods	3 pieces (1 oz)	110	2	410	23	—
Snack Mix	½ cup (1 oz)	140	6	330	18	—
Sticks	50 pieces (1 oz)	110	2	490	23	—
Seyfart's						
Butter Rods	1 oz	110	1	530	21	—
Snyder's						
Logs	1 oz	310	0	360	22	—
Minis	1 oz	310	0	460	22	—
Minis Unsalted	1 oz	310	0	70	22	—
Nibblers	1 oz	310	0	460	22	—
Oat Bran	1 oz	120	1	300	14	—
Old Fashioned Hard	1 oz	111	0	655	23	—
Old Fashioned Hard Unsalted	1 oz	100	0	89	23	—
Old Tyme	1 oz	310	0	310	22	—
Old Tyme Unsalted	1 oz	110	0	70	22	—
Rods	1 oz	310	0	320	22	—
Sourdough Hard Buttermilk Ranch	1 oz	130	5	250	19	0
Sourdough Hard Cheddar Cheese	1 oz	160	7	320	13	0
Sourdough Hard Honey Mustard & Onion	1 oz	130	5	250	19	0
Stix	1 oz	310	0	900	22	—
Very Thins	1 oz	310	0	720	22	—
Sunshine						
California Pretzels	1 oz	110	2	350	22	1
Ultra Slim-Fast						
Lite N' Tasty	1 oz	100	tr	460	21	[illegible]
Wege						
Sourdough	1 oz	102	tr	548	23	—
Unsalted	1 oz	102	tr	60	23	—
Whole Wheat	1 oz	109	1	25	21	—

FOOD	PORTION	CAL.	FAT	SOD.	CARB.	FIB.
Weight Watchers						
Oat Bran Nuggets	1 pkg (1.5 oz)	170	3	250	33	3
PRICKLYPEAR						
fresh	1	42	1	6	10	—
PRUNE JUICE						
canned	1 cup	181	tr	11	45	3
Del Monte						
Juice	8 fl oz	170	0	20	43	1
S&W						
Unsweetened	6 oz	120	0	20	31	—
PRUNES						
CANNED						
in heavy syrup	5	90	tr	2	24	—
in heavy syrup	1 cup	245	tr	6	65	—
DRIED						
cooked w/ sugar	½ cup	147	tr	2	39	7
cooked w/o sugar	½ cup	113	tr	2	30	6
dried	10	201	tr	3	53	6
dried	1 cup	385	1	6	101	12
Del Monte						
Pitted	¼ cup (1.4 oz)	120	0	5	29	3
Unpitted	⅓ cup (1.4 oz)	110	0	5	12	1
Mariani						
Pitted	¼ cup	140	1	—	—	—
Whole	¼ cup	140	1	—	—	—
Sonoma						
Pitted	¼ cup (1.4 oz)	120	0	5	29	3
Sunsweet						
Orange Essence Pitted Prunes	6 (1.4 oz)	100	0	5	26	3
PUDDING						
(*see also* CUSTARD, PUDDING POPS)						
HOME RECIPE						
bread pudding	1 recipe 6 serv (26.4 oz)	1266	44	1741	185	—
chocolate as prep w/ whole milk	½ cup (5.5 oz)	221	6	137	40	—
corn	⅔ cup	181	9	92	21	—
cornstarch	½ cup (4.4 oz)	137	5	—	20	—
rice	½ cup (5.3 oz)	217	4	85	40	—
yorkshire as prep w/ skim milk	3.5 oz	93	4	—	12	1

FOOD	PORTION	CAL.	FAT	SOD.	CARB.	FIB.
yorkshire as prep w/ whole milk	3.5 oz	104	5	—	12	1
MIX						
banana as prep w/ 2% milk	½ cup (4.9 oz)	142	2	232	26	—
banana as prep w/ whole milk	½ cup (4.9 oz)	157	4	231	25	—
chocolate as prep w/ 2% milk	½ cup (5 oz)	150	3	148	28	—
chocolate as prep w/ whole milk	½ cup (5 oz)	158	5	147	26	—
coconut cream as prep w/ 2% milk	½ cup (4.9 oz)	148	4	226	25	—
coconut cream as prep w/ whole milk	½ cup (4.9 oz)	160	4	227	25	—
instant banana as prep w/ 2% milk	½ cup (5.2 oz)	152	3	435	29	—
instant banana as prep w/ whole milk	½ cup (5.2 oz)	167	4	434	27	—
instant chocolate as prep w/ whole milk	½ cup (5.2 oz)	164	5	417	28	—
instant coconut cream as prep w/ 2% milk	½ cup (5.2 oz)	157	3	362	28	—
instant coconut cream as prep w/ whole milk	½ cup (5.2 oz)	172	5	360	28	—
instant lemon as prep w/ 2% milk	½ cup (5.2 oz)	155	4	394	30	—
instant lemon as prep w/ whole milk	½ cup (5.2 oz)	169	4	393	30	—
instant vanilla as prep w/ 2% milk	½ cup (5 oz)	147	2	407	28	—
instant vanilla as prep w/ whole milk	½ cup (5 oz)	181	4	406	28	—
instant chocolate as prep w/ 2% milk	½ cup (5.2 oz)	149	3	418	28	—
lemon	½ cup (5.1 oz)	163	2	94	36	—
rice as prep w/ 2% milk	½ cup (5.1 oz)	161	2	159	30	—
rice as prep w/ whole milk	½ cup (5.1 oz)	175	4	158	30	—
tapioca as prep w/ 2% milk	½ cup (5 oz)	147	2	172	28	—
tapioca as prep w/ whole milk	½ cup (5 oz)	161	4	171	28	—
vanilla as prep w/ 2% milk	½ cup (4.9 oz)	141	2	224	26	—
vanilla as prep w/ whole milk	½ cup (4.9 oz)	155	4	223	26	—

FOOD	PORTION	CAL.	FAT	SOD.	CARB.	FIB.
Emes						
Dietetic as prep w/ skim milk	½ cup (4 fl oz)	71	1	110	13	—
Jell-O						
Americana Rice as prep w/ skim milk	½ cup (5.2 oz)	140	0	160	29	0
Americana Tapioca as prep w/ skim milk	½ cup (5.1 oz)	130	0	180	28	0
Banana Cream as prep w/ 2% milk	½ cup (5.1 oz)	140	3	240	26	0
Butterscotch as prep w/ 2% milk	½ cup (5.2 oz)	160	3	190	30	0
Chocolate as prep w/ 2% milk	½ cup (5.2 oz)	150	3	170	28	tr
Chocolate Fudge as prep w/ 2% milk	½ cup (5.2 oz)	150	3	170	28	1
Coconut Cream as prep w/ 2% milk	½ cup (5.1 oz)	150	5	210	24	tr
Fat Free Chocolate as prep w/ skim milk	½ cup (5.2 oz)	130	0	170	29	0
Fat Free Vanilla as prep w/ skim milk	½ cup (5.1 oz)	130	0	200	28	0
Instant Banana Cream as prep w/ 2% milk	½ cup (5.2 oz)	150	3	410	29	0
Instant Butterscotch as prep w/ 2% milk	½ cup (5.2 oz)	150	3	450	29	0
Instant Chocolate as prep w/ 2% milk	½ cup (5.2 oz)	160	3	470	31	tr
Instant Chocolate Fudge as prep w/ 2% milk	½ cup (4.2 oz)	160	3	440	31	tr
Instant Coconut Cream as prep w/ 2% milk	½ cup (4.2 oz)	160	5	320	27	tr
Instant French Vanilla as prep w/ 2% milk	½ cup (4.2 oz)	150	3	410	29	0
Instant Lemon as prep w/ 2% milk	½ cup (4.2 oz)	150	3	370	29	0
Instant Pistachio as prep w/ 2% milk	½ cup (4.2 oz)	160	3	410	29	0
Instant Vanilla as prep w/ 2% milk	½ cup (4.2 oz)	150	3	410	29	0
Instant Fat Free Chocolate as prep w/ skim milk	½ cup (5.3 oz)	140	0	410	31	tr

FOOD	PORTION	CAL.	FAT	SOD.	CARB.	FIB.
Jell-O (CONT.)						
Instant Fat Free Devil's Food as prep w/ skim milk	½ cup (5.3 oz)	140	0	420	31	tr
Instant Fat Free Sugar Free Banana as prep w/ skim milk	½ cup (4.6 oz)	70	0	410	12	0
Instant Fat Free Sugar Free Butterscotch as prep w/ skim milk	½ cup (4.6 oz)	70	0	400	12	0
Instant Fat Free Sugar Free Chocolate Fudge as prep w/ skim milk	½ cup (4.7 oz)	80	0	390	14	tr
Instant Fat Free Sugar Free Chocolate as prep w/ skim milk	½ cup (4.6 oz)	80	0	390	14	tr
Instant Fat Free Sugar Free Vanilla as prep w/ skim milk	½ cup (4.6 oz)	70	0	400	12	0
Instant Fat Free Sugar Free White Chocolate as prep w/ skim milk	½ cup (4.6 oz)	70	0	400	12	0
Instant Fat Free Vanilla as prep w/ skim milk	½ cup (5.2 oz)	140	0	410	29	0
Instant Fat Free White Chocolate as prep w/ skim milk	½ cup (5.2 oz)	140	0	410	29	0
Lemon as prep	½ cup (4.4 oz)	140	2	75	29	0
Milk Chocolate as prep w/ 2% milk	½ cup (5.2 oz)	150	3	170	28	tr
Sugar Free Chocolate as prep w/ 2% milk	½ cup (4.6 oz)	90	3	170	13	tr
Sugar Free Vanilla as prep w/ 2% milk	½ cup (4.5 oz)	80	3	170	11	0
Vanilla as prep w/ 2% milk	½ cup (5.1 oz)	140	3	200	26	0
Knorr						
Creme Caramel Flan & Sauce as prep	½ cup + 1 tbsp sauce	190	4	70	34	—
*My*T*Fine*						
Butterscotch	mix for 1 serv	90	0	190	22	—
Chocolate	mix for 1 serv	100	0	135	23	0
Chocolate Almond	mix for 1 serv	100	1	135	23	—
Chocolate Fudge	mix for 1 serv	100	0	140	24	—

FOOD	PORTION	CAL.	FAT	SOD.	CARB.	FIB.
*My*T*Fine* (CONT.)						
Lemon	mix for 1 serv	90	0	170	22	—
Vanilla	mix for 1 serv	90	0	120	22	0
Vanilla Tapioca	mix for 1 serv	80	0	160	19	—
Royal						
Banana Cream	mix for 1 serv	80	0	110	20	0
Banana Cream Instant	mix for 1 serv	90	0	390	22	—
Butterscotch	mix for 1 serv	90	0	180	25	0
Butterscotch Instant	mix for 1 serv	90	0	400	22	—
Cherry Vanilla Instant	mix for 1 serv	90	0	300	23	0
Chocolate	mix for 1 serv	90	0	90	22	0
Chocolate Almond Instant	mix for 1 serv	120	1	440	26	—
Chocolate Chocolate Chip Instant	mix for 1 serv	110	1	590	26	0
Chocolate Instant	mix for 1 serv	110	0	450	23	0
Chocolate Peanut Butter Instant	mix for 1 serv	110	1	480	26	0
Chocolate Sugar Free Instant	mix for 1 serv	50	0	420	11	—
Dark 'n Sweet Chocolate	mix for 1 serv	90	0	95	22	1
Dark'N Sweet Instant	mix for 1 serv	110	0	460	25	0
Lemon Instant	mix for 1 serv	90	0	320	23	—
Pistachio Instant	mix for 1 serv	90	1	360	22	0
Strawberry Instant	mix for 1 serv	100	0	330	24	—
Toasted Coconut Instant	mix for 1 serv	100	2	450	22	—
Vanilla	mix for 1 serv	80	0	160	20	0
Vanilla Chocolate Chip Instant	mix for 1 serv	90	1	350	22	0
Vanilla Instant	mix for 1 serv	90	0	325	23	—
READY-TO-EAT						
banana	1 pkg (5 oz)	180	5	278	30	—
chocolate	1 pkg (5 oz)	189	6	183	32	—
lemon	1 pkg (5 oz)	177	4	199	36	—
rice	1 pkg (5 oz)	231	11	121	31	—
tapioca	1 pkg (5 oz)	169	5	168	28	—
vanilla	1 pkg (4 oz)	146	4	153	25	—
Del Monte						
Snack Cups Banana	1 serv (4 oz)	140	4	190	25	0
Snack Cups Butterscotch	1 serv (4 oz)	140	4	170	25	0
Snack Cups Chocolate	1 serv (4 oz)	160	4	130	27	0
Snack Cups Chocolate Fudge	1 serv (4 oz)	150	4	190	25	0

FOOD	PORTION	CAL.	FAT	SOD.	CARB.	FIB.
Del Monte (CONT.)						
Snack Cups Chocolate Peanut Butter	1 serv (4 oz)	160	4	270	28	0
Snack Cups Lite Chocolate	1 serv (4 oz)	100	1	140	19	0
Snack Cups Lite Vanilla	1 serv (4 oz)	90	1	190	18	0
Snack Cups Tapioca	1 serv (4 oz)	140	4	110	23	0
Snack Cups Vanilla	1 serv (4 oz)	150	4	150	26	0
Handi-Snacks						
Banana	1 serv (3.5 oz)	120	4	150	22	0
Butterscotch	1 serv (3.5 oz)	120	4	150	22	0
Chocolate	1 serv (3.5 oz)	130	4	125	23	tr
Chocolate Fudge	1 serv (3.5 oz)	130	4	130	23	tr
Fat Free Chocolate	1 serv (3.5 oz)	90	0	170	21	0
Hunt's						
Snack Pack Banana	1 (4 oz)	158	6	163	25	0
Snack Pack Butterscotch	1 (4 oz)	153	6	211	24	0
Snack Pack Chocolate	1 (4 oz)	167	6	173	25	0
Snack Pack Chocolate Fudge	1 (4 oz)	167	6	191	26	0
Snack Pack Chocolate Marshmallow	1 (4 oz)	155	6	124	23	0
Snack Pack Fat Free Chocolate	1 (4 oz)	96	tr	212	21	0
Snack Pack Fat Free Tapioca	1 (4 oz)	95	tr	185	21	0
Snack Pack Fat Free Vanilla	1 (4 oz)	93	tr	167	21	0
Snack Pack Lemon	1 (4 oz)	162	3	100	33	0
Snack Pack Swirl Chocolate Caramel	1 (4 oz)	168	6	176	26	0
Snack Pack Swirl Chocolate Peanut Butter	1 (4 oz)	166	6	165	25	0
Snack Pack Swirl Milk Chocolate	1 (4 oz)	164	6	175	26	0
Snack Pack Swirl Smores	1 (4 oz)	154	6	129	25	0
Snack Pack Tapioca	1 (4 oz)	151	6	134	23	0
Snack Pack Vanilla	1 (4 oz)	163	6	176	25	0
Imagine Foods						
Lemon Dream	1 (4 oz)	120	0	5	30	—
Jell-O						
Chocolate	1 serv (4 oz)	160	5	190	28	0

FOOD	PORTION	CAL.	FAT	SOD.	CARB.	FIB.
Jell-O (CONT.)						
Chocolate Marshmallow	1 serv (4 oz)	160	5	180	27	0
Chocolate Vanilla Swirls	1 serv (4 oz)	160	5	180	27	0
Free Chocolate	1 serv (4 oz)	100	0	190	23	tr
Free Chocolate Vanilla Swirl	1 serv (4 oz)	100	0	210	23	tr
Free Devil's Food	1 serv (4 oz)	100	0	210	23	tr
Free Rocky Road	1 serv (4 oz)	100	0	210	23	tr
Free Vanilla	1 serv (4 oz)	100	0	240	23	0
Tapioca	1 serv (4 oz)	140	4	160	26	0
Tapioca	1 serv (4 oz)	100	0	240	23	0
Vanilla	1 serv (4 oz)	160	5	170	25	0
Kozy Shack						
Banana	1 pkg (4 oz)	130	3	150	22	1
Chocolate	1 pkg (4 oz)	140	4	150	24	1
Light Chocolate	1 pkg (4 oz)	110	1	150	22	1
Light Vanilla	1 pkg (4 oz)	110	1	160	22	0
Rice	1 pkg (4 oz)	130	3	140	23	1
Tapioca	1 pkg (4 oz)	140	3	160	25	0
Vanilla	1 pkg (4 oz)	130	3	150	22	1
Matthew Walker						
Plum	3.5 oz	290	7	100	60	1
Snack Pack						
Banana	4.25 oz	145	6	180	22	0
Butterscotch	4.25 oz	170	6	210	27	0
Chocolate	4.25 oz	170	6	120	26	0
Chocolate Marshmallow	4.25 oz	165	6	125	26	0
Chocolate Fudge	4.25 oz	165	6	125	27	0
Lemon	4.25 oz	150	4	75	30	tr
Light Chocolate	4.25 oz	100	2	120	20	0
Light Tapioca	4.25 oz	100	2	105	18	0
Tapioca	4.25 oz	150	5	125	23	0
Vanilla	4.25 oz	170	6	150	27	0
Swiss Miss						
Butterscotch	4 oz	180	6	135	29	0
Chocolate	4 oz	180	6	160	29	0
Chocolate Fudge	4 oz	220	6	180	38	0
Chocolate Sundae	4 oz	220	7	140	36	0
Light Chocolate	4 oz	100	1	120	20	0
Light Chocolate Fudge	4 oz	100	1	120	20	0
Light Vanilla	4 oz	100	1	105	20	0
Light Vanilla Chocolate Parfait	4 oz	100	1	110	20	0
Tapioca	4 oz	160	5	170	27	0

FOOD	PORTION	CAL.	FAT	SOD.	CARB.	FIB.
Swiss Miss (CONT.)						
Vanilla	4 oz	190	7	140	30	0
Vanilla Parfait	4 oz	180	6	150	29	0
Vanilla Sundae	4 oz	200	7	180	36	0
Ultra Slim-Fast						
Butterscotch	4 oz	100	tr	230	21	2
Chocolate	4 oz	100	tr	240	21	2
Vanilla	4 oz	100	tr	230	21	2
TAKE-OUT						
blancmange	1 serv (4.7 oz)	154	5	—	25	tr
bread pudding	1 serv (6.7 oz)	564	18	—	94	6
bread pudding	½ cup (4.4 oz)	212	7	291	31	—
bread w/ raisins	½ cup	180	5	185	31	—
chocolate	½ cup (5.5 oz)	206	4	157	41	—
queen of puddings	1 serv (4.4 oz)	266	10	—	41	tr
rice pudding	1 serv (3 oz)	110	4	—	17	tr
rice w/ raisins	½ cup	246	6	270	42	4
tapioca	½ cup (5.3 oz)	189	7	288	26	—
vanilla	½ cup (4.3 oz)	130	4	113	20	—

PUDDING POPS

(*see also* ICE CREAM AND FROZEN DESSERTS, PUDDING)

FOOD	PORTION	CAL.	FAT	SOD.	CARB.	FIB.
chocolate	1 (1.6 oz)	72	2	77	12	—
vanilla	1 (1.6 oz)	75	2	50	13	—

PUMMELO

FOOD	PORTION	CAL.	FAT	SOD.	CARB.	FIB.
fresh	1	228	tr	7	59	—
sections	1 cup	71	tr	2	18	—

PUMPKIN

FOOD	PORTION	CAL.	FAT	SOD.	CARB.	FIB.
CANNED						
pumpkin	½ cup	41	tr	6	10	—
Libby						
Solid Pack	½ cup	60	1	5	15	4
Owatonna						
Pumpkin	½ cup	40	1	—	—	—
FRESH						
cooked mashed	½ cup	24	tr	2	6	—
flowers cooked	½ cup	10	tr	4	2	—
flowers raw	1	0	0	0	tr	—
leaves cooked	½ cup	7	tr	3	1	—
leaves raw	½ cup	4	tr	2	tr	—
raw cubed	½ cup	15	tr	1	4	—
SEEDS						
dried	1 oz	154	13	5	5	—

FOOD	PORTION	CAL.	FAT	SOD.	CARB.	FIB.
roasted	1 cup	1184	96	40	31	—
roasted	1 oz	148	12	5	4	—
salted & roasted	1 oz	148	12	144	4	—
salted & roasted	1 cup	1184	96	1294	31	—
whole roasted	1 oz	127	6	5	15	—
whole roasted	1 cup	285	12	12	34	—
whole salted roasted	1 cup	285	12	268	34	—
whole salted roasted	1 oz	127	6	191	15	—
PURSLANE						
cooked	1 cup	21	tr	51	4	—
raw	1 cup	7	tr	20	1	—
QUAHOGS						
(*see* CLAM)						
QUAIL						
breast w/o skin raw	1 (2 oz)	69	2	31	0	—
w/ skin raw	1 quail (3.8 oz)	210	13	58	0	—
w/o skin raw	1 quail (3.2 oz)	123	4	47	0	—
QUICHE						
HOME RECIPE						
lorraine	⅛ of 8 in pie	600	48	653	29	—
TAKE-OUT						
cheese	1 slice (3 oz)	283	20	—	16	1
lorraine	1 slice (3 oz)	352	25	—	18	1
mushroom	1 slice (3 oz)	256	18	—	17	1
QUINCE						
fresh	1	53	tr	4	14	—
QUINOA						
quinoa	½ cup	318	5	—	59	—
Arrowhead						
Quinoa	¼ cup (1.4 oz)	140	2	0	25	4
Eden						
Not Prep	¼ cup (1.6 oz)	170	3	0	31	3
RABBIT						
domestic w/o bone roasted	3 oz	167	7	40	0	—
wild w/o bone stewed	3 oz	147	3	38	0	—
RACCOON						
roasted	3 oz	217	12	—	0	—
RADICCHIO						
leaf	3.5 oz	18	tr	—	3	1
raw shredded	½ cup	5	tr	4	1	—

FOOD	PORTION	CAL.	FAT	SOD.	CARB.	FIB.
RADISHES						
DRIED						
chinese	½ cup	157	tr	161	37	—
daikon	½ cup	157	tr	161	37	—
FRESH						
chinese raw	1 (12 oz)	62	tr	71	14	—
chinese raw sliced	½ cup	8	tr	9	2	—
chinese sliced cooked	½ cup	13	tr	10	3	—
daikon raw	1 (12 oz)	62	tr	71	14	—
daikon raw sliced	½ cup	8	tr	9	2	—
daikon sliced cooked	½ cup	13	tr	10	3	—
red raw	10	7	tr	11	2	—
red sliced	½ cup	10	tr	14	2	—
white icicle raw	1 (½ oz)	2	tr	3	tr	—
white icicle raw sliced	½ cup	7	tr	8	1	—
Dole						
Radishes	7	20	0	35	3	0
SPROUTS						
raw	½ cup	8	tr	1	1	—
RAISINS						
chocolate coated	1 cup (6.7 oz)	741	28	68	130	—
chocolate coated	10 (0.4 oz)	39	2	4	7	—
golden seedless	1 cup	437	1	17	115	8
seedless	1 cup	434	1	17	115	8
seedless	1 tbsp	27	tr	—	7	—
sultanas	1 oz	88	0	—	23	2
Cinderella						
Seedless	½ cup	250	0	—	—	—
Del Monte						
Golden	¼ cup (1.4 oz)	130	0	10	31	2
Raisins	1 box (0.5 oz)	45	0	0	11	tr
Raisins	1 box (1.5 oz)	140	0	10	33	3
Raisins	¼ cup (1.4 oz)	130	0	10	31	2
Raisins	1 box (1 oz)	90	0	5	22	2
Yogurt Raisins Strawberry	1 pkg (0.9 oz)	110	3	25	20	tr
Yogurt Raisins Vanilla	1 pkg (1 oz)	120	3	25	22	tr
Yogurt Raisins Vanilla	3 tbsp (1 oz)	130	3	30	23	1
Yogurt Raisins Vanilla	1 pkg (0.9 oz)	110	3	25	20	tr
Dole						
Golden	½ cup	250	0	25	66	—
Seedless	½ cup	250	0	15	66	—
Sonoma						
Monukka Thompson	¼ cup (1.4 oz)	130	0	10	31	2

FOOD	PORTION	CAL.	FAT	SOD.	CARB.	FIB.
Tree Of Life						
Organic	¼ cup (1.4 oz)	130	0	10	31	2
RASPBERRIES						
CANNED						
in heavy syrup	½ cup	117	tr	4	30	—
FRESH						
raspberries	1 cup	61	1	0	14	—
raspberries	1 pint	154	2	0	36	—
Dole						
Raspberries	1 cup	45	0	0	10	9
FROZEN						
sweetened	1 cup	256	tr	1	65	—
sweetened	1 pkg (10 oz)	291	tr	1	74	—
Big Valley						
Raspberries	⅔ cup (4.9 oz)	80	0	0	18	3
Birds Eye						
Whole In Lite Syrup	½ cup	100	1	0	25	4
RASPBERRY JUICE						
Crystal Geyser						
Juice Squeeze Mountain Raspberry	1 bottle (12 fl oz)	135	0	20	32	—
Crystal Light						
Raspberry Ice Drink	1 serv (8 oz)	5	0	20	0	0
Raspberry Ice Drink Mix as prep	1 serv (8 oz)	5	0	0	0	0
Fresh Samantha						
Raspberry Dream	1 cup (8 oz)	120	1	0	30	2
Kool-Aid						
Drink Mix as prep	1 serv (8 oz)	60	0	0	17	0
Raspberry Drink as prep w/ sugar	1 serv (8 oz)	100	0	30	25	0
Splash Blue Raspberry Drink	1 serv (8 oz)	120	0	35	30	0
Smucker's						
Juice	8 oz	120	0	10	30	—
Juice Sparkler	10 oz	130	tr	5	32	—
RED BEANS						
CANNED						
Allen						
Red Beans	½ cup (4.5 oz)	160	1	310	19	9
Green Giant						
Red Beans	½ cup	90	1	340	19	5

FOOD	PORTION	CAL.	FAT	SOD.	CARB.	FIB.
Hunt's						
Small	½ cup (4.5 oz)	89	1	713	19	6
Van Camp's						
Red Beans	½ cup (4.6 oz)	90	0	560	20	5
DRIED						
Bean Cuisine						
Dried	½ cup	115	1	5	—	5
MIX						
Bean Cuisine						
Pasta & Beans Barcelona Red With Radiatore	½ cup	170	4	379	170	—
Mahatma						
Red Beans & Rice	1 cup	190	1	790	40	7
RELISH						
cranberry orange	½ cup	246	tr	44	64	—
hamburger	1 tbsp	19	tr	164	5	—
hamburger	½ cup	158	1	1338	42	—
hot dog	½ cup	111	1	1332	28	—
hot dog	1 tbsp	14	tr	164	4	—
piccalilli	1.4 oz	13	tr	—	2	1
sweet	1 tbsp	19	tr	122	5	—
sweet	½ cup	159	1	990	43	—
Claussen						
Pickle Relish	1 tbsp	14	tr	—	—	—
Del Monte						
Hamburger	1 tbsp (0.5 oz)	20	0	220	6	tr
Hot Dog	1 tbsp (0.5 oz)	15	0	140	4	tr
Sweet Pickle	1 tbsp (0.5 oz)	20	0	125	5	0
Hellman's						
Sandwich Spread	1 tbsp (15 g)	55	5	170	2	—
Old El Paso						
Jalapeno	1 tbsp (0.5 oz)	5	0	110	1	0
Vlasic						
Dill	1 oz	2	0	415	1	—
Hamburger	1 oz	40	0	255	9	—
Hot Dog	1 oz	40	1	255	8	—
Hot Piccalilli	1 oz	35	0	165	8	—
India	1 oz	30	0	205	8	—
Sweet	1 oz	30	0	220	8	—
RENNIN						
tablet	1 (0.9 g)	1	0	234	tr	—
RHUBARB						
fresh	½ cup	13	tr	2	3	—

FOOD	PORTION	CAL.	FAT	SOD.	CARB.	FIB.
frzn	½ cup	60	tr	1	3	—
frzn as prep w/ sugar	½ cup	139	tr	2	37	—

RICE

(*see also* BRAN, CEREAL, FLOUR, RICE CAKES, WILD RICE)

FOOD	PORTION	CAL.	FAT	SOD.	CARB.	FIB.
brown long grain cooked	½ cup	109	tr	5	23	2
brown medium grain cooked	½ cup	109	tr	1	23	—
glutinous cooked	½ cup	116	tr	6	25	—
starch	3½ oz	343	0	61	85	—
white long grain cooked	½ cup	131	tr	2	28	tr
white long grain instant cooked	½ cup	80	tr	2	17	tr
white long grain parboiled cooked	½ cup	100	tr	3	22	tr
white medium grain cooked	½ cup	132	tr	0	29	—
white short grain cooked	½ cup	133	tr	0	29	—
Arrowhead						
Basmati Brown	¼ cup (1.5 oz)	150	1	0	33	2
Basmati White	¼ cup (1.5 oz)	150	0	0	34	tr
Brown Quick Regular	⅓ cup (1.5 oz)	150	1	0	32	2
Brown Quick Spanish Style	¼ pkg (1.4 oz)	150	1	250	30	2
Brown Quick Vegetable Herb	¼ pkg (1.4 oz)	150	1	160	30	3
Brown Quick Wild Rice & Herb	¼ pkg (1.3 oz)	140	1	220	28	3
Birds Eye						
Rice & Broccoli Au Gratin	½ pkg	150	4	490	24	1
Budget Gourmet						
Oriental Rice With Vegetables	1 pkg (5.75 oz)	230	12	420	28	—
Rice Pilaf With Green Beans	1 pkg (5.5 oz)	230	11	510	30	—
Carolina						
Red Beans & Rice as prep	¼ pkg	190	1	790	40	6
Casbah						
Basmati as prep	1 cup	158	tr	—	36	—
Jambalaya	1 pkg (1.4 oz)	130	0	500	27	1
La Fiesta	1 pkg (1.59 oz)	170	1	400	34	0
Nutted Pilaf as prep	1 cup	220	3	460	40	1

FOOD	PORTION	CAL.	FAT	SOD.	CARB.	FIB.
Casbah (CONT.)						
Pilaf as prep	1 cup	200	tr	430	44	tr
Spanish Pilaf as prep	1 cup	200	1	430	44	1
Thai Yum	1 pkg (1.7 oz)	180	3	500	33	1
Chun King						
Fried Rice	1 pkg (8 oz)	290	6	1310	48	5
Fried Rice With Chicken	1 pkg (8 oz)	270	6	1330	44	4
Goodman's						
Rice & Vermicelli For Beef	¾ cup	160	1	860	33	0
Rice & Vermicelli For Chicken	¾ cup	160	1	920	33	1
Green Giant						
Garden Gourmet Asparagus Pilaf	1 pkg	190	4	610	37	3
Garden Gourmet Sherry Wild Rice	1 pkg	210	4	580	40	3
One Serve Rice 'N Broccoli In Cheese Sauce	1 pkg	180	6	550	25	—
One Serve Rice Peas & Mushrooms With Sauce	1 pkg	130	2	410	27	—
Rice Originals Italian Rice s Spinach In Cheese Sauce	½ cup	140	4	400	22	—
Rice Originals Pilaf	½ cup	110	1	530	21	—
Rice Originals Rice 'N Broccoli In Cheese Sauce	½ cup	120	4	510	18	—
Rice Originals Rice Medley	½ cup	100	1	310	19	—
Rice Originals White & Wild	½ cup	130	2	540	24	—
Hain						
Almondine	½ cup	130	5	260	17	—
Oriental 3-Grain Goodness	½ cup	120	5	300	15	—
Kikkoman						
Fried Rice Seasoning Mix	1 oz pkg	91	tr	—	—	—
Kitchen Del Sol						
Mediterranean Paella Costa Brava as prep	½ cup (1.2 oz)	130	2	312	23	1

FOOD	PORTION	CAL.	FAT	SOD.	CARB.	FIB.
Kitchen Del Sol (CONT.)						
Mediterranean Sunny Lemon Pilaf as prep	½ cup (1.2 oz)	110	1	210	22	1
Mediterranean Tomato & Basil With Pine Nuts	½ cup (1 oz)	110	4	270	18	1
Knorr						
Risotto Milanese With Saffron	½ cup	130	3	420	24	—
Risotto Tomato	½ cup	110	tr	460	23	—
Risotto With Mushrooms	½ cup	110	tr	430	24	—
Risotto With Onion	½ cup	110	tr	390	24	—
Risotto With Peas And Corn	½ cup	110	1	470	23	—
La Choy						
Chinese Fried Rice	¾ cup	190	1	820	41	tr
Lipton						
Golden Saute Beef	½ cup (2.1 oz)	230	4	930	43	1
Golden Saute Chicken	1 cup (2.2 oz)	240	5	920	44	1
Golden Saute Chicken Broccoli	½ cup (2.3 oz)	260	5	800	47	2
Golden Saute Fried Rice	½ cup (2.1 oz)	240	1	900	47	1
Golden Saute Herb & Butter	½ cup (2.1 oz)	240	5	870	42	1
Golden Saute Onion Mushroom	½ cup (2.1 oz)	240	4	850	45	2
Golden Saute Oriental	½ cup (2.1 oz)	240	5	910	43	1
Golden Saute Savory Herb	½ cup (2.1 oz)	240	5	900	43	1
Golden Saute Spanish	½ cup (2.3 oz)	250	5	910	46	2
Rice & Beans Cajun as prep	½ cup (2.5 oz)	260	1	540	53	7
Rice & Sauce Alfredo Broccoli as prep	½ cup (2.2 oz)	250	5	860	44	1
Rice & Sauce Beef Broccoli as prep	½ cup (2.1 oz)	230	1	940	46	2
Rice & Sauce Beef Flavor as prep	½ cup (2.2 oz)	230	1	940	47	2
Rice & Sauce Cajun as prep	½ cup (2.2 oz)	230	1	930	49	2
Rice & Sauce Cheddar Broccoli as prep	½ cup (2.2 oz)	250	3	940	48	1
Rice & Sauce Chicken Broccoli as prep	½ cup (2.2 oz)	250	2	940	48	2

FOOD	PORTION	CAL.	FAT	SOD.	CARB.	FIB.
Lipton (CONT.)						
Rice & Sauce Chicken Flavor as prep	½ cup (2.2 oz)	240	2	900	48	1
Rice & Sauce Chicken Risotto	½ cup (2.1 oz)	230	2	740	44	1
Rice & Sauce Creamy Chicken as prep	½ cup (2.2 oz)	260	5	770	46	2
Rice & Sauce Herb & Butter as prep	½ cup (2.1 oz)	240	4	920	43	1
Rice & Sauce Long Grain Mushroom	½ cup (2.2 oz)	250	2	550	50	1
Rice & Sauce Medley as prep	½ cup (2.1 oz)	240	2	810	46	2
Rice & Sauce Mushroom as prep	½ cup (2.1 oz)	220	1	890	45	1
Rice & Sauce Oriental as prep	½ cup (2.1 oz)	230	1	750	46	1
Rice & Sauce Original Long Grain as prep	½ cup (2.2 oz)	250	1	890	51	2
Rice & Sauce Pilaf as prep	½ cup (2.1 oz)	230	1	850	46	1
Rice & Sauce Spanish as prep	½ cup (2.2 oz)	230	1	940	47	2
Luigino's						
Fried Rice Chicken	1 pkg (8 oz)	250	5	640	38	2
Fried Rice Pork	1 pkg (8 oz)	250	7	830	37	2
Fried Rice Pork & Shrimp	1 pkg (8 oz)	250	5	890	39	2
Fried Rice Shrimp	1 pkg (8 oz)	220	4	730	38	2
Risotto Parmesano	1 pkg (8 oz)	360	20	740	30	2
Mahatma						
Broccoli & Cheese	1 cup	200	2	620	41	2
Jambalaya	1 cup (2 oz)	190	1	700	43	tr
Long Grain & Wild	1 cup (2 oz)	190	1	1240	41	2
Pilaf	1 cup (2 oz)	190	0	820	43	tr
Spanish	1 cup (2 oz)	180	1	760	42	2
Yellow Rice Mix	1 cup	190	0	970	43	tr
Minute						
Boil-In-Bag White as prep	1 cup (5.7 oz)	190	0	10	42	tr
Instant Brown as prep	1 cup (5.2 oz)	170	2	10	34	2
Instant White as prep	1 cup (5.7 oz)	160	0	5	36	tr
Long Grain & Wild Seasoned w/ Herbs as prep	1 cup (7.8 oz)	230	1	950	50	1

FOOD	PORTION	CAL.	FAT	SOD.	CARB.	FIB.
Near East						
Barley Pilaf as prep	1 cup	220	4	620	41	5
Beef Pilaf as prep	1 cup	220	5	850	42	1
Curry Rice as prep	1 cup	220	4	660	42	1
Lentil Pilaf as prep	1 cup	210	4	650	37	0
Long Grain & Wild as prep	1 cup	220	5	810	42	2
Pilaf Brown Rice as prep	1 cup	220	5	710	41	2
Pilaf Chicken as prep	1 cup	220	5	940	42	1
Pilaf Kosher as prep	1 cup	220	5	870	42	1
Spanish Pilaf as prep	1 cup	230	6	990	42	1
Old El Paso						
Mexican	½ cup (4 oz)	410	2	1350	90	3
Spanish	1 cup (8.6 oz)	130	1	1340	28	2
Pritikin						
Mexican	⅓ cup (2 oz)	200	2	105	43	—
Oriental	⅓ cup (2 oz)	190	2	260	43	—
Rice-A-Roni						
Beef	½ cup	140	4	610	24	—
Beef & Mushroom	½ cup	150	3	740	26	—
Chicken	½ cup	150	3	560	26	—
Chicken & Broccoli	½ cup	150	3	710	25	—
Chicken & Mushroom	½ cup	180	7	840	26	—
Chicken & Vegetables	½ cup	140	3	790	25	—
Fried Rice	½ cup	110	5	700	21	—
Herb & Butter	½ cup	130	4	790	22	—
Long Grain & Wild Chicken w/ Almonds	½ cup	140	4	690	24	—
Long Grain & Wild Original	½ cup	130	3	660	23	—
Long Grain & Wild Pilaf	½ cup	130	3	550	23	—
Pilaf	½ cup	150	4	620	25	—
Risotto	½ cup	200	6	1130	32	—
Spanish	½ cup	150	4	1090	25	—
Stroganoff	½ cup	200	8	810	27	—
Yellow Rice	½ cup	140	4	780	25	—
S&W						
Brown Quick Natural Long Grain	3.5 oz	110	0	0	25	—
Brown Quick Natural Long Grain cooked	3.5 oz	119	0	0	26	—
Long Grain cooked	3.5 oz	106	0	0	23	—
Success						
Beef Oriental	½ cup	190	1	920	43	2

FOOD	PORTION	CAL.	FAT	SOD.	CARB.	FIB.
Success (CONT.)						
Broccoli & Cheese	½ cup	200	2	690	41	2
Brown & Wild	½ cup	190	1	830	40	3
Classic Chicken	½ cup	150	1	720	32	1
Long Grain & Wild	½ cup	190	0	890	42	1
Pilaf	½ cup	200	0	630	44	2
Spanish	½ cup	190	1	780	43	1
Superfino						
Arborio	½ cup	100	0	5	22	—
Ultra Slim-Fast						
Oriental Style	2.3 oz	240	1	900	58	4
Rice & Chicken Sauce	2.3 oz	240	1	1080	56	4
Uncle Ben						
Boil-In-Bag	1 serv (0.9 oz)	94	tr	9	22	tr
Brown	1 serv (1.6 oz)	158	1	1	34	1
Brown & Wild Fast Cooking	1 serv (1.3 oz)	120	1	383	26	1
Country Inn Broccoli Almondine	1 serv (1.2 oz)	124	2	367	25	1
Country Inn Broccoli & White Cheddar	1 serv (1.2 oz)	131	3	288	24	1
Country Inn Broccoli Au Gratin	1 serv (1.1 oz)	116	2	342	22	1
Country Inn Chicken Stock	1 serv (1.2 oz)	123	1	269	24	1
Country Inn Chicken With Wild Rice	1 serv (1.1 oz)	108	1	359	23	1
Country Inn Creamy Chicken & Mushroom	1 serv (1.3 oz)	138	3	380	24	1
Country Inn Creamy Chicken & Wild Rice	1 serv (1.3 oz)	135	1	340	27	1
Country Inn Green Bean Almondine	1 serv (1.2 oz)	128	2	280	25	1
Country Inn Herbed Au Gratin	1 serv (1.2 oz)	119	2	361	24	1
Country Inn Homestyle Chicken & Vegetables	1 serv (1.3 oz)	139	3	298	24	1
Country Inn Rice Florentine	1 serv (1.2 oz)	212	2	354	24	1
Country Inn Vegetable Pilaf	1 serv (1.2 oz)	115	1	357	25	1
In An Instant	1 serv (1.1 oz)	111	tr	10	25	tr
Long Grain & Wild Chicken Stock Sauce	1 serv (1.3 oz)	133	2	601	25	1

FOOD	PORTION	CAL.	FAT	SOD.	CARB.	FIB.
Uncle Ben (CONT.)						
Long Grain & Wild Fast Cooking	1 serv (1 oz)	101	tr	450	22	1
Long Grain & Wild Garden Vegetable Blend	1 serv (1.3 oz)	128	1	601	26	1
Long Grain & Wild Original	1 serv (1 oz)	96	tr	363	21	1
White Converted	1 serv (1.2 oz)	123	tr	1	27	tr
Van Camp's						
Spanish	1 cup (9 oz)	180	3	1290	37	3
Watkins						
Brown & Wild	¼ cup (1.6 oz)	160	0	10	34	3
Calico Medley	¼ cup (1.6 oz)	160	0	30	37	4
East/West Medley	¼ cup (1.6 oz)	160	0	0	33	5
Heartland Medley	¼ cup (1.6 oz)	160	0	10	35	4
Minnesota Medley	¼ cup (1.6 oz)	160	0	10	34	2
White & Wild	¼ cup (1.6 oz)	160	0	5	34	1
TAKE-OUT						
pilaf	½ cup	84	3	362	11	3
risotto	6.6 oz	426	18	—	65	3
spanish	¾ cup	363	27	1339	19	—

RICE CAKES

(*see also* POPCORN CAKES)

FOOD	PORTION	CAL.	FAT	SOD.	CARB.	FIB.
brown rice	1 (0.3 oz)	35	tr	29	7	tr
brown rice & buckwheat	1 (0.3 oz)	34	tr	10	7	tr
brown rice & buckwheat unsalted	1 (0.3 oz)	34	tr	tr	7	tr
brown rice & corn	1 (0.3 oz)	35	tr	26	7	—
brown rice & rye	1 (0.3 oz)	35	tr	10	7	tr
brown rice & sesame seed	1 (0.3 oz)	35	tr	20	7	—
brown rice multigrain	1 (0.3 oz)	35	tr	23	7	—
brown rice multigrain unsalted	1 (0.3 oz)	35	tr	tr	7	—
brown rice unsalted	1 (0.3 oz)	35	tr	3	7	tr
Hain						
5-Grain	1	40	tr	10	8	—
Mini Apple Cinnamon	½ oz	60	tr	10	12	0
Mini Barbeque	½ oz	70	3	50	10	0
Mini Cheese	½ oz	60	2	100	10	0
Mini Honey Nut	½ oz	60	tr	30	11	0
Mini Nacho Cheese	½ oz	70	2	90	10	—
Mini Plain	½ oz	60	tr	20	12	0

FOOD	PORTION	CAL.	FAT	SOD.	CARB.	FIB.
Hain (CONT.)						
Mini Plain No Salt Added	½ oz	60	tr	5	12	0
Mini Ranch	½ oz	70	3	90	9	—
Mini Teriyaki	½ oz	50	tr	75	12	0
Plain	1	40	tr	10	8	—
Plain No Salt Added	1	40	tr	<5	8	—
Sesame	1	40	tr	10	8	—
Sesame No Salt	1	40	tr	<5	8	—
Ka-Me						
Cheese	16 pieces (1 oz)	120	2	180	24	0
Onion	16 pieces (1 oz)	120	1	75	25	0
Plain	16 pieces (1 oz)	120	2	15	25	0
Seaweed	16 pieces (1 oz)	120	2	100	25	0
Sesame	16 pieces (1 oz)	120	2	85	24	0
Unsalted	16 pieces (1 oz)	120	1	0	26	0
Lundberg						
Organic Lightly Salted	1	60	1	120	14	—
Organic Unsalted	1	60	1	3	14	—
Premium Lightly Salted	1	60	1	120	14	—
Premium Unsalted	1	60	1	3	14	—
Sesame Lightly Salted	1	59	0	6	16	—
Mother's						
Mini Apple	5 (0.5 oz)	50	0	40	12	0
Mini Caramel	5 (0.5 oz)	50	0	40	12	0
Mini Cinnamon	5 (0.5 oz)	50	0	40	12	0
Mini Plain Unsalted	7 (0.5 oz)	60	0	0	12	0
Multigrain Lightly Salted	1 (0.3 oz)	35	0	30	7	0
Rye Unsalted	1 (0.3 oz)	35	0	0	7	1
Wheat Unsalted	1 (0.3 oz)	35	0	0	7	1
Pritikin						
Mini Apple Crisp	5 (0.5 oz)	50	0	20	12	—
Multigrain	1 (0.3 oz)	35	0	20	7	—
Multigrain Unsalted	1 (0.3 oz)	35	0	0	7	—
Plain	1 (0.3 oz)	35	0	20	7	—
Plain Unsalted	1 (0.3 oz)	35	0	0	7	—
Sesame Low Sodium	1 (0.3 oz)	35	0	20	7	—
Sesame Unsalted	1 (0.3 oz)	35	0	0	7	—
Quaker						
Apple Cinnamon	1 (0.5 oz)	50	0	0	11	—
Banana Crunch	1 (0.5 oz)	50	0	45	11	—
Cinnamon Crunch	1 (0.5 oz)	50	0	25	11	—
Mini Apple Cinnamon	5 (0.5 oz)	50	0	0	12	—
Mini Banana Nut	5 (0.5 oz)	50	0	40	12	—
Mini Butter Popped Corn	6 (0.5 oz)	50	0	120	12	—

FOOD	PORTION	CAL.	FAT	SOD.	CARB.	FIB.
Quaker (CONT.)						
Mini Caramel Corn	5 (0.5 oz)	50	0	25	12	—
Mini Chocolate Crunch	5 (0.5 oz)	50	0	10	12	—
Mini Cinnamon Crunch	5 (0.5 oz)	50	0	25	12	—
Mini Honey Nut	5 (0.5 oz)	50	0	25	12	—
Mini Monterey Jack	6 (0.5 oz)	50	0	100	11	—
Mini White Cheddar	6 (0.5 oz)	50	0	120	11	—
Salt-Free	1 (0.3 oz)	35	0	0	7	—
Salted	1 (0.3 oz)	35	0	15	7	—
Tree Of Life						
Fat Free Mini Apple Cinnamon	15	60	0	5	13	0
Fat Free Mini Caramel	15	60	0	10	13	0
Fat Free Mini Honey Nut	15	60	0	0	13	0
Fat Free Mini Jalapeno	15	60	0	25	13	0
Fat Free Mini Plain	15	50	0	45	12	0
ROCKFISH						
pacific cooked	1 fillet (5.2 oz)	180	3	114	0	—
pacific cooked	3 oz	103	2	65	0	—
pacific raw	3 oz	80	1	51	0	—
ROE						
(*see also individual fish names*)						
fish	3.5 oz	39	2	—	tr	—
fresh baked	3 oz	173	7	—	2	—
fresh baked	1 oz	58	2	—	1	—
ROLL						
(*see also* BISCUIT, CROISSANT, ENGLISH MUFFIN, MUFFIN, POPOVER, SCONE)						
FROZEN						
Pepperidge Farm						
Cinnamon Roll	1 (2¼ oz)	220	14	190	34	—
Sara Lee						
All Butter Cinnamon Roll w/ Icing	1	280	11	220	43	—
All Butter Cinnamon Roll w/o Icing	1	230	11	220	31	—
Weight Watchers						
Glazed Cinnamon Rolls	1 (2.1 oz)	200	5	200	33	1
HOME RECIPE						
dinner as prep w/ 2% milk	1 (2½ in)	111	3	145	19	—
dinner as prep w/ whole milk	1 (2½ in)	112	3	145	19	—
raisin & nut	1 (2 oz)	196	7	185	30	—

FOOD	PORTION	CAL.	FAT	SOD.	CARB.	FIB.
MIX						
Dromedary						
Hot Roll Mix	2	239	5	410	41	—
Natural Ovens						
German Hard	1 (2.1 oz)	138	1	140	36	1
Gourmet Dinner	1 (1 oz)	50	1	140	15	2
Hearty Sandwich	1 (1.8 oz)	110	1	140	30	2
Pillsbury						
Hot Roll Mix	2	240	4	430	42	—
READY-TO-EAT						
brown & serve	1 (1 oz)	85	2	148	14	—
cheese	1 (2.3 oz)	238	12	236	29	—
cinnamon raisin	1 (2¾ in)	223	10	229	31	1
dinner	1 (1 oz)	85	2	148	14	—
egg	1 (2½ in)	107	2	191	18	1
french	1 (1.3 oz)	105	2	232	19	—
hamburger	1 (1½ oz)	123	2	241	22	—
hamburger multi-grain	1 (1½ oz)	113	2	197	19	2
hamburger reduced calorie	1 (1½ oz)	84	1	190	18	3
hard	1 (3½ in)	167	2	310	30	—
hot cross bun	1	202	4	—	38	1
hotdog	1 (1½ oz)	123	2	241	22	—
hotdog multi-grain	1 (1½ oz)	113	2	197	19	2
hotdog reduced calorie	1 (1½ oz)	84	1	190	18	3
kaiser	1 (3½ in)	167	2	310	30	—
oat bran	1 (1.2 oz)	78	2	136	13	1
rye	1 (1 oz)	81	1	253	15	—
submarine	1 (4.7 oz)	155	2	313	30	—
wheat	1 (1 oz)	77	2	96	13	—
whole wheat	1 (1 oz)	75	1	135	15	—
Alvarado St. Bakery						
Burger Buns	1 (2.2 oz)	140	2	290	27	3
Hot Dog Buns	1 (2.2 oz)	140	2	290	28	3
Arnold						
8-inch Francisco	1 (2.5 oz)	210	3	260	39	—
Augusto Pan Cubano	1	230	3	500	43	2
Bakery Light	1 (1.5 oz)	80	<2	190	21	4
Bran'nola Buns	1 (1.5 oz)	100	1	160	20	3
Deli Kaiser	1	170	2	—	34	—
Deli Onion	1	170	2	—	34	—
Dinner Plain	1 (0.7 oz)	50	1	80	9	1
Dinner Sesame	1 (0.7 oz)	50	1	80	9	1
Dutch Egg	1	130	3	180	21	2
French Francisco	1 (2.5 oz)	210	3	260	39	—

FOOD	PORTION	CAL.	FAT	SOD.	CARB.	FIB.
Arnold (CONT.)						
French Mini Francisco	1	130	2	140	24	—
Hamburger	1	120	2	190	20	2
Hot Dog	1 (1.5 oz)	110	2	160	21	1
Hot Dog Bran'nola	1 (1.5 oz)	110	2	170	18	1
Hot Dog New England Style	1	110	2	160	20	1
Italian 8-inch Savoni	1	210	3	—	38	3
Kaiser Francisco	1 (2 oz)	180	—	230	34	—
Onion Premium	1 (2.6 oz)	180	1	340	38	2
Onion Soft	1	140	—	200	28	2
Party Petite	2	70	2	70	10	1
Potato	1	140	2	210	25	2
Sandwich Soft Sesame	1	130	3	220	23	2
Sourdough Brown N' Serve	1 (1 oz)	100	1	120	19	—
Sourdough Francisco	1 (1 oz)	100	1	120	19	—
Wheat Old Fashioned	2	80	3	98	11	—
August Bros.						
Dinner	1	90	1	170	18	—
Kaiser	1	170	1	310	35	2
Onion	1	160	1	310	33	2
Sesame Cubano	1	170	1	310	35	2
Bread Du Jour						
Bavarian Cracked Wheat	1 (1.2 oz)	90	1	190	17	1
Crusty Italian	1 (1.2 oz)	80	1	190	16	tr
French Petite	1 (3.5 oz)	230	2	530	47	2
Rye	1 (1.2 oz)	90	2	230	16	1
Sourdough	1 (2.2 oz)	140	2	230	29	2
Country Kitchen						
Frankfurt	1	120	2	—	—	—
Dicarlo's						
Extra Sourdough	1 (1.6 oz)	100	1	230	20	1
French	1 (1 oz)	70	1	150	14	tr
Hollywood						
Dark Bread	1	40	tr	—	—	—
Dinner Light Pan Special Formula	1	60	tr	—	—	—
Sliced Light Special Formula	1	80	tr	—	—	—
Home Pride						
Dinner Wheat	1 (1.9 oz)	160	4	270	26	2
Hamburger Potato Bun	1 (1.9 oz)	130	2	270	27	2
Hot Dog Potato Bun	1 (1.9 oz)	130	2	270	27	2

FOOD	PORTION	CAL.	FAT	SOD.	CARB.	FIB.
Home Pride (CONT.)						
Sandwich Roll Wheat	1 (1.9 oz)	160	4	270	26	2
White	2 (1.6 oz)	130	4	230	22	1
Levy						
Sub Old Country	1	180	2	230	34	—
Martin's						
Big Marty Poppy	1	170	2	320	31	3
Big Marty Sesame	1	170	2	320	31	3
Hoagie	1	240	3	430	41	3
Hoagie Sesame	1	240	3	430	41	4
Potato Dinner	1	100	1	135	18	1
Potato Long	1	140	1	200	27	2
Potato Party	1	50	1	70	10	1
Potato Sandwich	1	140	1	200	26	2
Sandwich Whole Wheat 100% Stoneground	1	160	2	290	28	5
Matthew's						
Salad Roll	1	110	2	190	19	2
Sandwich	1	110	2	180	19	2
Pepperidge Farm						
Brown 'N Serve Club	1	100	1	190	19	1
Brown 'N Serve French	½ roll	180	2	380	36	1
Brown 'N Serve Hearth	1	50	1	100	10	tr
Dinner	1	60	2	95	8	tr
Dinner Country Style Classic	1	50	1	90	9	0
Finger Poppy Seed	1	50	2	80	8	tr
Finger Sesame Seed	1	60	2	85	9	tr
Frankfurter Dijon	1	160	5	230	23	2
Frankfurter Side Sliced	1	140	3	270	24	1
Frankfurter Top Sliced	1	140	3	270	24	1
Frankfurter w/ Poppy Seeds	1	130	2	280	23	1
French Style	1	100	1	230	20	1
Hamburger	1	130	2	240	22	1
Hamburger	1	130	2	240	22	1
Heat & Serve Butter Crescent	1	110	6	150	13	tr
Heat & Serve Golden Twist	1	110	5	150	14	tr
Hoagie Soft	1	210	5	320	34	1
Old Fashioned	1	50	2	85	7	tr
Parker House	1	60	1	80	9	tr
Party	1	30	1	50	5	tr

FOOD	PORTION	CAL.	FAT	SOD.	CARB.	FIB.
Pepperidge Farm (CONT.)						
Potato Sandwich	1	160	4	260	28	1
Sandwich Onion w/ Poppy Seeds	1	150	3	260	26	1
Sandwich Salad	1	110	4	150	16	—
Sandwich w/ Sesame Seeds	1	140	3	230	23	1
Soft Family	1	100	2	190	18	1
Sourdough French	1	100	1	240	19	1
Roman Meal						
Brown & Serve	2 (2 oz)	140	3	275	24	2
Dinner	2 (2 oz)	136	2	282	24	2
Hamburger	1 (1.6 oz)	111	2	229	19	2
Hotdog	1 (1.5 oz)	103	2	214	18	2
Sandwich	1 (2.7 oz)	181	3	392	31	3
Sandwich	1 (2.7 oz)	181	3	392	31	3
San Francisco						
Sourdough	1 (1.8 oz)	180	0	300	37	3
The Baker						
Honey Cinnamon Raisin	1 (2 oz)	150	2	115	31	4
Wonder						
Brown 'N Serve Buttermilk	1 (1 oz)	70	1	160	13	tr
Brown 'N Serve Wheat	1 (1 oz)	70	1	135	14	tr
Brown 'N Serve White	1 (1 oz)	70	1	135	14	tr
Dinner White Light	1 (1 oz)	60	1	150	9	4
Hamburger	1 (1.5 oz)	110	2	250	21	tr
Hamburger Light	1 (1.5 oz)	80	2	210	13	5
Hamburger Wheat	1 (2.2 oz)	170	3	370	31	1
Hot Dog	1 (1.5 oz)	110	2	250	21	tr
Hot Dog Light	1 (1.5 oz)	80	2	210	13	5
Tea Dinner Rolls	1 (1.5 oz)	80	1	210	19	5
REFRIGERATED						
cinnamon w/ frosting	1	109	4	250	17	—
crescent	1 (1 oz)	98	4	341	14	—
Pillsbury						
Best Quick Cinnamon Rolls w/ Icing	1	110	5	260	17	—
Butterflake	1	140	5	530	20	—
Crescent	1	100	6	230	11	—

ROSE APPLE

fresh	3½ oz	32	tr	—	7	—

ROSE HIP

fresh	3½ oz	91	0	146	19	—

FOOD	PORTION	CAL.	FAT	SOD.	CARB.	FIB.
ROSELLE						
fresh	1 cup	28	tr	3	6	—
ROSEMARY						
dried	1 tsp	4	tr	1	1	—
ROUGHY						
orange baked	3 oz	75	1	69	0	—
RUTABAGA						
CANNED						
Sunshine						
Diced	½ cup (4.2 oz)	30	0	220	7	3
FRESH						
cooked mashed	½ cup	41	tr	22	9	—
raw cubed	½ cup	25	tr	14	6	—
SABLEFISH						
baked	3 oz	213	17	61	0	—
fillet baked	5.3 oz	378	30	108	0	—
smoked	1 oz	72	6	206	0	—
smoked	3 oz	218	17	626	0	—
SAFFLOWER						
seeds dried	1 oz	147	11	—	10	—
SAFFRON						
saffron	1 tsp	2	tr	1	tr	—
SAGE						
ground	1 tsp	2	tr	tr	tr	—
Watkins						
Sage	¼ tsp (0.5 g)	0	0	0	0	0
SALAD						
(*see also* LETTUCE, PASTA SALAD)						
MIX						
Dole						
Caesar Salad	⅓ pkg (3.5 oz)	170	14	480	9	1
Classic Blend	3.5 oz	25	1	20	4	1
Coleslaw Blend	3.5 oz	30	1	35	5	2
French Blend	3.5 oz	25	1	15	4	1
Italian Blend	3.5 oz	25	1	45	3	1
Salad-In-A-Minute Oriental	3.5 oz	110	7	290	12	2
Salad-In-A-Minute Spinach	3.5 oz	180	9	660	19	3

FOOD	PORTION	CAL.	FAT	SOD.	CARB.	FIB.
Fresh Express						
American Salad	1½ cups (3 oz)	20	0	10	3	1
Caesar Salad	1½ cups (3 oz)	140	11	320	8	1
European Salad	1½ cups (3 oz)	20	0	10	3	1
Garden Salad	1½ cups (3 oz)	20	0	10	3	1
Italian Salad	1½ cups (3 oz)	20	0	0	3	1
Oriental Salad	1½ cups (3 oz)	120	8	330	11	1
Riviera Salad	1½ cups (3 oz)	10	0	0	2	1
Spinach Salad	1½ cups (3 oz)	130	3	430	23	3
Suddenly Salad						
Caesar Low Fat Recipe as prep	¾ cup	170	3	580	30	1
Caesar as prep	¾ cup	220	9	580	30	1
Italian Pepperoni Low Fat Recipe as prep	1 cup	180	2	700	35	2
Italian Pepperoni as prep	1 cup	200	4	700	35	1
Ranch & Bacon Low Fat Recipe as prep	¾ cup	180	2	530	31	1
Ranch & Bacon as prep	¾ cup	320	19	490	31	1
Weight Watchers						
Caesar Salad	1 serv (3.5 oz)	60	0	600	11	1
Caesar Salad w/ Cookies	1 pkg (4.3 oz)	160	3	670	29	3
European Salad	1 serv (3.5 oz)	60	0	530	13	2
European Salad w/ Cookies	1 pkg (4.3 oz)	160	3	620	31	2
Garden Salad	1 serv (3.5 oz)	60	0	270	12	1
Garden Salad w/ Cookies	1 pkg (4 oz)	120	2	340	24	2
TAKE-OUT						
caesar	2 cups (5 oz)	235	20	440	11	1
chef w/o dressing	1½ cups	386	28	279	9	—
tossed w/o dressing	¾ cup	16	0	27	3	—
tossed w/o dressing	1½ cups	32	tr	53	7	—
tossed w/o dressing w/ cheese & egg	1½ cups	102	6	119	5	—
tossed w/o dressing w/ chicken	1½ cups	105	2	209	4	—
tossed w/o dressing w/ pasta & seafood	1½ cups (14.6 oz)	380	21	1572	32	—
tossed w/o dressing w/ shrimp	1½ cups	107	2	487	7	—
waldorf	½ cup	79	6	49	6	1

SALAD DRESSING

FOOD	PORTION	CAL.	FAT	SOD.	CARB.	FIB.
HOME RECIPE						
french	1 tbsp	88	10	92	1	—
vinegar & oil	1 tbsp	72	8	tr	tr	—

FOOD	PORTION	CAL.	FAT	SOD.	CARB.	FIB.
MIX						
Good Seasons						
Cheese Garlic as prep	2 tbsp (1 oz)	140	16	330	1	0
Fat Free Honey Mustard as prep	2 tbsp (1.2 oz)	20	0	280	5	0
Fat Free Italian as prep	2 tbsp (1.1 oz)	10	0	290	2	0
Fat Free Ranch as prep	2 tbsp (1.2 oz)	20	0	250	5	0
Fat Free Zesty Herb as prep	2 tbsp (1.1 oz)	10	0	260	2	0
Garlic & Herbs as prep	2 tbsp (1 oz)	140	15	340	1	0
Gourmet Caesar as prep	2 tbsp (1.1 oz)	150	16	300	3	0
Gourmet Parmesan Italian as prep	2 tbsp (1.1 oz)	150	16	330	2	0
Honey French as prep	2 tbsp (1.2 oz)	160	15	250	5	0
Honey Mustard as prep	2 tbsp (1.1 oz)	150	15	240	3	0
Italian as prep	2 tbsp (1 oz)	140	15	320	1	0
Mexican Spice as prep	2 tbsp (1.1 oz)	140	15	310	2	0
Mild Italian as prep	2 tbsp (1.1 oz)	150	15	370	2	0
Oriental Sesame as prep	2 tbsp (1.1 oz)	150	16	360	3	0
Reduced Calorie Italian as prep	2 tbsp (1 oz)	50	5	280	2	0
Reduced Calorie Zesty Italian as prep	2 tbsp (1 oz)	50	5	260	2	0
Roasted Garlic as prep	2 tbsp (1.1 oz)	150	15	340	2	0
Zesty Italian as prep	2 tbsp (1 oz)	140	15	220	1	0
Hain						
No Oil 1000 Island	1 tbsp	12	0	150	3	—
No Oil Bleu Cheese	1 tbsp	14	1	190	1	—
No Oil Buttermilk	1 tbsp	11	tr	150	1	—
No Oil Caesar	1 tbsp	6	tr	200	1	—
No Oil French	1 tbsp	12	0	340	3	—
No Oil Garlic & Cheese	1 tbsp	6	tr	180	1	—
No Oil Herb	1 tbsp	2	0	140	1	—
No Oil Italian	1 tbsp	2	0	170	1	—
READY-TO-EAT						
blue cheese	1 tbsp	77	8	—	1	—
french	1 tbsp	67	6	214	3	—
french reduced calorie	1 tbsp	22	1	128	4	—
italian	1 tbsp	69	7	116	2	—
italian reduced calorie	1 tbsp	16	2	118	1	—
russian	1 tbsp	76	8	133	2	—
russian reduced calorie	1 tbsp	23	1	141	5	—
sesame seed	1 tbsp	68	7	153	1	—
thousand island	1 tbsp	59	6	109	2	—

FOOD	PORTION	CAL.	FAT	SOD.	CARB.	FIB.
thousand island reduced calorie	1 tbsp	24	2	153	3	—
Estee						
Blue Cheese	2 tbsp (1 oz)	15	1	80	1	—
Creamy French	2 tbsp (1 oz)	10	0	80	2	—
Creamy French Fat Free	1 pkg (0.5 oz)	5	0	40	1	—
Creamy Garlic	2 tbsp (1 oz)	60	0	80	2	—
Creamy Garlic Fat Free	1 pkg (0.5 oz)	5	0	40	1	—
Creamy Italian	2 tbsp (1 oz)	15	1	80	2	—
Fat Free Thousand Island	1 pkg (0.5 oz)	5	0	40	1	—
Italian	2 tbsp (1 oz)	5	0	80	1	—
Italian Fat Free	1 pkg (0.5 oz)	0	0	40	tr	—
Low Fat Blue Cheese	1 pkg (0.5 oz)	5	0	40	tr	—
Thousand Island	2 tbsp (1 oz)	10	0	80	2	—
Hain						
1000 Island	1 tbsp	50	5	85	0	—
Canola Garden Tomato	1 tbsp	60	6	150	1	—
Canola Italian	1 tbsp	50	5	150	1	—
Canola Spicy French Mustard	1 tbsp	50	5	190	1	—
Canola Tangy Citrus	1 tbsp	50	5	75	1	—
Creamy Caesar	1 tbsp	60	6	220	1	—
Creamy Caesar Low Salt	1 tbsp	60	6	15	1	—
Creamy French	1 tbsp	60	6	80	1	—
Creamy Italian	1 tbsp	80	8	100	0	—
Creamy Italian No Salt Added	1 tbsp	80	8	25	1	—
Cucumber Dill	1 tbsp	80	8	210	0	—
Dijon Vinaigrette	1 tbsp	50	5	180	0	—
Garlic & Sour Cream	1 tbsp	70	7	100	0	—
Honey & Sesame	1 tbsp	60	5	210	2	—
Italian Cheese Vinaigrette	1 tbsp	55	6	130	0	—
Old Fashioned Buttermilk	1 tbsp	70	7	100	0	—
Poppyseed Rancher's	1 tbsp	60	7	105	0	—
Savory Herb No Salt Added	1 tbsp	90	10	45	0	—
Swiss Cheese Vinaigrette	1 tbsp	60	7	160	0	—
Traditional Italian	1 tbsp	80	8	330	0	—
Traditional Italian No Salt Added	1 tbsp	60	6	20	1	—

FOOD	PORTION	CAL.	FAT	SOD.	CARB.	FIB.
Hollywood						
Caesar	1 tbsp	70	7	65	2	0
Creamy French	1 tbsp	70	7	45	2	0
Creamy Italian	1 tbsp	90	9	140	2	0
Dijon Vinaigrette	1 tbsp	60	6	40	2	0
Italian	1 tbsp	90	9	300	1	0
Italian Cheese	1 tbsp	80	8	60	2	0
Old Fashion Buttermilk	1 tbsp	75	8	40	1	0
Poppy Seed Rancher's	1 tbsp	75	8	35	1	0
Thousand Island	1 tbsp	60	6	15	3	0
Kraft						
⅓ Less Fat Catalina	2 tbsp (1.2 oz)	80	5	400	9	0
⅓ Less Fat Cucumber Ranch	2 tbsp (1.1 oz)	60	5	480	2	0
⅓ Less Fat Italian	2 tbsp (1.1 oz)	70	7	240	3	0
⅓ Less Fat Ranch	2 tbsp (1.1)	110	11	310	1	0
⅓ Less Fat Thousand Island	2 tbsp (1.2 oz)	70	5	340	7	0
Bacon & Tomato	2 tbsp (1.1 oz)	140	14	280	2	0
Buttermilk Ranch	2 tbsp (1.1 oz)	150	16	240	1	0
Caesar Italian	2 tbsp (1.1 oz)	100	10	480	2	0
Caesar Ranch	2 tbsp (1.1 oz)	110	11	290	1	0
Catalina	2 tbsp (1.1 oz)	120	10	390	7	0
Catalina With Honey	2 tbsp (1.1 oz)	130	11	320	7	0
Classic Caesar	2 tbsp (1.1 oz)	110	11	290	1	0
Coleslaw	2 tbsp (1.1 oz)	130	11	410	7	0
Creamy French	2 tbsp (1.1 oz)	160	15	270	5	0
Creamy Garlic	2 tbsp (1.1 oz)	110	11	360	2	0
Creamy Italian	2 tbsp (1.1 oz)	110	11	250	2	0
Cucumber Ranch	2 tbsp (1.1 oz)	140	15	220	2	0
Free Blue Cheese	2 tbsp (1.2 oz)	45	0	360	11	1
Free Caesar Italian	2 tbsp (1.2 oz)	25	0	480	4	0
Free Catalina	2 tbsp (1.2 oz)	35	0	320	8	tr
Free Classic Caesar	2 tbsp (1.2 oz)	45	0	360	11	tr
Free Creamy Italian	2 tbsp (1.2 oz)	50	0	330	12	tr
Free French	2 tbsp (1.2 oz)	45	0	300	11	tr
Free Garlic Ranch	2 tbsp (1.2 oz)	45	0	320	11	1
Free Honey Dijon	2 tbsp (1.2 oz)	45	0	330	10	1
Free Italian	2 tbsp (1.2 oz)	20	0	430	4	0
Free Peppercorn Ranch	2 tbsp (1.2 oz)	45	0	330	11	tr
Free Ranch	1 tbsp (1.2 oz)	50	0	350	11	1
Free Red Wine Vinegar	2 tbsp (1.1 oz)	15	0	410	3	0
Free Thousand Island	2 tbsp (1.2 oz)	40	0	280	9	1
Garlic Ranch	2 tbsp (1.1 oz)	180	19	270	1	0

FOOD	PORTION	CAL.	FAT	SOD.	CARB.	FIB.
Kraft (CONT.)						
Herb Vinaigrette	2 tbsp (1.1 oz)	140	15	250	tr	0
Honey Dijon	2 tbsp (1.1 oz)	110	10	210	6	0
Honey Mustard	2 tbsp (1.1 oz)	110	10	210	6	0
House Italian w/ Olive Oil Blend	2 tbsp (1.1 oz)	120	12	240	2	0
Peppercorn Ranch	2 tbsp (1 oz)	170	18	270	1	0
Pesto Italian	2 tbsp (1.1 oz)	90	9	310	2	0
Ranch	2 tbsp (1 oz)	170	18	280	1	0
Roka Blue Cheese	2 tbsp (1.1 oz)	130	13	310	2	tr
Russian	2 tbsp (1.2 oz)	130	10	310	10	0
Sour Cream & Onion Ranch	2 tbsp (1 oz)	170	18	250	1	0
Thousand Island	2 tbsp (1.1 oz)	110	10	310	5	0
Thousand Island With Bacon	2 tbsp (1.1 oz)	130	12	200	5	0
Tomato & Herb Italian	2 tbsp (1.1 oz)	100	9	340	3	0
Zesty Italian	2 tbsp (1.1 oz)	110	11	540	2	0
Marzetti						
Bacon Spinach Salad	2 tbsp	80	15	260	16	15
Blue Cheese	2 tbsp	160	17	230	0	0
Buttermilk & Herb	2 tbsp	180	20	260	1	0
Buttermilk Bacon Ranch	2 tbsp	180	19	270	1	0
Buttermilk Blue Cheese	2 tbsp	160	18	220	1	0
Buttermilk Parmesan Pepper	2 tbsp	170	18	310	1	0
Buttermilk Parmesan Ranch	2 tbsp	160	17	240	1	0
Buttermilk Ranch	2 tbsp	180	20	250	1	0
Buttermilk Veggie Dip	2 tbsp	170	18	240	1	0
Caesar	2 tbsp	150	16	390	1	0
Caesar Ranch	2 tbsp	190	20	300	2	0
California French	2 tbsp	160	13	240	11	0
Celery Seed	2 tbsp	160	13	180	10	0
Chunky Blue Cheese	2 tbsp	150	16	300	1	0
Classic Caesar Ranch	2 tbsp	190	20	300	2	0
Country French	2 tbsp	150	13	220	7	0
Cracked Peppercorn	2 tbsp	140	14	280	1	0
Creamy Garlic Italian	2 tbsp	160	17	140	1	0
Creamy Italian	2 tbsp	150	16	170	1	0
Crispy Celery Seed	2 tbsp	160	13	190	11	0
Dijon Honey Mustard	2 tbsp	140	13	180	6	0
Dijon Ranch	2 tbsp	170	18	190	2	0
Dutch Sweet'N Sour	2 tbsp	160	13	200	10	0

FOOD	PORTION	CAL.	FAT	SOD.	CARB.	FIB.
Marzetti (CONT.)						
Fat Free California French	2 tbsp	45	0	330	11	0
Fat Free Honey Dijon	2 tbsp	60	0	190	14	1
Fat Free Honey French	2 tbsp	45	0	330	11	0
Fat Free Italian	2 tbsp	15	0	450	3	0
Fat Free Peppercorn Ranch	2 tbsp	30	0	420	7	1
Fat Free Ranch	2 tbsp	30	0	430	7	1
Fat Free Raspberry	2 tbsp	70	0	150	18	0
Fat Free Slaw	2 tbsp	45	0	390	11	0
Fat Free Sweet & Sour	2 tbsp	45	0	290	14	0
Fat Free Thousand Island	2 tbsp	35	0	370	9	0
Garden Ranch	2 tbsp	180	19	250	1	0
Gusto Italian	2 tbsp	120	13	740	1	0
Honey Dijon	2 tbsp	140	13	170	6	0
Honey Dijon Ranch	2 tbsp	150	15	200	2	0
Honey French	2 tbsp	160	14	230	11	0
Honey French Blue Cheese	2 tbsp	160	13	260	11	0
House Caesar	2 tbsp	150	16	340	1	0
Italian With Olive Oil	2 tbsp	120	13	480	1	0
Light Blue Cheese	2 tbsp	60	6	650	4	0
Light Buttermilk Ranch	2 tbsp	90	9	280	3	0
Light California French	2 tbsp	80	6	360	8	0
Light Chunky Blue Cheese	2 tbsp	80	7	330	4	0
Light French	2 tbsp	40	2	320	6	0
Light French	2 tbsp	40	2	320	6	0
Light Honey French	2 tbsp	80	4	250	12	0
Light Italian	2 tbsp	60	5	570	3	0
Light Ranch	2 tbsp	90	8	430	7	0
Light Red Wine Vinegar & Oil	2 tbsp	20	1	490	3	0
Light Slaw	2 tbsp	60	7	380	10	0
Light Sweet & Sour	2 tbsp	100	6	260	11	0
Light Thousand Island	2 tbsp	70	5	350	6	0
Old Fashioned Poppyseed	2 tbsp	140	11	220	10	0
Olde Venice Italian	2 tbsp	130	13	490	2	0
Olde World Caesar	2 tbsp	150	16	340	1	0
Parmesan Pepper	2 tbsp	160	17	260	1	0
Peppercorn Ranch	2 tbsp	180	19	220	1	0
Poppyseed	2 tbsp	160	13	310	10	0

FOOD	PORTION	CAL.	FAT	SOD.	CARB.	FIB.
Marzetti (CONT.)						
Potato Salad Dressing	2 tbsp	120	13	300	7	0
Ranch	2 tbsp	180	20	260	1	0
Red Wine Vinegar & Oil	2 tbsp	130	14	460	2	0
Romano Cheese Caesar	2 tbsp	150	16	370	1	0
Romano Italian	2 tbsp	160	17	390	1	0
Savory Italian	2 tbsp	110	12	520	3	0
Slaw	2 tbsp	170	16	370	6	0
Southern Slaw	2 tbsp	100	11	210	14	0
Sweet & Saucy	2 tbsp	140	12	290	9	0
Sweet & Sour	2 tbsp	160	13	210	10	0
Thousand Island	2 tbsp	150	15	230	5	0
Vintage Champagne	2 tbsp	150	16	460	2	0
Wilde Raspberry	2 tbsp	150	12	65	12	0
Nasoya						
Creamy Dill	2 tbsp (1 oz)	63	5	145	3	tr
Creamy Italian	2 tbsp (1 oz)	60	5	187	3	tr
Garden Herb	2 tbsp (1 oz)	61	5	148	3	tr
Sesame Garlic	2 tbsp (1 oz)	63	5	137	3	tr
Thousand Island	2 tbsp (1 oz)	62	4	146	6	tr
Newman's Own						
Italian Light	1 tbsp (0.5 fl oz)	10	tr	170	tr	—
Olive Oil & Vinegar	1 tbsp (0.5 fl oz)	80	9	80	tr	—
Ranch	1 tbsp (0.5 fl oz)	90	9	80	1	—
Pfeiffer						
1000 Island	2 tbsp	140	14	220	4	0
California French	2 tbsp	140	12	290	9	0
French	2 tbsp	150	13	220	7	0
Honey Dijon	2 tbsp	140	13	170	6	0
Lite Italian	2 tbsp	50	5	410	3	0
Ranch	2 tbsp	180	20	260	1	0
Savory Italian	2 tbsp	110	12	520	3	0
Pritikin						
Dijon Balsamic Vinaigrette	2 tbsp (1 oz)	3	0	125	6	—
French	2 tbsp (1 oz)	35	0	130	8	—
Honey Dijon	2 tbsp (1 oz)	45	0	130	11	—
Honey French	2 tbsp (1 oz)	40	0	135	11	—
Italian	2 tbsp (1 oz)	20	0	115	5	—
Raspberry Vinaigrette	2 tbsp (1 oz)	45	0	70	11	—
Red Wing						
"K" Dressing	1 tbsp (0.5 oz)	70	7	90	4	0

FOOD	PORTION	CAL.	FAT	SOD.	CARB.	FIB.
Red Wing (CONT.)						
Chunky Blue Cheese	2 tbsp (1 oz)	130	13	290	3	0
Creamy Ranch	2 tbsp (1 oz)	150	15	280	2	0
French Traditional	2 tbsp (1 oz)	130	11	250	8	0
Italian Traditional	2 tbsp (1 oz)	100	9	550	4	0
Spicy Sweet French	2 tbsp (1 oz)	130	11	370	8	0
Thousand Island Thick & Rich	2 tbsp (1 oz)	110	9	270	8	0
S&W						
Blue Cheese Low Calorie	1 tbsp	25	2	200	2	—
Creamy Cucumber Low Calorie	1 tbsp	25	2	190	2	—
Creamy Italian Low Calorie	1 tbsp	10	1	180	1	—
French Low Calorie	1 tbsp	18	0	120	3	—
Italian No-Oil	1 tbsp	2	0	290	0	—
Russian Low Calorie	1 tbsp	25	1	120	4	—
Thousand Island Low Calorie	1 tbsp	25	2	105	2	—
Seven Seas						
⅓ Less Fat Creamy Italian	2 tbsp (1.1 oz)	60	5	500	2	0
⅓ Less Fat Italian w/ Olive Oil Blend	2 tbsp (1.1 oz)	45	4	460	2	0
⅓ Less Fat Ranch	2 tbsp (1.1 oz)	100	9	320	5	0
⅓ Less Fat Red Wine Vinegar & Oil	2 tbsp (1.1 oz)	45	4	320	3	0
⅓ Less Fat Viva Italian	2 tbsp (1.1 oz)	45	4	320	2	0
2 Cheese Italian	2 tbsp (1.1 oz)	70	7	240	3	0
Chunky Blue Cheese	2 tbsp (1.1 oz)	130	13	310	2	tr
Classic Caesar	2 tbsp (1.1 oz)	100	10	480	2	0
Creamy Italian	2 tbsp (1.1 oz)	120	12	510	1	0
Free Ranch	2 tbsp (1.2 oz)	45	0	330	11	1
Free Red Wine Vinegar	2 tbsp (1.1 oz)	15	0	410	3	0
Free Sour Cream & Onion Ranch	2 tbsp (1.2 oz)	50	0	300	11	1
Free Viva Italian	2 tbsp (1.1 oz)	10	0	480	2	1
Green Goddess	2 tbsp (1.1 oz)	130	13	260	1	0
Herbs & Spices	2 tbsp (1.1 oz)	90	9	290	1	0
Ranch	2 tbsp (1.1 oz)	160	17	260	2	0
Red Wine Vinegar & Oil	2 tbsp (1.1 oz)	90	9	500	2	0
Viva Italian	2 tbsp (1.1 oz)	90	9	370	2	0
Viva Russian	2 tbsp (1.1 oz)	150	16	210	3	0

FOOD	PORTION	CAL.	FAT	SOD.	CARB.	FIB.
Tree Of Life						
Cafe Venice	2 tbsp (1 oz)	100	12	170	2	0
Fat Free Blue Cheese	2 tbsp (1 oz)	15	1	260	2	—
Fat Free Honey French	2 tbsp (1 oz)	35	0	150	8	—
Fat Free Italian Garlic	2 tbsp (1 oz)	20	0	260	4	—
Fat Free Oriental Ginger	2 tbsp (1 oz)	15	0	310	3	—
Frisco's Raspberry	2 tbsp (1 oz)	120	11	80	5	0
Maison Caesar	2 tbsp (1 oz)	70	6	115	1	0
Shanghai Palace	2 tbsp (1 oz)	80	7	310	3	0
Ultra Slim-Fast						
French	1 tbsp	20	tr	150	4	0
Italian	1 tbsp	6	tr	170	1	0
W.J. Clark						
Ginger Orange Vinaigrette	1 tbsp	73	7	134	tr	0
Herbs & Romano	1 tbsp	67	6	111	2	0
Lemon Peppercorn	1 tbsp	72	7	135	tr	0
Lime Cilantro Vinaigrette	1 tbsp	73	8	147	tr	0
Poppy Seed	1 tbsp	75	6	106	3	0
Sweet Pepper Basil	1 tbsp	69	7	127	2	0
Tarragon Honey Mustard	1 tbsp	66	6	139	2	0
Walden Farms						
Fat Free Balsamic Vinaigrette	2 tbsp (1 oz)	15	0	360	3	0
Fat Free Bleu Cheese	2 tbsp (1 oz)	25	0	240	4	0
Fat Free Caesar	2 tbsp (1 oz)	25	0	360	4	0
Fat Free Creamy Italian With Parmesan	1 tbsp (1 oz)	25	0	360	4	0
Fat Free French Style	2 tbsp (1 oz)	25	0	360	4	0
Fat Free Honey Dijon	2 tbsp (1 oz)	25	0	240	6	0
Fat Free Italian	2 tbsp (1 oz)	10	0	290	2	0
Fat Free Ranch	2 tbsp (1 oz)	25	0	290	4	0
Fat Free Raspberry Vinaigrette	2 tbsp (1 oz)	20	0	290	4	0
Fat Free Russian	2 tbsp (1 oz)	30	0	240	6	0
Fat Free Sodium Free Italian	2 tbsp (1 oz)	10	0	0	2	0
Fat Free Sugar Free Italian	2 tbsp (1 oz)	0	0	290	0	0
Fat Free Thousand Island	2 tbsp (1 oz)	35	0	240	7	0
Italian With Sun Dried Tomato	2 tbsp (1 oz)	15	0	290	3	0
Ranch With Sun Dried Tomato	2 tbsp (1 oz)	25	0	290	4	0

FOOD	PORTION	CAL.	FAT	SOD.	CARB.	FIB.
Weight Watchers						
Fat Free Caesar	2 tbsp	10	0	390	1	0
Fat Free Caesar	1 pkg (0.75 oz)	5	0	290	1	0
Fat Free Creamy Italian	2 tbsp	30	0	360	7	0
Fat Free French Style	2 tbsp	40	0	200	9	0
Fat Free Honey Dijon	2 tbsp	45	0	150	11	0
Fat Free Italian	2 tbsp	10	0	360	2	0
Fat Free Ranch	2 tbsp	35	0	270	7	0
Fat Free Ranch	1 pkg (0.75 oz)	25	0	200	6	0
Wishbone						
Caesar Olive Oil	2 tbsp (1 oz)	90	10	400	2	0
Chunky Blue Cheese	2 tbsp (1 oz)	170	17	280	2	0
Classic House Italian	2 tbsp (1 oz)	140	14	360	2	0
Classic Olive Oil Italian	2 tbsp (1 oz)	70	6	400	4	0
Creamy Italian	2 tbsp (1 oz)	100	10	310	3	0
Creamy Roasted Garlic	2 tbsp (1 oz)	140	13	240	3	0
Deluxe French	2 tbsp (1 oz)	120	11	170	5	0
Fat Free Chunky Blue Cheese	2 tbsp (1 oz)	35	0	310	7	0
Fat Free Creamy Roasted Garlic	2 tbsp (1 oz)	40	0	280	9	0
Fat Free Honey Dijon	2 tbsp (1 oz)	45	0	270	10	0
Fat Free Italian	2 tbsp (1 oz)	15	0	280	2	0
Fat Free Ranch	2 tbsp (1 oz)	40	0	270	9	0
Fat Free Sweet & Spicy French	2 tbsp (1 oz)	30	0	220	7	0
Fat Free Thousand Island	2 tbsp (1 oz)	35	0	290	8	0
Honey Dijon	2 tbsp (1 oz)	130	10	390	9	0
Italian	2 tbsp (1 oz)	80	9	590	3	0
Lite Caesar With Olive Oil	2 tbsp	60	5	380	2	0
Lite Chunky Blue Cheese	2 tbsp (1 oz)	80	7	380	2	0
Lite Classic Dijon Vinaigrette	2 tbsp (1 oz)	60	5	400	3	0
Lite Creamy Italian	2 tbsp (1 oz)	60	4	240	7	0
Lite French	2 tbsp	50	2	250	9	0
Lite Italian	2 tbsp (1 oz)	24	1	380	2	0
Lite Ranch	2 tbsp (1 oz)	100	8	240	5	0
Lite Thousand Island	2 tbsp (1 oz)	80	5	250	7	0
Olive Oil Vinaigrette	2 tbsp (1 oz)	60	5	250	4	0
Ranch	2 tbsp (1 oz)	160	17	210	1	0
Robusto Italian	2 tbsp (1 oz)	100	10	610	4	0
Russian	2 tbsp (1 oz)	110	6	350	15	0
Santa Fe	2 tbsp (1 oz)	150	15	220	3	0

FOOD	PORTION	CAL.	FAT	SOD.	CARB.	FIB.
Wishbone (CONT.)						
Sierra	2 tbsp	150	16	260	2	0
Sweet 'N Spicy French	2 tbsp (1 oz)	130	12	330	6	0
Thousand Island	2 tbsp (1 oz)	130	12	340	7	0
SALMON						
CANNED						
chum w/ bone	3 oz	120	5	414	0	—
chum w/ bone	1 can (13.9 oz)	521	20	1797	0	—
pink w/ bone	3 oz	118	5	471	0	—
pink w/ bone	1 can (15.9 oz)	631	27	2514	0	—
sockeye w/ bone	3 oz	130	6	458	0	—
sockeye w/ bone	1 can (12.9 oz)	566	27	1987	0	—
Bumble Bee						
Keta	3.5 oz	160	8	490	0	—
Pink	3.5 oz	160	8	490	0	—
Pink Skinless & Boneless	3.25 oz	120	5	420	0	—
Red	3.5 oz	180	10	490	0	—
Red Skinless & Boneless	3.25 oz	130	6	420	0	—
Deming's						
Alaska Keta	½ cup	140	5	450	0	—
Alaska Pink	½ cup	140	6	450	0	—
Alaska Red Sockeye	½ cup	170	9	450	0	—
Double Q						
Alaska Pink	½ cup	140	6	450	0	—
Humpty Dumpty						
Alaska Chum	½ cup	140	2	450	0	—
Libby						
Keta	½ can (3.8 oz)	140	6	—	—	—
Pink	½ can (3.8 oz)	150	7	—	—	—
S&W						
Bluepack Fancy Diet	½ cup	188	11	45	0	—
Red Fancy Sockeye Bluepack	½ cup	190	10	590	0	—
FRESH						
atlantic baked	3 oz	155	7	48	0	—
chinook baked	3 oz	196	11	51	0	—
chum baked	3 oz	131	4	54	0	—
coho cooked	3 oz	157	6	50	0	—
coho cooked	½ fillet (5.4 oz)	286	12	91	0	—
coho raw	3 oz	124	5	39	0	—
pink baked	3 oz	127	4	73	0	—
roe raw	3.5 oz	207	10	—	1	—

FOOD	PORTION	CAL.	FAT	SOD.	CARB.	FIB.
sockeye cooked	3 oz	183	9	102	0	—
sockeye cooked	½ fillet (5.4 oz)	334	17	102	0	—
sockeye raw	3 oz	143	7	40	0	—
SMOKED						
chinook	1 oz	33	1	220	0	—
chinook	3 oz	99	4	666	0	—
Nathan's						
Nova	2 oz	80	3	1150	1	0
TAKE-OUT						
salmon cake	1 (3 oz)	241	15	602	6	—

SALSA

(*see also* KETCHUP, SAUCE, SPANISH FOODS)

FOOD	PORTION	CAL.	FAT	SOD.	CARB.	FIB.
Casa Fiesta						
Chili Salsa	1 oz	9	tr	117	2	—
Picante Mild	1 oz	9	tr	117	2	—
Chi-Chi's						
Hot	2 tbsp (1 oz)	10	0	160	1	0
Medium	1 tbsp (1 oz)	10	0	140	1	0
Mild	2 tbsp (1 oz)	10	0	150	1	0
Verde Medium	2 tbsp (1.2 oz)	15	0	180	3	0
Verde Mild	2 tbsp (1.2 oz)	15	0	180	3	0
Del Monte						
Mexicana	2 tbsp (1.1 oz)	5	0	200	2	1
Taquera	2 tbsp (1.1 oz)	5	0	220	2	1
Verde	2 tbsp (1.1 oz)	10	0	280	2	tr
Guiltless Gourmet						
Picante Hot	1 oz	6	0	133	1	tr
Picante Medium	1 oz	6	0	133	1	tr
Hain						
Hot	¼ cup	22	0	480	4	—
Mild	¼ cup	20	0	410	4	—
Heluva Good Cheese						
Cheese & Salsa	2 tbsp (1.1 oz)	80	6	210	3	0
Thick & Chunky Hot	2 tbsp (1.2 oz)	10	0	180	2	0
Thick & Chunky Mild	2 tbsp (1.2 oz)	10	0	180	2	0
Hot Cha Cha						
Medium	2 tbsp (1 oz)	5	0	0	2	—
Hunt's						
Alfresco Medium	2 tbsp (1.1 oz)	10	tr	199	2	tr
Alfresco Mild	2 tbsp (1.1 oz)	10	tr	199	2	tr
Hot	2 tbsp (1.1 oz)	27	tr	236	6	1
Medium	2 tbsp (1.1 oz)	27	tr	236	6	1
Mild	2 tbsp (1.1 oz)	27	tr	236	6	1

FOOD	PORTION	CAL.	FAT	SOD.	CARB.	FIB.
Hunt's (CONT.)						
Picante Medium	2 tbsp (1.1 oz)	11	tr	256	2	tr
Picante Mild	2 tbsp (1.1 oz)	11	tr	256	2	tr
Louise's						
Fat Free BBQ Black Bean	1 oz	10	0	110	2	0
Fat Free Black Bean	1 oz	10	0	110	2	0
Fat Free Medium	1 oz	10	0	80	3	1
Fat Free Mild	1 oz	10	0	80	3	1
Fat Free Nacho Queso	1 oz	15	0	45	3	0
Muir Glen						
Organic Fat Free Hot	2 tbsp (1.1 oz)	10	0	160	2	0
Organic Fat Free Medium	2 tbsp (1.1 oz)	10	0	160	2	0
Organic Fat Free Mild	2 tbsp (1.1 oz)	10	0	160	2	0
Newman's Own						
Bandito Hot	1 tbsp (0.7 oz)	6	tr	120	tr	—
Bandito Medium	1 tbsp (0.7 oz)	6	tr	45	tr	—
Bandito Mild	1 tbsp (0.7 oz)	6	tr	40	tr	—
Old El Paso						
Green Chili Medium	2 tbsp (1 oz)	10	0	110	2	tr
Homestyle	2 tbsp (1 oz)	5	0	110	1	0
Homestyle Mild	2 tbsp (1 oz)	5	0	110	1	0
Picante Hot	2 tbsp (1 oz)	10	0	230	2	0
Picante Medium	2 tbsp (1 oz)	10	0	230	2	0
Picante Mild	2 tbsp (1 oz)	10	0	230	2	0
Picante Thick'n Chunky Hot	2 tbsp (1 oz)	10	0	160	2	0
Picante Thick'n Chunky Medium	2 tbsp (1 oz)	10	0	140	2	0
Picante Thick'n Chunky Mild	2 tbsp (1 oz)	10	0	130	2	0
Pico De Gallo Hot	2 tbsp (1 oz)	5	0	260	2	tr
Pico De Gallo Medium	1 tbsp (1 oz)	5	0	260	2	tr
Salsa Verde	2 tbsp (1 oz)	10	0	95	2	0
Thick'n Chunky Hot	2 tbsp (1 oz)	10	0	130	2	0
Thick'n Chunky Medium	2 tbsp (1 oz)	10	0	140	2	0
Thick'n Chunky Mild	2 tbsp (1 oz)	10	0	140	2	0
Ortega						
Hot Green Chili	1 tbsp	6	0	190	2	—
Medium Green Chili	1 tbsp	6	0	190	1	—
Mild Green Chili	1 tbsp	8	0	190	2	—
Pace						
Picante	2 tbsp (1 fl oz)	7	0	294	2	tr
Thick & Chunky	2 tbsp (1 fl oz)	12	0	321	2	1

FOOD	PORTION	CAL.	FAT	SOD.	CARB.	FIB.
Progresso						
Italian Hot	2 tbsp (1 oz)	30	0	170	2	tr
Italian Medium	2 tbsp (1 oz)	10	0	170	2	tr
Italian Mild	2 tbsp (1 oz)	10	0	170	2	tr
Rosarita						
Chunky Hot	3 tbsp (1.5 oz)	25	tr	300	6	tr
Chunky Medium	3 tbsp (1.5 oz)	25	tr	350	6	tr
Chunky Mild	3 tbsp (1.5 oz)	25	tr	340	6	tr
Taco Salsa Chunky Medium	3 tbsp (1.5 oz)	25	tr	310	6	tr
Taco Salsa Chunky Mild	3 tbsp (1.5 oz)	25	tr	300	6	tr
Tabasco						
Picante	2 tbsp (1.5 oz)	17	tr	313	3	1
Taco Bell						
Smooth 'N Zesty Picante Medium	2 tbsp (1.1 oz)	15	0	190	3	tr
Smooth 'N Zesty Picante Mild	2 tbsp (1.1 oz)	15	0	190	3	tr
Thick 'N Chunky Salsa Hot	2 tbsp (1.1 oz)	15	0	240	2	tr
Thick 'N Chunky Salsa Medium	2 tbsp (1.1 oz)	15	0	240	2	tr
Thick 'N Chunky Salsa Mild	2 tbsp (1.1 oz)	15	0	240	3	tr
Tostitos						
Hot	2 tbsp (1 oz)	12	0	205	3	1
Medium	2 tbsp (1 oz)	12	0	205	3	1
Mild	2 tbsp (1 oz)	12	0	205	3	1
Tree Of Life						
Hot	2 tbsp (1 oz)	10	0	30	2	—
Medium	2 tbsp (1 oz)	10	0	30	2	—
Mild	2 tbsp (1 oz)	10	0	30	2	—
No Salt	2 tbsp (1 oz)	10	0	20	2	—
Watkins						
Salsa Seasoning Blend	⅛ tsp (0.5 g)	0	0	5	0	0
Tropical	2 tbsp (1 oz)	60	0	430	13	0
Wise						
Picante	2 tbsp	12	0	130	3	—
SALSIFY						
fresh sliced cooked	½ cup	46	tr	11	10	—
raw sliced	½ cup	55	tr	13	12	—
SALT/SEASONED SALT (*see also* SALT SUBSTITUTES)						
salt	1 tbsp (18 g)	0	0	6976	0	—

FOOD	PORTION	CAL.	FAT	SOD.	CARB.	FIB.
salt	1 tsp (6 g)	0	0	2325	0	—
Hain						
Sea Salt	1 tsp	0	0	2255	0	—
Sea Salt Iodized	1 tsp	0	0	2255	0	—
Morton						
Garlic	1 tsp	3	tr	—	—	—
Iodized	1 tsp	tr	0	—	—	—
Kosher	1 tsp	0	0	—	—	—
Lite	1 tsp	tr	0	—	—	—
Nature's Season Seasoning Blend	1 tsp	3	tr	—	—	—
Non-Iodized	1 tsp	0	0	—	—	—
Seasoned	1 tsp	4	tr	—	—	—
Watkins						
Bacon Cheese Salt	¼ tbsp (1 g)	0	0	280	0	0
Butter Salt	¼ tbsp (1 g)	0	0	330	0	0
Cheese Salt	¼ tbsp (1 g)	0	0	290	0	0
Garlic Salt	¼ tsp (1 g)	0	0	270	0	0
Salt & Vinegar Seasoning Blend	¼ tsp (1 g)	0	0	105	0	0
Seasoning Salt	¼ tsp (1 g)	0	0	270	0	0
Sour Cream & Onion Salt	¼ tbsp (1 g)	0	0	270	0	0
SALT SUBSTITUTES						
Cardia						
Salt Alternative	1 pkg (0.6 g)	0	0	135	0	—
Morton						
Salt Substitute	1 tsp	2	tr	—	—	—
Mrs. Dash						
Onion & Herb	⅛ tsp (0.02 oz)	2	0	1	tr	—
Papa Dash						
Lite Salt	½ tsp (1 g)	0	0	170	1	—
SANDWICH						
TAKE-OUT						
submarine w/ salami ham cheese lettuce tomato onion & oil	1	456	19	1650	51	—
SAPODILLA						
fresh	1	140	2	20	34	—
fresh cut up	1 cup	199	3	29	48	—
SAPOTES						
fresh	1	301	1	21	76	—

FOOD	PORTION	CAL.	FAT	SOD.	CARB.	FIB.
SARDINES						
CANNED						
atlantic in oil w/ bone	1 can (3.2 oz)	192	11	465	0	—
atlantic in oil w/ bone	2	50	3	121	0	—
pacific in tomato sauce w/ bone	1 can (13 oz)	658	44	1532	0	—
pacific in tomato sauce w/ bone	1	68	5	157	0	—
Del Monte						
In Tomato Sauce	1 fish (1.4 oz)	50	3	130	1	tr
Empress						
Skinless & Boneless Olive Oil	1 can (3.8 oz)	420	38	530	2	—
Skinless & Boneless Soy Oil	1 can (4.4 oz)	500	45	630	2	—
Port Clyde						
In Louisiana Hot Sauce	1 can (3.75 oz)	170	9	760	1	0
In Mustard Sauce	1 can (3.75 oz)	150	9	450	1	1
In Soybean Oil Select Small	1 can (3.3 oz)	220	17	360	0	0
In Soybean Oil With Hot Chilies	1 can (3.3 oz)	155	9	310	0	0
In Soybean Oil drained	1 can (3.3 oz)	220	17	360	0	0
In Spring Water	1 can (3.3 oz)	170	10	240	0	0
In Tomato Sauce	1 can (3.75 oz)	150	9	480	0	0
S&W						
Norwegian Brisling	1.5 oz	130	10	220	0	—
Underwood						
Brisling In Olive Oil	3.75 oz	260	20	450	1	—
In Mustard Sauce	3.75 oz	220	16	560	2	—
In Sild Oil drained	3.75 oz	460	42	120	1	—
In Soya Oil drained	3 oz	230	18	400	1	—
In Tomato Sauce	3.75 oz	220	16	500	2	—
With Tabasco Pepper Sauce drained	3 oz	220	16	400	1	—
Viking's Delight						
Brisling In Olive Oil	1 can (3.75 oz)	460	42	450	1	—
Brisling In Olive Oil drained	1 can (3.75 oz)	260	20	450	1	—
FRESH						
raw	3½ oz	135	5	100	0	—

SAUCE

(*see also* BARBECUE SAUCE, GRAVY, PIZZA, SALSA, SPAGHETTI SAUCE, TOMATO)

FOOD	PORTION	CAL.	FAT	SOD.	CARB.	FIB.
JARRED						
teriyaki	1 oz	30	0	1380	6	—
teriyaki	1 tbsp	15	0	690	3	—
Armour						
Chili Hot Dog	¼ cup (2.2 oz)	120	9	310	6	—
Meatless Sloppy Joe Sauce	¼ cup (2.2 oz)	30	0	430	7	—
Best Foods						
Tartar	1 tbsp (14 g)	70	8	190	tr	—
Bright Day						
Tartar	1 tbsp	50	5	—	—	—
Casa Fiesta						
Taco Mild	1 oz	9	tr	117	2	—
Cheez Whiz						
Cheese	2 tbsp (1.2 oz)	90	7	540	3	0
Cheese Jalapeno Pepper	2 tbsp (1.2 oz)	90	7	510	3	0
Cheese Mild Salsa	2 tbsp (1.2 oz)	100	7	530	3	0
Chi-Chi's						
Taco Thick & Chunky	1 tbsp (0.5 oz)	10	0	75	1	0
Contadina						
Sweet 'n Sour	2 tbsp	40	1	110	8	—
Del Monte						
Cocktail	¼ cup (2.7 oz)	100	0	910	24	0
Sloppy Joe Hickory Flavor	¼ cup (2.4 oz)	70	0	700	18	0
Sloppy Joe Italian Style	¼ cup (2.4 oz)	70	0	700	16	0
Sloppy Joe Original	¼ cup (2.4 oz)	70	0	680	16	0
El Molino						
Taco Red Mild	2 tbsp	10	0	170	2	—
Escoffier						
Diable	1 tbsp	20	0	160	4	—
Gebhardt						
Enchilada Sauce	3 tbsp (1.5 oz)	25	1	170	2	tr
Hot Dog Chili Sauce	2 tbsp	30	1	180	4	tr
Hot Sauce	½ tsp	tr	tr	55	tr	tr
Gold's						
Rib	1 oz	60	0	250	14	—
Golden Dipt						
Cajun Style	1 oz	90	8	360	5	—
Creole	1 oz	20	1	190	2	—
Dijonaise	1 oz	52	4	130	2	—
French White	1 oz	55	4	210	3	—
Ginger Teriyaki Marinade	1 oz	120	7	920	12	—
Lemon Butter Dill	1 oz	100	9	190	4	—

FOOD	PORTION	CAL.	FAT	SOD.	CARB.	FIB.
Golden Dipt (CONT.)						
Lemon Herb Marinade	1 oz	130	14	210	2	—
Seafood Cocktail	1 tbsp	20	0	210	5	—
Seafood Cocktail Extra Hot	1 tbsp	20	0	210	5	—
Tartar	1 tbsp	70	7	100	2	—
Tartar Lite	1 tbsp	50	4	40	4	—
Heinz						
Worcestershire	1 tbsp	6	0	170	1	—
Hellman's						
Tartar	1 tbsp (14 g)	70	8	190	tr	—
Heluva Good Cheese						
Cocktail	¼ cup (1.6 oz)	40	0	410	10	—
Hormel						
Not-So-Sloppy-Joe Sauce	¼ cup (2.2 oz)	70	0	720	15	1
House Of Tsang						
Bangkok Padang	1 tbsp (0.6 oz)	45	3	240	4	0
Hoisin	1 tsp (6 g)	15	0	105	3	0
Mandarin Marinade	1 tbsp (0.6 oz)	25	0	680	6	0
Saigon Sizzle	1 tbsp (0.6 oz)	40	1	350	8	0
Spicy Brown Bean	1 tsp (6 g)	15	0	125	3	0
Stir Fry Classic	1 tbsp (0.6 oz)	25	1	570	4	0
Stir Fry Sweet & Sour	1 tbsp (0.6 oz)	35	0	50	8	0
Stir Fry Szechuan Spicy	1 tbsp (0.6 oz)	20	1	490	4	0
Sweet & Sour Concentrate	1 tsp (6 g)	10	0	15	3	0
Teriyaki Korean	1 tbsp (0.6 oz)	30	1	430	6	0
Hunt's						
Chicken Sensations Barbecue Flavor	1 tbsp (0.5 oz)	35	3	308	3	tr
Chicken Sensations Italian Garlic	1 tbsp (0.5 oz)	30	3	326	1	1
Chicken Sensations Lemon Herb	1 tbsp (0.5 oz)	31	3	378	2	tr
Chicken Sensations South Western	1 tbsp (0.5 oz)	27	3	281	1	tr
Pepper Sauce Original	1 tsp (5.2 g)	1	tr	205	tr	0
Steak	1 tbsp (0.6 oz)	10	tr	256	2	tr
Just Rite						
Hot Dog	2 oz	60	3	220	6	tr
Ka-Me						
Black Bean Sauce	1 tbsp (0.5 oz)	10	0	550	2	1
Chili Sauce Hot Garlic	1 tbsp (0.5 oz)	15	0	115	4	1

FOOD	PORTION	CAL.	FAT	SOD.	CARB.	FIB.
Ka-Me (CONT.)						
Duck Sauce	2 tbsp (1 oz)	80	0	480	20	0
Fish Sauce	1 tbsp (0.5 fl oz)	10	0	1300	1	0
Hoisin Sauce	2 tbsp (1 oz)	45	0	620	10	1
Hot Sauce	1 tsp (5 g)	0	0	80	1	0
Lemon Sauce	1 tbsp (0.5 oz)	45	0	125	11	0
Mandarin Orange Sauce	2 tbsp (1 oz)	80	0	430	21	0
Oyster Sauce	1 tbsp (0.5 fl oz)	10	0	460	3	0
Plum	2 tbsp (1 fl oz)	80	0	420	19	0
Stir Fry Sauce	1 tbsp	10	0	570	1	0
Sweet & Sour	2 tbsp (1 fl oz)	50	0	270	13	0
Szechuan	1 tbsp (0.5 oz)	20	1	410	2	2
Tamari	1 tbsp (0.5 fl oz)	10	1	930	1	0
Tempura Sauce	2 tbsp (1 fl oz)	15	0	1790	3	0
Teriyaki Sauce	1 tbsp (0.5 fl oz)	10	0	480	2	0
Kikkoman						
Stir-Fry	1 tbsp	16	tr	369	3	1
Sweet & Sour	1 tbsp	19	tr	97	4	tr
Teriyaki	1 tbsp	15	0	626	3	0
Knorr						
Grilling And Broiling Chardonnay	1.6 oz	50	4	630	4	—
Grilling And Broiling Spicy Plum	1.7 oz	60	2	790	11	—
Grilling And Broiling Tequilla Lime	1.6 oz	50	3	690	6	—
Grilling And Broiling Tuscan Herb	1.6 oz	50	4	600	5	—
Microwave Hollandaise	1 oz	50	5	190	1	—
Microwave Mandarin Ginger	1.6 oz	50	4	690	5	—
Microwave Parmesano	1.6 oz	50	4	680	3	—
Microwave Vera Cruz	3.3 oz	70	3	580	9	—
Kraft						
Cocktail	¼ cup (2.3 oz)	60	1	800	13	1
Fat Free Tartar Sauce	2 tbsp (1.1 oz)	25	0	200	5	0
Lemon & Herb Tartar Sauce	2 tbsp (1 oz)	150	16	170	tr	0
Reduced Fat Sandwich Spread	1 tbsp (0.5 oz)	35	3	130	3	0
Sandwich Spread	1 tbsp (0.5 oz)	50	4	105	3	0
Sweet'n Sour	2 tbsp (1.2 oz)	60	0	125	14	0
Tartar	2 tbsp (1.1 oz)	90	9	170	4	2

FOOD	PORTION	CAL.	FAT	SOD.	CARB.	FIB.
La Choy						
Duck Sauce Sweet & Sour	1 tbsp	25	tr	40	7	tr
Sweet & Sour	1 tbsp	25	tr	40	7	tr
Lawry's						
Marinade Lemon Pepper	1 tbsp (0.5 oz)	10	1	380	1	—
Teriyaki Marinade	2 tbsp	72	tr	7100	11	tr
Lea & Perrins						
Steak	1 oz	40	tr	220	10	—
Worcestershire	1 tsp	5	tr	55	1	—
Worcestershire White Wine	1 tsp	4	tr	40	1	—
Manwich						
Bold	¼ cup (2.2 oz)	62	1	802	13	1
Burrito	¼ cup (2.2 oz)	25	tr	559	6	4
Mexican	¼ cup (2.2 oz)	27	tr	552	5	1
Original	¼ cup (2.2 oz)	32	tr	365	6	1
Taco	¼ cup (2.2 oz)	31	tr	587	7	1
Thick & Chunky	¼ cup (2.3 oz)	44	tr	737	9	1
Marzetti						
Teriyaki Stir-Fry	2 tbsp	80	2	820	14	0
McIlhenny						
7 Spice Chili	2 tbsp (1.1 fl oz)	16	tr	191	3	1
Sauce	2 tbsp (1.1 oz)	48	2	201	7	tr
Tabasco	1 tsp	1	tr	30	tr	tr
Mrs. Dash						
Steak	1 tbsp (0.4 oz)	17	tr	10	4	—
Newman's Own						
Bandito Diavalo Spicy	4 oz	70	2	530	11	—
Old El Paso						
Enchilada Hot	¼ cup (2 oz)	30	2	190	4	0
Enchilada Mild	¼ cup (2 oz)	25	1	160	4	0
Green Chili Enchilada Sauce	¼ cup (2.1 oz)	30	2	330	3	0
Taco Hot	1 tbsp (0.5 oz)	5	0	90	1	0
Taco Medium	1 tbsp (0.5 oz)	5	0	70	1	0
Taco Mild	1 tbsp (0.5 oz)	5	0	85	1	0
Taco Sauce	1 tbsp (0.5 oz)	5	0	85	1	0
Taco Sauce Extra Chunky Medium	1 tbsp (0.5 oz)	5	0	80	1	0
Taco Sauce Extra Chunky Mild	1 tbsp (0.5 oz)	5	0	80	1	0
Ortega						
Taco Thick & Smooth Hot	1 tbsp	8	0	105	2	0

FOOD	PORTION	CAL.	FAT	SOD.	CARB.	FIB.
Ortega (CONT.)						
Taco Thick & Smooth Mild	1 tbsp	8	0	115	2	0
Taco Western Style	1 oz	8	0	—	—	—
Progresso						
Alfredo	½ cup (4.4 oz)	310	27	670	5	0
Red Wing						
Chili Sauce	1 tbsp (0.6 oz)	20	0	220	5	0
Seafood Cocktail	¼ cup (2 oz)	90	1	830	22	0
Sauce Arturo						
Original	¼ cup (2.2 fl oz)	50	1	680	8	0
Simmer Chef						
Golden Honey Mustard	½ cup (4 fl oz)	150	2	400	30	1
Hearty Onion & Mushroom	½ cup (4 fl oz)	50	1	670	9	1
Snow's						
Newburg With Sherry	⅓ cup	120	8	520	10	—
Welsh Rarebit Cheese	½ cup	170	11	460	10	—
Taco Bell						
Taco Sauce Medium	2 tbsp (1.1 oz)	15	0	160	3	tr
Taco Sauce Mild	2 tbsp (1.1 oz)	15	0	160	3	tr
The Restaurant Hot Sauce	1 tsp (5 g)	0	0	50	0	0
Trappey						
Indi-Pep West Indian Style Pepper Sauce	1 tsp (0.1 oz)	1	tr	41	tr	tr
Mexi Pep Louisiana Hot Sauce	1 tsp (0.1 oz)	tr	tr	59	tr	tr
Pepper Sauce	1 tsp (0.2 oz)	1	tr	85	tr	tr
Red Devil Buffalo Style Hot Sauce	1 tsp (0.1 oz)	1	tr	59	tr	tr
Red Devil Cayenne Pepper Sauce	1 tsp (0.1 oz)	1	tr	44	tr	tr
Worcestershire Chef Magic	1 tsp (0.1 oz)	3	tr	39	1	tr
Watkins						
Inferno Hot Pepper Sauce	2 tbsp (1 oz)	35	0	930	8	1
Steak Sauce	1 tbsp (0.5 oz)	20	0	220	4	0
Wolf Brand						
Hot Dog	1.25 oz	44	2	199	4	—
MIX						
bearnaise as prep w/ milk & butter	1 cup	701	68	1265	18	—

FOOD	PORTION	CAL.	FAT	SOD.	CARB.	FIB.
cheese as prep w/ milk	1 cup	307	17	1566	23	—
curry as prep w/ milk	1 cup	270	15	1276	26	—
mushroom as prep w/ milk	1 cup	228	10	1533	24	—
sour cream as prep w/ milk	1 cup	509	30	1007	45	—
stroganoff as prep	1 cup	271	11	1829	34	—
sweet & sour as prep	1 cup	294	tr	779	73	—
teriyaki as prep	1 cup	131	1	4791	28	—
white as prep w/ milk	1 cup	241	13	796	21	—
Cajun King						
Etoufee Seasoning Mix	3.5 oz	383	6	1087	70	—
Jambalaya Seasoning Mix	3.5 oz	375	9	2855	61	—
Durkee						
A La King as prep	1 cup	60	4	800	8	0
Cheese as prep	¼ cup	25	2	260	4	0
Hollandaise as prep	2 tbsp	10	0	70	2	0
Nacho Cheese as prep	2 tbsp	25	2	180	2	0
White as prep	¼ cup	20	1	330	5	0
French's						
Cheese as prep	¼ cup	25	1	250	4	0
Hollandaise as prep	2 tbsp	10	0	75	2	0
Kikkoman						
Marinade For Meat	1 oz pkg	64	tr	—	—	—
Sweet & Sour	2⅛ oz pkg	228	tr	—	—	—
Teriyaki	1½ oz pkg	125	tr	—	—	—
Knorr						
Au Jus as prep	2 oz	8	tr	160	1	—
Bearnaise as prep	2 oz	170	17	340	5	—
Classic Brown Gravy as prep	2 oz	25	1	300	3	—
Demi-Glace as prep	2 oz	30	1	310	4	—
Hollandaise as prep	2 oz	170	18	310	5	—
Hunter as prep	2 oz	25	tr	340	4	—
Lyonnaise as prep	2 oz	20	tr	360	3	—
Mushroom as prep	2 oz	60	3	240	5	—
Napoli as prep	4 oz	100	3	960	17	—
Pepper as prep	2 oz	20	1	380	3	—
Watkins						
Beef Marinade	¼ tbsp (2 g)	5	0	160	1	0
Calypso Hot Pepper Sauce	1 tsp (5 g)	10	0	25	3	0
Caribbean Red Pepper Sauce	1 tsp (5 g)	10	0	25	3	0
Chicken & Pork Marinade	¼ tbsp (2 g)	5	0	280	2	0

FOOD	PORTION	CAL.	FAT	SOD.	CARB.	FIB.
Watkins (CONT.)						
Fish & Seafood Marinade	¼ tbsp (2 g)	10	0	100	1	0
Meat Magic	1 tsp (6 g)	10	0	190	2	0
SHELF-STABLE						
Cheez Whiz						
Cheese Sqeezable	2 tbsp (1.2 oz)	100	8	470	4	0
Fresh Gourmet						
Stir 'n Sauce Italian	1 tbsp (0.5 oz)	30	1	230	5	—

SAUERKRAUT

canned	½ cup	22	tr	780	5	—
Claussen						
Canned	½ cup	17	tr	—	—	—
Del Monte	½ cup (4.2 oz)	15	0	700	4	2
Eden						
Organic	½ cup (3.9 oz)	25	0	580	4	3
Hebrew National						
Gallon Kraut	½ cup	25	0	800	4	—
New Kraut	½ cup (3.1 oz)	50	1	550	11	—
Rosoff's						
Sauerkraut	½ cup (3.2 oz)	50	1	550	11	—
S&W						
Canned	½ cup	25	0	850	5	—
Schorr's						
New Kraut	½ cup (3.2 oz)	50	1	550	11	—
Seneca						
Canned	2 tbsp	5	0	192	0	1
SnowFloss						
Kraut	4 oz	28	0	780	4	1
Kraut Bavarian Style	4 oz	64	0	780	12	1
Vlasic						
Old Fashioned	1 oz	4	0	280	1	—

SAUERKRAUT JUICE

S&W						
Juice	4 oz	14	0	1120	3	—

SAUSAGE

(*see also* HOT DOG, SAUSAGE SUBSTITUTES)

bierschinken	3.5 oz	174	11	753	tr	—
bierwurst	3.5 oz	258	21	—	0	—
blutwurst uncooked	3½ oz	424	39	680	0	—
bockwurst	3.5 oz	276	25	700	0	—
bockwurst pork & veal raw	1 link (2.3 oz)	200	18	—	tr	—

FOOD	PORTION	CAL.	FAT	SOD.	CARB.	FIB.
bratwurst pork cooked	1 link (3 oz)	256	22	473	2	—
brotwurst pork	1 oz	92	8	315	1	—
brotwurst pork & beef	1 link (2.5 oz)	226	19	778	2	—
country-style pork cooked	1 link (½ oz)	48	4	168	tr	—
country-style pork cooked	1 patty (1 oz)	100	8	349	tr	—
fleischwurst	3.5 oz	305	29	829	0	—
gelbwurst uncooked	3½ oz	363	33	640	0	—
italian pork cooked	1 (2.4 oz)	216	17	618	1	—
italian pork cooked	1 (3 oz)	268	21	765	1	—
jagdwurst	3.5 oz	211	16	818	0	—
kielbasa pork	1 oz	88	8	305	1	—
knockwurst pork & beef	1 (2.4 oz)	209	19	687	1	—
knockwurst pork & beef	1 oz	87	8	286	1	—
mettwurst uncooked	3½ oz	483	45	1090	0	—
plockwurst uncooked	3½ oz	312	45	—	0	—
polish pork	1 (8 oz)	739	65	1989	4	—
polish pork	1 oz	92	8	248	tr	—
pork & beef cooked	1 link (½ oz)	52	5	105	tr	—
pork & beef cooked	1 patty (1 oz)	107	10	217	1	—
pork cooked	1 link (½ oz)	48	4	168	tr	—
pork cooked	1 patty (1 oz)	100	8	349	tr	—
regensburger uncooked	3½ oz	354	31	—	0	—
smoked beef cooked	1 sausage (1.4 oz)	134	12	—	—	—
smoked pork	1 link (2.4 oz)	265	22	1020	1	—
smoked pork	1 sm link (½ oz)	62	5	240	tr	—
smoked pork & beef	1 link (2.4 oz)	229	21	151	1	—
smoked pork & beef	1 sm link (½ oz)	54	5	151	tr	—
vienna canned	7 (4 oz)	315	28	1077	2	—
vienna canned	1 (½ oz)	45	4	152	tr	—
weisswurst uncooked	3½ oz	305	27	620	0	—
zungenwurst (tongue)	3.5 oz	285	24	—	0	—
Aidells						
Andouille Cajun Cooked	1 (3.5 oz)	220	17	770	1	—
Burmese Curry Cooked	1 (3.5 oz)	220	15	730	3	—
Chicken & Apple Fresh	1 (1.9 oz)	110	8	250	1	—
Chicken & Apple Smoked	1 (3.5 oz)	220	16	730	0	0
Chicken & Turkey New Mexico Smoked	1 (3.5 oz)	220	16	600	2	—
Chicken & Turkey Thai Fresh	1 (3.5 oz)	200	16	600	0	—
Chicken & Turkey Thai Smoked	1 (3.5 oz)	220	16	770	0	—

FOOD	PORTION	CAL.	FAT	SOD.	CARB.	FIB.
Aidells (CONT.)						
Chicken & Turkey With Sun-Dried Tomatoes & Basil Fresh	1 (3.5 oz)	200	15	550	1	—
Chicken & Turkey With Sun-Dried Tomatoes & Basil Smoked	1 (3.5 oz)	200	14	730	0	—
Creole Hot Cooked	1 (3.5 oz)	220	16	600	2	—
Duck & Turkey Smoked	1 (3.5 oz)	220	16	700	1	—
Hunter's Cooked	1 (3.5 oz)	240	19	720	0	—
Italian Hot Fresh	1 (3.5 oz)	230	18	550	0	—
Italian Mild Fresh	1 (3.5 oz)	230	18	550	0	—
Lamb & Beef With Rosemary Fresh	1 (3.5 oz)	220	16	600	2	—
Lemon Chicken Cooked	1 (3.5 oz)	220	16	700	1	—
Mexican Chorizo Beef Fresh	1 (3.5 oz)	400	37	550	3	—
Whiskey Fennel Cooked	1 (3.5 oz)	230	18	730	1	—
Armour						
Country Sausage Lower Salt	1 oz	110	11	—	—	—
Country Sausage Lower Salt Patties	1.5 oz	160	16	—	—	—
Country Sausage Lower Salt Links	1 oz	110	11	—	—	—
Pork	1 oz	110	11	—	—	—
Pork Links	1 oz	110	11	—	—	—
Pork Patties	1.5 oz	160	16	—	—	—
Vienna Sausage 25% Less Fat	3 (1.9 oz)	130	11	420	1	—
Vienna Sausage In BBQ Sauce	3 (2.1 oz)	160	14	550	4	—
Vienna Sausage In Beef Stock	3 (1.9 oz)	170	16	420	1	—
Vienna Sausage In Hot Sauce	3 (2.1 oz)	170	15	630	3	—
Vienna Sausage Smoked	3 (1.9 oz)	170	16	420	1	—
Banner						
Sausage Tripe	2 oz	90	5	430	2	—
Bilinski's						
Chicken & Vegetable	1 (3 oz)	80	2	530	2	tr
Chicken Italian With Peppers & Onions	1 (3 oz)	120	4	800	1	—

FOOD	PORTION	CAL.	FAT	SOD.	CARB.	FIB.
Golden Brown						
Beef	1	80	7	160	tr	—
Mild	1	100	10	150	tr	—
Spicy	1	100	9	150	tr	—
Healthy Choice						
Low Fat Smoked	2 oz	70	2	590	4	1
Low Fat Smoked Polska Kielbasa	2 oz	70	2	590	4	1
Hebrew National						
Beef Knocks	1 (3 oz)	260	25	670	—	—
Polish Beef	1 link	240	22	680	—	—
Hillshire						
Beer Bratwurst	1 (2 oz)	190	17	500	2	—
Bratwurst Fresh	1 (2 oz)	190	17	410	1	—
Bratwurst Light Fresh	1 (2 oz)	150	11	620	2	—
Bratwurst Spicy	1 (2 oz)	180	17	490	1	—
Flavorseal Kielbasa Polska	2 oz	190	17	540	2	—
Flavorseal Kielbasa Polska Beef	2 oz	190	17	550	2	—
Flavorseal Kielbasa Polska Lite	2 oz	130	11	512	1	—
Flavorseal Kielbasa Polska Mild	2 oz	190	17	530	2	—
Flavorseal Kielbasa Polska Turkey	2 oz	90	5	500	2	—
Flavorseal Smoked	2 oz	190	17	500	2	—
Flavorseal Smoked Beef	2 oz	180	16	490	2	—
Flavorseal Smoked Beef & Cheddar	2 oz	190	15	500	1	—
Flavorseal Smoked Country Recipe	2 oz	180	16	490	2	—
Flavorseal Smoked Hot	2 oz	180	16	510	2	—
Flavorseal Smoked Lite	2 oz	130	11	512	1	—
Flavorseal Smoked Turkey	2 oz	90	5	500	2	—
Flavorseal Smoked w/ Italian Seasoning	2 oz	200	18	500	1	—
Italian Mild	1 (2 oz)	190	17	490	1	—
Italian Mild Light	1 (2 oz)	150	11	620	2	—
Italian Hot	1 (2 oz)	180	17	500	1	—
Italian Hot Light	1 (2 oz)	150	11	620	2	—
Kielbasa Fresh Polska	1 (2 oz)	190	17	410	1	—
Kielbasa Fresh Polska Lower Fat	1 (2 oz)	150	11	620	2	-

FOOD	PORTION	CAL.	FAT	SOD.	CARB.	FIB.
Hillshire (CONT.)						
Links 80% Fat Free Cheddar Hots	2 oz	150	12	640	1	—
Links 80% Fat Free Kielbasa	2 oz	130	10	630	2	—
Links 80% Fat Free Smokies	2 oz	130	10	640	2	—
Links Brats Fully Cooked	2 oz	170	16	380	1	—
Links Bratwurst Smoked	2 oz	190	17	540	1	—
Links Bun Size Cheddarwurst	2 oz	200	18	480	1	—
Links Bun Size Kielbasa	2 oz	180	16	570	2	—
Links Bun Size Smoked	2 oz	180	16	570	2	—
Links Bun Size Smoked Beef	2 oz	180	16	570	2	—
Links Cheddarwurst	2 oz	190	17	480	1	—
Links Cheddarwurst Lite	1 link (2.7 oz)	190	15	680	2	—
Links Hot	2 oz	190	16	530	2	—
Links Hot Beef	2 oz	190	17	560	1	—
Links Hot Lite	1 link (2.7 oz)	190	15	690	2	—
Links Keilbasa Polska	2 oz	190	17	530	2	—
Links Keilbasa Polska Lite	1 link (2.7 oz)	190	15	610	2	—
Links Knockwurst Lite	2 oz	180	16	460	1	—
Links Lit'l Polskas	2 oz	180	16	600	2	—
Links Lit'l Smokies	2 oz	180	16	600	2	—
Links Lit'l Smokies Beef	2 oz	180	16	600	2	—
Links Lit'l Smokies Cheddar	2 oz	180	16	600	2	—
Links Lit'l Smokies Light	2 oz	120	8	600	1	—
Links Polish	2 oz	190	17	520	2	—
Links Smoked	2 oz	190	18	520	1	—
Mexican Style	1 (2 oz)	190	17	410	1	—
Mexican Style Lower Fat	1 (2 oz)	150	11	620	2	—
Hormel						
Light & Lean 97 Dinner Smoked	2 oz	60	2	640	2	0
Pickled Hot	6 (2 oz)	140	11	380	1	0
Pickled Smoked	6 (2 oz)	140	11	380	1	0
Vienna	2 oz	140	13	420	1	0
Vienna Chicken	2 oz	90	10	420	1	0
Jimmy Dean						
Brick Sausage	2.5 oz	270	25	550	0	0
Bulk	2.5 oz	300	28	490	0	0

FOOD	PORTION	CAL.	FAT	SOD.	CARB.	FIB.
Jimmy Dean (CONT.)						
Hickory Smoked Dinner Sausage	2 oz	170	14	500	2	0
Pattie Pre-Cooked	1 (1.9 oz)	230	22	520	0	0
Polska Kielbasa	2 oz	170	15	500	1	0
Sage Pattie	1 (2 oz)	200	19	340	0	0
Sausage Pattie Raw	1 (2 oz)	200	19	400	0	0
Skinless Link	2 (2 oz)	200	19	440	0	0
Skinless Link	4 (2 oz)	200	19	440	0	0
Jones						
Brown & Serve Bacon	1	90	8	140	tr	—
Brown & Serve Beef	1	90	9	190	tr	—
Brown & Serve Light	1	60	5	140	1	—
Brown & Serve Regular	1	100	10	150	tr	—
Cello Beef	1 slice (1 oz)	130	13	160	tr	—
Cello Hot Country	1 slice (1 oz)	110	10	170	tr	—
Cello Original	1 slice (1 oz)	100	10	180	tr	—
Dinner Link	1	280	28	310	tr	—
Golden Brown Light Links	1	60	5	130	1	—
Golden Brown Mild Pattie	1	150	14	220	tr	—
Italian	1	160	14	420	tr	—
Light Link	1	70	6	210	1	—
Little Link	1	140	14	170	tr	—
Patties	1	150	14	270	tr	—
Scrapple	1 slice	90	6	230	5	—
Scrapple	1 slice (1.5 oz)	90	6	230	5	—
Little Sizzlers						
Brown & Serve	2 patties (1.4 oz)	190	18	560	1	0
Brown & Serve	3 links (2.1 oz)	190	22	670	1	0
Cooked	2 patties (2 oz)	250	23	680	0	0
Cooked	3 links (1.4 oz)	210	20	570	0	0
Heat & Serve Pork cooked	3 links (1.4 oz)	210	20	570	0	0
Louis Rich						
Polska Kielbasa	2 oz	80	5	510	1	0
Smoked Sausage With Cheese cooked	1 (1 oz)	47	3	269	1	—
Turkey	2.5 oz	110	6	580	3	0
Turkey & Cheese Smoked	2 oz	90	5	550	2	0
Turkey Links	2 (2 oz)	90	6	470	0	0
Turkey Smoked	2 oz	90	5	510	2	0

FOOD	PORTION	CAL.	FAT	SOD.	CARB.	FIB.
Mr. Turkey						
Breakfast	2.5 oz	130	9	460	0	—
Hearty Blend Polish Kielbasa	1 oz	70	6	260	1	—
Hearty Blend Smoked	1 oz	70	6	260	1	—
Hot Smoked	1 oz	45	3	250	2	—
Italian Smoked	1 oz	45	3	250	2	—
Polish Kielbasa	1 oz	45	3	250	2	—
Smoked	1 oz	45	3	250	2	—
Old Smokehouse						
Summer Sausage	1 oz	110	10	400	1	0
Oscar Mayer						
Pork cooked	2 links (1.7 oz)	170	15	410	1	0
Smokies Beef	1 (1.5 oz)	120	11	430	1	0
Smokies Cheese	1 (1.5 oz)	130	12	450	1	0
Smokies Links	1 (1.5 oz)	130	12	430	1	0
Smokies Little	6 (2 oz)	170	16	580	1	0
Perdue						
Breakfast Links Turkey Cooked	2 links (2 oz)	100	6	430	0	—
Hot Italian Turkey Cooked	1 link (2.4 oz)	110	6	500	1	—
Sweet Italian Turkey Cooked	1 link (2.4 oz)	110	6	500	1	—
Rudy's Farm						
Italian Hot	2.5 oz	240	22	570	0	0
Italian Mild	2.5 oz	240	22	500	0	0
Italian Mild Natural Casing	1 (2 oz)	190	17	410	0	0
Morning Right Link	3 (2.9 oz)	150	10	260	0	0
Morning Right Pattie	2 (2.9 oz)	150	10	260	0	0
Pattie Pre-Cooked	1 (1.4 oz)	100	6	200	0	1
Smoked	4 (2.1 oz)	200	18	590	1	0
Sweet Link	1 (3.9 oz)	380	35	820	1	0
Shofar						
Knockwurst Beef	1 (3 oz)	260	23	620	tr	0
Tyson						
Country Pork	3.5 oz	320	29	905	1	—
Wampler Longacre						
Breakfast Links	1 (2.8 oz)	170	12	525	2	—
Italian Links	1 (2.8 oz)	170	12	520	2	—
Tinderlings Garlic & Pepper	1 (3.5 oz)	143	5	500	3	—
Turkey	1 pattie (2 oz)	120	8	380	4	—

FOOD	PORTION	CAL.	FAT	SOD.	CARB.	FIB.
Wampler Longacre (CONT.)						
Turkey	1 link (1 oz)	60	4	190	1	—
TAKE-OUT						
pork	1 link (0.5 oz)	48	4	168	tr	—
pork	1 patty (1 oz)	100	8	349	tr	—

SAUSAGE DISHES

FOOD	PORTION	CAL.	FAT	SOD.	CARB.	FIB.
Jimmy Dean						
Italian Sausage & Mozzarella Sandwich	1 (4.5 oz)	380	22	1030	28	2
Ovenstuffs						
French Roll Italian Sausage	1 (4.75 oz)	390	22	910	29	—
French Roll Pepperoni	1 (4.75 oz)	370	20	870	30	—
TAKE-OUT						
sausage roll	1 (2.3 oz)	311	24	—	22	1

SAUSAGE SUBSTITUTES

FOOD	PORTION	CAL.	FAT	SOD.	CARB.	FIB.
Knox Mountain Farm						
No-So-Sausage	1 serv (1/10 pkg)	120	1	696	6	2
LaLoma						
Linketts	2 (71 g)	140	8	320	2	—
Little Links	2 (46 g)	90	5	180	2	—
Lightlife						
Lean Links Breakfast	1.25 oz	69	3	250	4	—
Lean Links Italian	1.5 oz	83	3	300	5	—
Morningstar Farms						
Breakfast Links	2 (45 g)	90	5	300	3	—
Breakfast Patties	2 (76 g)	190	12	710	7	—
Country Crisp Patties	1 (71 g)	220	15	620	13	—
Grillers	1 (64 g)	180	12	350	5	—
White Wave						
Meatless Healthy Links	2 (1.6 oz)	140	10	450	5	3
Worthington						
Leanies	1 link (40 g)	100	6	440	2	—
Prosage Links	2 (45 g)	130	9	460	3	—
Saucettes	2 links (67 g)	150	11	430	3	—
Super-Links	1 (48 g)	100	7	440	3	—
Veja-Links	2 (62 g)	140	10	330	4	—

SAVORY

FOOD	PORTION	CAL.	FAT	SOD.	CARB.	FIB.
ground	1 tsp	4	tr	tr	1	—

SCALLOP

FOOD	PORTION	CAL.	FAT	SOD.	CARB.	FIB.
FRESH						
raw	3 oz	75	1	137	2	—

FOOD	PORTION	CAL.	FAT	SOD.	CARB.	FIB.
FROZEN						
Mrs. Paul's						
Fried	2 oz	160	7	320	18	—
HOME RECIPE						
breaded & fried	2 lg	67	3	144	3	—
TAKE-OUT						
breaded & fried	6 (5 oz)	386	19	919	38	—
SCONE						
apricot scone	1	232	7	201	39	—
Finnegan's						
Irish Raisin	1 (2.7 oz)	90	2	176	20	1
TAKE-OUT						
cheese	1 (1.75 oz)	182	9	—	22	1
fruit	1 (1.75 oz)	158	5	—	27	2
orange poppy	1 (3 oz)	260	6	400	47	2
plain	1 (1.75 oz)	181	7	—	27	1
SCROD						
Gorton's						
Microwave Entree Baked	1 pkg	320	18	420	18	—
SCUP						
fresh baked	3 oz	115	3	46	0	—
SEA BASS						
(*see* BASS)						
SEATROUT						
(*see* TROUT)						
SEAWEED						
agar dried	1 oz	87	tr	29	23	—
agar fresh	1 oz	tr	tr	3	2	—
irishmoss fresh	1 oz	14	tr	19	4	—
kelp fresh	1 oz	12	tr	66	3	—
kombu fresh	1 oz	12	tr	66	3	—
laver fresh	1 oz	10	tr	14	1	—
nori fresh	1 oz	10	tr	14	1	—
spirulina dried	1 oz	83	2	309	7	—
spirulina fresh	1 oz	7	tr	28	1	—
tangle fresh	1 oz	12	tr	66	3	—
wakame fresh	1 oz	13	tr	249	3	—
Eden						
Agar Agar Bars	1 tbsp (2.5 oz)	10	0	10	2	2
Agar Agar Flakes	1 tbsp (2.5 oz)	10	0	10	2	2
Arame	½ cup (0.3 oz)	30	0	120	7	7

FOOD	PORTION	CAL.	FAT	SOD.	CARB.	FIB.
Eden (CONT.)						
Hiziki	½ cup (0.3 oz)	30	0	160	6	6
Kombu	3.5 in piece (3.3 g)	10	0	90	2	1
Nori	1 sheet (2.5 g)	10	0	5	1	1
Sushi Nori	1 sheet (2.5 g)	10	0	5	1	1
Wakame	½ cup (0.3 oz)	25	0	660	4	4
Wakame Flakes	½ cup (0.3 oz)	25	0	720	4	4
Maine Coast						
Alaria	⅓ cup (7 g)	18	0	301	3	2
Dulse	⅓ cup (7 g)	18	0	122	3	2
Dulse Flakes	1 oz	75	1	493	13	9
Kelp	⅓ cup (7 g)	17	0	312	3	3
Kelp Crunch	1 bar (1 oz)	129	6	109	14	2
Kelp Crunch Peanut-Raisin	1 bar (1 oz)	129	6	109	14	2
Laver	⅓ cup (7 g)	22	0	113	3	3
Sea Seasoning Dulse	1 g	3	0	17	1	—
Sea Seasoning Dulse With Celery	1 g	3	0	17	1	—
Sea Seasoning Dulse With Garlic	1 g	3	0	13	1	—
Sea Seasoning Dulse With Sesame	1 g	3	0	6	1	—
Sea Seasoning Kelp	1 g	3	0	35	1	—
Sea Seasoning Kelp With Cayenne	1 g	3	0	35	1	—
Sea Seasoning Nori	1 g	3	0	8	1	—
Sea Seasoning Nori With Ginger	1 g	3	0	3	1	—

SEITAN

(*see* WHEAT)

SEMOLINA

FOOD	PORTION	CAL.	FAT	SOD.	CARB.	FIB.
dry	½ cup	303	tr	1	61	3

SESAME

FOOD	PORTION	CAL.	FAT	SOD.	CARB.	FIB.
seeds	1 tsp	16	2	1	tr	—
seeds dried	1 tbsp	52	5	1	2	—
seeds dried	1 cup	825	72	16	34	—
seeds roasted & toasted	1 oz	161	14	3	7	—
sesame butter	1 tbsp	95	8	2	4	1
sesame crunch candy	1 oz	146	9	—	14	—
sesame crunch candy	20 pieces (1.2 oz)	181	12	—	18	—
sesame sticks	1 oz	153	10	422	13	—

FOOD	PORTION	CAL.	FAT	SOD.	CARB.	FIB.
sesame sticks unsalted	1 oz	153	10	8	13	—
tahini from roasted & toasted kernels	1 tbsp	89	8	17	3	—
tahini from stone ground kernels	1 tbsp	86	7	11	4	—
tahini from unroasted kernels	1 tbsp	85	8	0	3	—
Arrowhead						
Sesame Tahini	1 oz	170	17	5	4	—
Casbah						
Tahini Sauce Mix as prep	¼ cup	160	13	160	10	tr
Eden						
Sesame Shake	½ tsp (1.5 g)	10	1	40	0	tr
Sesame Shake Garlic	½ tsp (1.5 g)	10	1	35	0	tr
Sesame Shake Organic Seaweed	½ tsp (1.5 g)	10	1	35	0	tr
Erewhon						
Sesame Butter	2 tbsp (32 g)	190	17	20	3	—
Sesame Tahini	2 tbsp (32 g)	200	18	65	3	—
Joyva						
Tahini	2 tbsp (1 oz)	200	18	25	3	1
Planters						
Nut Mix	1 oz	150	12	240	9	2
Stone-Buhr						
Seeds Raw	4 tsp (1 oz)	180	16	10	3	1
SESBANIA						
flower	1	1	0	0	tr	—
flowers	1 cup	5	tr	3	1	—
flowers cooked	1 cup	23	tr	11	5	—
SHAD						
american baked	3 oz	214	15	56	0	—
roe baked w/ butter & lemon	3.5 oz	126	3	73	2	—
roe raw	3½ oz	130	2	—	2	—
SHALLOTS						
dried	1 tbsp	3	0	1	1	—
raw chopped	1 tbsp	7	tr	1	2	—
SHARK						
batter-dipped & fried	3 oz	194	12	103	5	—
raw	3 oz	111	4	67	0	—
SHEEPSHEAD FISH						
cooked	1 fillet (6.5 oz)	234	3	136	0	—

FOOD	PORTION	CAL.	FAT	SOD.	CARB.	FIB.
cooked	3 oz	107	1	62	0	—
raw	3 oz	92	2	61	0	—
SHELLFISH						
(*see individual names,* SHELLFISH SUBSTITUTES)						
SHELLFISH SUBSTITUTES						
crab imitation	3 oz	87	1	715	1	—
scallop imitation	3 oz	84	tr	676	9	—
shrimp imitation	3 oz	86	1	599	8	—
surimi	1 oz	28	tr	40	2	—
surimi	3 oz	84	1	122	6	—
Louis Kemp						
Crab Delights Chunk Style	2 oz	54	tr	320	5	—
Lobster Delights	2 oz	60	tr	470	6	—
Maryland Style Cakes	2.5 oz	154	9	780	10	—
Ocean Magic						
Imitation King Crab	3 oz	80	tr	740	11	—
SHELLIE BEANS						
canned	½ cup	37	tr	408	8	—
SHERBET						
(*see also* ICES AND ICE POPS)						
orange	½ cup (4 fl oz)	132	2	44	29	—
orange	½ gal	2158	31	706	469	—
orange	1 bar (2.75 fl oz)	91	1	30	20	—
orange home recipe	½ cup	120	2	30	24	—
Borden						
Orange	½ cup	110	1	40	25	—
Bresler's						
All Flavors	3.5 oz	140	2	—	30	—
Hood						
Lime Orange Lemon	½ cup (3.1 oz)	120	1	35	26	0
Orange	½ cup (3.1 oz)	120	1	35	26	0
Rainbow Swirl	½ cup (3.1 oz)	120	1	30	26	0
Raspberry Orange Lime	½ cup (3.1 oz)	120	1	30	26	0
Sealtest						
Lime	½ cup (3 oz)	130	1	30	28	0
Orange	½ cup (3 oz)	130	1	30	28	0
Rainbow Orange Red Raspberry Lime	½ cup (3 oz)	130	1	25	28	0
Red Raspberry	½ cup (3 oz)	130	1	25	28	0
SHRIMP						
CANNED						
canned	3 oz	102	2	143	1	—

FOOD	PORTION	CAL.	FAT	SOD.	CARB.	FIB.
canned	1 cup	154	3	216	1	—
Robinson						
Canned Shrimp	2 oz	58	1	—	—	—
S&W						
Deveined Medium Whole Shrimp	2 oz	65	0	—	1	—
FRESH						
cooked	4 large	22	tr	49	0	—
cooked	3 oz	84	1	190	0	—
raw	4 large	30	tr	42	tr	—
raw	3 oz	90	1	126	1	—
FROZEN						
Cajun Cookin'						
Shrimp Creole	12 oz	390	11	1130	55	—
Shrimp Etouffee	17 oz	360	9	1170	52	—
Shrimp Jambalaya	12 oz	450	20	800	43	—
Gorton's						
Butterfly Shrimp	4 oz	160	tr	540	16	—
Microwave Crunchy Shrimp	5 oz	380	20	870	35	—
Microwave Entree Shrimp Scampi	1 pkg	390	30	470	21	—
Shrimp Crisps	4 oz	280	15	740	26	—
Mrs. Paul's						
Entrees Light Seafood & Clams With Linguini	10 oz	240	5	750	36	—
Van De Kamp's						
Breaded Butterfly	7 (4 oz)	280	14	580	28	2
Breaded Popcorn	20 (4 oz)	270	13	610	28	1
Breaded Whole	7 (4 oz)	240	10	520	26	2
TAKE-OUT						
breaded & fried	3 oz	206	10	292	10	—
breaded & fried	6 to 8 (6 oz)	454	25	1447	40	—
jambalaya	¾ cup	188	5	83	26	8

SMELT

FOOD	PORTION	CAL.	FAT	SOD.	CARB.	FIB.
rainbow cooked	3 oz	106	3	65	0	—
rainbow raw	3 oz	83	2	51	0	—

SNACKS

(*see also* CHIPS, FRUIT SNACKS, NUTS MIXED, POPCORN, PRETZELS)

FOOD	PORTION	CAL.	FAT	SOD.	CARB.	FIB.
oriental mix	1 oz	155	12	235	9	—
pork skins	1 oz	154	9	521	0	—
pork skins barbecue	1 oz	152	9	756	1	—
trail mix	1 cup (5.3 oz)	693	44	343	67	—

FOOD	PORTION	CAL.	FAT	SOD.	CARB.	FIB.
trail mix	1 oz	131	8	65	13	—
trail mix tropical	1 oz	115	5	3	19	—
trail mix w/ chocolate chips	1 oz	137	9	34	13	—
trail mix w/ chocolate chips	1 cup (5.1 oz)	707	47	177	66	—
Bakem-ets						
Hot'N Spicy	21 pieces (1 oz)	150	9	750	1	—
Snacks	21 pieces (1 oz)	160	10	850	2	—
Big Dipper						
Bagel Chips Lowfat Barbeque	12 (1 oz)	110	2	190	21	1
Bagel Chips Lowfat Garlic	12 (1 oz)	120	2	295	21	1
Bagel Chips Lowfat Original	12 (1 oz)	110	2	150	21	1
Bugles						
Nacho Cheese	1 oz	160	9	250	17	—
Ranch	1 oz	150	9	290	16	—
Snacks	1 oz	150	8	290	18	—
Cheetos						
Cheddar Valley	26 pieces (1 oz)	160	9	240	16	1
Crunchy	26 pieces (1 oz)	150	9	310	17	1
Curls	15 pieces (1 oz)	150	9	270	17	1
Flamin' Hot	26 pieces (1 oz)	150	9	240	16	1
Light	38 pieces (1 oz)	140	6	280	19	1
Paws	16 pieces (1 oz)	160	10	310	15	1
Puffed Ball	38 pieces (1 oz)	160	10	360	16	1
Puffs	33 pieces (1 oz)	160	9	330	16	1
Cheez Doodles						
Crunchy	1 oz	160	10	230	16	—
Puffed	1 oz	150	9	360	16	—
Cheez Waffies						
Snacks	1 oz	140	8	420	14	—
Chex						
Snack Mix Barbeque	½ cup (1.1 oz)	130	5	330	20	1
Snack Mix Cool Sour Cream And Onion	½ cup (1 oz)	130	4	310	21	2
Snack Mix Golden Cheddar	½ cup (1 oz)	130	4	310	20	1
Snack Mix Traditional	⅔ cup (1.2 oz)	150	5	410	23	2
Combos						
Cheddar Cheese Cracker	1 pkg (1.7 oz)	250	13	520	28	1
Cheddar Cheese Cracker	1 oz	140	8	300	16	0
Cheddar Cheese Pretzel	1 pkg (1.8 oz)	240	9	560	33	1
Cheddar Cheese Pretzel	1 oz	130	5	310	18	0

FOOD	PORTION	CAL.	FAT	SOD.	CARB.	FIB.
Combos (CONT.)						
Chili Cheese w/ Corn Shell	1 oz	140	6	420	17	1
Chili Cheese w/ Corn Shell	1 pkg (1.7 oz)	230	11	710	29	2
Mustard Pretzel	1 pkg (1.8 oz)	230	8	500	35	1
Mustard Pretzel	1 oz	130	4	270	19	1
Nacho Cheese Pretzel	1 pkg (1.7 oz)	230	8	580	34	1
Nacho Cheese Pretzel	1 oz	130	5	320	19	1
Nacho Cheese w/ Tortilla Shell	1 oz	140	6	380	17	1
Nacho Cheese w/ Tortilla Shell	1 pkg (1.7 oz)	230	11	640	30	1
Peanut Butter Cracker	1 oz	140	8	260	15	1
Pepperoni & Cheese Pizza	1 oz	140	7	280	17	0
Pepperoni & Cheese Pizza	1 pkg (1.7 oz)	240	11	480	30	1
Pizzeria Pretzel	1 pkg (1.8 oz)	230	8	520	35	1
Pizzeria Pretzel	1 oz	130	5	290	19	1
Tortilla Ranch	1 oz	140	7	350	17	1
Tortilla Ranch	1 bag (1.7 oz)	240	12	610	29	1
Cornnuts						
Barbecue	1 oz	120	4	270	22	2
Nacho Cheese	1 oz	120	4	180	22	2
Original	1 oz	120	4	170	22	2
Original	1 pkg (2 oz)	260	8	340	40	4
Picante	1 oz	120	4	260	22	2
Ranch	1 oz	120	4	190	20	2
Doo Dads						
Snacks	1 oz	130	6	360	17	—
Energy Food Factory						
Poprice Cheddar Cheese	½ oz	60	3	110	8	—
Poprice Herb & Garlic	½ oz	50	2	70	10	—
Poprice Lite	½ oz	50	2	70	9	—
Poprice Original No Salt	½ oz	45	0	1	11	—
Estee						
Snack Crisps Apple Cinnamon	27 crisps (1 oz)	130	3	110	24	1
Snack Crisps Apple Cinnamon	1 pkg (0.66 oz)	90	2	70	16	tr
Snack Crisps Chocolate	1 pkg (0.66 oz)	90	2	70	15	1
Snack Crisps Chocolate	30 crisps (1 oz)	130	3	110	23	2
Snack Crisps Lemon	1 pkg (0.66 oz)	90	2	70	16	tr

FOOD	PORTION	CAL.	FAT	SOD.	CARB.	FIB.
Estee (CONT.)						
Snack Crisps Lemon	30 (1 oz)	130	3	110	23	tr
Snack Crisps Ranch	1 pkg (0.6 oz)	90	2	135	15	0
Snack Crisps Ranch	30 (1 oz)	130	3	200	22	tr
Snack Crisps White Cheddar	1 pkg (0.6 oz)	90	2	135	14	tr
Snack Crisps With Cheddar	27 crisps (1 oz)	130	3	200	22	tr
Frito Lay						
Corn Nuggets Toasted	1.38 oz	170	5	265	29	—
Funyums						
Onion Rings	11 pieces (1 oz)	140	7	265	18	1
Hapi						
Chili Bits	½ cup (1 oz)	110	0	180	25	1
Health Valley						
Cheddar Lites	0.75 oz	40	2	35	4	tr
Cheddar Lites With Green Onion	0.75 oz	40	2	35	4	tr
Innovative Foods						
Roasted Sweet Corn	1 pkg (0.8 oz)	76	0	5	17	2
Lance						
Cheese Balls	1 pkg (32 g)	190	13	420	16	—
Crunchy Cheese Twists	1 pkg (42 g)	260	16	290	25	—
Gold-N-Chees	1 pkg (39 g)	180	9	410	23	—
Pork Skins	1 pkg (14 g)	80	5	270	0	—
Pork Skins BBQ	1 pkg (14 g)	80	5	400	0	—
Mr. Peanut						
Peanut Butter Crisps Graham	12 pieces (1.1 oz)	150	8	100	18	2
Munchos						
Snack	16 pieces (1 oz)	160	10	230	15	—
Pita Puffs						
Barbeque	35 (1 oz)	120	3	150	20	1
Lowfat Garlic	35 (1 oz)	110	1	125	22	1
Lowfat Original	35 (1 oz)	110	1	170	22	1
Lowfat Salsa	35 (1 oz)	110	1	290	21	1
Pizza	35 (1 oz)	120	2	230	21	1
Ranch	35 (1 oz)	120	2	195	21	1
Planters						
Cheez Balls	1 oz	150	10	300	15	1
Cheez Balls	1 pkg (1 oz)	150	10	330	15	1
Cheez Curls	1 oz	150	10	310	15	1
Cheez Curls	1 pkg (1.2 oz)	190	12	380	19	1
Heat Snack Mix	1 oz	140	8	230	13	2

FOOD	PORTION	CAL.	FAT	SOD.	CARB.	FIB.
Snyder's						
Cheddar Cheese Twists	1 oz	150	8	200	17	—
Kruncheez	1 oz	160	10	170	15	—
Onion Toasters	1 oz	150	8	280	17	3
Snack Mix	1 oz	170	8	410	11	tr
Sopaipillas Apple & Cinnamon	1 oz	150	8	15	18	1
Splurge						
Snack Mix Fat Free Original	⅔ cup (1 oz)	100	0	340	25	tr
Ultra Slim-Fast						
Lite N' Tasty Cheese Curls	1 oz	110	3	360	20	3
Weight Watchers						
Cheese Curls	1 pkg (0.5 oz)	70	3	85	10	0
SNAIL						
cooked	3 oz	233	1	350	13	—
raw	3 oz	117	tr	175	7	—
SNAPPER						
cooked	3 oz	109	1	48	0	—
cooked	1 fillet (6 oz)	217	3	96	0	—
raw	3 oz	85	1	54	0	—
SODA						
(*see also* DRINK MIXERS, MINERAL/BOTTLED WATER, SPORTS DRINKS)						
club	12 oz	0	0	75	0	—
cola	12 oz	151	tr	14	39	—
cream	12 oz	191	0	43	49	—
diet cola	12 oz	2	0	21	tr	—
diet cola w/ Equal	12 oz	2	0	21	tr	—
diet cola w/ saccharin	12 oz	2	0	57	tr	—
ginger ale	12 oz can	124	0	25	32	—
grape	12 oz	161	0	57	42	—
lemon lime	12 oz	149	0	41	38	—
orange	12 oz	177	0	49	46	—
pepper type	12 oz	151	tr	38	38	—
quinine	12 oz	125	0	15	32	—
root beer	12 oz	152	0	49	39	—
tonic water	12 oz	125	0	15	32	—
7 Up						
Cherry	1 oz	13	0	—	—	—
Cherry Diet	1 oz	tr	0	—	—	—
Diet	1 oz	tr	0	—	—	—

FOOD	PORTION	CAL.	FAT	SOD.	CARB.	FIB.
7 Up (CONT.)						
Gold	1 oz	13	0	—	—	—
Gold Diet	1 oz	tr	0	—	—	—
Original	1 oz	12	0	—	—	—
After The Fall						
Raspberry Ginger Ale	1 can (12 oz)	150	0	25	36	0
Barrelhead						
Root Beer	8 fl oz	110	0	25	27	0
Burst						
Cola Strawberry	8 fl oz	117	0	0	31	—
Canada Dry						
Birch Beer Brown	8 fl oz	110	0	40	27	0
Birch Beer Clear	8 fl oz	110	0	40	27	0
Black Cherry Wishniak	8 fl oz	130	0	40	32	0
Cactus Cooler	8 fl oz	110	0	40	27	0
California Strawberry	8 fl oz	110	0	45	27	0
Club	8 fl oz	0	0	60	0	0
Club Sodium Free	8 fl oz	0	0	0	0	0
Concord Grape	8 fl oz	120	0	45	29	0
Diet Ginger Ale	8 fl oz	0	0	60	0	0
Diet Ginger Ale Cherry	8 fl oz	0	0	60	0	0
Diet Ginger Ale Cranberry	8 fl oz	0	0	50	tr	0
Diet Ginger Ale Lemon	8 fl oz	5	0	60	0	0
Diet Tonic Water	8 fl oz	0	0	35	0	0
Diet Tonic Water Twist Of Lime	8 fl oz	0	0	45	0	0
Ginger Ale	8 fl oz	100	0	20	25	0
Ginger Ale Cherry	8 fl oz	110	0	25	27	0
Ginger Ale Cranberry	8 fl oz	100	0	15	25	0
Ginger Ale Golden	8 fl oz	100	0	10	24	0
Ginger Ale Lemon	8 fl oz	100	0	20	25	0
Half & Half	8 fl oz	110	0	25	27	0
Hi-Spot	8 fl oz	110	0	50	28	0
Island Lime	8 fl oz	140	0	15	33	0
Jamaica Cola	8 fl oz	110	0	10	27	0
Lemon Sour	8 fl oz	100	0	15	21	0
Peach	8 fl oz	120	0	40	30	0
Pina Pineapple	8 fl oz	110	0	40	26	0
Seltzer	8 fl oz	0	0	10	0	0
Seltzer Cherry	8 fl oz	0	0	10	0	0
Seltzer Cranberry Lime	8 fl oz	0	0	10	0	0
Seltzer Grapefruit	8 fl oz	0	0	10	0	0
Seltzer Lemon Lime	8 fl oz	0	0	10	0	0

FOOD	PORTION	CAL.	FAT	SOD.	CARB.	FIB.
Canada Dry (CONT.)						
Seltzer Mandarin Orange	8 fl oz	0	0	10	0	0
Seltzer Peach	8 fl oz	0	0	10	0	0
Seltzer Raspberry	8 fl oz	0	0	10	0	0
Seltzer Strawberry	8 fl oz	0	0	10	0	0
Seltzer Tropical	8 fl oz	0	0	10	0	0
Sunripe Orange	8 fl oz	140	0	45	35	0
Tahitian Treat	8 fl oz	150	0	45	36	0
Tonic Water	8 fl oz	100	0	15	24	0
Tonic Water Twist Of Lime	8 fl oz	100	0	20	24	0
Vanilla Cream	8 fl oz	120	0	40	30	0
Vichy Water	8 fl oz	0	0	490	0	0
Wild Cherry	8 fl oz	110	0	40	28	0
Clearly 2						
Black Cherry	8 fl oz	2	0	9	0	—
Key Lime	8 fl oz	2	0	9	0	—
Clearly Canadian						
Alpine Fruit & Berries	8 fl oz	90	0	9	23	—
Boysenberry Mist	8 fl oz	2	0	9	0	—
Coastal Cranberry	8 fl oz	90	0	9	22	—
Country Raspberry	8 fl oz	80	0	9	19	—
Green Apple	8 fl oz	80	0	9	19	—
Mountain Blackberry	8 fl oz	100	0	9	24	—
Orchard Peach Strawberry	8 fl oz	90	0	9	22	—
Soda	8 fl oz	0	0	5	0	—
Summer Strawberry	8 fl oz	80	0	9	19	—
Western Loganberry	8 fl oz	80	0	9	19	—
Wild Cherry	8 fl oz	90	0	9	23	—
Coca-Cola						
Cherry	8 fl oz	104	0	4	28	—
Classic	8 fl oz	97	0	9	27	—
Classic Caffeine-Free	8 fl oz	97	0	9	27	—
Coke II	8 fl oz	105	0	4	29	—
Diet	8 fl oz	1	0	4	tr	—
Diet Cherry	8 fl oz	1	0	4	tr	—
Diet Coke Caffeine-free	8 fl oz	1	0	4	tr	—
Cott						
Cola	8 fl oz	110	0	10	27	0
Ginger Ale	8 fl oz	90	0	20	20	0
Grape	8 fl oz	130	0	25	30	0
Orange	8 fl oz	140	0	25	33	0
Pineapple	8 fl oz	130	0	25	32	0

FOOD	PORTION	CAL.	FAT	SOD.	CARB.	FIB.
Cott (CONT.)						
Punch	8 fl oz	130	0	25	32	0
Seltzer	8 fl oz	0	0	0	0	0
Crush						
Cherry	8 fl oz	140	0	30	35	0
Grape	8 fl oz	110	0	—	—	0
Orange	8 fl oz	140	0	—	—	0
Orange Diet	8 fl oz	0	0	—	0	0
Pineapple	8 fl oz	140	0	30	35	0
Strawberry	8 fl oz	130	0	—	—	0
Tropical Fruit Punch	1 bottle (10 fl oz)	180	0	20	44	0
Tropical Fruit Punch	1 can (11.5 fl oz)	200	0	—	—	—
Diet Rite						
Black Cherry Salt/ Sodium Free	8 fl oz	2	0	0	1	—
Cola	8 fl oz	1	0	0	tr	—
Cola Caffeine/Sugar Free	8 fl oz	1	0	7	tr	—
Cola Salt/Sodium Free	8 fl oz	1	0	tr	tr	—
Fruit Punch Salt/Sodium Free	8 fl oz	2	0	0	tr	—
Golden Peach Salt/ Sodium Free	8 fl oz	2	0	0	tr	—
Key Lime Salt/Sodium Free	8 fl oz	7	0	0	2	—
Pink Grapefruit Salt/ Sodium Free	8 fl oz	2	0	0	1	—
Red Raspberry Salt/ Sodium Free	8 fl oz	3	0	tr	1	—
Tangerine Salt/Sodium Free	8 fl oz	2	0	0	tr	—
White Grape Salt/ Sodium Free	8 fl oz	1	0	0	tr	—
Dr Pepper						
Diet	1 oz	tr	0	—	—	—
Free	1 oz	12	0	—	—	—
Free Diet	1 oz	tr	0	—	—	—
Original	1 oz	13	0	—	—	—
Dr. Nehi						
Soda	8 fl oz	100	0	35	26	—
Fanta						
Ginger Ale	8 fl oz	86	0	4	23	—
Grape	8 fl oz	117	0	9	31	—
Orange	8 fl oz	118	0	9	32	—
Root Beer	8 fl oz	111	0	4	29	—

FOOD	PORTION	CAL.	FAT	SOD.	CARB.	FIB.
Fresca						
Soda	8 fl oz	3	0	1	tr	—
Health Valley						
Ginger Ale	12 oz	153	1	30	35	0
Rootbeer Old Fashioned	12 oz	120	1	12	26	—
Sarsaparilla Rootbeer	12 oz	153	1	27	35	—
Wild Berry	12 oz	142	1	27	33	—
Hires						
Cream	8 fl oz	130	0	30	0	0
Cream Soda Diet	8 fl oz	0	0	35	0	0
Original Mocha	8 fl oz	100	0	45	24	0
Original Mocha Diet	8 fl oz	5	0	45	0	0
Root Beer	8 fl oz	130	0	45	31	0
Root Beer Diet	8 fl oz	0	0	70	0	0
IBC						
Root Beer	8 oz	110	0	40	29	—
Kick						
Soda	8 fl oz	120	0	35	32	—
Like						
Cola	1 oz	13	0	—	—	—
Cola Sugar Free	1 oz	tr	0	—	—	—
Lucozade						
Soda	7 oz	136	0	—	36	0
Manischewitz						
Seltzer No Salt Added No Calories	8 fl oz	0	0	9	0	—
Mello Yellow						
Diet	8 fl oz	4	0	tr	tr	—
Soda	8 fl oz	119	0	9	32	—
Minute Maid						
Berry	8 fl oz	111	0	9	30	—
Diet Orange	8 fl oz	2	0	0	0	—
Fruit Punch	8 fl oz	117	0	10	32	—
Grape	8 fl oz	121	0	9	32	—
Grapefruit	8 fl oz	108	0	9	29	—
Orange	8 fl oz	118	0	0	32	—
Peach	8 fl oz	110	0	9	29	—
Pineapple	8 fl oz	109	0	9	30	—
Raspberry	8 fl oz	111	0	9	30	—
Soda	8 fl oz	110	0	11	29	—
Strawberry	8 fl oz	122	0	9	33	—
Mountain Dew						
Diet	8 fl oz	2	0	0	tr	—
Soda	8 fl oz	118	0	21	30	—

FOOD	PORTION	CAL.	FAT	SOD.	CARB.	FIB.
Mr. PiBB						
Diet	8 fl oz	1	0	2	tr	—
Soda	6 oz	97	0	7	26	—
Mug						
Cream	8 fl oz	122	0	21	32	—
Diet Cream	8 fl oz	2	0	29	0	—
Diet Root Beer	8 fl oz	1	0	26	tr	—
Root Beer	8 fl oz	141	0	26	29	—
Nehi						
Cream	8 fl oz	120	0	0	32	—
Fruit Punch	8 fl oz	120	0	35	34	—
Ginger Ale	8 fl oz	90	0	35	24	—
Grape	8 fl oz	120	0	35	32	—
Orange	8 fl oz	130	0	35	35	—
Peach	8 fl oz	130	0	35	34	—
Pineapple	8 fl oz	130	0	0	36	—
Quinine Water	8 fl oz	90	0	35	23	—
Root Beer	8 fl oz	120	0	35	32	—
Strawberry	8 fl oz	120	0	35	32	—
Wild Red	8 fl oz	120	0	33	32	—
Old Colony						
Grape	8 fl oz	140	0	40	32	0
Orangina						
Sparkling Citrus	6 fl oz	80	0	0	19	—
Pepsi						
Caffeine Free	8 fl oz	105	0	0	27	—
Diet	8 fl oz	1	0	tr	tr	—
Diet Caffeine Free	8 fl oz	1	0	tr	tr	—
Regular	8 fl oz	105	0	0	27	—
Ramblin' Root Beer						
Ramblin' Root Beer	8 fl oz	120	0	4	33	—
Razing Razberry						
Cola	8 fl oz	117	0	0	31	—
Royal Crown						
Caffeine Free Cola	8 fl oz	110	0	35	29	—
Cherry	8 fl oz	110	0	35	29	—
Cola	8 fl oz	100	0	35	28	—
Diet	8 fl oz	1	0	tr	tr	—
Diet Caffeine Free	8 fl oz	1	0	tr	tr	—
Diet Cranberry Apple Salt/Sodium Free	8 fl oz	2	0	1	tr	—
Diet Cranberry Salt/ Sodium Free	8 fl oz	2	0	1	tr	—

FOOD	PORTION	CAL.	FAT	SOD.	CARB.	FIB.
Royal Mistic						
'N Juice Black Cherry	12 fl oz	146	0	26	36	—
'N Juice Peach Vanilla	12 fl oz	146	0	18	36	—
'N Juice Tangerine Orange	12 fl oz	146	0	30	36	—
'N Juice Tropical Supreme	12 fl oz	152	0	14	38	—
'N Juice Wild Berry	12 fl oz	156	0	30	38	—
Caribbean Fruit Punch	16 fl oz	230	0	5	57	—
Grape Strawberry	16 fl oz	230	0	5	57	—
Sparkling Diet With Lime Kiwi	11.1 fl oz	0	0	<90	0	—
Sparkling Diet With Raspberry Boysenberry	11.1 fl oz	0	0	<90	0	—
Sparkling Diet With Royal Peach	11.1 fl oz	0	0	<90	0	—
Sparkling Diet With Wild Cherry	11.1 fl oz	0	0	<90	0	—
Sparkling With Lime Kiwi	11.1 fl oz	112	0	38	28	—
Sparkling With Mandarin Orange Pineappple	11.1 fl oz	120	0	18	30	—
Sparkling With Mango Passion	11.1 fl oz	112	0	34	28	—
Sparkling With Raspberry Boysenberry	11.1 fl oz	112	0	24	28	—
Sparkling With Royal Peach	11.1 fl oz	112	0	30	28	—
Sparkling With Wild Cherry	11.1 fl oz	112	0	28	28	—
Schweppes						
Bitter Lemon	8 fl oz	110	0	45	28	0
Club	8 fl oz	0	0	70	0	0
Club Sodium Free	8 fl oz	0	0	0	0	0
Diet Ginger Ale	8 fl oz	0	0	75	0	0
Diet Ginger Ale Dry Grape	8 fl oz	2	0	90	0	0
Diet Ginger Ale Raspberry	8 fl oz	0	0	75	0	0
Ginger Ale	8 fl oz	90	0	50	22	0
Ginger Ale Dry Grape	8 fl oz	100	0	50	26	0
Ginger Ale Raspberry	8 fl oz	100	0	50	26	0

FOOD	PORTION	CAL.	FAT	SOD.	CARB.	FIB.
Schweppes (CONT.)						
Ginger Beer	8 fl oz	100	0	90	25	0
Grape	8 fl oz	130	0	55	33	0
Grapefruit	8 fl oz	110	0	75	27	0
Lemon Sour	8 fl oz	110	0	25	26	0
Lemon-Lime	8 fl oz	100	0	75	25	0
Seltzer Black Berry	8 fl oz	0	0	10	0	0
Seltzer Lemon	8 fl oz	0	0	10	0	0
Seltzer Lemon Lime	8 fl oz	0	0	10	0	0
Seltzer Lime	8 fl oz	0	0	10	0	0
Seltzer Orange	8 fl oz	0	0	10	0	0
Seltzer Peaches & Cream	8 fl oz	0	0	10	0	0
Seltzer Raspberry	8 fl oz	0	0	0	0	0
Tonic Citrus	8 fl oz	90	0	25	20	0
Tonic Cranberry	8 fl oz	90	0	25	20	0
Tonic Raspberry	8 fl oz	90	0	25	20	0
Tonic Water Diet	8 fl oz	0	0	85	0	0
Shasta						
Black Cherry	1 can (12 oz)	170	0	54	41	0
Caffeine Free Cola	1 can (12 oz)	160	0	45	41	—
Cherry Cola	1 can (12 oz)	160	0	45	39	—
Club Soda	1 can (12 oz)	0	0	90	0	—
Cola	1 can (12 oz)	170	0	45	42	0
Creme	1 can (12 oz)	190	0	45	47	0
Diet Birch Beer	12 oz	4	0	—	—	—
Diet Black Cherry	1 can (12 oz)	0	0	55	0	0
Diet Caffeine Free Cola	1 can (12 oz)	0	0	55	0	0
Diet Cherry Cola	1 can (12 oz)	0	0	55	0	0
Diet Cola	1 can (12 oz)	0	0	45	0	0
Diet Creme	1 can (12 oz)	0	0	55	0	0
Diet Doc Shasta	1 can (12 oz)	0	0	45	0	0
Diet Ginger Ale	1 can (12 oz)	0	0	55	0	0
Diet Grape	1 can (12 oz)	0	0	55	0	0
Diet Grapefruit	1 can (12 oz)	0	0	55	0	0
Diet Grapefruit	1 can (12 oz)	0	0	45	0	0
Diet Kiwi-Strawberry	1 can (12 oz)	0	0	45	0	0
Diet Lemon-Lime Twist	1 can (12 oz)	0	0	55	0	0
Diet Orange	1 can (12 oz)	0	0	55	0	0
Diet Pineapple-Orange	1 can (12 oz)	0	0	55	0	0
Diet Raspberry Creme	1 can (12 oz)	0	0	45	0	0
Diet Red Pop	1 can (12 oz)	0	0	55	0	0
Diet Root Beer	1 can (12 oz)	0	0	55	0	0
Diet Strawberry	1 can (12 oz)	0	0	55	0	0

FOOD	PORTION	CAL.	FAT	SOD.	CARB.	FIB.
Shasta (CONT.)						
Diet Strawberry-Peach	1 can (12 oz)	0	0	55	0	0
Doc Shasta	1 can (12 oz)	160	0	45	39	0
Fruit Punch	1 can (12 oz)	200	0	45	50	0
Ginger Ale	1 can (12 oz)	130	0	45	32	0
Grape	1 can (12 oz)	190	0	45	48	0
Kiwi-Strawberry	1 can (12 oz)	170	0	45	43	0
Lemon-Lime Twist	1 can (12 oz)	150	0	45	38	0
Moon Mist	1 can (12 oz)	180	0	45	46	0
Orange	1 can (12 oz)	200	0	45	49	0
Peach	1 can (12 oz)	170	0	45	43	0
Pineapple	1 can (12 oz)	200	0	45	51	0
Pineapple-Orange	1 can (12 oz)	180	0	45	46	0
Quinine/Tonic	1 can (12 oz)	130	0	45	32	0
Raspberry Creme	1 can (12 oz)	170	0	45	44	0
Red Pop	1 can (12 oz)	170	0	45	43	0
Root Beer	1 can (12 oz)	170	0	45	42	0
Strawberry	1 can (12 oz)	190	0	45	46	0
Strawberry-Peach	1 can (12 oz)	170	0	45	42	0
Slice						
Diet Lemon Lime	8 fl oz	5	0	1	tr	—
Diet Mandarin	8 fl oz	5	0	10	tr	—
Lemon Lime	8 fl oz	100	0	10	26	—
Mandarin Orange	8 fl oz	128	0	10	33	—
Red	8 fl oz	128	0	10	33	—
Snapple						
Amazin' Grape	8 fl oz	120	0	5	28	—
Cherry Lime Ricky	8 fl oz	110	0	0	27	—
Creme D'Vanilla	8 fl oz	130	0	0	33	—
French Cherry	8 fl oz	120	0	0	29	—
Kiwi Peach	8 fl oz	120	0	0	29	—
Kiwi Strawberry	8 fl oz	130	0	5	33	—
Mango Madness	8 fl oz	130	0	5	33	—
Passion Supreme	8 fl oz	120	0	0	29	—
Peach Melba	8 fl oz	120	0	0	31	—
Raspberry	8 fl oz	120	0	0	31	—
Seltzer Black Cherry	8 fl oz	0	0	0	0	—
Seltzer Lemon Lime	8 fl oz	0	0	0	0	—
Seltzer Original	8 fl oz	0	0	0	0	—
Seltzer Tangerine	8 fl oz	0	0	0	0	—
Tru Root Beer	8 fl oz	110	0	0	29	—
Sprite						
Diet	8 fl oz	3	0	0	0	—
Soda	8 fl oz	100	0	31	26	—

FOOD	PORTION	CAL.	FAT	SOD.	CARB.	FIB.
Sundrop						
Cherry	8 fl oz	130	0	15	21	0
Diet	8 fl oz	5	0	65	0	0
Soda	8 fl oz	140	0	20	34	0
Sunkist						
Cactus Cooler	8 fl oz	110	0	40	27	0
Cherry	8 fl oz	140	0	35	35	0
Diet Citrus	8 fl oz	0	0	90	0	0
Diet Orange	8 fl oz	5	0	75	0	0
Fruit Punch	8 fl oz	130	0	35	33	0
Orange	8 fl oz	140	0	40	35	0
Peach	8 fl oz	120	0	40	30	0
Pineapple	8 fl oz	140	0	35	35	0
Strawberry	8 fl oz	140	0	35	34	0
TAB						
Soda	8 fl oz	1	0	4	tr	—
Tropical Chill						
Cola	8 fl oz	117	0	0	31	—
Diet	8 fl oz	1	0	0	tr	—
Upper 10						
Diet	8 fl oz	3	0	0	1	—
Diet Salt/Sodium Free	8 fl oz	3	0	0	1	—
Salt Free	8 fl oz	100	0	0	29	—
Soda	8 fl oz	100	0	35	28	—
Welch's						
Sparkling Apple	12 oz	180	0	—	—	—
Sparkling Grape	12 oz	180	0	—	—	—
Sparkling Orange	12 oz	180	0	—	—	—
Sparkling Strawberry	12 oz	180	0	—	—	—
Wink						
Diet	8 fl oz	5	0	95	1	0
Soda	8 fl oz	130	0	35	31	0
Yoo-Hoo						
Original	9 fl oz	150	tr	200	31	tr
SOLDIER BEANS						
Bean Cuisine						
Dried	½ cup	115	1	5	—	5
SOLE						
FRESH						
cooked	1 fillet (4.5 oz)	148	2	133	0	—
cooked	3 oz	99	1	89	0	—
lemon raw	3½ oz	85	1	80	0	—
raw	3½ oz	90	1	100	0	—

FOOD	PORTION	CAL.	FAT	SOD.	CARB.	FIB.
FROZEN						
Gorton's						
Fishmarket Fresh	5 oz	110	1	140	1	—
Microwave Entree In Lemon Butter	1 pkg	380	24	560	17	—
Microwave Entree In Wine Sauce	1 pkg	180	8	770	3	—
Mrs. Paul's						
Light Fillets	1 fillet	240	10	450	20	—
Van De Kamp's						
Lightly Breaded Fillets	1 (4 oz)	220	11	410	17	0
Natural Fillets	1 (4 oz)	110	2	125	0	0
TAKE-OUT						
battered & fried	3.2 oz	211	11	484	15	—
breaded & fried	3.2 oz	211	11	484	15	—

SORBET
(*see* ICES AND ICE POPS)

SORGHUM

FOOD	PORTION	CAL.	FAT	SOD.	CARB.	FIB.
sorghum	½ cup	325	3	—	72	—

SOUFFLE

FOOD	PORTION	CAL.	FAT	SOD.	CARB.	FIB.
cheese	3.5 oz	253	20	—	10	tr
grand marnier	1 cup	109	4	58	14	—
lemon chilled	1 cup	176	tr	108	34	—
raspberry chilled	1 cup	173	tr	108	34	—
spinach	1 cup	218	18	763	3	—

SOUP
(FAST FACT: Canned chicken noodle soup is the No. 1 selling food item in supermarkets. Three hundred and fifty million cans are purchased each year.)

FOOD	PORTION	CAL.	FAT	SOD.	CARB.	FIB.
CANNED						
asparagus cream of as prep w/ milk	1 cup	161	8	1041	16	—
asparagus cream of as prep w/ water	1 cup	87	4	981	11	—
beef broth ready-to-serve	1 cup	16	1	782	tr	—
beef broth ready-to-serve	1 can (14 oz)	27	1	1294	tr	—
beef noodle as prep w/ water	1 cup	84	3	952	9	—
black bean turtle soup	1 cup	218	1	922	40	—
black bean as prep w/water	1 cup	116	2	1198	20	—
celery cream of as prep w/ milk	1 cup	165	10	1010	15	—

FOOD	PORTION	CAL.	FAT	SOD.	CARB.	FIB.
celery cream of as prep w/ water	1 cup	90	6	949	9	—
celery cream of not prep	1 can (10¾ oz)	219	14	2308	21	—
cheese as prep w/ milk	1 cup	230	15	1020	16	—
cheese as prep w/ water	1 cup	155	10	959	11	—
cheese not prep	1 can (11 oz)	377	25	2331	26	—
chicken broth as prep w/ water	1 cup	39	1	776	1	—
chicken cream of as prep w/ milk	1 cup	191	11	1046	15	—
chicken cream of as prep w/ water	1 cup	116	7	986	9	—
chicken gumbo as prep w/ water	1 cup	56	1	955	8	—
chicken noodle as prep w/ water	1 cup	75	2	1107	9	—
chicken rice as prep w/ water	1 cup	251	2	814	7	—
clam chowder manhattan as prep w/ water	1 cup	77	2	1029	12	—
clam chowder new england as prep w/ water	1 cup	95	3	914	12	—
clam chowder new england as prep w/ milk	1 cup	163	7	992	17	—
consomme w/ gelatin not prep	1 can (10½ oz)	71	0	1550	4	—
consomme w/ gelatin as prep w/ water	1 cup	29	0	637	2	—
escarole ready-to-serve	1 cup	27	2	3865	2	—
french onion as prep w/ water	1 cup	57	2	1053	8	—
gazpacho ready-to-serve	1 cup	57	2	1183	1	—
minestrone as prep w/ water	1 cup	83	3	911	11	—
mushroom cream of as prep w/ milk	1 cup	203	14	1076	15	—
mushroom cream of as prep w/ water	1 cup	129	9	1031	9	—
oyster stew as prep w/ milk	1 cup	134	8	1040	10	—
oyster stew as prep w/ water	1 cup	59	4	980	4	—
pepperpot as prep w/ water	1 cup	103	5	970	9	—
potato cream of as prep w/ milk	1 cup	148	6	1060	17	—

FOOD	PORTION	CAL.	FAT	SOD.	CARB.	FIB.
potato cream of as prep w/ water	1 cup	73	2	1000	11	—
scotch broth as prep w/ water	1 cup	80	3	1012	9	—
split pea w/ ham as prep w/ water	1 cup	189	4	1008	28	—
tomato as prep w/ milk	1 cup	160	6	932	22	—
tomato as prep w/water	1 cup	86	2	872	17	—
vegetarian vegetable as prep w/ water	1 cup	72	2	823	12	—
vichyssoise	1 cup	148	6	1060	17	—
Campbell						
Asparagus Cream Of as prep	8 oz	80	4	820	10	—
Bean Homestyle as prep	8 oz	130	1	700	25	—
Bean With Bacon as prep	8 oz	140	4	840	21	—
Beef as prep	8 oz	80	2	830	10	—
Beef Broth as prep	8 oz	16	0	820	1	—
Beef Noodle Homestyle as prep	8 oz	80	4	810	7	—
Beef Noodle as prep	8 oz	70	3	830	7	—
Beefy Mushroom as prep	8 oz	60	3	960	5	—
Broccoli Cream Of as prep	8 oz	80	5	790	8	—
Broccoli Cream Of as prep w/ 2% milk	8 oz	140	7	850	14	—
Celery Cream Of as prep	8 oz	100	7	820	8	—
Cheddar Cheese as prep	8 oz	110	6	810	10	—
Chicken Alphabet as prep	8 oz	80	3	800	10	—
Chicken Noodle-O's as prep	8 oz	70	2	820	9	—
Chicken Vegetable as prep	8 oz	70	3	850	8	—
Chicken & Pasta With Garden Vegetables	1 cup (8.4 oz)	90	1	850	14	1
Chicken & Stars as prep	8 oz	60	2	870	7	—
Chicken 'n Dumplings as prep	8 oz	80	3	960	9	—
Chicken Barley as prep	8 oz	70	2	850	10	—
Chicken Broth as prep	8 oz	30	2	710	2	—
Chicken Broth & Noodles as prep	8 oz	45	1	860	8	—

FOOD	PORTION	CAL.	FAT	SOD.	CARB.	FIB.
Campbell (CONT.)						
Chicken Cream Of as prep	8 oz	110	7	810	9	—
Chicken Gumbo as prep	8 oz	60	2	900	8	—
Chicken Mushroom Creamy as prep	8 oz	120	8	920	8	—
Chicken Noodle Homestyle as prep	8 oz	70	3	880	8	—
Chicken Noodle as prep	8 oz	60	2	900	8	—
Chicken With Rice as prep	8 oz	60	3	790	7	—
Chili Beef as prep	8 oz	140	5	840	20	—
Chunky Chicken Nuggets w/ Vegetables & Noodles	10¾ oz	190	6	1060	24	—
Clam Chowder Manhattan Style as prep	8 oz	70	2	820	10	—
Clam Chowder New England as prep	8 oz	80	3	870	12	—
Clam Chowder New England as prep w/ whole milk	8 oz	150	7	930	17	—
Consomme as prep	8 oz	25	0	750	2	—
Curly Noodle With Chicken as prep	8 oz	80	3	800	11	—
French Onion as prep	8 oz	60	2	900	9	—
Green Pea as prep	8 oz	160	3	820	25	—
Healthy Request Bean With Bacon as prep	8 oz	140	4	470	22	—
Healthy Request Chicken Noodle as prep	8 oz	60	2	460	8	—
Healthy Request Chicken With Rice as prep	8 oz	60	3	480	7	—
Healthy Request Cream Of Mushroom as prep	8 oz	60	2	460	9	—
Healthy Request Cream Of Chicken	8 oz	70	2	490	11	—
Healthy Request Hearty Chicken Vegetable	8 oz	120	2	460	16	—
Healthy Request Ready-To-Serve Chicken Broth	8 oz	10	0	400	1	—

FOOD	PORTION	CAL.	FAT	SOD.	CARB.	FIB.
Campbell (CONT.)						
Healthy Request Ready-To-Serve Hearty Minestrone	8 oz	90	3	430	13	—
Healthy Request Ready-To-Serve Hearty Chicken Noodle	8 oz	80	2	470	7	—
Healthy Request Ready-To-Serve Hearty Chicken Rice	8 oz	110	2	400	15	—
Healthy Request Ready-To-Serve Hearty Vegetable	8 oz	110	3	480	17	—
Healthy Request Ready-To-Serve Hearty Vegetable Beef	8 oz	120	3	490	15	—
Healthy Request Tomato as prep	8 oz	90	2	430	17	—
Healthy Request Tomato as prep w/ skim milk	8 oz	130	2	490	22	—
Healthy Request Vegetable as prep	8 oz	90	2	500	14	—
Healthy Request Vegetable Beef as prep	8 oz	70	2	490	9	—
Home Cookin' Bean & Ham	10¾ oz	210	4	1000	29	—
Home Cookin' Beef With Vegetables & Pasta	10¾ oz	140	2	1060	18	—
Home Cookin' Chicken Minestone	10¾ oz	180	6	950	17	—
Home Cookin' Chicken Gumbo With Sausages	10¾ oz	140	4	1090	15	—
Home Cookin' Chicken Rice	10¾ oz	150	6	1090	10	—
Home Cookin' Chicken With Noodles	10¾ oz	140	4	1150	12	—
Home Cookin' Country Vegetable	10¾ oz	120	2	1070	20	—
Home Cookin' Garden Tomato	10¾ oz	150	3	930	29	—
Home Cookin' Hearty Lentil	10¾ oz	170	2	930	28	—

FOOD	PORTION	CAL.	FAT	SOD.	CARB.	FIB.
Campbell (CONT.)						
Home Cookin' Minestrone	10¾ oz	140	3	1220	22	—
Home Cookin' Split Pea With Ham	10¾ oz	230	1	1310	38	—
Home Cookin' Vegetable Beef	10¾ oz	140	3	1160	17	—
Minestrone as prep	8 oz	80	2	900	13	—
Mushroom Cream Of as prep	8 oz	100	7	820	8	—
Mushroom Golden as prep	8 oz	70	3	870	9	—
Nacho Cheese as prep	8 oz	110	8	740	8	—
Nacho Cheese as prep w/ milk	8 oz	180	12	800	13	—
Noodles & Ground Beef as prep	8 oz	90	4	820	10	—
Onion Cream Of as prep	8 oz	100	5	830	12	—
Onion Cream Of as prep w/ whole milk & water	8 oz	140	7	860	15	—
Oyster Stew as prep	8 oz	70	5	840	5	—
Oyster Stew as prep w/ whole milk	8 oz	140	9	890	10	—
Pepper Pot as prep	8 oz	90	4	970	9	—
Potato Cream Of as prep	8 oz	80	3	870	12	—
Potato Cream Of as prep w/ whole milk & water	8 oz	120	4	900	15	—
Ready-To-Serve Chunky Chili Beef	11 oz	290	7	1120	37	—
Ready-To-Serve Chunky Mediterranean Vegetable	9½ oz	170	6	1010	24	—
Ready-To-Serve Chunky Minestrone	9½ oz	160	4	870	24	—
Ready-To-Serve Chunky Beef	10¾ oz	200	5	1100	24	—
Ready-To-Serve Chunky Beef Stroganoff	10¾ oz	320	16	1230	28	—
Ready-To-Serve Chunky Chicken Corn Chowder	10¾ oz	340	21	1200	23	—
Ready-To-Serve Chunky Chicken Noodle	10¾ oz	200	7	1140	20	—
Ready-To-Serve Chunky Chicken Vegetable	9½ oz	170	6	1080	19	—

FOOD	PORTION	CAL.	FAT	SOD.	CARB.	FIB.
Campbell (CONT.)						
Ready-To-Serve Chunky Chicken With Rice	9½ oz	140	4	1060	16	—
Ready-To-Serve Chunky Creamy Chicken Mushroom	10½ oz	270	19	1280	13	—
Ready-To-Serve Chunky Creole Style	10¾ oz	240	8	910	31	—
Ready-To-Serve Chunky Ham 'n Butter Bean	10¾ oz	280	10	1180	34	—
Ready-To-Serve Chunky Manhattan Style Clam Chowder	10¾ oz	160	4	1110	24	—
Ready-To-Serve Chunky New England Clam Chowder	10¾ oz	290	17	1200	26	—
Ready-To-Serve Chunky Old Fashioned Chicken	10¾ oz	180	5	1220	21	—
Ready-To-Serve Chunky Old Fashioned Vegetable Beef	10¾ oz	190	6	1100	20	—
Ready-To-Serve Chunky Old Fashioned Bean w/ Ham	11 oz	290	9	1110	38	—
Ready-To-Serve Chunky Pepper Steak	10¾ oz	180	3	1050	24	—
Ready-To-Serve Chunky Sirloin Burger	10¾ oz	220	9	1240	23	—
Ready-To-Serve Chunky Split Pea w/ Ham	10¾ oz	230	6	1080	33	—
Ready-To-Serve Chunky Steak & Potato	10¾ oz	200	5	1140	24	—
Ready-To-Serve Chunky Turkey Vegetable	9⅜ oz	150	6	1060	16	—
Ready-To-Serve Low Sodium Chicken Vegetable Beef	10¾ oz	180	5	90	19	—
Ready-To-Serve Low Sodium Chicken Broth	10½ oz	30	1	85	2	—
Ready-To-Serve Low Sodium Chicken With Noodles	10¾ oz	170	5	90	17	—
Ready-To-Serve Low Sodium Mushroom Cream Of	10½ oz	210	14	55	18	—

FOOD	PORTION	CAL.	FAT	SOD.	CARB.	FIB.
Campbell (CONT.)						
Ready-To-Serve Low Sodium Split Pea	10¾ oz	230	4	30	37	—
Ready-To-Serve Low Sodium Tomato With Tomato Pieces	10½ oz	190	6	45	30	—
Scotch Broth as prep	8 oz	80	3	870	9	—
Shrimp Cream Of as prep	8 oz	90	6	810	8	—
Shrimp Cream Of as prep w/ whole milk	8 oz	160	10	860	13	—
Split Pea With Bacon as prep	8 oz	160	4	780	24	—
Teddy Bear as prep	8 oz	70	2	790	11	—
Tomato as prep	8 oz	90	2	680	17	—
Tomato as prep w/ 2% milk	8 oz	150	4	740	22	—
Tomato Bisque as prep	8 oz	120	3	820	22	—
Tomato Homestyle Cream Of as prep	8 oz	110	3	810	20	—
Tomato Homestyle Cream Of as prep w/ whole milk	8 oz	180	7	860	25	—
Tomato Rice Old Fashioned as prep	8 oz	110	2	730	22	—
Tomato Zesty as prep	8 oz	100	2	760	20	—
Turkey Vegetable as prep	8 oz	70	3	710	8	—
Turkey Noodle as prep	8 oz	70	2	880	9	—
Vegetable Homestyle as prep	8 oz	60	2	880	9	—
Vegetable as prep	8 oz	90	2	830	14	—
Vegetable Beef as prep	8 oz	70	2	780	10	—
Vegetable Old Fashioned as prep	8 oz	60	2	880	9	—
Vegetarian Vegetable as prep	8 oz	80	2	790	13	—
Won Ton as prep	8 oz	40	1	850	5	—
College Inn						
Beef Broth	½ can (7 oz)	16	0	960	1	—
Chicken Broth	½ can (7 oz)	35	3	990	0	0
Chicken Broth Lower Salt	½ can (7 oz)	20	2	550	0	0
Gold's						
Borscht	8 oz	100	0	1280	21	—

FOOD	PORTION	CAL.	FAT	SOD.	CARB.	FIB.
Gold's (CONT.)						
Borscht Lo-Cal	8 oz	20	tr	1160	5	—
Schav	8 oz	25	0	1380	4	—
Gorton's						
New England Clam Chowder as prep w/ whole milk	¼ can	140	5	740	17	—
Goya						
Black Bean	7.5 oz	160	4	720	29	9
Hain						
Chicken Broth	8.75 fl oz	70	6	870	0	—
Chicken Broth No Salt Added	8.75 fl oz	60	5	75	0	—
Chicken Noodle	9.5 fl oz	120	4	980	11	—
Chicken Noodle No Salt Added	9.5 fl oz	120	4	90	12	—
Creamy Mushroom	9.25 fl oz	110	4	740	16	—
Italian Vegetable Pasta	9.5 fl oz	160	5	910	25	—
Italian Vegetable Pasta Low Sodium	9.5 fl oz	140	6	90	22	—
Minestrone	9.5 fl oz	170	2	1060	27	—
Minestrone No Salt Added	9.5 fl oz	160	4	35	28	—
Mushroom Barley	9.5 fl oz	100	2	600	17	—
New England Clam Chowder	9.5 fl oz	180	4	780	26	—
Split Pea	9.5 fl oz	170	1	970	28	—
Split Pea No Salt Added	9.5 fl oz	170	1	40	29	—
Turkey Rice	9.5 fl oz	100	3	970	10	—
Turkey Rice No Salt Added	9.5 fl oz	120	4	85	13	—
Vegetable Chicken	9.5 fl oz	120	4	930	14	—
Vegetable Chicken No Salt Added	9.5 fl oz	130	4	100	14	—
Vegetable Broth	9.5 fl oz	45	0	1180	10	—
Vegetable Broth Low Sodium	9.5 fl oz	40	tr	85	8	—
Vegetable Split Pea	9.5 fl oz	170	1	970	28	—
Vegetable Split Pea No Salt Added	9.5 fl oz	170	1	70	27	—
Vegetarian Lentil	9.5 fl oz	160	3	690	25	—
Vegetarian Lentil No Salt Added	9.5 fl oz	160	3	65	24	—
Vegetarian Vegetable	9.5 fl oz	140	4	920	22	—

FOOD	PORTION	CAL.	FAT	SOD.	CARB.	FIB.
Hain (CONT.)						
Vegetarian Vegetable No Salt Added	9.5 fl oz	150	5	45	23	—
Health Valley						
Beef Broth	7.5 oz	10	tr	420	2	0
Beef Broth No Salt Added	7.5 oz	10	tr	5	2	0
Black Bean	7.5 oz	150	2	280	24	16
Black Bean No Salt Added	7.5 oz	150	2	20	24	16
Chicken Broth	7.5 oz	35	2	410	1	0
Chicken Broth No Salt Added	7.5 oz	35	2	0	1	0
Chunky Chicken Vegetable	7.5 oz	125	2	290	20	4
Chunky Five Bean Vegetable	7.5 oz	110	2	290	21	11
Chunky Five Bean Vegetable No Salt Added	7.5 oz	110	2	60	21	11
Chunky Vegetable Chicken No Salt Added	7.5 oz	125	2	60	20	4
Green Split Pea	7.5 oz	180	tr	290	34	15
Green Split Pea No Salt Added	7.5 oz	180	tr	25	34	15
Lentil	7.5 oz	220	4	290	33	10
Lentil No Salt Added	7.5 oz	220	4	25	4	10
Manhattan Clam Chowder	7.5 oz	110	2	290	15	2
Manhattan Clam Chowder No Salt Added	7.5 oz	110	2	60	15	2
Minestrone	7.5 oz	130	3	290	19	13
Minestrone No Salt Added	7.5 oz	130	3	90	19	13
Mushroom Barley	7.5 oz	100	2	290	2	9
Mushroom Barley No Salt Added	7.5 oz	100	2	20	16	9
Potato Leek	7.5 oz	130	2	290	23	7
Potato Leek No Salt Added	7.5 oz	130	2	20	23	7
Tomato	7.5 oz	130	3	290	21	1
Tomato No Salt Added	7.5 oz	130	3	40	21	1

FOOD	PORTION	CAL.	FAT	SOD.	CARB.	FIB.
Health Valley (CONT.)						
Vegetable	7.5 oz	110	1	300	20	8
Vegetable No Salt Added	7.5 oz	110	1	40	20	8
Healthy Choice						
Bean & Ham	1 cup (8.7 oz)	184	—	465	34	10
Beef & Potato	1 cup (8.5 oz)	119	2	635	18	3
Chicken Corn Chowder	1 cup (8.8 oz)	176	3	466	30	2
Chicken Pasta	1 cup (8.6 oz)	118	3	493	18	1
Chicken With Rice	1 cup (8.4 oz)	108	3	426	15	1
Chili Beef	1 cup (9.1 oz)	166	1	384	30	5
Clam Chowder	1 cup (8.8 oz)	123	1	481	23	2
Country Vegetable	1 cup (8.6 oz)	104	1	431	23	2
Cream Of Mushroom	1 cup (8.8 oz)	77	1	450	14	1
Cream Of Chicken With Mushrooms	1 cup (8.9 oz)	127	2	421	20	1
Cream Of Chicken With Vegetables	1 cup (8.9 oz)	127	2	384	21	1
Garden Vegetable	1 cup (8.6 oz)	118	1	405	26	3
Hearty Chicken	1 cup (8.7 oz)	132	3	461	20	1
Lentil	1 cup (8.7 oz)	146	1	419	28	5
Minestrone	1 cup (8.6 oz)	112	1	392	23	3
Old Fashion Chicken Noodle	1 cup (8.8 oz)	137	3	402	19	1
Split Pea & Ham	1 cup (8.8 oz)	155	2	399	26	2
Tomato Garden	1 cup (8.6 oz)	106	2	424	21	3
Turkey With Wild Rice	1 cup (8.4 oz)	92	2	355	13	1
Vegetable Beef	1 cup (8.8 oz)	130	1	422	22	2
Hormel						
Bean & Ham	1 cup (7.5 oz)	190	4	650	28	7
Beef Vegetable	1 cup (7.5 oz)	90	1	740	14	2
Broccoli Cheese With Ham	1 cup (7.5 oz)	170	13	700	10	1
Chicken & Rice	1 cup (7.5 oz)	110	3	900	17	1
Chicken Noodle	1 cup (7.5 oz)	110	3	690	13	1
New England Clam Chowder	1 cup (7.5 oz)	130	5	820	16	1
Potato Cheese With Ham	1 cup (7.5 oz)	190	13	730	16	1
Manischewitz						
Borscht Low Calorie	8 fl oz	20	0	725	4	—
Borscht With Beets	8 fl oz	80	0	660	20	—
Schav	1 cup	11	tr	4	—	—
Old El Paso						
Black Bean With Bacon	1 cup (8.6 oz)	160	2	960	26	7
Chicken Vegetable	1 cup (8.4 oz)	110	3	620	13	0

FOOD	PORTION	CAL.	FAT	SOD.	CARB.	FIB.
Old El Paso (CONT.)						
Chicken With Rice	1 cup (8.4 oz)	90	3	680	10	0
Garden Vegetable	1 cup (8.4 oz)	110	3	710	17	0
Hearty Beef	1 cup (8.4 oz)	120	3	690	14	0
Hearty Chicken Noodle	1 cup (8.4 oz)	110	3	720	10	0
Pritikin						
Chicken & Rice	1 cup (8.8 oz)	80	1	250	13	—
Chicken Broth	1 cup (8.5 oz)	15	0	290	1	—
Chicken Pasta	1 cup (8.6 oz)	100	1	290	18	—
Hearty Vegetable	1 cup (8.8 oz)	90	1	290	20	—
Lentil	1 cup (8.4 oz)	130	1	280	24	—
Minestrone	1 cup (8.8 oz)	90	1	290	19	—
Split Pea	1 cup (9.2 oz)	140	1	290	29	—
Three Bean Chili	½ cup (4.5 oz)	90	1	170	19	—
Vegetable Broth	1 cup (8.3 oz)	20	0	250	3	—
Vegetarian Vegetables	1 cup (9 oz)	100	0	290	23	—
Progresso						
Bean And Ham	1 cup (8.4 oz)	160	2	870	25	8
Beef	1 can (10.5 fl oz)	180	6	840	17	—
Beef Barley	1 cup (8.5 oz)	130	4	780	13	3
Beef Minestrone	1 cup (8.5 oz)	140	4	850	14	3
Beef Noodle	1 cup (8.5 oz)	140	4	950	15	1
Beef Vegetable & Rotini	1 cup (8 oz)	120	4	830	10	3
Broccoli & Shells	1 cup (8.5 oz)	70	1	720	14	3
Chickarina	1 cup (8.3 oz)	120	5	710	10	1
Chicken Minestrone	1 cup (8.4 oz)	120	4	790	12	2
Chicken Vegetables & Penne	1 cup (8.4 oz)	100	3	780	11	3
Chicken & Wild Rice	1 cup (8.4 oz)	100	2	820	15	2
Chicken Barley	1 cup (8.5 oz)	110	3	720	14	3
Chicken Broth	1 cup ((8.2 oz)	20	1	860	1	0
Chicken Noodle	1 can (10.5 oz)	110	3	910	10	1
Chicken Noodle	1 cup (8.4 oz)	80	2	730	8	1
Chicken Rice Vegetable	1 can (10.5 oz)	130	4	940	15	tr
Chicken Rice Vegetable	1 cup (8.4 oz)	110	3	750	12	tr
Clam & Rotini Chowder	1 cup (8.8 oz)	200	9	800	21	0
Corn Chowder	1 cup (8.6 oz)	180	10	780	20	2
Cream Of Chicken	1 cup (8.4 oz)	170	10	880	11	0
Cream Of Mushroom	1 cup (8.4 oz)	140	8	920	12	1
Creamy Tortellini	1 cup (8.4 oz)	210	15	830	15	0
Escarole In Chicken Broth	1 cup (8.1 oz)	25	1	980	2	0
Green Split Pea	1 cup (8.6 oz)	170	3	870	25	5
Healthy Classics Beef Barley	1 cup (8.5 oz)	140	2	490	20	3

FOOD	PORTION	CAL.	FAT	SOD.	CARB.	FIB.
Progresso (CONT.)						
Healthy Classics Beef Vegetable	1 cup (8.5 oz)	150	2	410	25	6
Healthy Classics Chicken Noodle	1 cup (8.3 oz)	80	2	480	10	1
Healthy Classics Chicken Rice With Vegetables	1 cup (8.4 oz)	90	2	450	12	1
Healthy Classics Cream Of Broccoli	1 cup (8.6 oz)	90	3	580	13	2
Healthy Classics Garlic & Pasta	1 cup (8.5 oz)	100	2	450	18	3
Healthy Classics Lentil	1 cup (8.5 oz)	120	3	510	20	1
Healthy Classics Minestrone	1 cup (8.5 oz)	120	3	510	20	1
Healthy Classics New England Clam Chowder	1 cup (8.6 oz)	120	2	530	20	1
Healthy Classics Split Pea	1 cup (8.9 oz)	180	3	420	30	5
Healthy Classics Tomato Garden Vegetable	1 cup (8.6 oz)	100	1	480	19	4
Healthy Classics Vegetable	1 cup (8.4 oz)	80	2	470	13	1
Hearty Minestrone With Shells	1 cup (8.4 oz)	120	2	700	20	4
Hearty Black Bean	1 cup (8.5 oz)	170	2	730	30	10
Hearty Chicken	1 can (10.5 fl oz)	120	3	1070	10	0
Hearty Chicken & Rotini	1 cup (8.4 oz)	90	2	860	8	0
Hearty Penne In Chicken Broth	1 cup (8.4 oz)	70	1	930	12	0
Hearty Tomato & Rotini	1 cup (8.4 oz)	90	1	820	16	3
Hearty Vegetable With Rotini	1 cup (8.4 oz)	110	1	720	20	3
Homestyle Chicken Vegetable	1 cup (8.4 oz)	100	3	680	10	1
Lentil	1 can (10.5 fl oz)	170	3	930	27	8
Lentil	1 cup (8.5 oz)	140	2	750	22	7
Lentil & Shells	1 cup (8.5 oz)	130	2	840	22	4
Lentil With Sausage	1 cup (8.5 oz)	170	7	780	19	5
Macaroni & Bean	1 cup (8.6 oz)	160	4	800	23	6
Manhattan Clam Chowder	1 cup (8.4 oz)	110	2	710	11	3
Meatballs & Pasta Pearls	1 cup (8.3 oz)	140	7	700	13	0
Minestrone	1 can (10.5 fl oz)	170	4	1190	27	6

FOOD	PORTION	CAL.	FAT	SOD.	CARB.	FIB.
Progresso (CONT.)						
Minestrone	1 cup (8.4 oz)	130	3	960	22	5
New England Clam Chowder	1 can (10.5 oz)	220	12	1050	21	2
New England Clam Chowder	1 cup (8.4 oz)	180	10	850	17	2
Spicy Chicken & Penne	1 cup (8.5 oz)	120	4	680	13	0
Split Pea With Ham	1 cup (8.5 oz)	160	4	830	20	5
Tomato	1 cup (8.5 oz)	90	2	990	15	4
Tomato Tortellini	1 cup (8.4 oz)	120	5	910	13	2
Tomato Beef & Rotini	1 cup (8.5 oz)	140	5	750	15	2
Tortellini In Chicken Broth	1 cup (8.3 oz)	80	2	750	10	2
Vegetable	1 cup (8.4 oz)	90	2	850	15	3
Zesty Minestrone	1 cup (8.3 oz)	150	6	790	17	4
Snow's						
Manhattan Clam Chowder as prep w/ water	7.5 fl oz	70	2	630	9	—
New England Clam Chowder as prep w/ milk	7.5 fl oz	140	6	670	13	—
New England Corn Chowder as prep w/ milk	7.5 fl oz	150	6	640	18	—
New England Fish Chowder as prep w/ milk	7.5 fl oz	130	6	620	11	—
New England Seafood Chowder as prep w/ milk	7.5 fl oz	130	6	690	11	—
Swanson						
Beef Broth	7¼ oz	18	1	750	1	—
Chicken Broth	7.25 oz	30	2	900	2	—
Natural Goodness Clear Chicken Broth	7¼ oz	20	1	580	1	—
Vegetable Broth	7.25 fl oz	20	1	920	3	—
Weight Watchers						
Chicken & Rice	1 can (10.5 oz)	110	2	720	17	4
Chicken Noodle	1 can (10.5 oz)	150	2	740	25	4
Minestrone	1 can (10.5 oz)	130	2	760	23	6
Vegetable	1 can (10.5 oz)	130	1	680	27	6
DRY						
asparagus cream of as prep w/ water	1 cup	59	2	801	9	—

FOOD	PORTION	CAL.	FAT	SOD.	CARB.	FIB.
beef broth	1 pkg (0.2 oz)	14	1	1019	1	—
beef broth as prep w/ water	1 cup	19	1	1368	2	—
beef broth cube	1 cube (3.6 g)	6	tr	864	1	—
beef broth cube as prep w/ water	1 cup	8	tr	1152	1	—
celery cream of as prep w/ water	1 cup	63	2	839	10	—
chicken broth	1 pkg (0.2 oz)	16	1	1116	1	—
chicken broth as prep w/ water	1 cup	21	1	1484	1	—
chicken broth cube	1 cube (4.8 g)	9	tr	1152	1	—
chicken broth cube, as prep w/ water	1 cup	13	tr	792	2	—
chicken cream of as prep w/ water	1 cup	107	5	1184	13	—
chicken noodle as prep w/ water	1 cup	53	1	1284	7	—
french onion not prep	1 pkg (1.4 oz)	115	2	3493	21	—
leek as prep w/ water	1 cup	71	2	966	11	—
onion as prep w/ water	1 cup	28	1	848	5	—
tomato as prep w/ water	1 cup	102	2	943	19	—
4C						
Noodle	8 oz	50	2	960	7	—
Onion Reduced Salt	8 oz	30	1	760	5	—
Armour						
Bouillon Cubes Beef	1 (4 g)	5	0	920	1	—
Bouillon Cubes Chicken	1 (4 g)	5	0	910	1	—
Arrowhead						
Bean & Barley	¼ cup (1.9 oz)	170	0	0	35	7
Bean Cuisine						
Bean Bouillabaisse	1 cup (7.5 fl oz)	174	tr	5	18	5
Island Black Bean	1 cup (8.7 fl oz)	210	4	504	33	10
Lots of Lentil	1 cup (7.7 oz)	166	tr	7	19	6
Mesa Maize	1 cup (9.2 fl oz)	179	tr	9	21	6
Rocky Mountain Red Bean	1 cup (8.6 oz)	202	tr	7	24	8
Sante Fe Corn Chowder	1 cup (9.2 oz)	179	tr	9	21	6
Thick As Fog Split Pea	1 cup (8.6 fl oz)	189	tr	13	21	1
Ultima Pasta E Fagioli	1 cup (8.6 fl oz)	179	tr	8	22	4
White Bean Provencal	1 cup (7.7 fl oz)	166	tr	7	19	6
Campbell						
Bean With Bacon 'n Ham Microwave	7½ oz	230	5	830	38	—
Chicken Noodle Microwave	7½ oz	100	4	870	11	—

FOOD	PORTION	CAL.	FAT	SOD.	CARB.	FIB.
Campbell (CONT.)						
Chicken Noodle as prep	8 oz	100	2	710	16	—
Chicken With Rice Microwave	7½ oz	100	4	820	14	—
Chili Beef Microwave	7½ oz	190	4	870	32	—
Hearty Noodle as prep	8 oz	90	1	840	15	—
Noodle as prep	8 oz	110	2	700	19	—
Onion as prep	8 oz	30	0	700	7	—
Vegetable as prep	8 oz	40	0	710	8	—
Vegetable Beef Microwave	7½ oz	100	2	830	16	—
Campbell's Cup						
Beef Noodle	1 (1.35 oz)	130	2	1270	23	—
Chicken Noodle	1 (1.35 oz)	140	3	1340	22	—
Chicken Noodle w/ White Meat as prep	6 oz	90	2	770	12	—
Creamy Chicken w/ White Meat as prep	6 oz	90	4	1020	12	—
Hearty Noodles With Vegetables	1 (1.7 oz)	180	2	1320	32	—
Noodle With Chicken Broth as prep	6 oz	90	2	910	15	—
Casbah						
Black Bean	1 pkg (1.7 oz)	170	2	530	30	9
Split Pea	1 pkg (2.3 oz)	230	1	500	40	10
Sweet Corn Chowder	1 pkg (1.2 oz)	125	1	440	26	2
Vegetarian Chili	1 pkg (1.8 oz)	170	2	430	31	7
Cup-A-Ramen						
Beef With Vegetables Low Fat as prep	8 oz	220	2	1600	44	—
Beef With Vegetables as prep	8 oz	270	10	1530	38	—
Chicken With Vegetables Low Fat as prep	8 oz	220	2	1500	44	—
Chicken With Vegetables as prep	8 oz	270	10	1470	38	—
Oriental With Vegetables Low Fat as prep	8 oz	220	2	1400	44	—
Oriental With Vegetables as prep	8 oz	270	10	1210	38	—
Shrimp With Vegetables Low Fat as prep	8 oz	230	2	1290	45	—
Shrimp With Vegetables as prep	8 oz	280	10	1190	40	—

FOOD	PORTION	CAL.	FAT	SOD.	CARB.	FIB.
Cup-A-Soup						
Chicken Vegetable as prep	1 pkg	50	1	520	10	0
Chicken Vegetable as prep	1 pkg	90	4	590	10	tr
Chicken Broth as prep	1 pkg	20	1	580	3	0
Chicken Noodle as prep	1 pkg	50	1	550	8	0
Cream Of Chicken as prep	1 pkg	70	3	650	11	0
Cream Of Mushroom as prep	1 pkg	60	2	590	10	0
Creamy Broccoli & Cheese as prep	1 pkg	70	3	550	8	1
Green Pea as prep	1 pkg	110	4	620	17	3
Hearty Chicken Noodle as prep	1 pkg	60	1	540	10	0
Hearty Chicken Supreme as prep	1 pkg	90	4	650	13	tr
Hearty Harvest Vegetable as prep	1 pkg	90	2	450	17	2
Ring Noodle as prep	1 pkg	50	1	560	9	0
Spring Vegetable as prep	1 pkg	50	1	500	21	1
Tomato as prep	1 pkg	90	2	490	19	1
Virginia Pea as prep	1 pkg	130	5	630	19	3
Emes						
Beef Base	1 tsp	18	tr	10	2	—
Chicken Base	1 tsp	18	tr	10	2	—
Fantastic						
Cha-Cha Chili Low Fat	1 pkg	220	1	470	37	13
George Washington						
Broth & Brown Seasoning	1 serv	6	0	—	—	—
Broth & Golden Seasoning	1 serv	6	0	—	—	—
Broth & Onion Seasoning	1 serv	12	0	—	—	—
Broth & Vegetable Seasoning	1 serv	12	0	—	—	—
Golden Dipt						
Lobster Bisque	¼ pkg	30	1	560	5	—
Manhattan Clam Chowder	¼ pkg	80	2	700	13	—
New England Clam Chowder	¼ pkg	24	2	680	12	—

FOOD	PORTION	CAL.	FAT	SOD.	CARB.	FIB.
Golden Dipt (CONT.)						
Seafood Chowder	¼ pkg	70	2	730	12	—
Shrimp Bisque	¼ pkg	30	1	570	5	—
Goodman's						
Cup Of Soup Beef	1 pkg (1½ cups)	180	3	1640	32	2
Cup Of Soup Chicken Noodle	1 pkg (1½ cups)	180	3	1360	31	2
Cup Of Soup Vegetable	1 pkg (1½ cups)	180	3	1500	32	2
Matzo Ball & Soup	1 cup	40	1	1040	9	1
Matzo Ball & Soup 50% Less Salt	1 serv	50	1	640	10	1
Noodleman	1 cup	45	1	990	9	0
Noodleman Low Sodium	1 cup	50	1	95	9	1
Onion	1 cup	30	1	1280	5	1
Onion Low Sodium	1 cup	30	1	115	6	1
Hain						
Cheese & Broccoli	¾ cup	310	22	980	19	—
Cheese Savory	¾ cup	250	16	890	20	—
Savory Lentil	¾ cup	130	2	810	20	—
Savory Minestrone	¾ cup	110	1	870	20	—
Savory Mushroom	¾ cup	210	15	710	11	—
Savory Mushroom No Salt Added	¾ cup	250	20	180	15	—
Savory Onion	¾ cup	50	2	900	6	—
Savory Onion No Salt Added	¾ cup	50	1	470	9	—
Savory Potato Leek	¾ cup	260	18	690	20	—
Savory Split Pea	¾ cup	310	10	940	16	—
Savory Tomato	¾ cup	220	14	770	19	—
Savory Vegetable	¾ cup	80	1	730	13	—
Savory Vegetable No Salt Added	¾ cup	80	1	330	13	—
Herb-Ox						
Beef Bouillon	1 cube (3.5 g)	10	0	700	1	0
Beef Instant Bouillon Powder	1 tsp (4 g)	10	0	750	1	0
Beef Instant Broth & Seasoning Pack	1 pkg (4.5 g)	10	0	900	1	0
Beef Instant Broth & Seasoning Pack Low Sodium	1 pkg (4 g)	15	0	5	2	0
Chicken Bouillon	1 cube (4 g)	10	0	1040	1	0
Chicken Instant Bouillon Powder	1 tsp (4 g)	10	0	1040	1	0

FOOD	PORTION	CAL.	FAT	SOD.	CARB.	FIB.
Herb-Ox (CONT.)						
Chicken Instant Broth & Seasoning Pack	1 pkg (5 g)	10	0	760	1	0
Chicken Instant Broth & Seasoning Pack Low Sodium	1 pkg (4 g)	15	0	20	1	0
Vegetable Bouillon	1 cube (4 g)	10	0	1000	1	0
Hodgson Mill						
13 Bean not prep	1.5 oz	100	1	0	14	12
Hurst						
15 Bean Soup Beef	1 serv (1.7 oz)	160	1	360	27	1
15 Bean Soup Cajun	1 serv (1.7 oz)	160	1	140	27	9
15 Bean Soup Chicken	1 serv (1.7 oz)	160	1	380	27	1
15 Bean Soup Chili	1 serv (1.7 oz)	160	1	240	27	1
15 Bean Soup Ham	1 serv (1.7 oz)	160	1	90	26	1
Spanish-American Black Bean	1 serv (1.3 oz)	120	1	280	22	8
Ka-Me						
Won Ton Chicken not prep	1 pkg (1.25 oz)	180	11	770	18	1
Won Ton Pork not prep	1 pkg (1.25 oz)	180	11	770	18	1
Knorr						
Black Bean Cup-A-Soup as prep	1 pkg	200	1	690	37	9
Broccoli as prep	8 fl oz	160	8	1050	16	—
Cauliflower as prep	8 fl oz	100	3	750	13	—
Chef's Series Wild Mushroom as prep	8 fl oz	100	3	800	14	—
Chick 'N Pasta as prep	8 fl oz	90	2	850	16	—
Chicken Bouillon as prep	8 fl oz	16	1	1200	tr	—
Chicken Flavored Noodle as prep	8 fl oz	100	2	710	18	—
Chicken Noodle Instant as prep	6 fl oz	25	tr	870	4	—
Fine Herb as prep	8 fl oz	130	6	990	15	—
Fish Bouillon as prep	8 fl oz	10	tr	1130	tr	—
French Onion as prep	8 fl oz	50	1	970	9	—
Hearty Minestrone Cup-A-Soup as prep	1 pkg	150	1	720	29	1
Lentil Cup-A-Soup as prep	1 pkg	220	0	900	40	6
Mushroom as prep	8 fl oz	100	4	870	12	—
Navy Bean Cup-A-Soup as prep	1 pkg	140	0	870	27	5

FOOD	PORTION	CAL.	FAT	SOD.	CARB.	FIB.
Knorr (CONT.)						
Oriental Hot And Sour as prep	8 fl oz	50	1	670	9	—
Oxtail Hearty Beef as prep	8 fl oz	70	2	1120	10	—
Potato Leek Cup-A-Soup as prep	1 pkg	120	0	970	24	1
Spinach as prep	8 fl oz	100	5	890	11	—
Spring Vegetable With Herbs as prep	8 fl oz	30	tr	710	6	—
Tomato Basil as prep	8 fl oz	90	3	940	14	—
Tortellini In Brodo as prep	8 fl oz	60	1	820	11	—
Vegetable Cup-A-Soup as prep	1 pkg	100	0	840	21	0
Vegetable as prep	8 fl oz	35	1	840	7	—
Vegetarian Vegetable Bouillon as prep	8 fl oz	16	1	990	1	—
Kojel						
Hearty Potato With Vegetables Instant	1 serv (6 fl oz)	60	0	650	15	2
Noodle Soup Chicken Flavor Instant	1 serv (6 fl oz)	70	1	590	11	2
Split Pea Instant	1 serv (6 fl oz)	60	tr	380	14	3
Tomato Instant	1 serv (6 fl oz)	50	0	540	15	1
Vegetable Chicken Couscous Instant	1 serv (6 fl oz)	80	1	530	18	2
Lipton						
Recipe Secrets Beefy Mushroom	2 tbsp	35	0	650	7	0
Recipe Secrets Beefy Onion	1 tbsp	25	1	610	5	0
Recipe Secrets Golden Herb With Lemon	2 tbsp	35	5	510	7	0
Recipe Secrets Golden Onion	2 tbsp	60	2	650	10	0
Recipe Secrets Italian Herb With Tomato	2 tbsp	40	1	520	9	0
Recipe Secrets Onion	1 tbsp	20	0	610	4	tr
Recipe Secrets Onion Mushroom	2 tbsp	35	1	620	6	0
Recipe Secrets Savory Herb With Garlic	1 tbsp	35	1	460	6	0
Recipe Secrets Vegetable	2 tbsp	30	0	580	7	1

FOOD	PORTION	CAL.	FAT	SOD.	CARB.	FIB.
Lipton (CONT.)						
Soup Secrets Chicken Noodle	1 serv	80	3	650	12	0
Soup Secrets Extra Noodle	1 serv	90	2	680	15	tr
Soup Secrets Giggle Noodle	1 serv	80	2	730	11	0
Soup Secrets Hearty Chicken Noodle	1 serv	80	2	670	14	0
Soup Secrets Hearty Noodle With Vegetables	1 serv	70	2	710	11	tr
Soup Secrets Noodle With Chicken Broth	1 serv	60	2	710	9	0
Soup Secrets Ring-O-Noodle	1 serv	70	2	710	10	0
Soup Secrets Ruffle Pasta	1 serv	60	1	670	10	0
Lite Line						
Beef Bouillon Instant Low Sodium	1 tsp	12	tr	5	2	—
Chicken Bouillon Instant Low Sodium	1 tsp	12	tr	5	2	—
Manischewitz						
Minestrone as prep	6 fl oz	50	tr	160	9	—
Split Pea as prep	6 fl oz	45	tr	320	9	—
Vegetable as prep	6 fl oz	50	tr	65	9	—
Maruchan						
Instant Lunch Oriental Noodles Beef	1 pkg (2.25 oz)	290	13	1260	37	—
Instant Lunch Oriental Noodles Chicken	1 pkg (2.25 oz)	290	13	1270	36	2
Instant Lunch Oriental Noodles Chicken Mushroom	1 pkg (2.25 oz)	280	13	1380	34	—
Instant Lunch Oriental Noodles Mushroom	1 pkg (2.25 oz)	290	13	1310	35	—
Instant Lunch Oriental Noodles Pork	1 pkg (2.25 oz)	290	13	1390	35	—
Instant Lunch Oriental Noodles Shrimp	1 pkg (2.25 oz)	290	13	1260	37	—
Instant Lunch Oriental Noodles Toast Onion	1 pkg (2.25 oz)	270	12	1290	34	—
Instant Lunch Oriental Noodles Vegetable Beef	1 pkg (2.25 oz)	290	12	1340	34	—

FOOD	PORTION	CAL.	FAT	SOD.	CARB.	FIB.
Maruchan (CONT.)						
Instant Wonton Chicken	1 pkg (1.49 oz)	200	12	1440	19	—
Instant Wonton Hot & Sour	1 pkg (1.49 oz)	200	11	1070	21	—
Instant Wonton Oriental	1 pkg (1.49 oz)	190	12	1340	19	—
Instant Wonton Pork	1 pkg (1.49 oz)	200	12	1450	19	—
Instant Wonton Shrimp	1 pkg (1.49 oz)	200	12	1120	19	—
Oriental Noodle Picante Style Beef	1 pkg (2.25 oz)	290	15	950	37	—
Oriental Noodle Picante Style Chicken	1 pkg (2.25 oz)	290	15	920	38	—
Oriental Noodle Picante Style Shrimp	1 pkg (2.25 oz)	300	16	1120	36	—
Ramen Beef	½ pkg (1.5 oz)	190	9	770	26	—
Ramen Chicken	½ pkg (1.5 oz)	190	8	780	20	—
Ramen Chicken Mushroom	½ pkg (1.5 oz)	190	8	780	25	—
Ramen Chili	½ pkg (1.5 oz)	190	9	710	26	—
Ramen Mushroom	½ pkg (1.5 oz)	190	9	910	25	—
Ramen Oriental	½ pkg (1.5 oz)	190	9	990	26	—
Ramen Pork	½ pkg (1.5 oz)	190	9	890	25	—
Ramen Shrimp	½ pkg (1.5 oz)	190	9	820	26	—
Wonton Beef	⅓ pkg (0.68 oz)	90	5	890	8	—
Wonton Chicken	⅓ pkg (0.67 oz)	90	5	810	8	—
Wonton Pork	⅓ pkg (0.68 oz)	90	5	930	9	—
Wonton Vegetable	⅓ pkg (0.7 oz)	90	6	980	9	—
Morga						
Vegetable Bouillon No Salt Added	½ cube (5 g)	25	2	115	1	0
Vegetable Broth Fat Free	1 tsp (4 g)	10	0	710	2	0
Nile Spice						
Couscous Almondine	1 pkg	200	3	490	37	2
Couscous Garbanzo	1 pkg	220	3	500	39	2
Couscous Lentil Curry	1 pkg	200	2	730	36	4
Couscous Minestrone	1 pkg	180	2	590	34	2
Couscous Parmesan	1 pkg	200	3	570	34	2
Homestyle Black Bean	1 pkg	190	2	570	34	2
Homestyle Chicken Flavored Vegetable	1 pkg	120	2	600	20	4
Homestyle Lentil	1 pkg	180	2	500	31	3
Homestyle Minestrone	1 pkg	160	2	550	29	4
Homestyle Red Beans & Rice	1 pkg	190	2	560	36	3
Homestyle Split Pea	1 pkg	200	2	710	35	6

FOOD	PORTION	CAL.	FAT	SOD.	CARB.	FIB.
Nile Spice (CONT.)						
Homestyle Sweet Corn Chowder	1 pkg	120	3	420	20	0
Italian Tomato	1 pkg	140	4	670	21	2
Potato Leek	1 pkg	150	6	490	21	2
Potato Romano	1 pkg	140	5	550	19	3
Ramen Noodle						
Beef Low Fat as prep	8 oz	160	1	890	32	—
Beef as prep	8 oz	190	8	1010	26	—
Chicken Low Fat as prep	8 oz	160	1	940	32	—
Chicken as prep	8 oz	190	8	970	26	—
Oriental Low Fat as prep	8 oz	150	1	940	31	—
Oriental as prep	8 oz	190	8	930	26	—
Pork Low Fat as prep	8 oz	150	1	1140	31	—
Pork as prep	8 oz	200	8	860	26	—
Ultra Slim-Fast						
Beef Noodle	6 oz	45	tr	700	7	2
Chicken Leek	6 oz	50	tr	1070	7	2
Chicken Noodle	6 oz	45	tr	970	6	2
Creamy Broccoli	6 oz	75	tr	800	14	2
Creamy Tomato	6 oz	60	tr	800	10	2
Hearty Vegetable	6 oz	50	tr	750	7	2
Onion	6 oz	45	tr	930	7	2
Potato Leek	6 oz	80	tr	780	15	2
Weight Watchers						
Instant Beef Broth	1 pkg (0.16 oz)	10	0	800	2	0
Instant Chicken Broth	1 pkg (0.16 oz)	10	0	830	2	0
Wyler's						
Beef Bouillon Instant	1 tsp	6	tr	930	1	—
Beef Bouillon Instant Cube	1	6	tr	930	1	—
Chicken Bouillon Instant	1 tsp	8	tr	900	1	—
Chicken Bouillon Instant Cube	1	8	tr	900	1	—
Onion Bouillon Instant	1 tsp	10	tr	910	1	—
Vegetable Bouillon Instant	1 tsp	6	tr	910	1	—
FROZEN						
Jaclyn's						
Barley & Mushroom	7.5 fl oz	90	1	234	16	–
Split Pea	7.5 fl oz	180	2	183	31	—
Vegetable	7.5 fl oz	90	1	195	18	—
Tabatchnick						
Barley Mushroom	1 serv (7.5 oz)	70	0	540	13	3

FOOD	PORTION	CAL.	FAT	SOD.	CARB.	FIB.
Tabatchnick (CONT.)						
Barley Mushroom No Salt Added	1 serv (7.5 oz)	70	0	98	13	3
Broccoli Cream Of	1 serv (7.5 oz)	90	4	740	12	3
Cabbage	1 serv (7.5 oz)	60	0	160	14	2
Chicken With Dumplings	1 serv (7.5 oz)	70	2	830	13	1
Corn Chowder	1 serv (7.5 oz)	150	6	650	22	1
Minestrone	1 serv (7.5 oz)	150	1	550	27	10
New England Potato	1 serv (7.5 oz)	150	6	540	21	2
New York Chicken	1 serv (7.5 oz)	35	0	850	6	0
Old Fashion Potato	1 serv (7.5 oz)	70	0	540	16	2
Pea	1 serv (7.5 oz)	180	2	520	31	11
Pea No Salt Added	1 serv (7.5 oz)	180	2	79	31	11
Spinach Cream Of	1 serv (7.5 oz)	90	4	630	11	2
Vegetable	1 serv (7.5 oz)	110	1	580	20	4
Vegetable No Salt Added	1 serv (7.5 oz)	110	1	77	20	4
Wisconsin Cheddar Vegetable	1 serv (7.5 oz)	140	9	930	12	1
Yankee Bean	1 serv (7.5 oz)	160	2	570	27	11
SHELF-STABLE						
Lunch Bucket						
Chicken Noodle	1 pkg (7.25 oz)	90	2	810	13	—
Country Vegetable	1 pkg (7.25 oz)	70	1	740	15	—
TAKE-OUT						
beef stew soup	1 cup (8.8 oz)	221	5	461	20	—
black bean turtle soup	1 cup	241	1	6	45	—
brunswick stew soup	1 cup (8.5 oz)	232	6	438	17	—
corn & cheese chowder	¾ cup	215	12	386	21	3
gazpacho	1 cup	46	tr	63	5	—
greek	¾ cup	63	2	386	7	2
hot & sour	1 serv (14 oz)	173	8	475	8	1
oxtail	5 oz	64	3	—	7	—
pasta e fagioli	1 cup (8.8 oz)	194	5	790	30	—
ratatouille	1 cup (7.5 oz)	266	25	329	12	—

SOUR CREAM

(*see also* SOUR CREAM SUBSTITUTES)

FOOD	PORTION	CAL.	FAT	SOD.	CARB.	FIB.
sour cream	1 tbsp (0.4 oz)	26	3	6	1	—
sour cream	1 cup (8 oz)	493	48	123	10	—
Breakstone's						
Free	2 tbsp (1.1 oz)	35	0	25	6	0
Reduced Fat	2 tbsp (1.1 oz)	45	4	20	2	0
Sour Cream	2 tbsp (1 oz)	60	5	15	1	0
Cabot						
Light	1 oz	33	2	72	2	—

FOOD	PORTION	CAL.	FAT	SOD.	CARB.	FIB.
Cabot (CONT.)						
Sour Cream	1 oz	60	6	15	1	—
Friendship						
Light	2 tbsp (1 oz)	35	3	30	2	0
Sour Cream	2 tbsp (1 oz)	60	5	15	2	0
Heluva Good Cheese						
Fat-Free	2 tbsp (1.1 oz)	20	0	45	3	0
Light	2 tbsp (1.1 oz)	40	3	20	3	0
Sour Cream	2 tbsp (1.1 oz)	60	5	15	2	0
Hood						
Fat Free	2 tbsp (1 oz)	20	0	25	3	0
Light	2 tbsp (1 oz)	40	3	20	2	0
Sour Cream	2 tbsp (1 oz)	60	5	20	2	0
Knudsen						
Free	2 tbsp (1.1 oz)	35	0	25	6	0
Free	2 tbsp (1.1 oz)	35	0	25	6	0
Hampshire	2 tbsp (1 oz)	60	6	15	1	0
Light	2 tbsp (1.1 oz)	50	3	10	2	0
Light	2 tbsp (1.1 oz)	40	3	20	2	0
Naturally Yours						
No Fat	2 tbsp (1 fl oz)	15	0	15	1	—
Sealtest						
Light	2 tbsp (1.1 oz)	40	3	20	2	0
SOUR CREAM SUBSTITUTES						
nondairy	1 cup	479	45	235	15	—
nondairy	1 oz	59	6	29	2	—
Pet						
Imitation	1 tbsp	25	2	25	tr	—
Tofutti						
Better Than Sour Cream Sour Supreme	1 oz	50	5	120	1	—
SOURSOP						
fresh	1	416	2	87	105	—
fresh cut up	1 cup	150	1	31	38	—
SOY						
(*see also* CHEESE SUBSTITUTES, ICE CREAM AND FROZEN DESSERTS, MILK SUBSTITUTES, MISO, SOY SAUCE, SOYBEANS, TEMPH, TOFU, AND YOGURT FROZEN)						
lecithin	1 tbsp	104	14	—	0	—
soy milk	1 cup	79	5	30	4	—
soya cheese	1.4 oz	128	11	—	tr	0
LaLoma						
Soyagen All Purpose	¼ cup	130	6	150	14	—

FOOD	PORTION	CAL.	FAT	SOD.	CARB.	FIB.
LaLoma (CONT.)						
Soyagen Carob	¼ cup	140	6	160	16	—
Soyagen No Sucrose	¼ cup	130	6	210	14	—
Worthington						
Soyamel	1 oz	130	7	150	11	—
SOY SAUCE						
shoyu	1 tbsp	9	tr	1029	2	—
soy sauce	1 tbsp	7	tr	1024	1	—
tamari	1 tbsp	11	tr	1005	1	—
Eden						
Shoyu Organic	1 tbsp (0.5 oz)	15	0	1040	2	0
Shoyu Traditional	1 tbsp (0.5 oz)	15	0	1010	2	0
Tamari Organic Domestic	1 tbsp (0.5 oz)	15	0	970	2	0
Tamari Organic Imported	1 tbsp (0.5 oz)	15	0	1130	2	0
House Of Tsang						
Dark	1 tbsp (0.6 oz)	10	0	860	1	0
Ginger Flavored Low Sodium	1 tbsp (0.6 oz)	10	0	280	2	0
Ginger Flavored	1 tbsp (0.6 oz)	20	0	730	4	0
Light	1 tbsp (0.6 oz)	5	0	900	0	0
Low Sodium	1 tbsp (0.6 oz)	5	0	280	0	0
Mushroom Flavored Low Sodium	1 tbsp (0.6 oz)	10	0	280	2	0
Ka-Me						
Chinese Dark	1 tbsp (0.5 fl oz)	10	0	1020	3	0
Chinese Light	1 tbsp (0.5 fl oz)	5	0	1170	1	0
Dark	1 tbsp (0.5 fl oz)	10	0	1020	3	0
Japanese	1 tbsp (0.5 fl oz)	5	0	520	1	0
Light	1 tbsp (0.5 oz)	5	0	1170	1	0
Mild	1 tbsp (0.5 fl oz)	5	0	490	0	0
Kikkoman						
Lite	1 tbsp	13	0	564	2	—
Soy Sauce	1 tbsp	12	0	938	2	0
La Choy						
Lite	½ tsp	1	tr	110	tr	tr
Soy Sauce	½ tsp	2	tr	230	tr	tr
Trappey						
Chef Magic	1 tbsp (0.5 oz)	23	tr	952	4	tr
Tree Of Life						
Shoyu	1 tbsp (0.5 oz)	15	0	960	1	—
Tamari Reduced Sodium	1 tbsp (0.5 oz)	20	0	700	1	—

FOOD	PORTION	CAL.	FAT	SOD.	CARB.	FIB.
Tree Of Life (CONT.)						
Tamari Wheat Free	1 tbsp (0.5 oz)	15	0	940	1	—

SOYBEANS

(*see also* MILK SUBSTITUTES, MISO, SOY, SOY SAUCE, TEMPEH, TOFU)

FOOD	PORTION	CAL.	FAT	SOD.	CARB.	FIB.
dried cooked	1 cup	298	15	1	17	—
dry-roasted	½ cup	387	19	2	28	—
green cooked	½ cup	127	6	13	10	4
honey toasted	¼ cup (1 oz)	130	4	45	19	0
roasted	½ cup	405	22	140	29	—
roasted & toasted	1 oz	129	7	1	9	—
roasted & toasted	1 cup	490	26	4	33	—
roasted & toasted salted	1 oz	129	7	54	9	—
roasted & toasted salted	1 cup	490	26	176	33	—
sprouts raw	½ cup	43	2	5	3	—
sprouts steamed	½ cup	38	2	5	3	—
sprouts stir fried	1 cup	125	7	14	9	—

SPAGHETTI

(*see* PASTA, PASTA DINNERS, PASTA SALAD, SPAGHETTI SAUCE)

SPAGHETTI SAUCE

(*see also* PIZZA, TOMATO)

FOOD	PORTION	CAL.	FAT	SOD.	CARB.	FIB.
JARRED						
marinara sauce	1 cup	171	8	1572	25	—
spaghetti sauce	1 cup	272	12	1236	40	—
Classico						
Beef & Pork	4 fl oz	80	4	540	7	—
Four Cheese	4 fl oz	70	4	440	7	—
Ripe Olives & Mushrooms	4 fl oz	50	2	470	7	—
Spicy Red Pepper	4 fl oz	50	2	250	6	—
Sweet Peppers & Onions	4 fl oz	50	4	360	7	—
Tomato & Basil	4 fl oz	60	3	340	6	—
Contadina						
Italian	¼ cup	15	0	320	4	1
Sauce	¼ cup	20	0	280	4	tr
Thick & Zesty	¼ cup	15	0	330	4	1
Del Monte						
Traditional	½ cup (4.4 oz)	80	1	470	15	tr
Traditional No Sugar Added	½ cup (4.4 oz)	60	1	470	11	tr
With Garlic & Onion	½ cup (4.4 oz)	70	1	440	15	tr
With Green Peppers & Mushrooms	½ cup (4.4 oz)	70	1	320	13	tr

FOOD	PORTION	CAL.	FAT	SOD.	CARB.	FIB.
Del Monte (CONT.)						
With Meat	½ cup (4.4 oz)	40	2	390	13	tr
With Mushrooms	½ cup (4.4 oz)	80	2	520	15	tr
Eden						
Organic	½ cup (4.4 oz)	80	3	320	12	3
Organic No Salt Added	½ cup (4.4 oz)	80	3	10	12	3
Enrico's						
Fat Free Organic Basil	½ cup (4 oz)	50	0	220	8	4
Fat Free Organic Garlic	½ cup (4 oz)	50	0	340	9	5
Fat Free Organic Hot Pepper	½ cup (4 oz)	50	0	350	8	5
Fat Free Organic Mushroom	½ cup (4 oz)	60	0	400	10	7
Fat Free Organic Traditional	½ cup (4 oz)	45	0	280	4	6
Healthy Choice						
Extra Chunky Garlic & Onion	½ cup (4.4 oz)	43	tr	368	8	1
Extra Chunky Italian Vegetable	½ cup (4.4 oz)	39	tr	380	8	1
Extra Chunky Mushroom	½ cup (4.4 oz)	41	tr	352	8	1
Garlic & Herbs	½ cup (4.4 oz)	47	1	391	10	2
Super Chunky Mushroom & Sweet Peppers	½ cup (4.4 oz)	44	tr	366	9	1
Super Chunky Tomato, Mushroom & Garlic	½ cup (4.4 oz)	46	tr	411	9	2
Super Chunky Vegetable Primavera	½ cup (4.4 oz)	46	tr	358	9	1
Traditional	½ cup (4.4 oz)	47	1	391	10	2
With Meat	½ cup (4.4 oz)	47	1	384	8	2
With Mushrooms	½ cup (4.4 oz)	47	1	391	10	3
Hunt's						
Chunky Marinara	½ cup (4.4 oz)	60	2	526	12	2
Chunky Tomato Garlic & Onion	½ cup (4.4 oz)	61	1	526	13	2
Chunky Vegetable	½ cup (4.4 oz)	63	1	528	13	2
Classic Garlic & Onion	½ cup (4.4 oz)	58	2	598	10	2
Classic Tomato & Basil	½ cup (4.4 oz)	48	2	613	8	4
Classic Italian With Parmesan	½ cup (4.4 oz)	50	2	634	8	2
Home Style With Meat	½ cup (4.4 oz)	56	2	596	7	2
Home Style With Mushrooms	½ cup (4.4 oz)	56	2	586	7	2

FOOD	PORTION	CAL.	FAT	SOD.	CARB.	FIB.
Hunt's (CONT.)						
Homestyle Traditional	½ cup (4.4 oz)	56	3	596	7	2
Italian Cheese & Garlic	½ cup (4.5 oz)	65	2	690	9	2
Italian Sausage	½ cup (4.5 oz)	77	3	596	12	2
Old Country Garlic & Herbs	½ cup (4.4 oz)	63	3	522	9	3
Old Country Italian Style Vegetables	½ cup (4.4 oz)	64	3	616	9	3
Old Country Traditional	½ cup (4.4 oz)	53	3	542	7	3
Old Country With Meat	½ cup (4.4 oz)	56	3	474	7	3
Old Country With Mushrooms	½ cup (4.4 oz)	53	3	542	7	3
Original Traditional	½ cup (4.4 oz)	65	2	621	11	4
Original With Meat	½ cup (4.4 oz)	65	2	604	11	2
Original With Mushrooms	½ cup (4.4 oz)	65	2	604	11	2
Mama Rizzo's						
Mushroom Onion	½ cup (4.3 oz)	60	2	290	9	1
Pepper Mushroom Onion	½ cup (4.3 oz)	60	2	290	9	1
Pepper Primavera Vegetable	½ cup (4.2 oz)	50	2	220	8	2
Pepper Tomato Basil Garlic	½ cup (4.7 oz)	60	2	490	10	1
Primavera Vegetable	½ cup (4.2 oz)	50	2	220	8	2
Tomato Basil Garlic	½ cup (4.6 oz)	60	2	500	8	2
Muir Glen						
Organic Cabernet Marinara	½ cup (4.4 oz)	45	0	350	10	2
Organic Chunky Style	½ cup (4.5 oz)	80	2	300	13	3
Organic Fat Free Tomato Basil	½ cup (4.3 oz)	50	0	300	10	2
Organic Garlic Onion	½ cup (4.3 oz)	50	0	300	11	3
Organic Garlic Roasted Garlic	½ cup (4.4 oz)	45	0	350	10	2
Organic Green Pepper & Mushroom	½ cup (4.5 oz)	70	2	360	10	4
Organic Italian Herb	½ cup (4.5 oz)	60	0	300	13	2
Organic Romano Cheese	½ cup (4.5 oz)	90	3	300	14	4
Organic Sun Dried Tomato	½ cup (4.4 oz)	40	0	360	9	2
Organic Sweet Pepper Onion	½ cup (4.4 oz)	40	0	300	8	1
Organic Tomato Basil	½ cup (4.3 oz)	50	0	300	10	2

FOOD	PORTION	CAL.	FAT	SOD.	CARB.	FIB.
Newman's Own						
Marinara	4 oz	70	2	560	11	—
Marinara With Mushrooms	4 oz	70	2	560	11	—
Sockarooni	4 oz	70	2	560	11	—
Prego						
Chunky Sausage & Green Peppers	4 oz	160	8	500	19	—
Extra Chunky Garden Combination	4 oz	80	2	420	14	—
Extra Chunky Mushroom & Tomato	4 oz	110	5	500	14	—
Extra Chunky Mushroom & Green Pepper	4 oz	100	4	410	14	—
Extra Chunky Mushroom & Onion	4 oz	100	4	490	13	—
Extra Chunky Mushroom With Extra Spice	4 oz	100	3	450	17	—
Extra Chunky Tomato & Onion	4 oz	110	5	490	14	—
Marinara	4 oz	100	6	620	10	—
Meat Flavored	4 oz	140	6	660	20	—
Mushroom	4 oz	130	5	630	20	—
Onion & Garlic	4 oz	110	4	510	16	—
Regular	4 oz	130	5	630	20	—
Three Cheese	4 oz	100	2	410	17	—
Tomato & Basil	4 oz	100	2	370	18	—
Pritikin						
Chunky Garden	½ cup (4 oz)	50	1	30	12	—
Marinara	½ cup (4 oz)	60	0	260	13	—
Original	½ cup (4 oz)	60	1	30	13	—
Progresso						
Marinara	½ cup (4.3 oz)	90	5	480	8	2
Meat Flavored	½ cup (4.4 oz)	100	5	610	12	3
Mushroom	½ cup (4.4 oz)	100	5	580	12	4
Sauce	½ cup (4.4 oz)	100	5	620	12	2
Ragu						
Fino Italian Garden Medley	½ cup (4.5 oz)	90	3	580	14	2
Fino Italian Garlic & Basil	½ cup (4.5 oz)	90	3	580	15	2
Fino Italian Parmesan	½ cup (4.5 oz)	100	3	580	15	2
Fino Italian Sliced Mushroom	½ cup (4.5 oz)	90	3	580	14	2

FOOD	PORTION	CAL.	FAT	SOD.	CARB.	FIB.
Ragu (CONT.)						
Fino Italian Tomato & Herb	½ cup (4.5 oz)	90	3	580	15	2
Fino Italian Zesty Tomato	½ cup (4.5 oz)	90	3	580	14	2
Gardenstyle Chunky Garden Combination	½ cup (4.5 oz)	120	4	540	18	3
Gardenstyle Chunky Green & Red Pepper	½ cup (4.5 oz)	120	4	570	19	2
Gardenstyle Chunky Mushroom & Green Pepper	½ cup (4.5 oz)	120	4	570	18	3
Gardenstyle Chunky Mushroom & Onion	½ cup (4.5 oz)	120	4	560	19	3
Gardenstyle Chunky Tomato Garlic & Onion	½ cup (4.5 oz)	120	4	550	19	3
Gardenstyle Super Mushroom	½ cup (4.5 oz)	120	4	540	19	3
Gardenstyle Super Vegetable Primavera	½ cup (4.5 oz)	110	4	480	17	4
Homestyle Mushroom	½ cup (4.5 oz)	120	4	650	18	3
Homestyle Tomato & Herb	½ cup (4.5 oz)	120	4	650	18	3
Homestyle With Meat	½ cup (4.5 oz)	130	4	650	18	3
Light Chunky Mushroom	½ cup (4.4 oz)	50	0	410	10	2
Light Garden Harvest	½ cup (4.4 oz)	50	0	410	11	2
Light No Sugar Added	½ cup (4.4 oz)	60	0	410	9	3
Light Tomato & Herb	½ cup (4.4 oz)	50	0	410	10	2
Old World Style Marinara	½ cup (4.4 oz)	90	5	820	9	3
Old World Style Mushrooms	½ cup (4.4 oz)	80	3	820	10	3
Old World Style Traditional	½ cup (4.4 oz)	80	3	820	10	3
Old World Style With Meat	½ cup (4.4 oz)	90	5	820	9	3
Sauce	4 fl oz	80	4	740	9	—
Thick & Hearty Mushroom	½ cup (4.5 oz)	120	3	580	19	3
Thick & Hearty Spaghetti Sauce	4 oz	100	3	460	15	—
Thick & Hearty Tomato & Herb	½ cup (4.5 oz)	120	3	580	19	3
Thick & Hearty With Meat	1.2 cup (4.5 oz)	130	5	580	19	3

FOOD	PORTION	CAL.	FAT	SOD.	CARB.	FIB.
Tree Of Life						
Pasta Sauce	½ cup (4 oz)	50	2	290	9	—
Pasta Sauce Calabrese	½ cup (3.9 oz)	60	3	310	9	—
Pasta Sauce Fat Free Classic	½ cup (3.9 oz)	40	0	250	8	0
Pasta Sauce Fat Free Mushroom & Basil	½ cup (3.9 oz)	30	0	300	7	0
Pasta Sauce Fat Free Onion & Garlic	½ cup (3.9 oz)	30	0	240	7	0
Pasta Sauce Fat Free Sweet Pepper	½ cup (3.9 oz)	30	0	280	7	0
Pasta Sauce No Salt	½ cup (3.9 oz)	50	2	0	9	—
MIX						
Durkee						
American Style as prep	½ cup	15	0	170	6	0
Family Style as prep	½ cup	20	0	560	4	0
Spaghetti Sauce as prep	½ cup	15	0	390	5	0
With Mushrooms as prep	½ cup	15	0	520	4	0
Zesty as prep	½ cup	20	0	350	5	0
French's						
All American as prep	½ cup	20	0	200	7	0
Italian as prep	½ cup	16	0	390	5	0
Mushroom as prep	½ cup	20	1	760	4	0
Thick as prep	½ cup	10	0	630	4	0
Zesty Pasta as prep	½ cup	20	0	350	5	0
REFRIGERATED						
Contadina						
Alfredo	½ cup (4.2 fl oz)	400	38	510	8	0
Four Cheese Sauce With White Wine & Shallots	½ cup (4.2 fl oz)	320	25	480	8	0
Light Alfredo	½ cup (4.2 fl oz)	190	13	560	10	0
Light Chunky Tomato	½ cup (4.4 fl oz)	45	0	470	8	3
Light Garden Vegetable	½ cup (4.4 fl oz)	45	1	540	8	3
Marinara	½ cup (4.4 fl oz)	80	4	470	8	2
Pesto With Basil	¼ cup (2 oz)	310	30	440	5	0
Pesto With Sun Dried Tomatoes	¼ cup (2 oz)	250	24	520	6	3
Plum Tomato With Basil	½ cup (4.4 fl oz)	70	3	450	8	3
Spicy Italian Sausage & Bell Pepper	½ cup (4.4 fl oz)	100	5	540	9	3
Di Giorno						
Alfredo	¼ cup (2.2 oz)	180	18	600	3	0
Basil Pesto	¼ cup (2.2 oz)	320	31	530	2	tr

FOOD	PORTION	CAL.	FAT	SOD.	CARB.	FIB.
Di Giorno (CONT.)						
Four Cheese	¼ cup (2.2 oz)	160	15	410	3	0
Garlic Pesto	¼ cup (2.1 oz)	340	33	540	3	tr
Light Alfredo Sauce	¼ cup (2.4 oz)	140	9	600	9	0
Marinara	½ cup (4.5 oz)	70	0	220	15	2
Plum Tomato Cream Sauce	½ cup (4.4 oz)	160	13	370	8	2
Plum Tomato & Mushroom	½ cup (4.4 oz)	60	0	260	13	2
Roasted Red Bell Pepper Cream Sauce	¼ cup (2.3 oz)	140	10	510	8	0
TAKE-OUT						
bolognese	5 oz	195	15	—	4	tr

SPANISH FOOD

(*see also* BEANS, CHIPS, CHILI, DINNER, PEPPERS, SALSA, SNACKS, SAUCE, TORTILLA)

FOOD	PORTION	CAL.	FAT	SOD.	CARB.	FIB.
CANNED						
Chi-Chi's						
Picante Hot	2 tbsp (1 oz)	10	0	270	2	0
Picante Medium	2 tbsp (1 oz)	10	0	200	2	0
Picante Mild	2 tbsp (1 oz)	10	0	210	2	0
Pico De Gallo	2 tbsp (1.2 oz)	10	0	170	2	0
Derby						
Tamales	2	160	7	570	15	1
El Molino						
Enchilada Sauce Hot	2 tbsp	16	1	100	2	—
Green Chili Sauce Mild	2 tbsp	10	0	210	2	—
Gebhardt						
Enchiladas	2	310	24	460	20	2
Tamales	2	290	22	730	19	2
Tamales Jumbo	2	400	30	1025	26	3
Guiltless Gourmet						
Picante Mild	1 oz	6	0	133	1	tr
Queso Mild Cheddar	1 oz	22	tr	150	5	tr
Hormel						
Tamales Beef	3 (7.5 oz)	280	21	1010	20	3
Tamales Chicken	3 (7.5 oz)	210	10	1020	22	2
Tamales Hot Spicy Beef	3 (7.5 oz)	280	21	1010	20	3
Tamales Jumbo Beef	2 (6.9 oz)	270	20	940	18	3
Old El Paso						
Tamales	3 (7.2 oz)	330	19	590	31	5
Rosarita						
Enchilada Sauce Mild	2.5 oz	25	1	230	3	tr

FOOD	PORTION	CAL.	FAT	SOD.	CARB.	FIB.
Rosarita (CONT.)						
Picante Chunky Hot	3 tbsp (2 fl oz)	18	tr	515	4	tr
Picante Chunky Medium	3 tbsp (2 fl oz)	16	tr	650	4	tr
Picante Chunky Mild	3 tbsp (2 oz)	25	tr	630	5	tr
Van Camp's						
Tamales	2 (5.1 oz)	210	13	610	20	3
Wolf Brand						
Tamales	7.5 oz	328	25	1181	25	—
FROZEN						
Amy's Organic						
Enchilada Cheese	1 (4.7 oz)	210	9	390	16	2
Banquet						
Beef Enchilada	1 pkg (11 oz)	320	12	1330	54	10
Chimichanga Meal	1 pkg (9.5 oz)	470	23	1180	56	9
Enchilada Cheese	1 pkg (11 oz)	350	6	1500	56	9
Enchilada Chicken	1 pkg (11 oz)	360	10	1580	54	9
Family Entree Beef Enchilada w/ Cheese	1 serv (4.67 oz)	130	4	690	19	3
El Charrito						
Enchiladas 4 Grande Beef	1 pkg (16.5 oz)	890	47	—	—	—
Healthy Choice						
Beef Burrito Ranchero Medium	1 (5.4 oz)	290	7	500	44	6
Beef Burrito Ranchero Mild	1 (5.4 oz)	300	7	480	45	7
Beef Enchilada Rio Grande	1 meal (13.4 oz)	410	8	480	70	9
Burrito Chicken Con Queso	1 (5.4 oz)	280	6	600	43	5
Chicken Enchilada Supreme	1 meal (13.4 oz)	390	9	390	60	8
Enchiladas Suiza Chicken	1 meal (10 oz)	270	4	440	43	5
Fiesta Chicken Fajitas	1 meal (7 oz)	260	4	410	36	5
Jimmy Dean						
Burrito Breakfast Bacon	1 (4 oz)	260	8	680	37	1
Burrito Breakfast Sausage	1 (4 oz)	250	8	580	36	2
Le Menu						
Entree LightStyle Enchiladas Chicken	8 oz	280	8	530	32	—
Lean Cuisine						
Chicken Enchilada Suiza w/ Mexican Style Rice	1 pkg (9 oz)	280	5	520	48	3

FOOD	PORTION	CAL.	FAT	SOD.	CARB.	FIB.
Life Choice						
Burrito Black Bean	1 meal (13.2 oz)	410	2	570	86	13
Vegetable Enchilada Sonora	1 meal (14 oz)	420	2	600	89	11
Lightlife						
Vegetarian Taco	2 oz	51	1	280	4	—
Old El Paso						
Burrito Bean & Cheese	1 (4.9 oz)	290	9	840	44	3
Burrito Beef & Bean Hot	1 (5 oz)	320	10	850	45	3
Burrito Beef & Bean Medium	1 (5 oz)	320	10	800	46	3
Burrito Beef & Bean Mild	1 (5 oz)	330	9	690	48	4
Chimichanga Beef	1 (4.5 oz)	370	20	470	37	3
Chimichanga Chicken	1 (4.5 oz)	350	16	540	39	2
Patio						
Burrito Bean & Cheese	1 (5 oz)	270	5	530	46	7
Burrito Chicken	1 (5 oz)	260	4	740	44	3
Burrito Red Chili	1 (5 oz)	270	6	850	42	6
Burritos Beef & Bean	1 (5 oz)	280	7	660	45	7
Burritos Beef & Bean Green Chili	1 (5 oz)	260	5	890	44	7
Burritos Beef & Bean Red Chili	1 (5 oz)	260	5	640	42	7
Enchilada Beef Dinner	1 meal (12 oz)	320	8	1810	52	9
Enchilada Cheese Dinner	1 meal (12 oz)	330	8	1570	52	10
Enchilada Chicken	1 pkg (12 oz)	380	9	1470	58	9
Family Entree Beef Enchilada	2 (5.7 oz)	170	4	940	27	5
Family Entree Enchilada Beef	2 (5.3 oz)	250	7	1350	35	8
Family Entree Enchilada Beef & Cheese	2 (5.3 oz)	250	6	1130	35	9
Family Entree Enchilada Cheese	2 (5.7 oz)	170	4	880	26	4
Fiesta Dinner	1 meal (12 oz)	340	9	1760	51	11
Mexican Dinner	1 meal (13.25 oz)	440	15	1840	59	13
Salis Con Queso	1 pkg (11 oz)	390	20	1570	33	10
Patio Britos						
Beef & Bean	10 (6 oz)	420	19	800	51	7
Nacho Beef	10 (6 oz)	410	18	1050	48	5
Nacho Cheese	10 (6 oz)	360	13	500	52	3
Spicy Chicken	10 (6 oz)	400	16	640	52	3
Rudy's Farm						
Burrito Beef/Bean	1 (5 oz)	326	12	765	43	5

FOOD	PORTION	CAL.	FAT	SOD.	CARB.	FIB.
Rudy's Farm (CONT.)						
Burrito Hot Beef/Bean	1 (5 oz)	305	9	844	44	5
Senor Felix's						
Burrito Black Bean	1 (10 oz)	540	18	510	70	7
Burrito Black Bean Soy	1 (5 oz)	240	7	360	36	3
Burrito Chicken	1 (10 oz)	520	20	1240	51	3
Burrito Hot Potato	1 (10 oz)	560	24	470	67	5
Burrito Soy Hot	1 (10 oz)	520	20	470	70	5
Burritos Charbroiled Chicken	1 + 4 tsp sauce (6.7 oz)	320	11	910	40	7
Burritos Sonora Style	1 + 4 tsp sauce (6.7 oz)	280	8	240	45	3
Burritos Yucatan Style	1 + 4 tsp sauce (6.7 oz)	310	9	500	46	5
Empanadas Chicken	1 (4.7 oz)	340	15	650	41	13
Empanadas Corn & Rice	1 (4.7 oz)	280	13	530	37	6
Empanadas Pumpkin & Mushroom	1 (4.7 oz)	260	11	520	32	6
Empanadas Spinach & Ricotta	1 (4.7 oz)	260	12	520	32	6
Enchilada Red Pepper	1 (10 oz)	420	19	640	51	8
Enchilada Soy Verda	1 (10 oz)	430	24	1230	41	6
Enchilada Supreme Soy Cheese	1 (10 oz)	460	23	490	48	6
Enchilada Verde	1 (5 oz)	423	23	1140	41	6
Tamales Blue Corn & Soy Cheese	2 + 4 tsp sauce (5.7 oz)	240	10	830	28	3
Tamales Chicken	2 + 4 tsp sauce (5.7 oz)	240	9	480	30	8
Tamales Gourmet Vegetarian	2 + 4 tsp sauce	240	9	480	30	8
Taquitos Blue Corn Soy	3 + 4 tsp sauce (5.2 oz)	230	11	560	27	3
Taquitos Chicken	2 + 4 tsp sauce (5.7 oz)	240	10	830	28	3
Stouffer's						
Cheese Enchilada	1 pkg (9.75 oz)	370	14	890	48	5
Chicken Enchilada	1 serv (4.8 oz)	230	11	530	25	3
Swanson						
Enchiladas Beef	13¾ oz	480	21	1350	55	—
Mexican Style Combination	14¼ oz	490	18	1760	62	—
Mexican Style Hungry Man	20¼ oz	820	41	2080	88	—

FOOD	PORTION	CAL.	FAT	SOD.	CARB.	FIB.
Today's Tamales						
Cheese & Chili	1 pkg (7 oz)	390	21	630	38	6
Del Sol	1 pkg (6.5 oz)	310	15	650	40	15
Original Bean	1 pkg (7 oz)	330	11	520	49	10
Spicy Taco	1 pkg (7 oz)	310	15	570	41	10
Tyson						
Fajita Kit Beef	3.84 oz	160	4	240	21	—
Fajita Kit Chicken	4 oz	80	2	240	2	—
Weight Watchers						
Smart Ones Chicken Enchiladas Suiza	1 pkg (9 oz)	270	9	540	33	4
Smart Ones Santa Fe Style Rice & Beans	1 pkg (10 oz)	290	8	670	41	10
MIX						
Gebhardt						
Menudo Mix	1 tsp	5	tr	310	1	tr
Hain						
Taco Seasoning Mix	1/10 pkg	10	0	200	2	—
Old El Paso						
Burrito Seasoning Mix	2 tsp (6 g)	20	0	290	3	1
Dinner Kit Burrito as prep	1	280	7	840	35	3
Dinner Kit Soft Taco as prep	2	380	10	1340	45	3
Dinner Kit Taco as prep	2	270	13	910	21	4
Enchilada Sauce Mix	2 tsp (4 g)	10	0	540	2	tr
Taco Mix 40% Less Sodium	2 tsp (6 g)	20	0	330	4	0
Taco Seasoning Mix	2 tsp (6 g)	20	0	550	5	0
Ortega						
Taco Meat Seasoning Mix Mild	1 filled taco	90	1	999	18	—
Quaker						
Masa Harina De Maiz	2 tortillas	137	2	5	28	3
Masa Trigo	2 tortillas	149	4	794	25	1
Taco Bell						
Home Originals Chicken Fajita Dinner as prep	2 (6.9 oz)	340	9	1120	45	3
Home Originals Soft Taco Dinner as prep	2 (6.3 oz)	410	18	1090	41	2
READY-TO-EAT						
taco shell baked	1 med (0.5 oz)	61	3	48	8	tr
taco shell baked w/o salt	1 med (1/2 oz)	61	3	2	8	tr

FOOD	PORTION	CAL.	FAT	SOD.	CARB.	FIB.
Casa Fiesta						
Taco Shells	3.5 oz	480	23	10	60	—
Chi-Chi's						
Taco Shells White Corned	2 (1 oz)	130	6	0	17	2
Gebhardt						
Taco Shells	1	50	2	tr	7	tr
Old El Paso						
Taco Shells Mini	7 (1.1 oz)	160	10	130	18	2
Taco Shells Regular	3 (1.1 oz)	170	10	130	18	2
Taco Shells Super	2 (1.3 oz)	190	12	150	21	2
Taco Shells White Corn	3 (1.1 oz)	170	10	30	18	2
Tostaco Shells	1 (0.8 oz)	130	7	10	14	1
Tostada Shells	3 (1.1 oz)	160	10	220	19	2
Rosarita						
Taco Shells	1 shell (11 g)	50	2	tr	7	tr
Tostada Shells	1 shell (14 g)	60	3	tr	8	tr
TAKE-OUT						
burrito w/ apple	1 sm (2.6 oz)	231	10	211	35	—
burrito w/ apple	1 lg (5.4 oz)	484	20	443	73	—
burrito w/ beans	2 (7.6 oz)	448	14	986	71	—
burrito w/ beans & cheese	2 (6.5 oz)	377	12	1166	55	—
burrito w/ beans & chili peppers	2 (7.2 oz)	413	15	1043	58	—
burrito w/ beans & meat	2 (8.1 oz)	508	18	1335	66	—
burrito w/ beans cheese & beef	2 (7.1 oz)	331	13	990	40	—
burrito w/ beans cheese & chili peppers	2 (11.8 oz)	663	23	2060	85	—
burrito w/ beef	2 (7.7 oz)	523	21	1492	59	—
burrito w/ beef & chili peppers	2 (7.1 oz)	426	17	1116	49	—
burrito w/ beef cheese & chili peppers	2 (10.7 oz)	634	25	2091	64	—
burrito w/ cherry	1 sm (2.6 oz)	231	10	211	35	—
burrito w/ cherry	1 lg (5.4 oz)	484	20	443	73	—
chimichanga w/ beef	1 (6.1 oz)	425	20	910	43	—
chimichanga w/ beef & cheese	1 (6.4 oz)	443	23	956	39	—
chimichanga w/ beef & red chili peppers	1 (6.7 oz)	424	19	1169	46	—
chimichanga w/ beef cheese & red chili peppers	1 (6.3 oz)	364	18	895	38	—

FOOD	PORTION	CAL.	FAT	SOD.	CARB.	FIB.
enchilada eggplant	1	142	5	—	—	—
enchilada w/ cheese	1 (5.7 oz)	320	19	784	29	—
enchilada w/ cheese & beef	1 (6.7 oz)	324	18	1320	30	—
enchirito w/ cheese beef & beans	1 (6.8 oz)	344	16	1251	34	—
frijoles w/ cheese	1 cup (5.9 oz)	226	8	882	29	—
nachos w/ cheese	6 to 8 (4 oz)	345	19	816	36	—
nachos w/ cheese & jalapeno peppers	6 to 8 (7.2 oz)	607	34	1736	60	—
nachos w/ cheese beans ground beef & peppers	6 to 8 (8.9 oz)	568	31	1800	56	—
nachos w/ cinnamon & sugar	6 to 8 (3.8 oz)	592	36	439	63	—
taco	1 sm (6 oz)	370	21	802	27	—
taco salad	1½ cups	279	15	763	24	—
taco salad w/ chili con carne	1½ cups	288	13	886	27	—
tostada w/ beans & cheese	1 (5.1 oz)	223	10	543	27	—
tostada w/ beans beef & cheese	1 (7.9 oz)	334	17	870	30	—
tostada w/ beef & cheese	1 (5.7 oz)	315	16	896	23	—
tostada w/ guacamole	2 (9.2 oz)	360	23	789	32	—
SPARE RIBS						
(*see* PORK)						
SPELT						
Arrowhead						
Spelt	1 oz	83	1	1	20	4
SPICES						
(*see* HERBS/SPICES, *individual names*)						
SPINACH						
CANNED						
spinach	½ cup	25	1	29	4	—
Del Monte						
50% Less Salt	½ cup (4 oz)	30	0	180	4	2
Chopped	½ cup (4 oz)	30	0	360	4	2
No Salt Added	½ cup (4 oz)	30	0	85	4	2
Whole Leaf	½ cup (4 oz)	30	0	360	4	2
Popeye						
Chopped	½ cup (4.1 oz)	40	1	310	6	4
Leaf	½ cup (4.2 oz)	45	1	310	7	4
Low Sodium	½ cup (4.2 oz)	35	1	35	4	3

FOOD	PORTION	CAL.	FAT	SOD.	CARB.	FIB.
S&W						
Northwest Premium	½ cup	25	0	395	3	—
Sunshine						
Chopped	½ cup (4.1 oz)	40	1	310	6	4
FRESH						
cooked	½ cup	21	tr	63	3	2
mustard chopped cooked	½ cup	14	tr	—	3	—
mustard raw chopped	½ cup	17	tr	—	3	—
new zealand chopped cooked	½ cup	11	tr	97	2	—
new zealand raw	½ cup	4	tr	36	1	—
raw chopped	½ cup	6	tr	22	1	1
raw chopped	1 pkg (10 oz)	46	1	160	7	—
Dole						
Spinach	3 oz	9	tr	107	tr	8
Fresh Express						
Spinach	1½ cups (3 oz)	40	0	160	10	5
FROZEN						
cooked	½ cup	27	tr	82	5	—
Birds Eye						
Chopped	½ cup	20	0	90	3	3
Creamed	½ cup	90	5	320	9	1
Leaf	½ cup	20	0	90	4	3
Budget Gourmet						
Au Gratin	1 pkg (5.5 oz)	160	11	600	9	—
Fresh Like						
Cut Leaf	3.5 oz	21	tr	81	4	1
Green Giant						
Creamed	½ cup	70	3	480	10	—
Cut Leaf In Butter Sauce	½ cup	40	2	380	6	4
Harvest Fresh	½ cup	25	0	170	5	3
Spinach	½ cup	25	0	100	6	5
Stouffer's						
Creamed	½ cup (2.25 oz)	150	12	380	8	2
Souffle	½ cup (4 oz)	150	10	480	9	—
Tabatchnick						
Creamed	7.5 oz	60	2	270	8	2
TAKE-OUT						
indian saag	1 serv	28	2	44	2	1
spanakopita spinach pie	1 cup (6 oz)	196	3	590	35	4

SPINACH JUICE

juice	3½ oz	7	0	73	1	—

FOOD	PORTION	CAL.	FAT	SOD.	CARB.	FIB.
SPORTS DRINKS						
(*see also* NUTRITIONAL SUPPLEMENTS)						
Gatorade						
Citrus Cooler	1 cup (8 oz)	50	0	110	14	—
Fruit Punch	1 cup (8 oz)	50	0	110	14	—
Grape	1 cup (8 oz)	50	0	110	14	—
Iced Tea Cooler	1 cup (8 oz)	50	0	110	14	—
Lemon-Lime	1 cup (8 oz)	50	0	110	14	—
Lemonade	1 cup (8 oz)	50	0	110	14	—
Orange	1 cup (8 fl oz)	50	0	110	14	—
Tropical Fruit	1 cup (8 oz)	50	0	110	14	—
PowerAde						
Fruit Punch	8 fl oz	72	0	28	19	—
Grape	8 fl oz	73	0	28	19	—
Lemon-Lime	8 fl oz	72	0	28	19	—
Orange	8 fl oz	72	0	28	19	—
Slice						
All Sport Diet Lemon Lime	8 fl oz	1	0	40	0	—
All Sport Lemon Lime	8 fl oz	72	0	55	19	—
All Sport Orange	8 fl oz	74	0	55	19	—
All Sport Punch	8 fl oz	81	0	55	22	—
Snapple						
Sport Fruit	1 bottle	80	0	60	20	—
Sport Lemon	1 bottle	80	0	60	20	—
Sport Lemon Lime	1 bottle	80	0	60	20	—
Sport Orange	1 bottle	80	0	60	20	—
Ultra Fuel						
Lemon Lime	16 fl oz	400	0	55	100	—
SPOT						
baked	3 oz	134	5	32	0	—
SQUAB						
breast w/o skin raw	1 (3.5 oz)	135	5	—	0	—
w/ skin raw	1 squab (6.9 oz)	584	47	—	0	—
w/o skin raw	1 squab (5.9 oz)	239	13	—	0	—
SQUASH						
(*see also* ZUCCHINI)						
CANNED						
crookneck sliced	½ cup	14	tr	5	3	—
Allen						
Yellow	½ cup (4.2 oz)	25	0	160	5	2
Sunshine						
Yellow	½ cup (4.2 oz)	25	0	160	5	2

FOOD	PORTION	CAL.	FAT	SOD.	CARB.	FIB.
FRESH						
acorn cooked mashed	½ cup	41	tr	3	11	3
acorn cubed baked	½ cup	57	tr	4	15	2
butternut baked	½ cup	41	tr	4	11	2
crookneck raw sliced	½ cup	12	tr	1	3	1
crookneck sliced cooked	½ cup	18	tr	1	4	1
hubbard baked	½ cup	51	tr	8	11	3
hubbard cooked mashed	½ cup	35	tr	6	8	3
scallop raw sliced	½ cup	12	tr	1	3	1
scallop sliced cooked	½ cup	14	tr	1	3	1
spaghetti cooked	½ cup	23	tr	14	5	2
Nature's Pasta						
Spaghetti Squash	1 cup (5.5 oz)	20	0	30	4	2
FROZEN						
butternut cooked mashed	½ cup	47	tr	2	12	3
crookneck sliced cooked	½ cup	24	tr	6	5	—
Birds Eye						
Winter Cooked	½ cup	45	0	0	11	2
Southland						
Butternut	4 oz	45	0	—	—	—
Prepared Squash	3.6 oz	80	2	—	—	—
SEEDS						
dried	1 oz	154	13	5	5	—
dried	1 cup	747	63	24	25	—
roasted	1 cup	1184	96	40	31	—
roasted	1 oz	148	12	5	4	—
salted & roasted	1 oz	148	12	5	4	—
salted & roasted	1 cup	1184	96	1294	31	—
whole roasted	1 oz	127	6	5	15	—
whole roasted	1 cup	285	12	12	34	—
whole salted roasted	1 oz	127	6	191	15	—
whole salted roasted	1 cup	285	12	368	34	—
SQUID						
fried	3 oz	149	6	260	7	—
raw	3 oz	78	1	37	3	—
SQUIRREL						
roasted	3 oz	147	4	102	0	—
STAR FRUIT						
fresh	1	42	tr	2	10	—
Sonoma						
Dried	7-9 pieces (1.4 oz)	140	0	0	34	0
STRAWBERRIES						
CANNED						
in heavy syrup	½ cup	117	tr	5	30	—

FOOD	PORTION	CAL.	FAT	SOD.	CARB.	FIB.
FRESH						
strawberries	1 cup	45	1	2	10	4
strawberries	1 pint	97	1	4	22	—
Dole						
Strawberries	8	50	0	0	13	3
FROZEN						
sweetened sliced	1 cup	245	tr	8	66	—
sweetened sliced	1 pkg (10 oz)	273	tr	9	74	—
unsweetened	1 cup	52	tr	3	14	—
whole sweetened	1 cup	200	tr	3	54	—
whole sweetened	1 pkg (10 oz)	223	tr	3	60	—
Big Valley						
Strawberries	⅔ cup (4.9 oz)	50	0	0	12	2
Birds Eye						
Halved In Delicious Syrup	½ cup	120	0	0	30	2
Halved In Lite Syrup	½ cup	90	0	5	22	2
Whole In Lite Syrup	½ cup	80	0	0	20	2

STRAWBERRY JUICE

FOOD	PORTION	CAL.	FAT	SOD.	CARB.	FIB.
Capri Sun						
Strawberry Cooler Drink	1 pkg (7 oz)	90	0	20	25	0
Juice Works						
Drink	6 oz	100	0	—	—	—
Kern's						
Nectar	6 fl oz	110	0	0	28	—
Kool-Aid						
Drink as prep w/ sugar	1 serv (8 oz)	100	0	30	25	0
Drink Mix as prep	1 serv (8 oz)	60	0	0	16	0
Libby						
Nectar	1 can (11.5 fl oz)	210	0	10	52	—
Smucker's						
Juice	8 oz	130	0	10	31	—

STUFFING/DRESSING

FOOD	PORTION	CAL.	FAT	SOD.	CARB.	FIB.
HOME RECIPE						
bread as prep w/ water & fat	½ cup	251	15	627	25	—
bread as prep w/ water egg & fat	½ cup	107	7	319	9	—
MIX						
bread dry as prep	½ cup	178	9	543	22	3
cornbread as prep	½ cup	179	9	455	22	—
Arnold						
All Purpose Seasoned	½ oz	50	0	200	9	1

FOOD	PORTION	CAL.	FAT	SOD.	CARB.	FIB.
Arnold (CONT.)						
Corn	½ oz	50	1	140	9	1
Herb Seasoned	½ oz	50	tr	150	2	1
Sage & Onion	½ oz	50	tr	230	9	1
Brownberry						
Corn	1 oz	103	2	350	19	2
Herb	1 oz	100	1	297	19	2
Sage & Onion	1 oz	97	1	450	18	2
Golden Grain						
Bread Stuffing Chicken	½ cup	180	9	730	20	—
Bread Stuffing Corn Bread	½ cup	180	9	870	21	—
Bread Stuffing Herb & Butter	½ cup	180	9	810	20	—
Bread Stuffing With Wild Rice	½ cup	180	9	710	21	—
Kellogg's						
Croutettes	1 cup (1.2 oz)	120	0	460	25	0
Pepperidge Farm						
Corn Bread	1 oz	110	1	320	22	—
Country Style	1 oz	100	1	400	21	—
Cube	1 oz	110	1	400	22	—
Distinctive Apple Raisin	1 oz	110	1	410	21	—
Distinctive Classic Chicken	1 oz	110	1	410	20	—
Distinctive Country Garden Herb	1 oz	120	4	300	18	—
Distinctive Vegetable & Almond	1 oz	110	3	250	19	—
Distinctive Wild Rice & Mushroom	1 oz	130	5	310	17	—
Herb Seasoned	1 oz	110	1	380	22	—
Stove Top						
Chicken as prep w/ margarine	½ cup (3.6 oz)	170	9	510	20	tr
Cornbread as prep w/ margarine	½ cup (3.6 oz)	170	8	580	21	1
Flexible Serve Chicken as prep w/ margarine	½ cup (3.3 oz)	170	8	520	19	tr
Flexible Serve Cornbread as prep w/ margarine	½ cup (3.3 oz)	160	8	560	19	1
Flexible Serve Homestyle Herb as prep w/ margarine	½ cup (3.3 oz)	170	8	500	19	1

FOOD	PORTION	CAL.	FAT	SOD.	CARB.	FIB.
Stove Top (CONT.)						
For Beef as prep w/ margarine	½ cup (3.7 oz)	180	9	540	22	1
For Pork as prep w/ margarine	½ cup (3.6 oz)	170	9	530	20	1
For Turkey as prep w/ margarine	½ cup (3.6 oz)	170	9	530	20	tr
Long Grain & Wild Rice as prep w/ margarine	½ cup (3.7 oz)	180	9	500	22	tr
Lower Sodium Chicken as prep w/ margarine	½ cup (3.6 oz)	180	9	340	21	tr
Microwave Chicken as prep w/ margarine	½ cup (3.5 oz)	160	7	480	20	tr
Microwave Homestyle Cornbread as prep w/ margarine	½ cup (3 oz)	160	7	480	20	tr
Mushroom & Onion as prep w/ margarine	½ cup (3.6 oz)	180	9	480	20	tr
San Francisco Style as prep w/ margarine	½ cup (3.6 oz)	170	9	530	20	1
Savory Herb as prep w/ margarine	½ cup (3.6 oz)	170	9	530	20	1
Traditional Sage as prep w/ margarine	½ cup (3.6 oz)	180	9	530	21	1
Wonder						
Seasoned Stuffing	1 cup (0.9 oz)	60	1	135	12	tr
TAKE-OUT						
bread	½ cup (3½ oz)	195	8	534	26	3
sausage	½ cup	292	11	258	40	1
STURGEON						
cooked	3 oz	115	4	—	0	—
raw	3 oz	90	3	—	0	—
roe raw	3.5 oz	207	10	—	1	—
smoked	1 oz	48	1	—	0	—
smoked	3 oz	147	4	—	0	—
SUCKER						
white baked	3 oz	101	3	44	0	—
SUGAR						
(*see also* FRUCTOSE, SUGAR SUBSTITUTES, SYRUP)						
brown packed	1 cup (7.7 oz)	828	0	86	214	—
brown unpacked	1 cup (5.1 oz)	546	0	57	141	—
maple	1 piece (1 oz)	100	tr	3	26	—

FOOD	PORTION	CAL.	FAT	SOD.	CARB.	FIB.
powdered	1 tbsp (0.3 oz)	31	0	0	8	—
powdered unsifted	1 cup (4.2 oz)	467	tr	2	119	—
white	1 cup (7 oz)	773	0	3	200	—
white	1 tbsp	45	0	tr	12	—
white	1 packet (6 g)	25	0	tr	6	—
white	1 tsp (4 g)	15	0	0	4	—
C&H						
White	1 tsp	16	0	—	4	—
Domino						
White	1 tsp	16	0	0	4	—
Hain						
Turbinado	1 tbsp	50	0	0	12	—
Hollywood						
Turbinado	1 tbsp	50	0	0	12	—
SUGAR SUBSTITUTES						
(*see also* FRUCTOSE)						
Equal						
Packet	1 pkg	4	0	0	tr	—
Mrs. Bateman's						
Sugarlike	1 tsp (4 g)	4	0	0	4	0
NatraTaste						
Packet	1 pkg (1 g)	0	0	0	1	—
S&W						
Liquid Table Sweetener	1/8 tsp	0	0	0	0	—
Sprinkle Sweet						
Sugar Substitute	1 tsp	2	0	1	tr	—
Sweet One						
Packet	1 pkg (1 g)	4	0	0	1	—
Sweet'N Low						
Granulated	1 pkg (1g)	4	0	1	—	—
*Sweet*10*						
Granular	1/8 tsp	0	0	2	0	—
Weight Watchers						
Sweetner	1 serv (1 g)	5	0	30	1	0
SUGAR-APPLE						
fresh	1	146	tr	15	37	—
fresh cut up	1 cup	236	1	24	59	—
SUNCHOKE						
fresh raw sliced	1/2 cup	57	tr	—	13	—
SUNDAE TOPPINGS						
(*see* ICE CREAM TOPPINGS)						
SUNFISH						
pumpkinseed baked	3 oz	97	1	87	0	—

FOOD	PORTION	CAL.	FAT	SOD.	CARB.	FIB.
SUNFLOWER						
seeds dried	1 oz	162	14	1	5	—
seeds dried	1 cup	821	71	4	27	—
seeds dry roasted	1 oz	165	14	1	7	—
seeds dry roasted	1 cup	745	64	4	31	—
seeds dry roasted salted	1 cup	745	64	975	31	—
seeds dry roasted salted	1 oz	165	14	195	7	—
seeds oil roasted	1 cup	830	78	4	20	—
seeds oil roasted salted	1 cup	830	78	804	20	—
seeds oil roasted salted	1 oz	175	16	201	4	—
seeds toasted	1 oz	176	16	1	6	—
seeds toasted	1 cup	826	76	4	28	—
seeds toasted salted	1 cup	826	76	817	28	—
seeds toasted salted	1 oz	176	16	204	6	—
sunflower butter	1 tbsp	93	8	82	4	—
sunflower butter w/o salt	1 tbsp	93	8	1	4	—
Erewhon						
Sunflower Seed Butter	2 tbsp (32 g)	200	18	20	3	—
Fisher						
Seeds Oil Roasted	1 oz	170	15	170	6	—
Seeds Salted In Shell shelled	1 oz	160	14	100	6	—
Seeds Salted In Shell unshelled	1 oz	170	15	110	6	—
Frito Lay						
Seeds	1 oz	160	14	265	6	—
Planters						
Kernels	1 pkg (2 oz)	340	29	310	11	8
Kernels	1 pkg (1.7 oz)	290	25	260	9	7
Kernels Barbecue	1 pkg (1.7 oz)	290	25	180	10	6
Kernels Honey Roasted	1 pkg (1.7 oz)	280	22	105	15	6
Kernels Salted	1 oz	170	14	140	4	4
Munch'N Go Singles Dry Roasted	1 pkg	120	11	70	4	1
Nuts Dry Roasted	¼ cup (1.1 oz)	190	17	230	6	4
Original With Shell Dry Roasted	¾ cup	160	15	35	5	2
Stone-Buhr						
Seeds Raw	4 tsp (1 oz)	170	14	10	6	6
SUSHI						
TAKE-OUT						
california roll	1 piece (0.8 oz)	28	1	37	4	—
kim chi	⅓ cup (5.8 oz)	18	tr	2143	4	—

FOOD	PORTION	CAL.	FAT	SOD.	CARB.	FIB.
sashimi	1 serv (6 oz)	198	7	718	4	—
tuna roll	1 piece (0.7 oz)	23	tr	33	3	—
vegetable roll	1 piece (1.2 oz)	27	1	47	5	—
vinegared ginger	⅓ cup (1.6 oz)	48	tr	6	12	—
wasabi	2 tsp (0.3 oz)	5	tr	124	1	—
yellowtail roll	1 piece (0.6 oz)	25	1	32	3	—
SWAMP CABBAGE						
chopped cooked	½ cup	10	tr	60	2	—
raw chopped	1 cup	11	tr	63	2	—
SWEET POTATO (*see also* YAM)						
CANNED						
in syrup	½ cup	106	tr	38	25	—
pieces	1 cup	183	tr	107	42	—
Princella						
Mashed	⅔ cup (5.1 oz)	120	1	30	28	3
Royal Prince						
Candied	½ cup (4.9 oz)	210	1	50	50	2
Halves	3 pieces (5.7 oz)	190	1	40	46	4
Orange Pineapple	½ cup (4.8 oz)	210	1	30	43	3
Sugary Sam						
Mashed	⅔ cup (5.1 oz)	120	1	30	28	3
FRESH						
baked w/ skin	1 (3½ oz)	118	tr	12	28	3
leaves cooked	½ cup	11	tr	4	2	—
mashed	½ cup	172	tr	21	40	3
FROZEN						
cooked	½ cup	88	tr	7	21	—
Mrs. Paul's						
Candied Sweet Potatoes	4 oz	170	0	40	42	—
Candied Sweets 'N Apples	4 oz	160	0	60	38	—
TAKE-OUT						
candied	3½ oz	144	3	73	29	—
SWEETBREADS						
beef braised	3 oz	230	15	51	0	—
lamb braised	3 oz	199	13	44	0	—
veal braised	3 oz	218	12	—	0	—
SWISS CHARD						
cooked	½ cup	18	tr	158	4	—
raw chopped	½ cup	3	tr	38	1	—

FOOD	PORTION	CAL.	FAT	SOD.	CARB.	FIB.
SWORDFISH						
cooked	3 oz	132	4	98	0	—
raw	3 oz	103	3	76	0	—
SYRUP						
(*see also* ICE CREAM TOPPINGS, PANCAKE/WAFFLE SYRUP)						
corn	2 tbsp	122	0	19	32	—
corn dark	1 tbsp (0.7 oz)	56	0	31	15	—
corn dark	1 cup (11.5 oz)	925	tr	608	251	—
corn light	1 cup (11.5 oz)	925	tr	395	251	—
corn light	1 tbsp (0.7 oz)	56	0	24	15	—
malt	1 tbsp (0.8 oz)	76	0	8	17	—
malt	1 cup (13 oz)	1222	tr	134	274	—
maple	1 cup (11.1 oz)	824	1	27	212	—
maple	1 tbsp (0.8 oz)	52	0	2	13	—
raspberry	3.5 oz	267	0	2	66	—
rose hip	3.5 oz	33	0	—	8	0
sorghum	1 tbsp (0.7 oz)	61	0	2	16	—
sorghum	1 cup (11.6 oz)	957	0	28	247	—
Eden						
Barley Malt Organic Syrup	1 tbsp (0.7 fl oz)	60	0	0	14	0
Estee						
Blueberry Lite	¼ cup (2.4 oz)	80	0	70	20	—
Home Brands						
Maple Rich	1 oz	110	0	—	—	—
Karo						
Corn Syrup Dark	1 tbsp (21 g)	60	0	40	15	—
Corn Syrup Dark	1 cup (331 g)	975	0	610	243	—
Corn Syrup Light	1 tbsp (21 g)	60	0	30	15	—
Corn Syrup Light	1 cup (331 g)	960	0	480	241	—
McIlhenny						
Cane	2 tbsp (1.4 oz)	130	0	20	32	tr
Quik						
Strawberry	2½ tsp (0.75 oz)	80	0	0	21	—
Strawberry	1 ⅔ tbsp	100	0	0	24	—
Red Wing						
Strawberry	2 tbsp (1.4 oz)	110	0	5	28	0
S&W						
Blueberry Diet	1 tbsp	4	0	25	1	—
Maple Flavored Diet	1 tbsp	4	0	25	1	—
Strawberry Diet	1 tbsp	4	0	25	1	—
Smucker's						
All Flavors Fruit Syrup	2 tbsp	100	0	<10	26	—

FOOD	PORTION	CAL.	FAT	SOD.	CARB.	FIB.
Tree Of Life						
Maple	1/4 cup (2.1 oz)	200	0	7	53	—
Rice Syrup	2 tbsp (1 oz)	120	1	5	29	—
Whistling Wings						
Blueberry	1 oz	45	tr	1	10	tr
Raspberry	1 oz	60	tr	2	14	0
TACO						
(*see* SPANISH FOOD)						
TAHINI						
(*see* SESAME)						
TAMARIND						
fresh	1	5	tr	1	1	—
fresh cut up	1 cup	287	1	33	75	—
TANGERINE						
CANNED						
in light syrup	1/2 cup	76	tr	8	20	—
juice pack	1/2 cup	46	tr	7	12	—
FRESH						
sections	1 cup	86	tr	3	22	—
tangerine	1	37	tr	1	9	—
Dole						
Tangerine	2	70	1	2	19	2
TANGERINE JUICE						
canned sweetened	1 cup	125	1	2	30	—
fresh	1 cup	106	tr	2	25	—
frzn sweetened as prep	1 cup	110	tr	2	27	—
frzn sweetened not prep	6 oz	344	1	7	83	—
After The Fall						
Juice	1 can (12 oz)	170	0	35	40	0
Dole						
Mandarin frzn as prep	8 fl oz	140	0	30	35	0
Fresh Samantha						
Fresh Juice	1 cup (8 oz)	106	1	0	24	1
Minute Maid						
Frozen	8 fl oz	120	0	0	29	—
TAPIOCA						
pearl dry	1/3 cup	174	0	0	45	1
starch	3 1/2 oz	344	tr	4	85	—
Minute						
Minute Tapioca	1 1/2 tsp (6 g)	20	0	0	5	0

FOOD	PORTION	CAL.	FAT	SOD.	CARB.	FIB.
TARO						
chips	1 oz	141	7	97	19	—
chips	10 (0.8 oz)	115	6	79	16	—
leaves cooked	½ cup	18	tr	2	3	—
raw sliced	½ cup	56	tr	6	14	—
shoots sliced cooked	½ cup	10	tr	1	2	—
sliced cooked	½ cup (2.3 oz)	94	tr	10	23	—
tahitian sliced cooked	½ cup	30	tr	37	5	—
TARRAGON						
ground	1 tsp	5	tr	1	1	—
TEA/HERBAL TEA						
(*see also* ICED TEA)						
(FAST FACT: On a typical day, one half of the U.S. population drinks tea. Sixty percent of all tea is from tea bags.)						
HERBAL						
Bigelow						
Almond Orange	5 fl oz	tr	tr	tr	tr	—
Apple Orchard	5 fl oz	5	tr	tr	1	—
Apple Spice	5 fl oz	tr	tr	1	tr	—
Chamomile	5 fl oz	tr	tr	2	—	—
Chamomile Mint	5 fl oz	tr	tr	1	tr	—
Cinnamon Orange	5 fl oz	tr	tr	tr	tr	—
Early Riser	5 fl oz	3	tr	tr	1	—
Feeling Free	5 fl oz	1	tr	1	tr	—
Fruit & Almond	5 fl oz	1	tr	tr	tr	—
Hibiscus & Rose Hips	5 fl oz	1	tr	1	tr	—
I Love Lemon	5 fl oz	1	tr	tr	tr	—
Lemon & C	5 fl oz	tr	tr	tr	tr	—
Looking Good	5 fl oz	1	tr	1	1	—
Mint Blend	5 fl oz	tr	tr	3	tr	—
Mint Medley	5 fl oz	1	tr	3	tr	—
Orange & C	5 fl oz	tr	tr	tr	tr	—
Orange & Spice	5 fl oz	1	tr	1	tr	—
Peppermint	5 fl oz	tr	tr	2	tr	—
Roasted Grains & Carob	5 fl oz	3	tr	1	1	—
Spearmint	5 fl oz	tr	tr	tr	tr	—
Sweet Dreams	5 fl oz	1	tr	1	tr	—
Take-A-Break	5 fl oz	3	tr	1	1	—
Celestial Seasonings						
Almond Sunset	8 fl oz	3	tr	2	1	—
Bengal Spice	8 fl oz	5	tr	3	tr	—
Caffeine Free	8 fl oz	2	tr	5	1	—
Chamomile	8 fl oz	2	tr	1	1	—

FOOD	PORTION	CAL.	FAT	SOD.	CARB.	FIB.
Celestial Seasonings (CONT.)						
Cinnamon Apple Spice	8 fl oz	<3	tr	1	tr	—
Cinnamon Rose	8 fl oz	<4	tr	1	1	—
Country Peach Spice	8 fl oz	3	tr	1	1	—
Cranberry Cove	8 fl oz	2	tr	1	1	—
Emperor's Choice	8 fl oz	4	tr	2	1	—
Ginseng Plus	8 fl oz	3	tr	4	1	—
Grandma's Tummy Mint	8 fl oz	2	tr	7	tr	—
Lemon Mist	8 fl oz	3	tr	3	tr	—
Lemon Zinger	8 fl oz	4	tr	1	1	—
Mama Bear's Cold Care	8 fl oz	6	tr	2	tr	—
Mandarin Orange Spice	8 fl oz	5	tr	2	1	—
Mellow Mint	8 fl oz	2	tr	5	tr	—
Mint Magic	8 fl oz	1	tr	13	tr	—
Orange Zinger	8 fl oz	6	tr	1	1	—
Peppermint	8 fl oz	2	tr	9	1	—
Raspberry Patch	8 fl oz	4	tr	1	1	—
Red Zinger	8 fl oz	4	tr	2	1	—
Roastaroma	8 fl oz	10	tr	3	2	—
Sleepytime	8 fl oz	4	tr	2	1	—
Spearmint	8 fl oz	5	1	6	tr	—
Strawberry Fields	8 fl oz	4	tr	1	1	—
Sunburst C	8 fl oz	3	tr	6	1	—
Tropical Escape	8 fl oz	1	tr	7	tr	—
Wild Forest Blackberry	8 fl oz	2	tr	1	1	—
Lipton						
Tea Bag Almond Pleasure as prep	1 cup	0	0	0	tr	0
Tea Bag Cinnamon Apple as prep	1 cup	0	0	0	0	0
Tea Bag Cinnamon Spice as prep	1 cup	0	0	0	tr	0
Tea Bag Country Cranberry as prep	1 cup	0	0	0	0	0
Tea Bag Gentle Orange as prep	1 cup	0	0	0	tr	0
Tea Bag Ginger Twist as prep	1 cup	0	0	0	0	0
Tea Bag Golden Honey & Lemon as prep	1 cup	0	0	0	tr	0
Tea Bag Lemon Mint Refresher as prep	1 cup	0	0	0	0	0
Tea Bag Lemon Smoother as prep	1 cup	0	0	0	0	0

FOOD	PORTION	CAL.	FAT	SOD.	CARB.	FIB.
Lipton (CONT.)						
Tea Bag Moonlight Mint as prep	1 cup	0	0	0	0	0
Tea Bag Mountain Berry	1 cup	0	0	0	tr	0
Tea Bag Orange Refresher as prep	1 cup	0	0	0	tr	0
Tea Bag Peppermint as prep	1 cup	0	0	0	0	0
Tea Bag Quietly Chamomile as prep	1 cup	0	0	0	tr	0
Tea Bag Wildflower & Honey as prep	1 cup	0	0	0	tr	—
REGULAR						
brewed tea	6 oz	2	0	5	tr	—
instant unsweetened as prep w/ water	8 oz	2	0	8	tr	—
Bigelow						
Chinese Fortune	5 fl oz	1	tr	tr	tr	—
Cinnamon Stick	5 fl oz	1	tr	tr	tr	—
Constant Comment	5 fl oz	1	tr	tr	tr	—
Darjeeling Blend	5 fl oz	1	tr	tr	tr	—
Earl Gray	5 fl oz	1	tr	tr	tr	—
English Teatime	5 fl oz	1	tr	tr	tr	—
Lemon Lift	5 fl oz	1	tr	tr	tr	—
Orange Pekoe	5 fl oz	1	tr	tr	tr	—
Peppermint Stick	5 fl oz	1	tr	1	tr	—
Plantation Mint	5 fl oz	1	tr	1	tr	—
Raspberry Royale	5 fl oz	1	tr	tr	tr	—
Celestial Seasonings						
Cinnamon Vienna	8 fl oz	2	tr	1	1	—
Earl Grey Extraordinary	8 fl oz	3	tr	tr	1	—
English Breakfast Classic	8 fl oz	3	tr	tr	tr	—
Lemon	8 fl oz	7	tr	1	1	—
Mint	8 fl oz	4	tr	1	tr	—
Morning Thunder	8 fl oz	3	tr	1	tr	—
Naturally Decaffeinated	8 fl oz	10	1	1	tr	—
Orange Spice	8 fl oz	7	tr	1	1	—
Orange Spice Decaff	8 fl oz	7	tr	1	1	—
Organically Grown	8 fl oz	12	tr	1	1	—
Raspberry	8 fl oz	7	tr	1	1	—
General Foods						
International Instant Tea Decaffeinated English Breakfast Creme	1 serv (8 oz)	70	2	105	13	0

FOOD	PORTION	CAL.	FAT	SOD.	CARB.	FIB.
General Foods (CONT.)						
International Instant Tea Decaffeinated Viennese Cinnamon Creme	1 serv (8 oz)	70	2	105	13	0
International Instant Tea English Breakfast Creme as prep	1 serv (8 oz)	70	2	65	13	0
International Instant Tea English Raspberry Creme as prep	1 serv (8 oz)	70	2	65	13	0
International Instant Tea Island Orange Creme as prep	1 serv (8 oz)	70	2	65	13	0
International Instant Tea Viennese Cinnamon Creme as prep	1 serv (8 oz)	70	2	65	13	0
Lipton						
English Blend as prep	1 cup	0	0	0	0	0
Family Size Bags Decaf as prep	1 qt	0	0	0	0	0
Family Size Bags as prep	1 qt	0	0	0	0	0
Instant as prep	1 serv	0	0	0	0	0
Instant Decaf as prep	1 serv	0	0	0	0	0
Instant Lemon as prep	1 serv	0	0	0	0	0
Special Blends Amaretto as prep	1 cup	0	0	0	0	0
Special Blends Blackberry as prep	1 cup	0	0	0	0	0
Special Blends Cinnamon as prep	1 cup	0	0	0	0	0
Special Blends Earl Grey as prep	1 cup	0	0	0	0	0
Special Blends English Breakfast as prep	1 cup	0	0	0	0	0
Special Blends Honey & Cinnamon as prep	1 cup	0	0	0	0	0
Special Blends Honey & Lemon as prep	1 cup	0	0	0	0	0
Special Blends Honey & Orange as prep	1 cup	0	0	0	0	0
Special Blends Mint as prep	1 cup	0	0	0	0	0
Special Blends Orange & Spice as prep	1 cup	0	0	0	0	0

FOOD	PORTION	CAL.	FAT	SOD.	CARB.	FIB.
Lipton (CONT.)						
Special Blends Peach as prep	1 cup	0	0	0	0	0
Special Blends Raspberry	1 cup	0	0	0	0	0
Tea Bag Decaf as prep	1	0	0	0	0	0
Tea Bag Green Tea as prep	1	0	0	0	0	0
Tea Bag as prep	1	0	0	0	0	0
Natural Touch						
Kaffree	8 fl oz	0	0	<1	0	—
Nestea						
Tea Bag as prep	6 oz	0	0	0	0	—
TEFF						
Arrowhead						
Whole Grain	¼ cup (1.6 oz)	160	1	5	32	6
TEMPEH						
tempeh	½ cup	165	6	5	14	—
Lightlife						
Garden Vege	4 oz	142	4	125	9	2
Tempeh	4 oz	182	6	10	9	—
White Wave						
Burger	1 patty (3 oz)	110	3	270	10	6
Lemon Broil	1 patty (2 oz)	130	6	340	11	4
Organic Wild Rice	⅓ block (2.7 oz)	140	4	10	12	6
Teriyaki Burger	1 patty (3 oz)	110	2	340	11	6
THYME						
ground	1 tsp	4	tr	1	1	-
Watkins						
Thyme	¼ tsp (0.5 oz)	0	0	0	0	0
TILEFISH						
cooked	½ fillet (5.3 oz)	220	7	88	0	—
cooked	3 oz	125	4	50	0	—
raw	3 oz	81	2	45	0	—
TOFU						
firm	¼ block (3 oz)	118	7	11	3	1
firm	½ cup	183	11	17	5	2
fresh fried	1 piece (0.5 oz)	35	3	2	1	tr
fuyu salted & fermented	1 block (⅓ oz)	13	1	316	1	tr
koyadofu dried frozen	1 piece (½ oz)	82	5	1	2	tr
okara	½ cup	47	1	6	8	1

FOOD	PORTION	CAL.	FAT	SOD.	CARB.	FIB.
regular	¼ block (4 oz)	88	6	8	2	1
regular	½ cup	94	6	9	2	1
Azumaya						
Blue Label	3.5 oz	46	1	2	4	—
Green Label	3.5 oz	68	2	2	4	—
Name Age Fried	3.5 oz	144	4	2	9	—
Red Label	3.5 oz	68	1	3	5	—
Casbah						
Gyro as prep w/ tofu	1 patty (2 oz)	105	3	480	15	tr
Jaclyn's						
Grilled In Black Bean Sauce	10.75 oz	270	8	170	45	—
Grilled In Peanut Sauce	10.75 oz	260	9	145	44	—
Mori-Nu						
Extra Firm	1 in slice (3 oz)	55	2	60	2	—
Firm	1 in slice (3 oz)	50	3	30	2	—
Lite Extra Firm	1 in slice (3 oz)	35	1	80	1	—
Lite Firm	1 in slice (3 oz)	35	1	70	1	—
Soft	1 in slice (3 oz)	45	3	5	2	—
Nasoya						
Chinise 5 Spice	¼ block (3 oz)	68	4	121	1	1
Extra Firm	⅕ block (3.2 oz)	92	5	9	1	tr
Firm	⅕ block (3.2 oz)	76	4	8	2	tr
French Country	⅕ block (3 oz)	68	4	130	1	1
Silken	⅕ block (3.2 oz)	48	2	12	2	tr
Soft	⅕ block (3.2 oz)	63	3	6	2	tr
Spring Creek						
Baked Barbeque	2 oz	88	4	234	7	—
Baked Cajun	2 oz	87	4	228	5	—
Baked Teriyaki	2 oz	84	4	393	3	—
Great Balls Of Tofu!	2 (3 oz)	107	5	485	5	—
Nigari Firm	4 oz	140	8	30	tr	3
Tofu Salads !Onion Dip	2 oz	46	14	155	6	—
Tofu Salads !Taco Dip	2 oz	46	14	175	6	—
Tofu Salads Missing Egg	2 oz	49	14	167	6	—
Tree Of Life						
Baked	⅕ block (3.2 oz)	150	8	310	5	0
Firm	⅕ block (3.2 oz)	100	5	5	2	0
Raw Firm	⅕ block (3.2 oz)	100	5	5	2	0
Ready Ground Hot & Spicy	⅓ pkg (3 oz)	60	4	10	2	0
Ready Ground Original	⅓ pkg (3 oz)	60	4	10	2	0
Ready Ground Savory Garlic	⅓ pkg (3 oz)	60	4	10	2	0

FOOD	PORTION	CAL.	FAT	SOD.	CARB.	FIB.
Tree Of Life (CONT.)						
Reduced Fat	⅕ block (3.2 oz)	90	4	5	4	2
Savory Baked	⅕ block (3.2 oz)	140	8	310	4	0
Smoked Hot'N Spicy	½ block (3 oz)	120	5	120	3	0
Smoked Original	½ block (3 oz)	120	5	120	3	0
White Wave						
Baked Tofus Teriyaki Oriental Style	¼ block (2 oz)	120	6	240	3	1
Hard	4 oz	120	7	15	1	—
International Baked Italian Garlic Herb	¼ pkg (2 oz)	120	6	240	3	1
International Baked Mexican Jalapeno	¼ pkg (2 oz)	120	6	240	3	1
International Baked Oriental Teriyaki	¼ pkg (2 oz)	120	6	240	3	1
International Baked Thai Sesame Peanut	¼ pkg (2 oz)	120	6	240	3	1
Soft	4 oz	120	7	15	1	—
YOGURT						
Stir Fruity						
Black Cherry	6 oz	141	2	51	25	—
Blueberry	6 oz	140	1	43	26	—
Lemon Chiffon	6 oz	152	3	43	26	—
Mixed Berry	6 oz	149	2	34	26	—
Orange	6 oz	143	2	51	26	—
Peach	6 oz	160	3	34	27	—
Pina Colada	6 oz	162	3	43	28	—
Raspberry	6 oz	155	2	34	29	—
Spiced Apple	6 oz	167	2	43	31	—
Strawberry	6 oz	140	2	51	25	—
Tropical Fruit	6 oz	170	2	43	32	—

TOMATILLO

fresh	1 (1.2 oz)	11	tr	0	2	—
fresh chopped	½ cup	21	1	1	4	—

TOMATO

(*see also* PIZZA, SPAGHETTI SAUCE)

CANNED						
paste	½ cup	110	1	86	25	6
puree	1 cup	102	tr	532	25	6
puree w/o salt	1 cup	102	tr	49	25	6
red whole	½ cup	24	tr	195	5	—
sauce	½ cup	37	tr	738	9	2
sauce spanish style	½ cup	40	tr	—	9	2

FOOD	PORTION	CAL.	FAT	SOD.	CARB.	FIB.
sauce w/ mushrooms	½ cup	42	tr	552	10	—
sauce w/ onion	½ cup	52	tr	672	12	—
stewed	½ cup	34	tr	325	8	—
w/ green chiles	½ cup	18	tr	481	4	—
wedges in tomato juice	½ cup	34	tr	285	8	—
Claussen						
Kosher	1	9	tr	—	—	—
Contadina						
California Sliced	½ cup	40	tr	—	—	—
Crushed	¼ cup	20	0	150	4	1
Italian Paste	2 tbsp	40	1	320	7	1
Italian Style Pear	½ cup	25	0	220	4	1
Italian Style Stewed	½ cup	40	0	260	8	1
Mexican Style Stewed	½ cup	40	0	220	9	1
Pasta Ready Primavera	½ cup	50	2	600	8	1
Pasta Ready Tomatoes	½ cup	50	2	550	7	1
Pasta Ready With Crushed Red Pepper	½ cup	60	3	690	8	1
Pasta Ready With Mushrooms	½ cup	50	2	640	9	1
Pasta Ready With Olives	½ cup	60	3	640	8	1
Pasta Ready With Three Cheeses	½ cup	70	4	650	8	tr
Paste	2 tbsp	30	0	20	6	1
Peeled Whole	½ cup	25	0	220	4	1
Puree	¼ cup	20	0	15	4	tr
Recipe Ready	½ cup	25	0	200	5	3
Stewed	½ cup	40	0	250	9	1
Del Monte						
Paste	2 tbsp (1.2 oz)	30	0	25	7	2
Peeled Diced	½ cup (4.4 oz)	25	0	160	6	2
Puree	¼ cup (2.2 oz)	30	0	25	7	1
Sauce	¼ cup (2.1 oz)	20	0	340	4	tr
Sauce No Salt Added	¼ cup (2.1 oz)	20	0	20	4	tr
Stewed Cajun Style	½ cup (4.4 oz)	35	0	460	9	2
Stewed Chunky Chili	½ cup (4.5 oz)	30	0	600	8	2
Stewed Chunky Pasta	½ cup (4.5 oz)	45	0	560	11	2
Stewed Chunky Pizza	½ cup (4.5 oz)	35	0	670	9	2
Stewed Chunky Salsa	½ cup (4.5 oz)	35	0	560	8	2
Stewed Italian Style	½ cup (4.4 oz)	30	0	420	8	2
Stewed Mexican Style	½ cup (4.4 oz)	35	0	400	9	2
Stewed Original	½ cup (4.4 oz)	35	0	360	9	2
Stewed Original No Salt Added	½ cup (4.4 oz)	35	0	50	9	2

FOOD	PORTION	CAL.	FAT	SOD.	CARB.	FIB.
Del Monte (CONT.)						
Wedges	½ cup (4.4 oz)	35	0	380	9	2
Whole Peeled	½ cup (4.4 oz)	25	0	160	6	2
Eden						
Crushed Organic	¼ cup (2.1 oz)	20	0	0	3	1
Sauce Lightly Seasoned	¼ cup (2.1 oz)	25	0	45	5	1
Health Valley						
Sauce	1 cup	70	1	460	13	tr
Sauce Low Sodium	1 cup	70	1	35	13	1
Hebrew National						
Pickled	⅓ tomato (1 oz)	4	0	280	1	—
Hunt's						
Choice Cut	½ cup (4.2 oz)	22	tr	325	5	1
Choice Cut Diced Tomatoes & Green Chiles	2 tbsp (0.4 oz)	1	0	24	tr	tr
Choice Cut Diced Tomatoes & Italian Herb	½ cup (4.2 oz)	24	—	600	5	1
Choice Cut Diced Tomatoes & Roasted Garlic	½ cup (4.2 oz)	24	0	505	5	1
Crushed	½ cup (4.2 oz)	29	tr	286	7	2
Crushed Angela Mia	½ cup (4.2 oz)	27	tr	380	6	2
Paste	2 tbsp (1.2 oz)	30	tr	88	6	2
Paste Italian	2 tbsp (1.2 oz)	27	tr	264	6	2
Paste No Salt Added	2 tbsp (1.2 oz)	30	tr	7	6	2
Paste With Garlic	2 tbsp (1.2 oz)	28	tr	281	6	2
Pear Shaped	½ cup (4.6 oz)	20	tr	360	4	1
Puree	¼ cup (2.2 oz)	24	tr	98	5	2
Ready Sauce Chunky Chili	¼ cup (2.2 oz)	22	tr	320	4	1
Ready Sauce Chunky Italian	¼ cup (2.2 oz)	26	tr	251	5	1
Ready Sauce Chunky Mexican	¼ cup (2.2 oz)	21	tr	390	4	1
Ready Sauce Chunky Special	¼ cup (2.2 oz)	21	tr	144	4	1
Ready Sauce Chunky Tomato	¼ cup (2.2 oz)	15	0	403	3	1
Ready Sauce Country Herb	¼ cup (2.2 oz)	33	1	255	5	1
Ready Sauce Garlic	¼ cup (2.2 oz)	29	1	269	5	2
Ready Sauce Garlic & Herb	¼ cup (2.2 oz)	26	tr	202	5	1

FOOD	PORTION	CAL.	FAT	SOD.	CARB.	FIB.
Hunt's (CONT.)						
Ready Sauce Meatloaf Fixins	¼ cup (2.2 oz)	23	tr	600	4	1
Ready Sauce Original	¼ cup (2.2 oz)	30	1	179	4	1
Ready Sauce Salsa	¼ cup (2.2 oz)	18	tr	357	3	1
Sauce	¼ cup (2.2 oz)	16	tr	366	3	1
Sauce Italian	¼ cup (2.2 oz)	32	1	210	5	1
Sauce No Salt Added	¼ cup (2.2 oz)	16	tr	12	3	1
Sauce With Herb	¼ cup (2.2 oz)	32	1	271	5	1
Stewed	½ cup (4.2 oz)	33	tr	357	7	2
Stewed Italian	4 oz	40	tr	370	9	tr
Tomatoes	½ cup (4.2 oz)	33	tr	31	7	2
Whole	2 (5.2 oz)	22	tr	403	4	1
Muir Glen						
Organic Chunky Sauce	¼ cup (2.3 oz)	20	0	160	4	1
Organic Crushed With Basil	¼ cup (2.3 oz)	25	0	85	4	1
Organic Diced	½ cup (4.5 oz)	25	0	290	4	1
Organic Diced No Salt Added	½ cup (4.5 oz)	25	0	45	4	1
Organic Ground Peeled	¼ cup (2.3 oz)	10	0	100	2	1
Organic Italian Style Diced	½ cup (4.4 oz)	25	0	290	4	1
Organic Paste	2 tbsp (1.2 oz)	30	0	20	6	1
Organic Puree	¼ cup (2.2 oz)	20	0	20	5	1
Organic Sauce	¼ cup (2.2 oz)	20	0	190	5	1
Organic Sauce No Salt Added	¼ cup (2.2 oz)	20	0	30	5	1
Organic Stewed	½ cup (4.5 oz)	30	0	290	7	tr
Organic Stewed Italian Style	½ cup (4.4 oz)	30	0	290	7	tr
Organic Stewed Mexican Style	½ cup (4.4 oz)	30	0	290	7	tr
Organic Whole Peeled	½ cup (4.6 oz)	30	0	260	5	1
Old El Paso						
Tomatoes & Jalapenos	¼ cup (2 oz)	15	0	290	3	1
Tomatoes & Green Chilies	¼ cup (2 oz)	10	0	310	2	0
Progresso						
Crushed	¼ cup (2.1 oz)	20	0	95	4	1
Paste	2 tbsp (1.2 oz)	30	0	20	6	1
Peeled Whole	½ cup (4.2 oz)	25	0	220	4	1
Peeled w/ Basil	½ cup (4.2 oz)	25	0	220	4	1
Puree	¼ cup (2.2 oz)	25	0	15	5	1

FOOD	PORTION	CAL.	FAT	SOD.	CARB.	FIB.
Progresso (CONT.)						
Puree Thick Style	¼ cup (2.2 oz)	30	0	15	5	1
Sauce	¼ cup (2.1 oz)	20	0	260	4	1
Ro-Tel						
Diced Tomatoes & Green Chilies	½ cup (4.4 oz)	20	0	370	4	1
Rosoff's						
Pickled	⅓ tomato (1 oz)	5	0	290	1	—
S&W						
Aspic Supreme	½ cup	60	0	860	16	—
Diced In Rich Puree	½ cup	35	0	290	8	—
Italian Stewed Sliced	½ cup	35	0	355	9	—
Italian Style w/ Basil	½ cup	25	0	220	5	—
Paste	6 oz	150	0	100	35	—
Peeled Ready Cut	½ cup	25	0	220	6	—
Puree	½ cup	60	0	35	14	—
Sauce	½ cup	40	0	620	9	—
Sauce Chunky	½ cup	45	0	615	10	—
Stewed 50% Salt Reduced	½ cup	35	0	180	9	—
Stewed Mexican Style	½ cup	40	0	360	8	—
Stewed Sliced	½ cup	35	0	355	9	—
Whole Diet	½ cup	25	0	20	5	—
Whole Peeled	½ cup	25	0	220	6	—
Schorr's						
Pickled	⅓ tomato (1 oz)	4	0	280	1	—
Sonoma						
Dried Spice Medley oil drained	1 tbsp (0.5 oz)	50	4	200	3	1
Pesto	¼ cup (2 oz)	110	9	125	6	1
Tapenade	1 tbsp (0.7 oz)	70	6	5	4	1
Tree Of Life						
Sauce	¼ cup (2 oz)	20	0	9	4	—
DRIED						
sun dried	1 piece	5	tr	42	1	—
sun dried	1 cup	140	2	1131	30	—
sun dried in oil	1 cup (4 oz)	235	15	293	26	—
sun dried in oil	1 piece (3 g)	6	tr	8	1	—
Sonoma						
Bits	2-3 tsp (5 g)	15	0	5	3	1
Dried	2-3 halves (5 g)	15	0	5	3	1
Halves	2-3 halves (5 g)	15	0	5	3	1
Julienne	7-9 pieces (5 g)	15	0	5	3	1
Pasta Toss	½ cup (0.7 oz)	70	0	75	13	3

FOOD	PORTION	CAL.	FAT	SOD.	CARB.	FIB.
Sonoma (CONT.)						
Season It	2-3 tsp (5 g)	20	0	25	3	1
FRESH						
cooked	½ cup	32	1	13	7	—
green	1	30	tr	16	6	—
red	1 (4.5 oz)	26	tr	11	6	2
red chopped	1 cup	35	tr	16	8	2
TAKE-OUT						
stewed	1 cup	80	3	460	13	—

TOMATO JUICE

FOOD	PORTION	CAL.	FAT	SOD.	CARB.	FIB.
beef broth & tomato	5½ oz	61	tr	220	14	—
clam & tomato	1 can (5½ oz)	77	tr	664	18	—
tomato juice	6 oz	32	tr	658	8	—
tomato juice	½ cup	21	tr	441	5	—
Campbell						
Juice	6 oz	40	0	540	8	—
Del Monte						
Snap-E-Tom	8 fl oz	50	0	670	11	2
Snap-E-Tom	10 fl oz	60	0	840	13	2
Snap-E-Tom	6 fl oz	40	0	500	8	1
Hunt's						
Juice	8 fl oz	22	tr	452	5	1
No Salt Added	8 fl oz	34	tr	12	8	2
Libby						
Juice	6 oz	35	0	450	35	—
Mott's						
Beefamato	8 fl oz	80	0	780	20	1
Clamato	8 fl oz	100	0	720	24	2
Clamato Caesar	8 fl oz	100	0	780	24	0
Muir Glen						
Organic	8 oz	40	0	550	7	tr
S&W						
California	6 oz	35	0	600	8	—
Diet	½ cup	35	0	20	8	—

TONGUE

FOOD	PORTION	CAL.	FAT	SOD.	CARB.	FIB.
beef simmered	3 oz	241	18	51	tr	—
lamb braised	3 oz	234	17	57	0	—
pork braised	3 oz	230	16	93	0	—

TOPPINGS

(*see* ICE CREAM TOPPINGS)

TORTILLA

(*see also* CHIPS TORTILLA, SPANISH FOOD)

FOOD	PORTION	CAL.	FAT	SOD.	CARB.	FIB.
corn	1 (6 in diam)	56	1	40	12	1

FOOD	PORTION	CAL.	FAT	SOD.	CARB.	FIB.
corn w/o salt	1-6 in diam (.9 oz)	56	1	3	12	1
flour w/o salt	1-8 in diam (1.2 oz)	114	3	167	20	1
Alvarado St. Bakery						
Burrito Size	1 (2.2 oz)	170	4	480	30	1
Fajita Size	1 (1.6 oz)	130	3	370	23	1
El Charrito						
Corn	2	95	1	—	—	—
Flour	2	170	4	—	—	—
Mariachi						
Tortilla	1	112	3	174	20	—
Old El Paso						
Flour	1 (1.4 oz)	150	3	340	27	0
Soft Taco Tortilla	2 (1.8 oz)	180	4	410	33	0
Tyson						
Burrito Style Flour	1	170	4	40	29	—
Burrito Style Hand Stretched Small Flour	1	106	2	50	19	—
Burrito Style Heat Pressed Large Flour	1	182	4	90	33	—
Enchilada Style Corn	1	54	tr	4	11	—
Fajito Style Flour	1	89	2	21	15	—
Soft Taco Flour	1	121	3	28	20	—
Whole Wheat	1	120	3	32	20	—
Wonder						
Low Fat Wheat	1 (1.4 oz)	120	2	280	24	1
Low Fat White	1 (1.4 oz)	110	2	280	22	1
Zapata						
Tortilla	1 (1.2 oz)	100	2	250	18	tr

TORTILLA CHIPS
(*see* CHIPS)

TREE FERN

chopped cooked	½ cup	28	tr	3	8	—

TRITICALE

dry	½ cup	323	2	5	69	17
triticale not prep	3.5 oz	329	2	26	64	7

TROUT

baked	3 oz	162	7	57	0	—
rainbow cooked	3 oz	129	4	29	0	—
seatrout baked	3 oz	113	4	63	0	—
Clear Springs						
Rainbow	3.5 oz	140	7	35	tr	—

FOOD	PORTION	CAL.	FAT	SOD.	CARB.	FIB.
TRUFFLES						
fresh	3½ oz	25	1	77	17	—
TUMERIC						
ground	1 tsp	8	tr	1	1	—
TUNA						
(*see also* TUNA DISHES)						
CANNED						
light in oil	3 oz	169	7	301	0	—
light in oil	1 can (6 oz)	399	14	606	0	—
light in water	1 can (5.8 oz)	192	1	558	0	—
light in water	3 oz	99	1	287	0	—
white in oil	3 oz	158	7	336	0	—
white in oil	1 can (6.2 oz)	331	14	704	0	—
white in water	1 can (6 oz)	234	4	673	0	—
white in water	3 oz	116	2	333	0	—
Bumble Bee						
Chunk Light In Oil	2 oz	160	12	250	0	—
Chunk Light In Water	2 oz	60	1	250	0	—
Chunk White In Oil	2 oz	160	12	250	0	—
Chunk White In Water	2 oz	70	2	250	0	—
Chunk White In Water Diet	2 oz	60	1	30	0	—
Solid White In Oil	2 oz	130	8	250	0	—
Solid White In Water	2 oz	70	2	250	0	—
Empress						
Chunk Light	2 oz	60	1	310	0	—
Chunk Light Tongol	2 oz	50	1	55	0	—
Solid White	2 oz	70	2	310	0	—
Progresso						
In Olive Oil	¼ cup (2 oz)	160	12	250	0	0
S&W						
Chunk Light Fancy In Oil	2 oz	140	10	450	0	—
Chunk Light Fancy In Water	2 oz	60	1	500	0	—
Fancy White Albacore in Oil	2 oz	160	12	450	0	—
Tree Of Life						
Tongol In Spring Water	2 oz	60	0	310	0	0
Tongol In Spring Water No Salt Water	2 oz	70	0	95	0	0
FRESH						
bluefin cooked	3 oz	157	5	43	0	—
bluefin raw	3 oz	122	4	33	0	—

FOOD	PORTION	CAL.	FAT	SOD.	CARB.	FIB.
skipjack baked	3 oz	112	1	40	0	—
yellowfin baked	3 oz	118	1	40	0	—
TUNA DISHES						
FROZEN						
Chefwich						
Tuna Melt	5 oz	360	14	—	—	—
Mrs. Paul's						
Microwave Tuna Sandwich	1	200	6	590	23	—
MIX						
Bumble Bee						
Tuna Mix-ins Classic Italian	⅓ pkg (0.17 oz)	25	0	5	5	—
Tuna Mix-ins Garden & Herb	⅓ pkg (0.17 oz)	25	0	5	5	—
Tuna Mix-ins Lemon Herb	⅓ pkg (0.17 oz)	25	0	5	6	—
Tuna Mix-ins Zesty Tomato	⅓ pkg (0.17 oz)	25	0	5	5	—
Tuna Helper						
AuGratin 50% Less Fat Recipe as prep	1 cup	250	6	870	36	1
AuGratin as prep	1 cup	310	12	930	36	1
Cheesy Pasta 50% Less Fat Recipe as prep	1 cup	230	5	850	32	tr
Cheesy Pasta as prep	1 cup	280	11	890	32	tr
Creamy Broccoli 50% Less Fat Recipe as prep	1 cup	240	5	820	35	1
Creamy Broccoli as prep	1 cup	280	11	880	35	1
Creamy Pasta 50% Less Fat Recipe as prep	1 cup	230	6	840	31	1
Creamy Pasta as prep	1 cup	300	13	910	31	1
Fettuccine Alfredo 50% Less Fat Recipe as prep	1 cup	240	6	870	32	1
Fettuccine Alfredo as prep	1 cup	310	14	950	32	1
Garden Cheddar 50% Less Fat Recipe as prep	1 cup	250	6	980	35	1
Garden Cheddar as prep	1 cup	310	12	1040	35	1
Pasta Salad Low Fat Recipe as prep	⅔ cup	230	2	790	26	1

FOOD	PORTION	CAL.	FAT	SOD.	CARB.	FIB.
Tuna Helper (CONT.)						
Pasta Salad as prep	⅔ cup	380	27	730	26	1
Tetrazzini 50% Less Fat Recipe as prep	1 cup	240	5	930	33	1
Tetrazzini as prep	1 cup	310	12	1010	33	1
Tuna Melt Reduced Fat Recipe as prep	1 cup	240	6	870	34	0
Tuna Melt as prep	1 cup	300	12	930	34	0
Tuna Pot Pie as prep	1 cup	440	24	1080	40	1
Tuna Romanoff 50% Less Fat Recipe as prep	1 cup	240	3	740	38	1
Tuna Romanoff as prep	1 cup	280	8	800	38	1
READY-TO-EAT						
The Spreadables						
Tuna Salad	¼ can	90	6	—	—	—
Wampler Longacre						
Salad	1 oz	60	4	130	3	—
TAKE-OUT						
tuna salad	1 cup	383	19	824	19	—
tuna salad	3 oz	159	8	342	8	—
tuna salad submarine sandwich w/ lettuce & oil	1	584	28	1294	55	—

TURBOT

european baked	3 oz	104	3	163	0	—

TURKEY

(*see also* DINNER, HOT DOG, TURKEY DISHES, TURKEY SUBSTITUTES)

CANNED						
w/ broth	½ can (2.5 oz)	116	5	332	0	—
w/ broth	1 can (5 oz)	231	10	663	0	—
Armour						
Turkey Loaf	2 oz	110	8	390	1	—
Hormel						
Chunk	2 oz	70	3	340	0	0
Chunk Turkey Ham	2 oz	70	4	600	0	0
Chunk White	2 oz	60	1	320	0	0
Swanson						
White	2½ oz	80	1	260	1	—
Underwood						
Chunky Light	2.08 oz	75	2	330	2	—
FRESH						
back w/ skin roasted	½ back (9 oz)	637	38	191	0	—
breast w/ skin roasted	4 oz	212	8	70	0	—

FOOD	PORTION	CAL.	FAT	SOD.	CARB.	FIB.
dark meat w/ skin roasted	3.6 oz	230	12	79	0	—
dark meat w/o skin roasted	1 cup (5 oz)	262	10	110	0	—
dark meat w/o skin roasted	3 oz	170	7	72	0	—
ground cooked	3 oz	188	11	68	0	—
leg w/ skin roasted	1 (1.2 lbs)	1133	54	420	0	—
leg w/ skin roasted	2.5 oz	147	7	55	0	—
light meat w/ skin roasted	4.7 oz	268	11	85	0	—
light meat w/ skin roasted	from ½ turkey (2.3 lbs)	2069	87	658	0	—
light meat w/o skin roasted	4 oz	183	4	75	0	—
neck simmered	1 (5.3 oz)	274	11	84	0	—
skin roasted	1 oz	141	13	17	0	—
skin roasted	from ½ turkey (9 oz)	1096	98	132	0	—
w/ skin roasted	½ turkey (4 lbs)	3857	181	1269	0	—
w/ skin roasted	8.4 oz	498	23	164	0	—
w/ skin neck & giblets roasted	½ turkey (8.8 lbs)	4123	190	1358	1	—
w/o skin roasted	7.3 oz	354	10	147	0	—
w/o skin roasted	1 cup (5 oz)	238	7	99	0	—
wing w/ skin roasted	1 (6.5 oz)	426	23	114	0	—
Butterball						
Ground All White Meat	3 oz	100	3	55	tr	—
Louis Rich						
Ground	3 oz	140	9	105	0	0
Mr. Turkey						
Ground 85% Fat Free	3.5 oz	210	16	90	0	—
Ground 91% Fat Free	3.5 oz	170	10	90	1	—
Perdue						
Breast Tenderloins Cooked	3 oz	110	1	35	0	—
Breast Boneless Cooked	3 oz	110	1	35	0	—
Breast Cutlets Thin Sliced Cooked	1 (2.5 oz)	90	1	25	0	—
Breast Fillets Cooked	3 oz	110	1	50	0	—
Burger Cooked	1 (3 oz)	170	9	65	0	—
Cubed Steak Cooked	3 oz	120	3	60	0	—
Dark Cooked	3 oz	200	14	55	0	—
Drumsticks Roasted	3 oz	150	7	70	0	—
Drumsticks Cooked	3 oz	150	7	70	0	—
Ground Cooked	3 oz	170	9	65	0	—
Ground Breast Cooked	3 oz	110	2	40	0	—
Half Breast Cooked	3 oz	170	8	35	0	—
Thighs Cooked	3 oz	180	11	55	0	—

FOOD	PORTION	CAL.	FAT	SOD.	CARB.	FIB.
Perdue (CONT.)						
Tom Wings Cooked	3 oz	160	8	90	0	—
White Cooked	3 oz	170	9	35	0	—
Whole Breast Cooked	3 oz	170	8	30	0	—
Wings Roasted	1 (3 oz)	180	10	60	0	—
Wings Drummettes Roasted	1 (3.5 oz)	180	9	65	0	—
Shady Brook						
Breast Prime Young	3 oz	140	7	—	—	—
Wings	3 oz	130	6	—	—	—
Swift-Eckrich						
Ground All White	3 oz	100	3	55	tr	—
The Turkey Store						
Seasoned Cuts Turkey Breast Roast	4 oz	110	1	530	4	—
Wampler Longacre						
Ground raw	1 oz	60	4	20	0	—
FROZEN						
roast boneless seasoned light & dark meat roasted	1 pkg (1.7 lbs)	1213	45	5320	24	—
Empire						
Patties	1 (3.1 oz)	200	10	280	14	1
READY-TO-EAT						
bologna	1 oz	57	4	249	tr	—
breast	1 slice (0.75 oz)	23	tr	301	0	—
diced light & dark seasoned	1 oz	39	2	241	tr	—
diced light & dark seasoned	½ lb	313	14	1928	2	—
ham thigh meat	1 pkg (8 oz)	291	12	2260	1	—
ham thigh meat	2 oz	73	3	565	tr	—
pastrami	2 oz	80	4	698	1	—
pastrami	1 pkg (8 oz)	320	14	2372	4	—
patties battered & fried	1 (3.3 oz)	266	17	752	15	—
patties battered & fried	1 (2.3 oz)	181	12	512	10	—
patties breaded & fried	1 (3.3 oz)	266	17	752	15	—
patties breaded & fried	1 (2.3 oz)	181	12	512	10	—
poultry salad sandwich spread	1 tbsp	109	2	49	1	—
poultry salad sandwich spread	1 oz	238	4	107	2	—
prebasted breast w/ skin roasted	½ breast (1.9 lbs)	1087	30	3434	0	—

FOOD	PORTION	CAL.	FAT	SOD.	CARB.	FIB.
prebasted breast w/ skin roasted	1 breast (3.8 lbs)	2175	60	6868	0	—
prebasted thigh w/ skin roasted	1 thigh (11 oz)	494	27	1371	0	—
roll light & dark meat	1 oz	42	2	166	1	—
roll light meat	1 oz	42	2	139	2	—
salami cooked	1 pkg (8 oz)	446	31	2278	1	—
salami cooked	2 oz	111	8	569	tr	—
turkey loaf breast meat	1 pkg (6 oz)	187	3	2433	0	—
turkey loaf breast meat	2 slices (1.5 oz)	47	1	608	0	—
turkey sticks battered & fried	1 stick (2.3 oz)	178	11	536	11	—
turkey sticks breaded & fried	1 stick (2.3 oz)	178	11	536	11	—
Alpine Lace						
Breast Fat Free	2 oz	50	0	290	0	—
Carl Buddig						
Honey Turkey	1 oz	40	2	360	1	—
Turkey	1 oz	50	3	340	1	0
Turkey Ham	1 oz	40	2	430	1	0
Empire						
Barbecue Whole	5 oz	250	12	320	0	0
Bologna	3 slices (1.8 oz)	90	6	430	3	0
Oven Prepared Breast Slices	3 slices (1.8 oz)	50	1	200	1	0
Pastrami	3 slices (1.8 oz)	60	2	270	0	1
Salami	3 slices (1.8 oz)	70	4	350	1	0
Smoked Breast Slices	3 slices (1.8 oz)	40	0	350	0	0
Falls						
BBQ	3 oz	140	8	300	—	—
Gourmet Breast	3 oz	80	1	320	—	—
Premium Cooked Breast	3 oz	100	2	240	—	—
Hansel n'Gretel						
Breast Gourmet	1 oz	28	1	170	1	—
Breast Gourmet Smoked	1 oz	31	1	170	tr	—
Breast Honey	1 oz	28	1	170	1	—
Breast Lessalt Cooked	1 oz	25	1	140	tr	—
Breast Oven Cooked	1 oz	26	tr	180	tr	—
Doubledecker Turkey Corned Beef	1 oz	30	1	195	1	—
Doubledecker Turkey Ham	1 oz	30	1	185	1	—
Healthy Choice						
Deli-Thin Honey Roast & Smoked	6 slices (2 oz)	70	2	410	2	0

FOOD	PORTION	CAL.	FAT	SOD.	CARB.	FIB.
Healthy Choice (CONT.)						
Deli-Thin Roasted Breast	6 slices (2 oz)	60	2	550	1	0
Deli-Thin Smoked Breast	6 slices (2 oz)	60	2	420	1	0
Deli-Thin Turkey Ham	6 slices (2 oz)	60	2	550	1	0
Fresh-Trak Honey Roast & Smoked Breast	1 slice (1 oz)	35	1	200	1	0
Fresh-Trak Oven Roasted Breast	1 slice (1 oz)	35	1	270	1	0
Honey Roasted & Smoked	1 slice (1 oz)	35	1	220	1	0
Oven Roasted Breast	1 slice (1 oz)	35	1	270	1	0
Smoked Breast	1 slice (1 oz)	30	1	230	0	0
Variety Pack Regular	3 slices (2.2 oz)	70	2	530	2	0
Hebrew National						
Deli Thin Hickory Smoked	1.8 oz	55	1	310	—	—
Deli Thin Lemon Garlic	1.8 oz	50	1	400	—	—
Deli Thin Oven Roasted	1.8 oz	80	1	420	—	—
Hillshire						
Deli Select Honey Roasted Breast	1 slice	10	tr	90	tr	—
Deli Select Oven Roasted Breast	1 slice	10	tr	105	tr	—
Deli Select Smoked Breast	1 slice	10	tr	100	tr	—
Deli Select Turkey Ham	1 slice	10	tr	95	tr	—
Flavor Pack 90-99% Fat Free Honey Roasted Breast	1 slice (0.75 oz)	20	tr	200	1	—
Flavor Pack 90-99% Fat Free Oven Roasted Breast	1 slice (0.75 oz)	20	tr	230	1	—
Flavor Pack 90-99% Fat Free Smoked Breast	1 slice (0.75 oz)	20	tr	220	tr	—
Honey Cured Breast	1 oz	35	1	340	2	—
Lunch 'N Munch Smoked Turkey/ Cheddar	1 pkg (4.5 oz)	350	21	1130	20	—
Lunch 'N Munch Smoked Turkey/ Cheddar/ Brownie	1 pkg (4.5 oz)	400	22	1240	34	—
Lunch 'N Munch Turkey/ Cheddar/ Brownie/ Hi-C	1 pkg (4.5 oz + 6 fl oz)	500	22	1260	58	—

FOOD	PORTION	CAL.	FAT	SOD.	CARB.	FIB.
Hillshire (CONT.)						
Smoked Breast	1 oz	35	1	340	1	—
Hormel						
Light & Lean 97 Breast Sliced	1 slice (1 oz)	30	1	360	0	0
Light & Lean 97 Breast Smoked	3 oz	80	1	780	1	0
Light & Lean 97 Cuts	16 pieces (1 oz)	30	1	460	1	0
Light & Lean 97 Cuts Smoked	16 pieces (1 oz)	30	1	460	1	0
Jordan's						
Healthy Trim Fat Free Oven Roasted Breast	1 slice (1 oz)	20	0	180	0	0
Healthy Trim Fat Free Oven Roasted Smoked Breast	1 slice (1 oz)	20	0	180	0	0
Louis Rich						
Bologna	1 slice (28 g)	50	4	250	1	0
Breaded Nuggets	4 (3.2 oz)	260	15	640	15	0
Breaded Patties	1 (3 oz)	220	13	550	13	0
Breaded Sticks	3 (3 oz)	230	15	580	12	0
Carving Board Oven Roasted Breast	2 slices (1.6 oz)	40	1	560	0	0
Carving Board Oven Roasted Thin Carved Breast	6 slices (2.1 oz)	60	1	740	0	0
Carving Board Smoked Breast	2 slices (1.6 oz)	40	1	560	0	0
Chopped Ham	1 slice (1 oz)	46	3	290	0	0
Cotto Salami	1 slice (28 g)	40	3	290	0	0
Deli-Thin Smoked Breast	4 slices (1.8 oz)	50	1	490	1	0
Fat Free Hickory Smoked Breast	1 slice (1 oz)	25	0	300	1	0
Fat Free Oven Roasted Breast	1 slice (28 g)	25	0	310	1	0
Ham Round	1 slice (28 g)	34	1	300	0	0
Ham Square	3 slices (2.2 oz)	70	3	710	1	0
Hickory Smoked Dinner Slices Breast	1 slice (2.8 oz)	80	1	1060	2	0
Honey Cured Turkey Ham	3 slices (2.2 oz)	70	2	660	2	0
Honey Roasted Breast	1 slice (1 oz)	30	1	320	1	0
Honey Roasted Dinner Slices Breast	1 slice (2.8 oz)	80	1	940	3	0

FOOD	PORTION	CAL.	FAT	SOD.	CARB.	FIB.
Louis Rich (CONT.)						
Oven Roasted Breast	2 oz	60	2	640	2	0
Oven Roasted Breast	1 slice (1 oz)	30	1	310	1	0
Oven Roasted Deli-Thin Breast	4 slices (1.8 oz)	50	1	580	2	0
Oven Roasted Dinner Slices Breast	1 slice (2.8 oz)	70	1	910	1	0
Pastrami	2 slices (1.6 oz)	45	2	520	0	0
Salami	1 slice (28 g)	45	3	290	0	0
Skinless Barbecued Breast	2 oz	60	1	680	2	0
Skinless Hickory Smoked Breast	2 oz	60	1	760	1	0
Skinless Honey Roasted Breast	2 oz	60	1	690	2	0
Skinless Oven Roasted Breast	2 oz	50	1	650	1	0
Smoked Breast	1 slice (1 oz)	25	1	260	0	0
Smoked White	1 slice (1 oz)	30	1	290	0	0
Turkey Ham	4 slices (1.8 oz)	60	2	580	0	0
Mr. Turkey						
Deli Cuts Hardwood Smoked Breast	3 slices	30	1	340	1	—
Deli Cuts Honey Roasted Breast	3 slices	30	1	310	2	—
Deli Cuts Oven Roasted Breast	3 slices	30	1	270	2	—
Deli Cuts Turkey Ham	3 slices	35	2	310	1	—
Deli Cuts Turkey Pastrami	3 slices	35	1	255	1	—
Hardwood Smoked Breast	1 slice	30	1	280	2	—
Hardwood Smoked Turkey Ham	1 slice	35	2	320	0	—
Honey Cured Turkey Ham	1 slice	30	1	320	1	—
Oven Roasted Breast	1 slice	30	1	270	2	—
Smoked Breakfast Turkey Ham	1 oz	30	1	325	1	—
Turkey Bologna	1 slice	70	5	370	1	—
Turkey Cotto Salami	1 slice	50	4	240	1	—
Turkey Ham	1 slice	35	2	320	0	—
Turkey Pastrami	1 slice	30	1	290	1	—
Oscar Mayer						
Deli-Thin Roast	4 slices (1.8 oz)	50	1	560	2	0

FOOD	PORTION	CAL.	FAT	SOD.	CARB.	FIB.
Oscar Mayer (CONT.)						
Deli-Thin Smoked Honey Roasted	4 slices (1.8 oz)	60	1	520	2	0
Free Oven Roasted Breast	4 slices (1.8 oz)	40	0	610	2	—
Free Smoked Breast	4 slices (1.8 oz)	40	0	550	2	—
Healthy Favorites Oven Roasted Breast	4 slices (1.8 oz)	40	0	610	2	0
Healthy Favorites Smoked Breast	4 slices (1.8 oz)	40	0	550	2	0
Lunchables Fun Pack Turkey/Pacific Cooler	1 pkg (11.2 oz)	460	21	1310	53	tr
Lunchables Fun Pack Turkey/Surger Cooler	1 pkg (11.2 oz)	440	16	1220	60	0
Lunchables Turkey Oven Roasted/Green Onion Cheese	1 pkg (4.5 oz)	380	20	1270	36	1
Lunchables Turkey Smoked/ Ranch & Herb Cheese	1 pkg (4.5 oz)	380	20	1280	36	1
Lunchables Turkey/ Cheddar	1 pkg (4.5 oz)	360	22	1650	20	1
Perdue						
Nuggets Dinosaur	3 (3 oz)	200	12	390	15	2
Sara Lee						
Hardwood Smoked Breast Of Turkey	2 oz	60	1	550	0	—
Hardwood Smoked Turkey Ham	2 oz	60	2	620	1	—
Honey Roasted Breast Of Turkey	2 oz	60	0	550	2	—
Honey Roasted Turkey Ham	2 oz	70	3	660	2	—
Mesquite Smoked Breast Of Turkey	2 oz	60	2	510	0	—
Oven Roasted Breast Of Turkey	2 oz	60	2	370	0	—
Peppered Breast Of Turkey	2 oz	50	0	420	2	—
Seasoned Breast Of Turkey Pastrami	2 oz	60	1	510	2	—
Tyson						
Breast	1 slice	20	tr	136	tr	—
Ham	1 slice	23	tr	182	1	—

FOOD	PORTION	CAL.	FAT	SOD.	CARB.	FIB.
Wampler Longacre						
Bologna	1 oz	60	5	260	tr	—
Breast Chops	1 serv (4 oz)	120	1	90	0	—
Breast Sliced	1 slice (1 oz)	35	tr	310	1	—
Breast Sliced Smoked	1 slice (0.75 oz)	20	tr	210	1	—
Burger	1 (4 oz)	230	17	90	0	—
Burger	1 (3 oz)	170	13	70	0	—
Burger Barbecue	1 (4 oz)	240	17	280	4	—
Chef Select Breast Skinless	1 oz	35	tr	220	tr	-
Chef Select Breast Smoked	1 oz	35	1	240	1	-
Chunk Dark Smoked Cured	1 oz	45	3	300	1	-
Chunk Ham 12% Water Smoked	1 oz	45	3	200	tr	—
Chunk Ham 20% Water	1 oz	40	2	370	2	—
Chunk Pastrami	1 oz	35	2	280	tr	—
Cook-In-The-Bag Breast	1 oz	30	1	125	1	—
Cook-In-The-Bag Breast Mini	1 oz	30	1	105	tr	—
Cook-In-The-Bag Combo Roast	1 oz	35	1	125	tr	—
Cook-In-The-Bag Thigh Roast	1 oz	40	2	130	1	—
Dark Smoked Cured	1 oz	45	3	3000	1	—
Deli Chef Breast And White Meat No Skin	1 oz	40	2	240	1	—
Gourmet Breast	1 oz	35	1	300	1	—
Gourmet Breast Mini	1 oz	35	1	300	1	—
Gourmet Breast Mini Smoked	1 oz	35	1	240	1	—
Gourmet Breast Smoked	1 oz	30	tr	230	1	—
Gourmet Brown & Glazed Breast	1 oz	35	1	240	1	—
Gourmet Brown & Roasted Breast	1 oz	35	1	260	1	—
Gourmet Honey Cured Breast	1 oz	30	1	210	1	—
Lean-Lite Breast Skinless	1 oz	35	tr	160	0	—
Lean-Lite Deli Breast	1 oz	35	1	160	0	—
Lean-Lite Deli Breast Smoked	1 oz	35	1	170	1	—

FOOD	PORTION	CAL.	FAT	SOD.	CARB.	FIB.
Wampler Longacre (CONT.)						
Old Fashioned Brown & Roasted Breast	1 oz	35	tr	160	tr	—
Pastrami	1 oz	35	2	280	tr	—
Premium Breast Skinless	1 oz	30	tr	250	1	—
Premium Brown & Roasted Breast Skinless	1 oz	16	1	300	1	—
Roll Combo	1 oz	44	3	187	tr	—
Roll Sliced Breast	1 slice (0.75 oz)	30	tr	250	1	—
Roll White	1 oz	45	3	200	tr	—
Salami	1 oz	50	3	280	1	—
Salt Watchers Breast Skinless	1 oz	35	1	20	0	—
Seasoned Roast	1 oz	40	2	90	0	—
Sliced Salami	1 slice (0.8 oz)	45	3	240	1	—
Tenderlings BBQ	1 serv (4 oz)	110	tr	520	0	—
Tenderlings Cajun	1 serv (4 oz)	110	tr	560	0	—
Tenderlings Garlic & Pepper	1 serv (4 oz)	110	tr	600	0	—
Tenderlings Original	1 serv (4 oz)	110	tr	480	0	—
Turkey Ham 12% Water Baked	1 oz	45	3	200	tr	—
Turkey Ham 20% Water Baked	1 oz	40	2	370	1	—
Unseasoned Roast	1 oz	40	2	15	0	—
Whole Browned & Roasted	1 oz	60	3	100	tr	—
Weight Watchers						
Deli Thin Smoked Breast	5 slices (1/3 oz)	10	tr	80	tr	—
Oven Roasted Breast	2 slices (3/4 oz)	25	1	200	tr	—
Oven Roasted Turkey Ham	2 slices (3/4 oz)	25	1	210	tr	—
Roasted & Smoked Breast	2 slices (3/4 oz)	25	1	170	tr	—

TURKEY DISHES

(*see also* DINNER, TURKEY SUBSTITUTES)

FOOD	PORTION	CAL.	FAT	SOD.	CARB.	FIB.
CANNED						
Dinty Moore						
Stew	1 cup (8.5 oz)	140	3	850	19	2
FROZEN						
gravy & turkey	1 pkg (5 oz)	95	4	786	7	—

FOOD	PORTION	CAL.	FAT	SOD.	CARB.	FIB.
gravy & turkey	1 cup (8.4 oz)	160	6	1328	11	—
Hot Pocket						
Stuffed Sandwich Turkey & Ham With Cheese	1 (4.5 oz)	320	13	680	38	1
Lean Pockets						
Stuffed Sandwich Turkey & Ham With Cheddar	1 (4.5 oz)	260	7	810	35	4
Stuffed Sandwich Turkey Broccoli & Cheese	1 (4.5 oz)	260	8	710	35	4
Luigino's						
Gravy Dressing & Turkey	1 pkg (8 oz)	340	15	910	36	2
Ovenstuffs						
Turkey Turnover	1 (4.75 oz)	350	16	700	35	—
READY-TO-EAT						
Spreadables						
Turkey Salad	¼ can	100	6	—	—	—
Wampler Longacre						
Meatloaf Italian	1 serv (4 oz)	114	5	640	5	—
Meatloaf Mexican	1 serv (4 oz)	114	5	680	4	—
Meatloaf Original	1 serv (4 oz)	126	5	620	10	—
Salad	1 oz	60	4	140	3	—
Salad Turkey Ham	1 oz	50	4	190	3	—
Teriyaki	1 serv (4 oz)	112	tr	640	14	—
SHELF-STABLE						
Dinty Moore						
Microwave Cup Stew	1 cup (7.5 oz)	130	3	760	16	2

TURKEY SUBSTITUTES

FOOD	PORTION	CAL.	FAT	SOD.	CARB.	FIB.
Harvest Direct						
TVP Poultry Chunks	3.5 oz	280	1	15	32	18
TVP Poultry Ground	3.5 oz	280	1	15	32	18
Soy Is Us						
Turkey Not!	½ cup (1.75 oz)	140	2	5	15	9
White Wave						
Meatless Sandwich Slices	2 slices (1.6 oz)	80	0	400	7	1
Worthington						
Smoked Turkey Slices	4 slices (76 g)	180	12	820	5	—
Turkee Slices	2 slices (63 g)	130	9	430	3	—

TURNIPS

FOOD	PORTION	CAL.	FAT	SOD.	CARB.	FIB.
CANNED						
greens	½ cup	17	tr	325	3	—

FOOD	PORTION	CAL.	FAT	SOD.	CARB.	FIB.
Allen						
Chopped Greens And Diced Turnip	½ cup (4.2 oz)	30	1	20	5	tr
Greens	½ cup (4.2 oz)	25	1	15	3	2
Luck's						
Turnip Greens w/ Diced Turnips Seasoned w/ Pork	7.5 oz	90	6	—	—	—
Sunshine						
Chopped Greens And Diced Turnip	½ cup (4.2 oz)	30	1	20	5	tr
Greens	½ cup (4.2 oz)	25	1	15	3	2
FRESH						
cooked mashed	½ cup (4.2 oz)	47	tr	25	10	—
cubed cooked	½ cup (3 oz)	33	tr	17	7	—
greens chopped cooked	½ cup	15	tr	21	3	2
greens raw chopped	½ cup	7	tr	11	2	1
raw cubed	½ cup (2.4 oz)	25	tr	14	6	—
FROZEN						
greens cooked	½ cup	24	tr	12	4	2
Southland						
Mashed	3.6 oz	90	6	—	—	—
Rutabaga Yellow Turnips	4 oz	50	0	—	—	—
TURTLE						
raw	3½ oz	85	1	—	0	—
TUSK FISH						
raw	3½ oz	79	tr	113	0	—
VANILLA						
Hershey						
Vanilla Milk Chips	¼ cup	240	14	65	25	—
Virginia Dare						
Vanilla Extract	1 tsp	10	0	—	—	—
VEAL						
(*see also* DINNER, VEAL DISHES)						
FRESH						
cutlet lean only braised	3 oz	172	4	57	0	—
cutlet lean only fried	3 oz	156	4	65	0	—
ground broiled	3 oz	146	6	70	0	—
loin chop w/ bone lean & fat braised	1 chop (2.8 oz)	227	14	64	0	—
loin chop w/ bone lean only braised	1 chop (2.4 oz)	155	6	58	0	—

FOOD	PORTION	CAL.	FAT	SOD.	CARB.	FIB.
shoulder w/ bone lean only braised	3 oz	169	5	83	0	—
sirloin w/ bone lean & fat roasted	3 oz	171	9	71	0	—
sirloin w/ bone lean only roasted	3 oz	143	5	72	0	—
VEAL DISHES						
TAKE-OUT						
parmigiana	4.2 oz	279	18	545	6	2
VEGETABLE JUICE						
vegetable juice cocktail	6 fl oz	34	tr	664	8	—
vegetable juice cocktail	½ cup	22	tr	442	6	—
Mott's						
Vegetable Juice as prep	8 fl oz	60	0	800	13	2
Muir Glen						
Organic	8 oz	70	0	620	15	3
Organic Reduced Sodium	8 oz	70	0	465	15	3
Odwalla						
Vegetable Cocktail	8 fl oz	70	0	290	18	2
Smucker's						
Vegetable Juice Hearty	8 fl oz	58	tr	714	13	—
Vegetable Juice Hot & Spicy	8 fl oz	58	tr	650	13	—
V8						
No Salt Added	6 fl oz	35	0	45	8	—
Original	6 fl oz	35	0	560	8	—
Spicy Hot	6 fl oz	35	0	650	8	—
VEGETABLES MIXED (*see also* VEGETABLE JUICE)						
CANNED						
mixed vegetables	½ cup	39	tr	122	8	—
peas & carrots	½ cup	48	tr	332	11	—
peas & carrots low sodium	½ cup	48	tr	332	11	—
peas & onions	½ cup	30	tr	265	5	—
succotash	½ cup	102	1	325	23	—
Allen						
Green Beans And Potatoes	½ cup (4.2 oz)	35	0	220	7	2
Okra & Tomatoes	½ cup (4 oz)	25	0	380	5	3
Okra Tomatoes & Corn	½ cup (4.1 oz)	30	0	280	6	4
Chi-Chi's						
Diced Tomatoes & Green Chilies	¼ cup (2.5 oz)	20	0	340	4	0

FOOD	PORTION	CAL.	FAT	SOD.	CARB.	FIB.
Del Monte						
Mixed	½ cup (4.4 oz)	40	0	360	8	2
Peas And Carrots	½ cup (4.5 oz)	60	0	360	11	2
Green Giant						
Garden Medley	½ cup	40	tr	290	9	1
Hanover						
Mixed	½ cup	110	0	—	—	—
Vegetable Salad	½ cup	90	0	—	—	—
House Of Tsang						
Vegetables & Sauce Cantonese Classic	½ cup (4.2 oz)	70	1	930	13	1
Vegetables & Sauce Hong Kong Sweet & Sour	½ cup (4.5 oz)	160	0	580	40	0
Vegetables & Sauce Szechuan Hot & Spicy	½ cup (4.2 oz)	70	1	1090	14	1
Vegetables & Sauce Tokyo Teriyaki	½ cup (4.4 oz)	100	0	1240	22	0
Ka-Me						
Stir Fry	½ cup (4.5 oz)	20	0	10	4	2
La Choy						
Chop Suey Vegetables	½ cup	10	tr	320	2	tr
S&W						
Garden Salad Marinated	½ cup	60	0	670	11	—
Mixed Vegetables Old Fashion Harvest Time	½ cup	35	0	380	6	—
Peas & Carrots Water Pack	½ cup	35	0	5	7	—
Succotash Country Style	½ cup	80	1	250	16	—
Sweet Peas & Diced Carrots	½ cup	50	0	310	9	—
Sweet Peas w/ Tiny Pearl Onions	½ cup	60	1	490	10	—
Seneca						
Peas & Carrots	½ cup	60	0	408	9	4
Succotash	½ cup	90	0	240	18	2
Sunshine						
Green Beans And Potatoes	½ cup (4.2 oz)	35	0	220	7	2
Trappey						
Okra & Tomatoes	½ cup (4 oz)	25	0	380	5	3
Okra Tomatoes & Corn	½ cup (4.1 oz)	30	0	280	6	4
FROZEN						
mixed vegetables cooked	½ cup	54	tr	32	12	2

FOOD	PORTION	CAL.	FAT	SOD.	CARB.	FIB.
peas & carrots cooked	½ cup	38	tr	55	8	—
peas & onions cooked	½ cup	40	tr	—	8	—
succotash cooked	½ cup	79	1	38	17	—
Big Valley						
California Blend	¾ cup (3 oz)	25	0	20	6	3
Italian Blend	¾ cup (3 oz)	30	0	20	5	2
Oriental Blend	¾ cup (3 oz)	25	0	10	5	3
Stew Vegetables	⅔ cup (3 oz)	40	0	30	10	2
Winter Blend	¾ cup (3 oz)	25	0	15	4	2
Birds Eye						
Broccoli Cauliflower And Carrots With Cheese Sauce	½ pkg	80	4	390	7	4
Farm Fresh Broccoli And Cauliflower	¾ cup	30	0	25	5	3
Farm Fresh Broccoli Carrots And Water Chestnuts	¾ cup	40	0	35	8	3
Farm Fresh Broccoli Cauliflower And Carrots	¾ cup	35	0	40	7	3
Farm Fresh Broccoli Cauliflower And Red Peppers	¾ cup	30	0	25	5	3
Farm Fresh Broccoli Corn And Red Peppers	⅔ cup	60	1	15	14	3
Farm Fresh Broccoli Green Beans Pearl Onions and Red Peppers	¾ cup	35	0	15	7	3
Farm Fresh Broccoli Red Peppers Onions And Mushrooms	¾ cup	30	0	20	6	3
Farm Fresh Brussels Sprouts Cauliflower And Carrots	¾ cup	40	0	30	8	4
Farm Fresh Cauliflower Carrots And Snow Peas	⅔ cup	35	0	30	8	4
In Butter Sauce Broccoli Cauliflower And Carrots	½ cup	40	2	180	6	2

FOOD	PORTION	CAL.	FAT	SOD.	CARB.	FIB.
Birds Eye (CONT.)						
In Sauce Peas And Pearl Onions With Seasonings	½ cup	70	0	440	13	3
Internationals Austrian	3.3 oz	70	3	390	6	1
Internationals Bavarian	3.3 oz	90	5	260	11	2
Internationals California	3.3 oz	90	4	200	10	3
Internationals French Country	3.3 oz	70	4	230	6	2
Internationals Italian	3.3 oz	80	5	250	8	2
Internationals Japanese	3.3 oz	60	3	270	6	2
Internationals New England	3.3 oz	100	5	280	12	2
Mixed	⅔ cup (3 oz)	60	1	40	11	2
Peas And Potatoes With Cream Sauce	½ cup	100	3	420	16	1
Polybag	½ cup	60	0	40	12	2
Budget Gourmet						
Mandarin Vegetables	1 pkg (5.25 oz)	160	11	440	13	—
New England Recipe Vegetables	1 pkg (5.5 oz)	230	13	380	21	—
Spring Vegetables In Cheese Sauce	1 pkg (5 oz)	130	8	370	9	—
Fresh Like						
California Blend	3.5 oz	31	tr	21	7	1
Chuckwagon Blend	3.5 oz	71	1	5	17	1
Italian Blend	3.5 oz	33	tr	21	7	1
Midwestern Blend	3.5 oz	42	tr	32	9	1
Mixed	3.5 oz	69	tr	48	14	1
Oriental Blend	3.5 oz	26	tr	11	5	1
Peas & Carrots	3.5 oz	63	tr	63	12	1
Winter Blend	3.5 oz	26	tr	26	5	1
Green Giant						
American Mixtures California	½ cup	25	0	40	6	2
American Mixtures Heartland	½ cup	25	0	35	6	2
American Mixtures New England	½ cup	70	1	75	14	4
American Mixtures San Francisco	½ cup	25	0	35	7	2
American Mixtures Sante Fe	½ cup	70	1	0	16	2
American Mixtures Seattle	½ cup	25	0	35	7	2

FOOD	PORTION	CAL.	FAT	SOD.	CARB.	FIB.
Green Giant (CONT.)						
Broccoli Cauliflower And Carrots In Butter Sauce	½ cup	30	1	240	4	—
Broccoli Cauliflower And Carrots In Cheese Sauce	½ cup	60	2	490	9	2
Harvest Fresh Mixed Vegetables	½ cup	40	0	125	9	2
Mixed	½ cup	40	0	40	9	2
Mixed In Butter Sauce	½ cup	60	2	300	11	2
One Serve Broccoli Carrots & Rotini In Cheese Sauce	1 pkg	120	3	520	20	—
One Serve Broccoli Cauliflower And Carrots	1 pkg	25	0	45	7	3
Valley Combinations Broccoli & Cauliflower	½ cup	60	2	340	9	—
Hanover						
Broccoli Cut & Cauliflower Cut	½ cup	20	0	—	—	—
Caribbean Blend	½ cup	20	0	—	—	—
Garden Medley	½ cup	20	0	—	—	—
Mixed	½ cup	50	0	—	—	—
Oriental Blend	½ cup	25	0	—	—	—
Succotash	½ cup	80	0	—	—	—
Summer Vegetables	½ cup	35	0	—	—	—
Vegetables For Soup	½ cup	60	0	—	—	—
La Choy						
Mixed Fancy	½ cup	12	tr	30	2	1
Ore Ida						
Stew Vegetables	⅔ cup (3 oz)	50	0	50	11	tr
Soglowek						
Golden Vegetarian Nuggets	4 pieces (2.5 oz)	190	11	220	9	1
Southland						
Peppers & Onions	2 oz	15	0	—	—	—
Soup Mix Vegetables	3.2 oz	50	0	—	—	—
Stew Vegetables	4 oz	60	0	—	—	—
Tree Of Life						
Mixed	½ cup (3 oz)	65	0	60	13	3
Veg-All						
Country Wisconsin Blend	3.5 oz	52	tr	16	13	1

FOOD	PORTION	CAL.	FAT	SOD.	CARB.	FIB.
Veg-All (CONT.)						
Scandinavian Blend	3.5 oz	48	tr	32	9	1
Vegetables For Soup (Eight)	3.5 oz	34	tr	44	12	1
Vegetables For Soup (Potatoes)	3.5 oz	53	tr	44	12	1
Vegetables For Stew 4-Way	3.5 oz	51	tr	42	12	1
Vegetables For Stew 5-Way	3.5 oz	54	tr	42	12	1
SHELF-STABLE						
Pantry Express						
Corn Green Beans Carrots Pasta In Tomato Sauce	½ cup	80	2	330	17	3
Green Beans Potatoes And Mushrooms In A Seasoned Sauce	½ cup	50	2	430	9	2
Mixed Vegetables	½ cup	35	tr	300	8	1
TAKE-OUT						
caponata	¼ cup	28	1	—	—	—
curry	1 serv (7.7 oz)	398	33	—	22	—
gyoza potstickers vegetable	8 (4.9 oz)	210	4	500	34	5
pakoras	1 (2 oz)	108	5	—	12	3
ratatouille	8.8 oz	190	16	—	10	5
samosa	2 (4 oz)	519	46	—	25	3
succotash	½ cup	111	1	16	23	—

VENISON

FOOD	PORTION	CAL.	FAT	SOD.	CARB.	FIB.
roasted	3 oz	134	3	46	0	—
Broken Arrow Ranch						
Antelope Chili Meat	3.5 oz	115	2	76	1	—
Antelope Ground Venison	3.5 oz	110	2	69	tr	—
Antelope Stew Meat	3.5 oz	110	2	54	2	—
Nilgai Chili Meat	3.5 oz	115	2	76	1	—
Nilgai Leg	3.5 oz	100	1	55	1	—
Nilgai Stew Meat	3.5 oz	110	2	54	2	—
Venison & Beef Smoked Sausage	6 oz	432	30	—	4	—
Venison Meat Chunks	6 oz	175	2	—	0	—
Venison Salami	6 oz	252	8	—	0	—

VINEGAR

FOOD	PORTION	CAL.	FAT	SOD.	CARB.	FIB.
balsamic	1 tbsp (0.5 oz)	5	0	0	2	—

FOOD	PORTION	CAL.	FAT	SOD.	CARB.	FIB.
cider	1 tbsp	tr	0	tr	1	—
Hain						
Cider	1 tbsp	2	0	1	4	—
Ka-Me						
Chinese Seasoned	1 tbsp (0.5 fl oz)	5	0	60	1	0
Rice Wine Chinese	1 tbsp (0.5 fl oz)	5	0	0	1	0
Rice Wine Japanese	1 tbsp (0.5 oz)	0	0	0	1	0
Seasoned Rice Japanese	1 tbsp (0.5 fl oz)	10	0	180	3	0
Nakano						
Rice	1 tbsp	0	0	1	0	—
Regina						
Red Wine	1 oz	4	0	0	0	—
Tree Of Life						
Apple Cider Organic	1 tbsp (0.5 oz)	0	0	0	tr	—
Brown Rice	1 tbsp (0.5 oz)	2	0	45	0	—
Victoria						
Balsamic	1 tbsp (0.5 oz)	5	0	0	2	—
White House						
Apple Cider	2 tbsp	2	0	0	1	0
Red Wine	2 tbsp	4	0	5	2	—

WAFFLES

FROZEN

FOOD	PORTION	CAL.	FAT	SOD.	CARB.	FIB.
buttermilk	1 4 in sq (1.2 oz)	88	3	262	14	1
plain	1 4 in sq (1.2 oz)	88	3	262	14	1
Aunt Jemima						
Blueberry	2 (2.5 oz)	190	7	530	28	1
Buttermilk	2 (2.5 oz)	170	6	410	27	1
Cinnamon	2 (2.5 oz)	180	6	470	28	1
Oatmeal	2 (2.5 oz)	170	7	660	27	3
Whole Grain	2 (2.5 oz)	170	7	450	24	2
Belgian Chef						
Belgian	2 (2.5 oz)	140	3	340	24	1
Downyflake						
Blueberry	2	180	4	570	32	—
Buttermilk	2	190	5	750	32	—
Multi-Grain	2	250	14	500	28	4
Oat Bran	2	260	13	650	30	3
Regular	2	120	3	420	20	—
Regular Jumbo	2	170	4	570	30	—
Rice Bran	2	210	11	230	25	4
Roman Meal	2	280	14	680	33	3
Waffles	2	180	6	620	27	—
Eggo						
Apple Cinnamon	2 (2.7 oz)	220	8	450	33	0

FOOD	PORTION	CAL.	FAT	SOD.	CARB.	FIB.
Eggo (CONT.)						
Blueberry	2 (2.7 oz)	220	8	450	33	0
Buttermilk	2 (2.7 oz)	220	8	480	30	0
Common Sense Oat Bran	2 (2.7 oz)	200	7	350	27	3
Common Sense Oat Bran With Fruit & Nut	2 (2.9 oz)	220	8	340	32	4
Homestyle	2 (2.7 oz)	220	8	470	30	0
Minis Blueberry	12 (3 oz)	240	8	510	37	0
Minis Cinnamon Toast	12 (3.2 oz)	280	9	470	40	0
Minis Homestyle	12 (1.8 oz)	240	8	520	34	0
Nut & Honey	2 (2.7 oz)	240	10	480	32	0
Nutri-Grain	2 (2.7 oz)	190	6	430	30	4
Nutri-Grain Multi-Bran	2 (2.7 oz)	180	6	400	32	6
Nutri-Grain Raisin & Bran	2 (3 oz)	210	6	390	36	5
Special K	2 (2 oz)	140	0	250	29	0
Strawberry	2 (2.7 oz)	220	8	460	32	0
Great Starts						
Belgian Waffles And Sausage	2.85 oz	280	19	420	21	—
Belgian Waffles Strawberries And Sausage	3.5 oz	210	8	240	31	—
Waffle With Bacon	2.2 oz	230	14	710	19	—
Van's						
7 Grain Belgian	2	152	4	160	9	8
Belgian Original	2	145	4	108	30	2
Belgian Original Toaster	2	145	4	92	24	2
Blueberry Toaster	2	157	4	92	24	2
Blueberry Wheat Free Toaster	2	225	5	390	32	5
Fat Free	2	155	2	230	30	7
Mini	4	107	4	275	18	6
Multigrain Toaster	2	160	4	135	25	6
Organic Whole Wheat	2	190	5	230	30	6
Organic Whole Wheat Blueberry	2	190	5	230	30	6
Wheat Free Cinnamon Apple Toaster	2	220	5	390	32	5
Wheat Free Toaster	2	220	5	390	32	5
HOME RECIPE						
plain	1 (7 in diam)	218	11	383	25	—

FOOD	PORTION	CAL.	FAT	SOD.	CARB.	FIB.
MIX						
plain as prep	1 7 in diam (2.6 oz)	218	10	458	26	1
WALNUTS						
black dried	1 oz	172	16	0	3	1
black dried chopped	1 cup	759	71	2	15	—
english dried	1 oz	182	18	3	5	1
english dried chopped	1 cup	770	74	12	22	6
Planters						
Black	1 pkg (2 oz)	340	31	0	8	3
Gold Measure Halves	1 pkg (2 oz)	380	38	0	8	2
Halves	⅓ cup (1.2 oz)	220	22	0	5	1
Pieces	¼ cup (1 oz)	190	20	0	4	1
WATER						
(*see* MINERAL/BOTTLED WATER)						
WATER CHESTNUTS						
CANNED						
chinese sliced	½ cup	35	tr	6	9	—
Empress						
Sliced	2 oz	14	0	10	3	—
Whole	2 oz	14	0	10	3	—
Ka-Me						
Whole In Water	½ cup (4.5 oz)	45	0	10	11	4
La Choy						
Sliced	¼ cup	18	tr	3	4	tr
Whole	4	14	tr	2	4	tr
FRESH						
sliced	½ cup	66	tr	9	15	—
WATERCRESS						
(*see also* CRESS)						
raw chopped	½ cup	2	tr	7	tr	tr
WATERMELON						
FRESH						
cut up	1 cup	50	1	3	11	1
wedge	1/16	152	2	10	35	2
SEEDS						
dried	1 oz	158	13	28	4	—
dried	1 cup	602	51	28	17	—
WATERMELON JUICE						
Kool-Aid						
Splash Drink	1 serv (8 oz)	110	0	35	30	0
WAX BEANS						
CANNED						
Del Monte						
Cut Golden	½ cup (4.3 oz)	20	0	360	4	2

FOOD	PORTION	CAL.	FAT	SOD.	CARB.	FIB.
Owatonna						
Cut	½ cup	20	0	—	—	—
S&W						
Golden Cut Premium	½ cup	20	0	385	5	—
Seneca						
Cuts Natural Pack	½ cup	25	0	0	6	2
Wax Beans	½ cup	25	0	360	6	2
WHALE						
raw	3.5 oz	134	3	100	0	—
WHEAT						
(*see also* BULGUR, BRAN, CEREAL, COUSCOUS, FLOUR, WHEAT GERM)						
sprouted	⅓ cup	71	tr	6	15	—
starch	3½ oz	348	tr	2	86	—
Arrowhead						
Kamut Grain	¼ cup (1.7 oz)	140	1	0	32	5
Seitan Quick Mix	⅓ cup (1.4 oz)	150	1	20	14	2
Hodgson Mill						
Vital Wheat Gluten Plus Ascorbic Acid	1 tbsp (0.3 oz)	30	0	0	2	1
Near East						
Taboule Salad Mix as prep	⅔ cup	120	3	340	23	3
Wheat Pilaf as prep	1 cup	220	5	690	42	5
Sonoma						
Wheat Nuts Salted	2 tbsp (0.5 oz)	60	3	140	8	1
White Wave						
Seitan	½ pkg (4 oz)	140	0	240	4	1
Seitan Fajita Strips	⅓ cup (1.8 oz)	60	0	105	2	1
Seitan Marinated Slices	3 slices (1.8 oz)	60	0	105	2	1
WHEAT GERM						
plain toasted	¼ cup	108	3	1	14	4
plain toasted	1 cup	431	12	4	56	—
plain untoasted	¼ cup	104	3	4	15	4
w/ brown sugar & honey toasted	1 cup	426	9	3	69	—
w/ brown sugar & honey toasted	1 oz	107	2	1	17	—
Arrowhead						
Wheat Germ	3 tbsp (0.5 oz)	50	1	0	10	2
Hodgson Mill						
Wheat Germ	2 tbsp (0.5 oz)	55	1	0	7	4
Kretschmer						
Honey Crunch	¼ cup	105	3	2	15	3

FOOD	PORTION	CAL.	FAT	SOD.	CARB.	FIB.
Kretschmer (CONT.)						
Original	¼ cup	103	3	2	12	3
Stone-Buhr						
Untoasted	2 tbsp (0.5 oz)	58	2	0	7	2
WHEY						
acid dry	1 tbsp (3 g)	10	tr	28	2	
acid fluid	1 cup (8 fl oz)	59	tr	118	13	–
sweet dry	1 tbsp (8 g)	26	tr	80	6	
sweet fluid	1 cup (8 fl oz)	66	1	132	13	—
whey cheese	3.5 oz	440	27	511	33	0
WHIPPED TOPPINGS (*see also* CREAM)						
cream pressurized	1 cup (2.1 oz)	154	13	78	7	-
cream pressurized	1 tbsp (3 g)	8	tr	4	tr	—
nondairy frzn	1 tbsp	13	1	1	1	—
nondairy powdered as prep w/ whole milk	1 cup	151	10	53	13	–
nondairy powdered as prep w/ whole milk	1 tbsp (4 g)	8	tr	3	1	
nondairy pressurized	1 tbsp (4 g)	11	1	2	1	
nondairy pressurized	1 cup	184	16	43	11	—
Cool Whip						
Extra Creamy	2 tbsp (0.3 oz)	25	2	5	2	0
Free	2 tbsp (0.3 oz)	15	0	5	3	0
Lite	2 tbsp (0.3 oz)	20	1	0	2	0
Original	2 tbsp (0.3 oz)	25	2	0	2	0
Dream Whip						
Mix as prep	2 tbsp (0.3 oz)	20	1	5	2	0
Estee						
Whipped Topping Sugar Free as prep	2 tbsp	10	1	5	1	—
Hood						
Instant	2 tbsp	20	2	0	1	0
Light Instant	2 tbsp	15	1	0	1	0
Kraft						
Dairy Whip Light Cream	2 tbsp (0.2 oz)	10	1	0	tr	0
La Creme						
Topping	1 tbsp	16	1	5	1	—
Pet						
Whip	1 tbsp	14	1	0	1	—
Reddiwip						
Lite	2 tbsp (8 g)	15	1	5	2	—
Non-Dairy	2 tbsp (8 g)	20	2	5	2	—

FOOD	PORTION	CAL.	FAT	SOD.	CARB.	FIB.
Reddiwip (CONT.)						
Real Whipped Heavy Cream	2 tbsp (8 g)	30	3	0	tr	—
Real Whipped Light Cream	2 tbsp (8 g)	20	2	0	tr	—
WHITE BEANS						
CANNED						
white beans	1 cup	306	1	13	58	—
Goya						
Spanish Style	7.5 oz	130	1	990	29	12
Progresso						
Cannellini	½ cup (4.6 oz)	100	1	270	18	5
DRIED						
regular cooked	1 cup	249	1	11	45	—
small cooked	1 cup	253	1	4	46	—
WHITEFISH						
baked	3 oz	146	6	56	0	—
smoked	1 oz	39	tr	285	0	—
smoked	3 oz	92	1	866	0	—
WHITING						
cooked	3 oz	98	1	113	0	—
raw	3 oz	77	1	61	0	—
WILD RICE						
cooked	½ cup	83	tr	3	18	—
Haddon House						
Extra Fancy	¼ cup (1.6 oz)	170	1	0	35	2
WINE						
(*see also* CHAMPAGNE, WINE COOLERS)						
madeira	3.5 oz	169	0	—	10	0
port	3.5 oz	156	0	4	11	0
red	3½ oz	74	0	6	2	—
rosé	3½ oz	73	0	5	2	—
sherry	2 oz	84	0	—	5	—
sweet dessert	2 oz	90	0	5	7	—
vermouth dry	3½ oz	105	0	—	1	—
vermouth sweet	3½ oz	167	0	—	12	—
white	3½ oz	70	0	5	1	—
Boone's						
Country Kwencher	1 fl oz	24	0	1	3	—
Delicious Apple	1 fl oz	21	0	1	3	—
Sangria	1 fl oz	22	0	1	3	—

FOOD	PORTION	CAL.	FAT	SOD.	CARB.	FIB.
Boone's (CONT.)						
Snow Creek Berry	1 fl oz	18	0	tr	3	—
Strawberry Hill	1 fl oz	22	0	1	3	—
Sun Peak Peach	1 fl oz	18	0	1	3	—
Wild Island	1 fl oz	18	0	tr	3	—
Carlo Rossi						
Blush	1 fl oz	21	0	1	1	—
Burgundy	1 fl oz	22	0	1	tr	—
Chablis	1 fl oz	21	0	1	tr	—
Paisano	1 fl oz	23	0	3	tr	—
Red Sangria	1 fl oz	24	0	1	2	—
Rhine	1 fl oz	21	0	1	1	—
Vin Rosé	1 fl oz	21	0	1	1	—
White Grenache	1 fl oz	20	0	tr	1	—
Fairbanks						
Cream Sherry	1 fl oz	42	0	1	4	—
Port	1 fl oz	44	0	1	4	—
Sherry	1 fl oz	34	0	2	2	—
White Port	1 fl oz	44	0	1	4	—
Gallo						
Blush Chablis	1 fl oz	22	0	2	1	—
Burgundy	1 fl oz	22	0	1	tr	—
Cabernet Sauvignon	1 fl oz	22	0	tr	0	—
Chablis Blanc	1 fl oz	20	0	1	tr	—
Chardonnay	1 fl oz	23	0	1	tr	—
Classic Burgundy	1 fl oz	21	0	tr	0	—
French Colombard	1 fl oz	21	0	1	1	—
Hearty Burgundy	1 fl oz	22	0	1	tr	—
Johannisberg Riesling '88	1 fl oz	20	0	1	1	—
Pink Chablis	1 fl oz	20	0	1	1	—
Red Rosé	1 fl oz	23	0	2	1	—
Rhine	1 fl oz	22	0	1	1	—
Sauvignon Blanc '90	1 fl oz	20	0	1	tr	—
White Grenache '92	1 fl oz	20	0	1	1	—
White Grenache New Vintage	1 fl oz	20	0	tr	1	—
White Zinfandel '91	1 fl oz	18	0	1	tr	—
White Zinfandel New Vintage	1 fl oz	18	0	1	tr	—
Zinfandel '87	1 fl oz	23	0	tr	0	—
Ka-Me						
Chinese Cooking	2 tbsp (1 fl oz)	20	0	170	5	0

FOOD	PORTION	CAL.	FAT	SOD.	CARB.	FIB.
Sheffield Cellars						
Sherry	1 fl oz	44	0	1	4	—
Tawny Port	1 fl oz	45	0	2	4	—
Vermouth Extra Dry	1 fl oz	28	0	1	1	—
Vermouth Sweet	1 fl oz	43	0	2	4	—
Very Dry Sherry	1 fl oz	32	0	2	1	—

WINE COOLERS

FOOD	PORTION	CAL.	FAT	SOD.	CARB.	FIB.
Bartles & Jaymes						
Berry	12 fl oz	210	0	0	32	—
Margarita	12 fl oz	260	0	40	46	—
Original	12 fl oz	190	0	10	28	—
Peach	12 fl oz	210	0	5	33	—
Pina Colada	12 fl oz	280	0	0	49	—
Planter's Punch	12 fl oz	230	0	0	36	—
Strawberry	12 fl oz	210	0	0	32	—
Strawberry Daquiri	12 fl oz	230	0	5	37	—
Tropical	12 fl oz	230	0	0	38	—

WINGED BEANS

FOOD	PORTION	CAL.	FAT	SOD.	CARB.	FIB.
dried cooked	1 cup	252	10	22	26	—

WOLFFISH

FOOD	PORTION	CAL.	FAT	SOD.	CARB.	FIB.
atlantic baked	3 oz	105	3	93	0	—

YAM

(*see also* SWEET POTATO)

CANNED

FOOD	PORTION	CAL.	FAT	SOD.	CARB.	FIB.
Allen						
Cut	⅔ cup (5.8 oz)	160	1	35	40	3
Bruce						
Cut	½ cup	139	1	27	20	—
Mashed	½ cup	130	1	50	29	—
Vacuum Pack	½ cup	122	1	30	28	—
Whole	½ cup	139	1	27	31	—
Princella						
Cut	⅔ cup (5.8 oz)	160	1	40	40	3
Royal Prince						
Whole	4 pieces (5.9 oz)	200	1	40	48	4
S&W						
Candied	½ cup	180	0	355	44	—
Southern Whole In Extra Heavy Syrup	½ cup	139	1	27	31	—
Sugary Sam						
Cut	⅔ cup (5.8 oz)	160	1	35	40	3

FOOD	PORTION	CAL.	FAT	SOD.	CARB.	FIB.
Trappey						
Whole	4 pieces (5.9 oz)	200	1	40	48	4
FRESH						
mountain yam hawaii cooked	½ cup	59	tr	9	14	—
yam cubed cooked	½ cup	79	tr	6	19	—
YAMBEAN						
cooked	¾ cup	38	tr	4	9	—
YARDLONG BEANS						
dried cooked	1 cup	202	1	9	36	—
YEAST						
baker's compressed	1 cake (0.6 oz)	18	tr	5	3	2
baker's dry	1 pkg (¼ oz)	21	tr	—	3	—
baker's dry	1 tbsp	35	1	—	5	3
brewer's dry	1 tbsp	25	tr	10	3	—
Fleischmann's						
Active Dry	1 pkg (¼ oz)	20	0	10	3	—
Fresh Active	1 pkg (0.6 oz)	15	0	5	2	—
Household Yeast	½ oz	15	0	5	2	—
RapidRise	1 pkg (¼ oz)	20	0	10	3	—
Red Star						
Yeast	4 tbsp (0.5 oz)	47	tr	5	5	4
Yeast Flakes	3 tbsp (0.5 oz)	47	tr	5	5	4
YELLOW BEANS						
canned	½ cup	13	tr	170	3	1
canned low sodium	½ cup	13	tr	1	3	1
dried cooked	1 cup	254	2	8	45	—
fresh cooked	½ cup	22	tr	2	5	—
fresh raw	½ cup	17	tr	3	4	—
frozen cooked	½ cup	18	tr	9	4	—
YELLOWEYE BEANS						
CANNED						
B&M						
Baked	½ cup (4.6 oz)	170	2	460	28	7
DRIED						
Bean Cuisine						
Dried	½ cup	115	1	5	—	5
YELLOWTAIL						
baked	3 oz	159	6	42	0	—
YOGURT (*see also* YOGURT FROZEN)						
coffee lowfat	8 oz	194	3	149	31	—

FOOD	PORTION	CAL.	FAT	SOD.	CARB.	FIB.
fruit lowfat	4 oz	113	1	60	21	—
fruit lowfat	8 oz	225	3	121	42	—
plain	8 oz	139	7	105	11	—
plain lowfat	8 oz	144	4	159	16	—
plain no fat	8 oz	127	tr	174	17	—
vanilla lowfat	8 oz	194	3	149	31	—
Breyers						
Blended Blueberry	4.4 oz	130	1	60	25	0
Blended Peach	4.4 oz	130	1	65	26	0
Light Nonfat Apple Pie A La Mode	8 oz	120	0	105	22	0
Light Nonfat Berry Banana Split	8 oz	120	0	105	21	0
Light Nonfat Black Cherry Jubilee	8 oz	120	0	100	23	0
Light Nonfat Blueberries N' Cream	8 oz	120	0	100	23	0
Light Nonfat Cherry Bon-Bon	8 oz	120	0	105	22	0
Light Nonfat Cherry Vanilla Cream	8 oz	120	0	105	22	0
Light Nonfat Classic Strawberry	8 oz	120	0	100	22	0
Light Nonfat Key Lime Pie	8 oz	120	0	100	22	0
Light Nonfat Lemon Chiffon	8 oz	120	0	100	22	0
Light Nonfat Peaches N' Cream	8 oz	120	0	115	22	0
Light Nonfat Raspberries N' Cream	8 oz	120	0	105	22	0
Light Nonfat Strawberry Cheesecake	8 oz	120	0	100	22	tr
Lowfat Black Cherry	8 oz	240	3	125	44	0
Lowfat Blueberry	8 oz	230	3	125	43	0
Lowfat Mixed Berry	8 oz	320	3	125	43	0
Lowfat Peach	8 oz	240	3	125	43	0
Lowfat Pineapple	8 oz	240	3	125	45	0
Lowfat Red Raspberry	8 oz	230	3	125	43	2
Lowfat Strawberry	8 oz	230	3	125	43	0
Lowfat Strawberry Banana	8 oz	240	3	125	44	tr
Lowfat Vanilla	8 oz	220	3	135	38	0
Smooth & Creamy Apple Cobbler	8 oz	230	2	140	46	0

FOOD	PORTION	CAL.	FAT	SOD.	CARB.	FIB.
Breyers (CONT.)						
Smooth & Creamy Black Cherry Parfait	8 oz	240	2	130	46	0
Smooth & Creamy Black Cherry Parfait	4.4 oz	130	1	70	26	0
Smooth & Creamy Blueberries 'N Cream	4.4 oz	130	1	70	26	0
Smooth & Creamy Blueberries 'N Cream	8 oz	240	2	125	46	0
Smooth & Creamy Classic Strawberry	4.4 oz	130	1	70	25	0
Smooth & Creamy Classic Strawberry	8 oz	230	2	125	45	0
Smooth & Creamy Orange Vanilla Cream	8 oz	230	2	125	45	0
Smooth & Creamy Peaches 'N Cream	8 oz	230	2	125	46	0
Smooth & Creamy Peaches 'N Cream	4.4 oz	130	1	70	25	0
Smooth & Creamy Raspberries 'N Cream	8 oz	230	2	135	45	0
Smooth & Creamy Strawberry Banana Split	8 oz	240	2	125	48	tr
Smooth & Creamy Strawberry Cheesecake	8 oz	240	2	125	46	0
Cabot						
All Flavors	8 oz	220	3	120	42	—
Plain	8 oz	140	4	160	16	—
Colombo						
Banana Strawberry	8 oz	210	4	110	39	0
Black Cherry	8 oz	200	4	115	36	0
Blueberry	8 oz	200	4	110	36	0
Fat Free Apples 'n Spice	8 oz	190	0	130	39	0
Fat Free Apricot	8 oz	190	0	130	39	0
Fat Free Banana Strawberry	8 oz	200	0	130	42	0
Fat Free Blueberry	8 oz	190	0	130	39	0
Fat Free Cappuccino	8 oz	180	0	140	35	0
Fat Free Cherry	8 oz	190	0	135	39	0
Fat Free Cranberry Strawberry	8 oz	200	0	120	43	0
Fat Free French Roast	8 oz	180	0	140	35	0

FOOD	PORTION	CAL.	FAT	SOD.	CARB.	FIB.
Colombo (CONT.)						
Fat Free Fruit Cocktail	8 oz	190	0	130	39	0
Fat Free Lemon	8 oz	170	0	150	33	0
Fat Free Peach	8 oz	190	0	130	33	0
Fat Free Plain	8 oz	110	0	170	16	0
Fat Free Raspberry	8 oz	190	0	130	39	0
Fat Free Strawberry	8 oz	190	0	130	39	0
Fat Free Strawberry Pineapple Orange	8 oz	190	0	125	38	0
Fat Free Vanilla	8 oz	170	0	150	32	0
French Vanilla	8 oz	180	4	130	29	0
Light 100 Blueberry	8 oz	100	0	140	16	0
Light 100 Cherry Vanilla	8 oz	100	0	120	16	0
Light 100 Coffee & Cream	8 oz	100	0	120	16	0
Light 100 Creamy Vanilla	8 oz	100	0	130	16	0
Light 100 Fruit Medley	8 oz	100	0	120	16	0
Light 100 Juicy Peach	8 oz	100	0	140	16	0
Light 100 Lemon Creme	8 oz	100	0	160	16	0
Light 100 Mandarin Orange	8 oz	100	0	120	16	0
Light 100 Mixed Berries	8 oz	100	0	110	16	0
Light 100 Raspberry	8 oz	100	0	140	16	0
Light 100 Strawberry	8 oz	100	0	140	16	0
Peach Melba	8 oz	200	4	115	36	0
Plain	8 oz	120	5	150	12	0
Raspberry	8 oz	200	4	115	36	0
Strawberry	8 oz	200	4	110	36	0
Dannon						
Blended Nonfat Blueberry	6 oz	160	0	105	33	0
Blended Nonfat French Vanilla	6 oz	160	0	100	31	0
Blended Nonfat Lemon Chiffon	6 oz	150	0	110	31	0
Blended Nonfat Peach	6 oz	150	0	100	31	0
Blended Nonfat Raspberry	6 oz	160	0	100	32	0
Blended Nonfat Strawberry	6 oz	150	0	105	31	0
Blended Nonfat Strawberry Banana	6 oz	150	0	105	31	0
Daniamls Lowfat Tropical Punch	4.4 oz	140	2	85	25	0

FOOD	PORTION	CAL.	FAT	SOD.	CARB.	FIB.
Dannon (CONT.)						
Danimals Lowfat Blueberry	4.4 oz	140	2	90	25	0
Danimals Lowfat Grape Lemonade	4.4 oz	130	2	80	23	0
Danimals Lowfat Lemon Ice	4.4 oz	130	2	90	22	0
Danimals Lowfat Orange Banana	4.4 oz	140	2	80	24	0
Danimals Lowfat Strawberry	4.4 oz	140	2	85	24	0
Danimals Lowfat Vanilla	4.4 oz	140	2	80	24	0
Danimals Lowfat Wild Raspberry	4.4 oz	130	2	80	22	0
Fruit On The Bottom Lowfat Apple Cinnamon	8 oz	240	3	140	46	1
Fruit On The Bottom Lowfat Blueberry	8 oz	240	3	140	46	1
Fruit On The Bottom Lowfat Boysenberry	8 oz	240	3	150	45	1
Fruit On The Bottom Lowfat Cherry	8 oz	240	3	135	46	1
Fruit On The Bottom Lowfat Mixed Berries	8 oz	240	3	150	45	1
Fruit On The Bottom Lowfat Orange	8 oz	240	3	135	45	0
Fruit On The Bottom Lowfat Peach	8 oz	240	3	140	45	1
Fruit On The Bottom Lowfat Pear	8 oz	240	3	135	45	0
Fruit On The Bottom Lowfat Raspberry	8 oz	240	3	150	45	1
Fruit On The Bottom Lowfat Strawberry	8 oz	240	3	135	46	1
Fruit On The Bottom Lowfat Strawberry Banana	8 oz	240	3	140	43	1
Light Nonfat Banana Cream Pie	4.4 oz	60	0	80	9	0
Light Nonfat Cherry Vanilla	1 cup (3.5 oz)	110	0	160	19	0
Light Nonfat Lemon Chiffon	4.4 oz	60	0	75	9	0

FOOD	PORTION	CAL.	FAT	SOD.	CARB.	FIB.
Dannon (CONT.)						
Light Nonfat Peach	4.4 oz	50	0	70	8	0
Light Nonfat Strawberry	4.4 oz	50	0	70	8	0
Light Nonfat Strawberry	1 cup (3.5 oz)	110	0	160	19	0
Light Nonfat Vanilla	1 cup (3.5 oz)	110	0	160	18	0
Light 'N Crunchy Nonfat Cappuccino w/ Chocolate	1 pkg	150	0	170	27	0
Light 'N Crunchy Nonfat Caramel Apple Crunch	1 pkg	150	0	180	28	0
Light 'N Crunchy Nonfat Lemon Chiffon w/ Blueberry	1 pkg	140	0	150	26	0
Light 'N Crunchy Nonfat Raspberry w/ Granola	1 pkg	150	0	135	17	0
Light 'N Crunchy Nonfat Vanilla w/ Chocolate	1 pkg	150	0	170	26	1
Light Nonfat Banana Cream Pie	8 oz	100	0	150	17	0
Light Nonfat Blueberry	8 oz	100	0	140	20	0
Light Nonfat Creme Caramel	8 oz	100	0	125	15	0
Light Nonfat Lemon	8 oz	100	0	140	17	0
Light Nonfat Peach	8 oz	100	0	140	18	0
Light Nonfat Raspberry	8 oz	100	0	150	18	0
Light Nonfat Strawberry	8 oz	100	0	140	18	0
Light Nonfat Strawberry Banana	8 oz	100	0	140	18	0
Light Nonfat Tropical Fruit	8 oz	100	0	140	19	0
Light Nonfat Vanilla	8 oz	100	0	140	17	0
Lowfat Coffee	1 cup (8.7 oz)	230	4	170	39	0
Lowfat Coffee	8 oz	210	3	160	36	0
Lowfat Cranberry Raspberry	8 oz	210	3	160	36	0
Lowfat Lemon	8 oz	210	3	160	36	0
Lowfat Lemon	1 cup (8.7 oz)	230	4	170	39	0
Lowfat Plain	1 cup (8.7 oz)	150	4	170	17	0
Lowfat Plain	8 oz	140	4	150	16	0
Lowfat Vanilla	1 cup (8.7 oz)	230	4	170	39	0
Lowfat Vanilla	8 oz	210	3	160	36	0
Minipack Blended Nonfat Blueberry	4.4 oz	120	0	105	23	0
Minipack Blended Nonfat Cherry	4.4 oz	110	0	75	23	0

FOOD	PORTION	CAL.	FAT	SOD.	CARB.	FIB.
Dannon (CONT.)						
Minipack Blended Nonfat Peach	4.4 oz	110	0	75	23	0
Minipack Blended Nonfat Raspberry	4.4 oz	120	0	75	23	0
Minipack Blended Nonfat Strawberry	4.4 oz	110	0	105	23	0
Minipack Blended Nonfat Strawberry Banana	4.4 oz	110	2	105	23	0
Nonfat Plain	1 cup (8.7 oz)	120	0	170	17	0
Nonfat Plain	8 oz	110	0	150	16	0
Nonfat Light Cherry Vanilla	8 oz	100	0	140	17	0
Nonfat Light Strawberry Fruit Cup	8 oz	100	0	140	18	0
Sprinkl'ins Banana	4.1 oz	140	3	85	24	0
Sprinkl'ins Cherry Vanilla	4.1 oz	140	3	95	24	0
Sprinkl'ins Crazy Crunch Cherry w/ Honey Grahams	4.4 oz	170	3	150	30	0
Sprinkl'ins Crazy Crunch Grape w/ Chocolate Grahams	4.4 oz	160	3	170	29	0
Sprinkl'ins Crazy Crunch Vanilla w/ Chocolate Grahams	4.4 oz	160	3	140	29	0
Sprinkl'ins Crazy Crunch Vanilla w/ Honey Grahams	4.4 oz	170	3	135	30	0
Sprinkl'ins Strawberry	4.1 oz	140	3	95	24	0
Sprinkl'ins Strawberry Banana	4.1 oz	140	3	95	24	0
Tropifruta Nonfat Banana	6 oz	150	0	105	31	0
Tropifruta Nonfat Guava	6 oz	150	0	105	29	0
Tropifruta Nonfat Mango	6 oz	150	0	105	31	0
Tropifruta Nonfat Papaya Pineapple	6 oz	150	0	105	30	0
Tropifruta Nonfat Pina Colada	6 oz	150	0	105	30	0
Tropifruta Nonfat Strawberry	6 oz	150	0	105	31	0
Tropifruta Nonfat Strawberry Banana	6 oz	150	0	105	31	0

FOOD	PORTION	CAL.	FAT	SOD.	CARB.	FIB.
Dannon (CONT.)						
Tropifruta Nonfat Strawberry Kiwi	6 oz	150	0	105	30	0
With Fruit Toppings Banana Creme Strawberry	6 oz	170	3	90	30	1
With Fruit Toppings Bavarian Creme Raspberry	6 oz	170	3	115	31	0
With Fruit Toppings Cheesecake Cherry	6 oz	170	3	90	31	0
With Fruit Toppings Cheesecake Strawberry	6 oz	170	3	90	30	1
With Fruit Toppings Vanilla Peach & Apricot	6 oz	170	3	90	30	0
With Fruit Toppings Vanilla Strawberry	6 oz	170	3	90	30	1
Friendship						
Coffee	8 oz	210	3	170	30	0
Fruit Crunch Blueberry	6 oz	190	4	125	32	0
Fruit Crunch Peach	6 oz	190	5	125	31	0
Fruit Crunch Strawberry	6 oz	190	5	125	31	0
Fruit Crunch Strawberry Banana	6 oz	190	4	125	32	0
Plain	8 oz	150	3	190	13	0
Hood						
Fat Free Blueberry	1 (8 oz)	190	0	120	40	1
Fat Free Cherry	1 (8 oz)	190	0	120	40	1
Fat Free Peach	1 (8 oz)	190	0	120	40	1
Fat Free Plain	1 (8 oz)	130	0	190	18	0
Fat Free Raspberry	1 (8 oz)	190	0	120	40	1
Fat Free Strawberry	1 (8 oz)	190	0	120	39	1
Fat Free Strawberry Banana	1 (8 oz)	190	0	120	40	1
Fat Free Vanilla	1 (8 oz)	190	0	170	34	1
Fat Free Swiss Blueberry	1 (8 oz)	210	0	110	45	0
Fat Free Swiss Lemon	1 (8 oz)	210	0	110	45	0
Fat Free Swiss Raspberry	1 (8 oz)	210	0	110	45	0
Fat Free Swiss Strawberry	1 (8 oz)	210	0	105	45	0
Fat Free Swiss Strawberry Banana	1 (8 oz)	210	0	110	45	0

FOOD	PORTION	CAL.	FAT	SOD.	CARB.	FIB.
Hood (CONT.)						
Fat Free Swiss Vanilla	1 (8 oz)	210	0	105	45	0
Jell-O						
Lowfat Cherry	4.4 oz	130	1	65	25	0
Lowfat Grape	4.4 oz	130	1	65	25	0
Lowfat Raspberry	4.4 oz	130	1	65	25	0
Lowfat Tropical Berry Twist	4.4 oz	130	1	65	25	0
Lowfat Tropical Punch	4.4 oz	130	1	65	25	0
Lowfat Watermelon	4.4 oz	130	1	65	25	0
Lowfat Wild Berry	4.4 oz	130	1	65	25	0
Lowfat Wild Strawberry	4.4 oz	130	1	65	25	0
La Yogurt						
French Style Banana	6 oz	180	3	100	32	0
French Style Blueberry	6 oz	180	3	100	32	1
French Style Cherry	6 oz	180	3	100	32	0
French Style Cherry Vanilla	6 oz	190	3	95	35	0
French Style Guava	6 oz	180	3	100	32	1
French Style Key Lime	6 oz	180	3	100	32	0
French Style Mango	6 oz	180	3	100	32	0
French Style Mixed Berry	6 oz	180	3	100	32	0
French Style Nonfat Blueberry	6 oz	70	0	90	12	0
French Style Nonfat Cherry	6 oz	75	0	90	13	0
French Style Nonfat Raspberry	6 oz	70	0	90	12	0
French Style Nonfat Strawberry	6 oz	70	0	90	12	0
French Style Nonfat Strawberry Banana	6 oz	70	0	90	12	0
French Style Peach	6 oz	180	3	100	32	0
French Style Pina Colada	6 oz	180	3	100	32	0
French Style Raspberry	6 oz	180	3	100	32	1
French Style Strawberry	6 oz	180	3	100	32	0
French Style Strawberry Banana	6 oz	180	3	100	32	0
French Style Strawberry Fruit Cup	6 oz	180	3	100	32	0
French Style Tropical Orange	6 oz	180	4	100	32	0
French Style Vanilla	6 oz	170	3	110	28	0
Latin Style Banana	6 oz	190	3	105	34	0

FOOD	PORTION	CAL.	FAT	SOD.	CARB.	FIB.
La Yogurt (CONT.)						
Latin Style Guava	6 oz	190	3	105	34	0
Latin Style Mango	6 oz	190	3	105	34	0
Latin Style Papaya	6 oz	190	3	105	34	0
Latin Style Passion Fruit	6 oz	190	3	105	34	0
Latin Style Strawberry Kiwi	6 oz	180	3	100	32	0
Light N'Lively						
Free Blueberry	4.4 oz	70	0	55	13	0
Free Peach	4.4 oz	70	0	65	12	0
Free Strawberry	4.4 oz	70	0	55	12	0
Free Strawberry Banana Cream	4.4 oz	70	0	55	13	0
Free Strawberry Fruit Cup	4.4 oz	70	0	55	13	0
Lowfat Blueberry	4.4 oz	130	1	60	25	0
Lowfat Peach	4.4 oz	130	1	65	26	0
Lowfat Pineapple	4.4 oz	130	1	60	26	0
Lowfat Red Raspberry	4.4 oz	120	1	65	23	0
Lowfat Strawberry	4.4 oz	130	1	60	26	0
Lowfat Strawberry Banana Cream	4.4 oz	130	1	60	25	0
Lowfat Strawberry Fruit Cup	4.4 oz	130	1	60	25	0
Lite Line						
Swiss Style Cherry Vanilla	1 cup	240	2	150	45	—
Swiss Style Peach	1 cup	230	2	150	42	—
Swiss Style Plain	1 cup	140	2	150	16	—
Swiss Style Strawberry	1 cup	240	2	150	46	—
Meadow Gold						
Plain	1 cup	160	5	160	16	—
Sundae Style Raspberry	1 cup	250	4	160	42	—
Mountain High						
Blueberry	1 cup	220	6	140	31	—
Plain	1 cup	200	9	140	16	—
Weight Watchers						
Ultimate 90 Blueberries 'n Creme	1 cup	90	0	140	14	3
Ultimate 90 Cappuccino	1 cup	90	0	140	14	0
Ultimate 90 Cherries Jubilee	1 cup	90	0	140	14	3
Ultimate 90 Cranberry Raspberry	1 cup	90	0	140	14	0

FOOD	PORTION	CAL.	FAT	SOD.	CARB.	FIB.
Weight Watchers (CONT.)						
Ultimate 90 Lemon Chiffon	1 cup	90	0	140	14	1
Ultimate 90 Plain	1 cup	90	0	150	14	0
Ultimate 90 Raspberries 'n Creme	1 cup	90	0	140	14	0
Ultimate 90 Strawberry	1 cup	90	0	140	14	2
Ultimate 90 Strawberry Banana	1 cup	90	0	140	14	2
Ultimate 90 Vanilla	1 cup	90	0	140	14	0
Utlimate 90 Peach	1 cup	90	0	140	14	0
Yoplait						
Custard Style Banana	6 oz	190	4	95	32	—
Custard Style Blueberry	6 oz	190	4	95	32	—
Custard Style Cherry	6 oz	180	4	95	30	—
Custard Style Lemon	6 oz	190	4	95	32	—
Custard Style Mixed Berry	6 oz	180	4	95	30	—
Custard Style Raspberry	6 oz	190	4	95	32	—
Custard Style Strawberry	4 oz	130	3	60	21	—
Custard Style Strawberry	6 oz	190	4	95	32	—
Custard Style Strawberry Banana	6 oz	190	4	95	32	—
Custard Style Strawvberry Banana	4 oz	130	3	60	21	—
Custard Style Vanilla	6 oz	180	4	110	30	—
Custard Style Vanilla	4 oz	130	3	70	20	—
Fat Free Blueberry	6 oz	150	0	95	31	—
Fat Free Cherry	6 oz	150	0	95	31	—
Fat Free Mixed Berry	6 oz	150	0	95	31	—
Fat Free Peach	6 oz	150	0	95	31	—
Fat Free Raspberry	6 oz	150	0	95	31	—
Fat Free Strawberry	6 oz	150	0	95	31	—
Fat Free Strawberry Banana	6 oz	150	0	95	31	—
Light Blueberry	4 oz	60	0	75	9	—
Light Blueberry	6 oz	80	0	80	13	—
Light Cherry	4 oz	60	0	75	9	—
Light Cherry	6 oz	80	0	80	13	—
Light Peach	4 oz	60	0	75	9	—
Light Peach	6 oz	80	0	80	13	—
Light Raspberry	4 oz	60	0	75	9	—
Light Raspberry	6 oz	80	0	80	13	—
Light Strawberry	4 oz	60	0	75	9	—

FOOD	PORTION	CAL.	FAT	SOD.	CARB.	FIB.
Yoplait (CONT.)						
Light Strawberry	6 oz	80	0	110	13	—
Light Strawberry Banana	4 oz	60	0	75	9	—
Light Strawberry Banana	6 oz	80	0	80	13	—
Nonfat Plain	8 oz	120	0	160	18	—
Nonfat Vanilla	8 oz	180	0	140	35	—
Original Apple	6 oz	190	3	110	32	—
Original Blueberry	6 oz	190	3	110	32	—
Original Blueberry	4 oz	120	2	75	21	—
Original Boysenberry	6 oz	190	3	110	32	—
Original Cherry	6 oz	190	3	110	32	—
Original Lemon	6 oz	190	3	110	32	—
Original Mixed Berry	6 oz	190	3	110	32	—
Original Orange	6 oz	190	3	110	32	—
Original Peach	4 oz	120	2	75	21	—
Original Peach	6 oz	190	3	110	32	—
Original Pina Colada	6 oz	190	3	110	32	—
Original Pineapple	6 oz	190	3	110	32	—
Original Plain	6 oz	130	3	140	15	—
Original Raspberry	6 oz	190	3	110	32	—
Original Raspberry	4 oz	120	2	75	21	—
Original Strawberry	6 oz	190	3	110	32	—
Original Strawberry	4 oz	120	2	75	21	—
Original Strawberry Banana	6 oz	190	3	110	32	—
Original Strawberry Rhubarb	6 oz	190	3	110	32	—
Original Vanilla	6 oz	180	3	120	29	—
YOGURT FROZEN (*see also* TOFU YOGURT)						
chocolate soft serve	½ cup (4 fl oz)	115	4	71	18	—
vanilla soft serve	½ cup (4 fl oz)	114	4	63	17	—
Bee-Lite						
Chocolate	4 oz	100	tr	55	23	—
Vanilla	4 oz	110	tr	55	23	—
Ben & Jerry's						
Cherry Garcia	½ cup (3.7 oz)	170	3	70	31	0
Chocolate Fudge Brownie	½ cup (3.7 oz)	190	4	130	35	2
Coffee Almond Fudge	½ cup (3.7 oz)	200	7	85	30	1
English Toffee Crunch	½ cup (3.7 oz)	190	6	110	32	0
No Fat Cappuccino	½ cup (3.3 oz)	140	0	85	32	0
Pop Cherry Garcia	1 (3.8 oz)	290	16	60	34	2

FOOD	PORTION	CAL.	FAT	SOD.	CARB.	FIB.
Borden						
Strawberry	½ cup	100	2	50	19	—
Bresler's						
All Flavors	5 oz	145	2	—	28	—
All Flavors Lite	5 oz	135	0	—	30	—
Breyers						
Chocolate	½ cup (2.7 oz)	150	4	45	25	1
Light Fat Free Apple Pie A La Mode	1 cup (8 oz)	130	0	110	23	tr
Light Fat Free Black Cherry Jubilee	1 cup (8 oz)	130	0	110	23	tr
Light Fat Free Blueberries n' Cream	1 cup (8 oz)	130	0	110	23	tr
Light Fat Free Cherry Chocolate	1 cup (8 oz)	130	0	110	23	tr
Light Fat Free Classic Strawberry	1 cup (8 oz)	130	0	110	23	tr
Light Fat Free Key Lime Pie	1 cup (8 oz)	130	0	110	23	tr
Light Fat Free Lemon Chiffon	1 cup (8 oz)	130	0	110	23	tr
Light Fat Free Peaches n'Cream	1 cup (8 oz)	130	0	110	23	tr
Light Fat Free Strawberry Cheesecake	1 cup (8 oz)	130	0	110	23	tr
Red Raspberry	½ cup (2.7 oz)	140	4	40	24	0
Strawberry Banana	½ cup (2.7 oz)	140	3	40	24	0
Vanilla	½ cup (2.7 oz)	140	4	45	24	0
Dannon						
Coco-Nut Fudge	½ cup (3 oz)	160	3	70	28	0
Light Cappuccino	½ cup (2.8 oz)	80	0	70	19	0
Light Cherry Vanilla Swirl	½ cup (2.8 oz)	90	0	65	21	0
Light Chocolate	½ cup (2.7 oz)	80	0	60	21	1
Light Lemon Chiffon	½ cup (2.8 oz)	90	0	65	22	0
Light Peach Raspberry Melba	½ cup (2.8 oz)	90	0	65	21	0
Light Strawberry Cheesecake	½ cup (2.8 oz)	90	0	60	22	0
Light Vanilla	½ cup (2.8 oz)	80	0	65	21	0
Light Nonfat Cappuccino	8 oz	100	0	140	17	0
Light'N Crunchy Banana Cream Pie	½ cup (2.8 oz)	110	1	65	24	0

FOOD	PORTION	CAL.	FAT	SOD.	CARB.	FIB.
Dannon (CONT.)						
Light'N Crunchy Mocha Chocolate Chunk	½ cup (2.8 oz)	110	1	60	26	0
Light'N Crunchy Peanut Chocolate Crunch	½ cup (2.8 oz)	110	0	65	29	0
Light'N Crunchy Triple Chocolate	½ cup (2.8 oz)	110	0	60	28	0
Light'N Crunchy Vanilla Blueberry Swirl	½ cup (2.8 oz)	110	1	65	26	0
Pure Indulgence Cherry Chocolate Cherry	½ cup (3 oz)	150	3	85	26	0
Pure Indulgence Chunky Chocolate Nut	½ cup (3 oz)	150	3	65	25	0
Pure Indulgence Cookies'n Cream	½ cup (3 oz)	150	3	105	24	0
Pure Indulgence Crunchy Expresso	½ cup (3 oz)	150	3	85	26	0
Pure Indulgence Heath Toffee Crunch	½ cup (3 oz)	150	3	105	25	0
Pure Indulgence Vanilla Raspberry Truffle	½ cup (3 oz)	150	3	70	25	1
Desserve						
All Flavors	4 oz	70	0	57	16	—
Dutch Chocolate	4 oz	80	0	62	18	—
Edy's						
Banana Strawberry	3 oz	80	1	40	15	—
Blueberry	3 oz	80	1	40	15	—
Cherry	3 oz	80	1	40	15	—
Chocolate	3 oz	80	1	40	15	—
Chocolate Chip	3 oz	100	1	55	20	—
Citrus Heights	3 oz	80	1	40	15	—
Cookies'N'Cream	3 oz	100	1	55	20	—
Marble Fudge	3 oz	100	1	55	20	—
Perfectly Peach	3 oz	80	1	40	15	—
Raspberry	3 oz	80	1	40	15	—
Raspberry Vanilla Swirl	3 oz	80	1	45	15	—
Strawberry	3 oz	80	1	40	15	—
Vanilla	3 oz	80	1	50	15	—
Elan						
Blueberry	4 oz	130	3	50	23	—
Caramel Almond Praline	4 oz	150	4	90	26	—
Chocolate	4 oz	130	3	50	24	—
Chocolate Almond	4 oz	160	6	50	22	—
Coffee	4 oz	130	3	60	22	—

FOOD	PORTION	CAL.	FAT	SOD.	CARB.	FIB.
Elan (CONT.)						
Coffee Decaffeinated	4 oz	130	3	60	22	—
Peach	4 oz	130	3	50	23	—
Rum Raisin	4 oz	135	3	55	25	—
Strawberry	4 oz	125	3	50	22	—
Vanilla	4 oz	130	3	60	22	—
Fi-Bar						
Chocolate	1	190	7	160	26	4
Strawberry	1	190	7	150	26	4
Vanilla	1	190	7	150	26	4
Friendly's						
Apple Bettie	½ cup (2.6 oz)	140	3	75	25	0
Fabulous Fudge Swirl	½ cup (2.6 oz)	140	3	80	23	0
Fudge Berry Swirl	½ cup (2.6 oz)	150	4	75	25	0
Lowfat Perfectly Peach	½ cup (2.6 oz)	110	2	55	21	0
Lowfat Purely Chocolate	½ cup (2.6 oz)	120	3	65	20	0
Lowfat Raspberry Delight	½ cup (2.6 oz)	120	3	60	21	0
Lowfat Simply Vanilla	½ cup (2.6 oz)	120	3	70	19	0
Lowfat Strawberry Patch	½ cup (2.6 oz)	110	2	55	20	0
Mint Chocolate Chip	½ cup (2.6 oz)	130	4	65	21	0
Strawberry Cheesecake Blast	½ cup (2.6 oz)	140	4	75	22	0
Toffee Almond Crunch	½ cup (2.6 oz)	160	5	85	24	tr
Good Humor						
Creamsicle Raspberry	1 (2.8 oz)	100	1	20	23	0
Frista Cup	1 (6.2 oz)	220	5	125	38	1
Haagen-Dazs						
Banana Nut Blast	½ cup (3.5 oz)	220	8	65	29	1
Bars Cherry Chocolate Fudge	1 (2.6 oz)	240	13	45	26	1
Bars Peach	1 (2.5 oz)	90	1	20	19	0
Bars Pina Colada	1 (2.5 oz)	100	1	45	19	0
Bars Raspberry & Vanilla	1 (2.5 oz)	90	1	25	19	0
Bars Strawberry Daiquiri	1 (2.5 oz)	90	1	20	18	0
Chocolate	½ cup (3.4 oz)	160	3	60	26	tr
Coffee	½ cup (3.4 oz)	160	3	55	26	0
Fat Free Bar Raspberry & Vanilla	1 (2.5 oz)	90	0	15	20	0
Fat Free Cherry Vanilla	½ cup (3.3 oz)	140	0	40	30	0
Fat Free Chocolate	½ cup (3.3 oz)	140	0	45	28	tr
Fat Free Coffee	½ cup (3.3 oz)	140	0	45	29	0
Fat Free Vanilla	½ cup (3.3 oz)	140	0	45	29	0
Fat Free Vanilla Fudge	½ cup (3.3 oz)	160	0	100	34	0

FOOD	PORTION	CAL.	FAT	SOD.	CARB.	FIB.
Haagen-Dazs (CONT.)						
Orange Tango	½ cup (3.5 oz)	130	1	25	26	0
Pina Colada	½ cup (3.4 oz)	130	2	25	26	0
Raspberry Randevous	½ cup (3.5 oz)	130	2	25	26	1
Strawberry Cheesecake Craze	½ cup (3.6 oz)	220	8	140	31	0
Strawberry Duet	½ cup (3.4 oz)	130	2	25	26	tr
Vanilla	½ cup (3.4 oz)	160	3	55	26	0
Hood						
Bavarian Truffle & Twist	½ cup (2.6 oz)	150	4	60	26	0
Coffee Toffee Chunk Sundae	½ cup (2.6 oz)	150	4	75	27	0
Combo Bars	1 (2.2 oz)	90	2	40	17	0
Cookies & Cream	½ cup (2.6 oz)	140	4	75	25	0
Grandma's Raisin Oatmeal Cookie Dough	½ cup (2.6 oz)	140	3	75	25	0
Mixed Berry Swirl	½ cup (2.6 oz)	120	2	45	24	0
Natural Strawberry	½ cup (2.6 oz)	110	3	50	21	0
Natural Strawberry Banana	½ cup (2.6 oz)	110	3	50	21	0
Natural Vanilla	½ cup (2.6 oz)	120	3	55	22	0
Nonfat Caramel & Brownie Sundae	½ cup (2.6 oz)	120	0	60	28	0
Nonfat Chocolate Marshmallow	½ cup (2.6 oz)	110	0	60	26	0
Nonfat Double Raspberry	½ cup (2.6 oz)	120	0	55	26	0
Nonfat Mocha Fudge	½ cup (2.6 oz)	120	0	55	27	0
Nonfat Olde Fashioned Vanilla	½ cup (2.6 oz)	110	0	55	24	0
Nonfat Peach Cobbler A La Mode	½ cup (2.6 oz)	110	0	50	25	0
Nonfat Strawberry	½ cup (2.6 oz)	100	0	50	23	0
Nonfat Vanilla Fudge	½ cup (2.6 oz)	120	0	55	27	0
Raspberry Swirl	½ cup (2.6 oz)	130	2	55	25	0
Sundae Cups Chocolate & Strawberry	1 (2.2 oz)	110	2	55	24	1
Vanilla Chocolate Strawberry	½ cup (2.6 oz)	120	3	50	22	0
Vanilla Swiss Almond Sundae	½ cup (2.6 oz)	150	4	60	25	0
Just 10						
All Flavors	1 oz	10	0	14	3	—

FOOD	PORTION	CAL.	FAT	SOD.	CARB.	FIB.
Kissed With Honey						
Chocolate	3.5 oz	100	3	50	18	—
Nonfat Chocolate	3.5 oz	85	tr	60	19	—
Nonfat Vanilla	3.5 oz	85	tr	50	18	—
Vanilla	3.5 oz	100	3	75	17	—
Meadow Gold						
Strawberry	½ cup	100	2	50	19	—
Sealtest						
Chocolate	½ cup (2.7 oz)	120	2	45	24	tr
Mocha Fudge	½ cup (2.6 oz)	130	2	45	25	tr
Vanilla	½ cup (2.6 oz)	120	2	45	24	0
Tofutti						
Better Than Yogurt Chocolate Fudge	4 fl oz	120	2	98	25	0
Better Than Yogurt Coffee Mashmallow Swirl	4 fl oz	100	1	77	24	0
Better Than Yogurt Passion Island Fruit	4 fl oz	100	1	100	21	0
Better Than Yogurt Peach Mango	4 fl oz	100	1	102	23	0
Better Than Yogurt Strawberry Banana	4 fl oz	100	1	92	23	0
Better Than Yogurt Vanilla Fudge	4 fl oz	120	2	90	24	0
Turkey Hill						
Chocolate Cherry Cordial	½ cup (2.6 oz)	130	3	60	22	0
Chocolate Chip Cookie Dough	½ cup (2.6 oz)	140	5	120	23	0
Death By Chocolate	½ cup (2.6 oz)	150	4	90	25	0
Nonfat Chocolate Cherry Cordial	½ cup (2.4 oz)	100	0	70	24	0
Nonfat Chocolate Marshmallow	½ cup (2.4 oz)	130	0	40	30	0
Nonfat Coffee Cappuccino	½ cup (2.4 oz)	110	0	60	23	0
Nonfat Mint Cookie 'N Cream	½ cup (2.4 oz)	110	0	80	24	0
Nonfat Neapolitan	½ cup (2.4 oz)	100	0	50	22	0
Nonfat Raspberry Chocolate Bliss	½ cup (2.4 oz)	110	0	100	25	0
Nonfat Southern Lemon Pie	½ cup (2.4 oz)	110	0	90	25	0
Nonfat Vanilla Fudge	½ cup (2.4 oz)	110	0	80	24	0

FOOD	PORTION	CAL.	FAT	SOD.	CARB.	FIB.
Turkey Hill (CONT.)						
Peach Raspberry	½ cup (2.6 oz)	110	2	60	20	0
Strawberry	½ cup (2.6 oz)	110	2	60	20	0
Tin Roof Sundae	½ cup (2.6 oz)	140	5	100	21	0
Vanilla & Chocolate	½ cup (2.6 oz)	110	3	70	19	0
Vanilla Bean	½ cup (2.6 oz)	110	3	70	17	0
ZUCCHINI						
CANNED						
italian style	½ cup	33	tr	427	8	—
Del Monte						
With Italian Tomato Sauce	½ cup (4.2 oz)	30	0	490	7	1
Progresso						
Italian Style	½ cup (4.2 oz)	40	2	400	7	2
S&W						
Italian Style	½ cup	45	1	467	7	—
FRESH						
baby raw	1 (0.5 oz)	3	tr	0	1	tr
raw sliced	½ cup	9	tr	2	2	1
sliced cooked	½ cup	14	tr	2	4	1
FROZEN						
cooked	½ cup	19	tr	2	4	—
Big Valley						
Zucchini	¾ cup (3 oz)	10	0	0	2	1
Empire						
Breaded	1 (2.9 oz)	100	0	280	18	1
Southland						
Zucchini Sliced	3.2 oz	15	0	—	—	—
TAKE-OUT						
indian paalkora	1 serv	46	2	141	7	2

Annette B. Natow, Ph.D., R.D. and Jo-Ann Heslin, M.A., R.D., are the authors of twenty-two books on nutrition. Both are former faculty members of Adelphi University and State University of New York, Downstate Medical Center. They are editors of the *Journal of Nutrition for the Elderly,* serve as editorial board members for the *Environmental Nutrition Newsletter* and *Vitality,* and are frequent contributors to magazines and journals.

Annette B. Natow, Ph.D., R.D. and Jo-Ann Heslin, M.A., R.D. are the authors of twenty-two books on nutrition, both are former faculty members of Adelphi University and State University of New York Downstate Medical Center. They are editors of the [illegible] of Nutrition for the Elderly, serve as advisory board members to the Environmental Nutrition Newsletter, and are frequent contributors to magazines and journals.